Complications in Foot and Ankle Surgery

Michael S. Lee • Jordan P. Grossman
Editors

Complications in Foot and Ankle Surgery

Management Strategies

Springer

Editors
Michael S. Lee
Capital Orthopedics and Sports Medicine
Clive, IA, USA

Jordan P. Grossman
Akron General Orthopedics, Inc.
Akron, OH, USA

ISBN 978-3-319-53684-2 ISBN 978-3-319-53686-6 (eBook)
DOI 10.1007/978-3-319-53686-6

Library of Congress Control Number: 2017942783

Printed on acid-free paper

This Springer imprint is published by Springer Nature
The registered company is Springer International Publishing AG
The registered company address is: Gewerbestrasse 11, 6330 Cham, Switzerland

Foreword

Complication-

> "The unfavorable evolution or consequence of a disease, a health condition or a therapy."
>
> "An unanticipated problem that arises following, and is a result of, a procedure, treatment, or illness. A complication is so named because it complicates the situation."

Surgical procedures of the foot and ankle carry the potential for adverse events and complications. Dealing with the sequelae of complications and errors that arise in the course of normal practice is part and parcel of a surgeon's working life. It is crucial to focus on the needs of patients and their families when complications occur. Surgeons must respond to the challenge of providing effective patient care and may also need to deal with the reactions of the patient's family, the judgment of colleagues, and, in some cases, with disciplinary or legal action. Complications can keep us awake at night, undermine our confidence and ability to function, and even affect our enjoyment of life. The ability to manage complications is therefore paramount to what we do.

We have witnessed a stunning evolution in the advancement of foot and ankle surgery. The volume of research that has resulted in evidence-based medicine, as well as technological advancements in our field, has been remarkable. Furthermore, the dissemination of information through all sorts of learning vehicles has exploded. This information is at our fingertips and can be easily accessed. We have huge volumes of information to assist and guide us in our decision-making. Surgeons can develop a plan for virtually any procedure with precision and accuracy. However, there is often a paucity of information when it comes to dealing with complications of foot and ankle surgery. It can be difficult to find information to help us deliver effective patient care in these situations. Obtaining information to help us deal with complications often requires cumbersome searches that provide little guidance. This textbook on complications of foot and ankle surgery is the first of its kind and is long overdue. It will serve as a resource to help us properly evaluate and institute appropriate therapy for complications.

This textbook by Michael Lee and Jordan Grossmann is a great starting point for those of us looking to deal with complications in a practical and effective manner. The text provides insight on how complications develop and evolve. It discusses major perioperative complications such as deep venous thrombosis, nonunions, incisional problems, surgical infections, and adverse effects associated with comorbid conditions. The text also reviews complications following specific surgical procedures. The authors in each section discuss evaluation and management of specific complications, as well as potential pitfalls with each procedure. Drs. Lee and Grossman have gathered a diverse group of authors who share their experience and techniques.

I am honored and privileged to provide the foreword for this complete, comprehensive and timely textbook on complications of foot and ankle surgery. I commend Drs. Lee and Grossman, recognized leaders in our profession, as well as my former residents and dear friends, for their dedication to this project. This will become an authoritative textbook on complications. Thanks for making me proud!

We must dedicate ourselves to deliver responsible, patient-centered care in a safe environment that includes equitable treatment and full disclosure to all patients. We must address surgical complications by providing effective, evidence-based patient care. These principles represent the way forward in our specialty and will define how well we are able to truly advance our profession. As such, it is imperative that we develop the requisite skills necessary to deal with complications. This textbook is a great STARTING point.

Alan Catanzariti

Acknowledgments

We would like to thank our *friends* and colleagues for their time, dedication, and efforts toward the completion of this book. This list of contributors is representative of the hardworking and thoughtful portion of our profession that have and will continue to advance the field of foot and ankle surgery. Completing a chapter is a daunting task as there are always other projects and expectations that manage to consume our day. We are grateful and appreciate these authors for finding the time to complete their respective chapters.

To that end, and equally important, we'd like to thank our own families for allowing us to find that precious time to dedicate to this worthy project. Your love and support has never wavered, and for that we are thankful. Finally, thanks to Alan Catanzariti, for his mentoring and friendship of both of us. Cats' dedication to the profession, his patients, his residents, and his family is an example for everyone—we are forever thankful and incredibly proud to be products of his West Penn family.

Contents

Contributors

Eric A. Barp, DPM, FACFAS Foot and Ankle Surgery, The Iowa Clinic, West Des Moines, IA, USA

Michelle Butterworth, DPM Pee Dee Foot Center, Kingstree, SC, USA

Glenn Weinraub Department of Orthopedic Surgery, Kaiser Permanente, San Leandro, CA, USA

Alan Catanzariti, DPM, FACFAS West Penn Hospital, The Foot and Ankle Institute, Pittsburgh, PA, USA

Gage M. Caudell Fort Wayne Orthopedics, Fort Wayne, IN, USA

Thomas J. Chang, DPM Redwood Orthopedic Surgery Associates, Inc., Santa Rosa, CA, USA

Luke D. Cicchinelli, DPM Centro Clinico Quirurgico, Vigo, Spain

J. Randolph Clements, DPM Carilion Clinic Orthopaedics, Virginia Tech Carilion School of Medicine, Roanoke, VA, USA

Richard Derner, DPM, FACFAS Past President, American College of Foot and Ankle Surgeons, Department of Orthopedics INOVA Fairfax Medical Campus, Falls Church, VA, USA

Brian T. Dix Sanford Health, Thief River Falls, MN, USA

Lawrence A. Di Domenico, DPM Ankle and Foot Care Centers, Youngstown, OH, USA

Kent State University, College of Podiatric Medicine, Cleveland, OH, USA

Michael W. Downey Fellowship Trained Trauma and Reconstruction Foot/Ankle Surgeon, Trinity Foot and Ankle Specialists, Texas Health Harris Southwest Hospital, Fort Worth, TX, USA

Mindi Feilmeier, DPM School- Des Moines University, College of Podiatric Medicine and Surgery, Des Moines, IA, USA

Justin J. Fleming, DPM Aria 3B Orthopaedics, Philadelphia, PA, USA

Lawrence A. Ford, DPM, FACFAS Department of Orthopedics and Podiatric Surgery, Kaiser Permanente Medical Center, Oakland, CA, USA

Kaiser San Francisco Bay Area Foot and Ankle Residency Program, Oakland, CA, USA

Michael Gentile, DPM Westside Foot and Ankle Specialists,Tigard, OR

Sean T. Grambart, DPM, FACFAS Carle Physician Group, Champaign, IL, USA

David Granger OSS Health, York, PA, USA

Graham A. Hamilton, DPM, FACFAS Department of Orthopedics and Podiatric Surgery, Kaiser Permanente Medical Center, Antioch, CA, USA

Kaiser San Francisco Bay Area Foot and Ankle Residency Program, Oakland, CA, USA

Matthew J. Hentges, DPM The Foot and Ankle Institute of Western Pennsylvania, Pittsburgh, PA, USA

Mark H. Hofbauer, DPM Monongahela Valley Hospital, Monongahela, PA, USA

Byron Hutchinson, DPM Department of Ortho, CHI/Fransiscan Health System, Spine and Foot and Ankle, Saint Francis Hospital, Federal Way, WA, USA

Christopher F. Hyer, DPM, MS, FACFAS Orthopedic Foot and Ankle Center, Westerville, OH, USA

Allen M. Jacobs, DPM St. Louis, MO, USA

Meagan M. Jennings, DPM Orthopedics and Podiatry, Palo Alto Foundation Medical Group, Mountain View, CA, USA

Erin E. Klein, DPM, MS Department of Surgery, Weil Foot and Ankle Institute, Des Plaines, IL, USA

Kwasi Y. Kwaadu, DPM Temple University School of Podiatric Medicine, Philadelphia, PA, USA

Bradley M. Lamm, DPM Foot and Ankle Deformity Center, Paley Orthopedic and Spine Institute, St. Mary's Medical Center & Palm Beach Children's Hospital, West Palm Beach, FL, USA

Guido LaPorta, DPM, FACFAS LaPorta and Associates, PC, Dunmore, PA, USA

George Tye Liu, DPM Department of Orthopaedic Surgery, University of Texas Southwestern Medical Center, Dallas, TX, USA

Frank A. Luckino Ankle and Foot Care Centers, Youngstown, OH , USA

Chrisitne P. Miller, DPM, DMM Department of Orthopaedics-Division of Foot and Ankle, University of Florida College of Medicine-Jacksonville, Jacksonville, FL, USA

Kyle Moore, DPM West Penn Hospital, The Foot and Ankle Institute, Pittsburgh, PA, USA

Trevor Payne, DPM Augusta Foot and Ankle, Evans, GA, USA

Ellianne M. Nasser, DPM Geisinger Health System, Scranton, PA, USA

Kyle S. Peterson, DPM Suburban Orthopaedics, Bartlett, IL, USA

Jason A. Piraino, DPM, MS, FACFAS Department of Orthopaedics-Division of Foot and Ankle, University of Florida College of Medicine-Jacksonville, Jacksonville, FL, USA

Rachael Poore Podiatric Medicine and Surgery, Unity Point Health-Des Moines, Des Moines, IA, USA

Christopher L. Reeves, DPM Orlando Foot and Ankle Clinic, Teaching Faculty, Florida Hospital East Orlando Residency Program, Orlando, FL, USA

Laurence G. Rubin, DPM, FACFAS Mechanicsville, VA, USA

D. Scot Malay, DPM, MSCE, FACFAS Director Podiatric Education and Staff Surgeon, Penn Presbyterian Medical Center, Philadelphia, PA, USA

Amber M. Shane, DPM, FACFAS Orlando Foot and Ankle Clinic, Teaching Faculty, Florida Hospital East Orlando Residency Program, Orlando, FL, USA

Naohiro Shibuya, DPM, MS, FACFAS Texas A&M University, Health Science Center, College of Medicine, Temple, TX, USA

Surgical Services, Central Texas VA Health Care System, Veterans Hospital, Temple, TX, USA

Department of Surgery, Baylor Scott and White Health Care System, Temple, TX, USA

Alan Sue Orthopedics and Podiatry, Palo Alto Foundation Medical Group, Mountain View, CA, USA

James Thomas, DPM The Orthopaedic Clinic, Auburn, AL, USA

Joshua D. Thun Monongahela Valley Hospital, Monongahela, PA, USA

Nicholas Todd, DPM Orthopedics and Podiatry, Palo Alto Foundation Medical Group, Mountain View, CA, USA

Lowell S. Weil, DPM Department of Surgery, Weil Foot and Ankle Institute, Des Plaines, IL, USA

Collin M. Zdenek, DPM Mountain View Center, Palo Alto Medcal Foundation, Mountain View, CA, USA

"Anatomy" of Complications

1

Allen M. Jacobs

Introduction

Complications are an inevitable occurrence in the performance of foot and ankle surgery. With reference to surgery, a variety of definitions have been offered to define the term "complication."

Sokol and Wilson [1] defined a complication as "any undesirable, unintended, and direct result of surgery affecting the patient which would not had occurred had the surgery gone as well as could reasonably be hoped." Classification systems for evaluation of foot and ankle surgical clinical outcomes, such as those advocated by the American College of Foot and Ankle Surgeons [2] or the American Orthopedic Foot and Ankle Society [3], examine postoperative results in terms of function, overall health of the patient, quality of life, and activity scores. Sink et al. [4] noted that no standard exists for reporting complication rates, and as a result, reported outcomes of surgical procedures such as surgery are incomplete without a standardized, objective, complication grading scheme applied concurrently with reporting outcome studies. As a result, the lack of an established basis for grading and reporting complications renders comparisons between studies ineffective. As an example, the impact of a nonunion following attempted arthrodesis of an interdigital joint for hammertoe surgery is considerably different from the impact of a nonunion following ankle joint arthrodesis.

Generally, clinical outcome studies describe complications in subjective terms, such as mild, moderate, or severe, without a standardized classification systems or consistency in definition.

A.M. Jacobs, DPM & Associates (✉)
6400 Clayton Road, Suite 402, St. Louis, MO 63117, USA
e-mail: drjacobs0902@sbcglobal.net

Definitions

Surgical complications should be differentiated from other postoperative occurrences such as failure of treatment (i.e., failure to cure), operative sequela, or surgical error. As an example, a patient continuing to demonstrate pain or limited range of motion following a cheilectomy or implant arthroplasty of the great toe performed for hallux rigidus is a failure to cure, or a procedure cure, but is not a complication. A failure of the operative intervention to provide a satisfactory outcome is per se not a complication, but rather a failure of the surgical procedure to have produced the desired outcome. Conversely, nonunion of a great toe arthrodesis for the correction of a hallux rigidus deformity is a complication and not a "failure to cure."

Postoperative sequelae are known, generally predictable, possible consequences of surgery. For example, the development of osteoarthritis of the ankle following subtalar joint fusion or triple arthrodesis is a known potential sequela of the arthrodesis, and is not a complication. The requirement for hardware removal, following ORIF of an ankle fracture, is a known potential sequela of the surgical procedure.

Surgical errors, or mistakes, may occur even when care is rendered by an outstanding foot or ankle surgeon. Surgical error may be associated with medical negligence in some circumstances. A mistake is negligence only when a reasonably careful practitioner would not have made the same mistake under similar circumstances [5]. A relationship may exist between complications and surgical error. In a review of 9830 surgical procedures, a complication rate of 3.4% was noted which included an identifiable error in 78.3% of those patients incurring a complication. The errors included most commonly error in surgical technique, judgment error, and attention to detail, or an incomplete understanding of the patient's clinical status [6].

M.S. Lee, J.P. Grossman (eds.), *Complications in Foot and Ankle Surgery*, DOI 10.1007/978-3-319-53686-6_1

Complication Classification Systems

At the present time, there is no generally recognized classification system for complications following foot and ankle surgery. Complications are accepted in the surgical literature as an important outcome measure and useful indicator for measuring quality. Efforts have been made to classify complications, such as general surgical complications, following abdominal surgery, as well as some orthopedic surgical procedures.

With reference to general surgery, one of the most commonly employed classification systems is that of Clavien-Dindo [7]. A modification of this classification system has been described for some orthopedic interventions [4], gastroenterology surgery [8], urologic surgery [9], and nephrology [10].

Presently, there are no accepted classification systems or postoperative complications subsequent to foot and ankle surgery. The lack of such classification systems results in unreliability when comparing clinical outcomes reported for the same or comparative procedures. For example, nonunion following first MPJ arthrodesis, or following first metatarsal-cuneiform arthrodesis, is frequently associated with little or no symptomatology. The nonunion rate reported for the Lapidus procedure may be greater than the nonunion rate for alternative surgical interventions, such as the Austin or scarf procedures utilized in the correction of hallux valgus and bunion deformity. However, the clinical impact of a nonunion of a procedure other than the Lapidus employed as an alternate procedure may be of greater impact on quality of life and may be associated with a greater need for operative intervention.

Table 1.1 contains a proposed adaptation of the Clavien-Dindo system for the classification of complications following foot and ankle surgery.

Table 1.1 Classification of complications following foot and ankle surgery (Jacobs-Babette)

Grade I

Any deviation from the normal postoperative course without the need for additional medical therapy, physical therapy, or surgical interventions. Such complications require no treatment and have no significant clinical relevance

Examples:

- Nonsymptomatic persistent edema following digital surgery
- Nonpainful hypertrophic scar formation
- Nonsymptomatic limited motion following bunion surgery

Grade II

A deviation from the normal postoperative course requiring unplanned physical therapy, or pharmacologic therapy

Examples:

- Symptomatic limited motion following total ankle joint replacement requiring physical therapy
- Postoperative infection requiring antibiotic therapy
- Transfer metatarsalgia requiring orthotic or shoe therapy

Grade III

A deviation from the normal postoperative course requiring surgical intervention

Examples:

- Postoperative infection requiring incision and drainage
- Osteotomy malalignment requiring revision
- Revision of a symptomatic arthrodesis or osteotomy nonunion
- Symptomatic nerve entrapment requiring operative intervention

A. Not requiring general anesthesia
B. Requiring general anesthesia

Grade IV

A deviation from the normal postoperative course which is limb threatening

Examples:

- Necrotizing fascial infection requiring extensive incision and debridement
- Acute vascular compromise to the foot or leg
- Compartment syndrome requiring fasciotomies

Grade V

A deviation from the normal postoperative course which is threatening to quality of life

Examples:

- Postoperative complex regional pain syndrome
- Significant limb shortening following total ankle joint infection and revision

Grade VI

A deviation from the normal postoperative course which is potentially life-threatening

Examples:

- DVT ± pulmonary embolism
- Malignant hyperthermia
- Organ failure (e.g., renal failure, cardiac failure)

Complication and the Surgical Patient

A ubiquity of complications may occur in association with foot and ankle surgery. There are virtually no surgical procedures without the potential for complication. Ingrown toenail correction, for example, can be associated with persistent pain or swelling, chemical burns, contact allergy, primary irritant sensitivity, infection, regrowth of the nail, spiculization, or acosmetically displeasing result.

Not infrequently, complications may result in a request for medical records by the patient and result in an allegation of malpractice. It is imperative that all patients have a clear understanding of the potential for complications to occur even when the best care has been rendered.

In some cases, the evaluation and treatment of complications following surgery will result in significant unanticipated inconvenience to the patient and considerable increased cost associated with care, again, unanticipated by the patient. These factors are superimposed on what may be a less than optimal outcome than had been perceived by the patient.

It is important that the surgeon appropriately recognize complications and appropriately treat such complications. It is equally important that the surgeon communicate with the patient regarding the nature of the complication and potential impact of the complication and express to the patient an understanding of the effects of additional delay in healing and financial burdens.

An acknowledgment of the complication should be made by the surgeon to the patient/family. Studies have demonstrated that a patient is more likely to seek medical-legal action against a provider if that physician does not disclose the complication and effectively communicate this information to the patient [11]. It should always be recalled that in most instances, a complication does not imply negligent care. However, when a complication does occur, the question of negligence arises when such complications are not recognized in a timely manner and treated in an appropriate manner.

In the case of surgical error or complication, an acknowledgment of the patient's emotions and increased physical as well as financial burden is helpful in maintaining the ability to assist the patient in resolving such complications.

In discussing the etiology of malpractice litigation, Nisselle discussed three major factors: poor patient rapport, unmet expectations, and a "big bill" [12]. Similarly, in a review of those factors leading patients to sue their doctors, insensitive handling of the incident, poor communication following the incident, and a less than satisfactory explanation are the most commonly cited factors [13]. Studies have demonstrated that a problematic doctor-patient relationship, a sense that the surgeon was abandoning the patient in the face of a complication, a devaluation of the patient and family views, a poor informational delivery, and a failure of the surgeon to understand the perspective of the patient and family are recognized as causes a patient with complications to seek litigation [14]. It is critical that faced with a complication, the surgeon communicate with and work closely with the patient.

Complications and Surgical Consent Forms

Because complications, failure to achieve the desired surgical outcome, or known common sequela may occur following any surgical procedure, the process of informed consent is required for surgical procedures.

The process of informed consent is more than obtaining a signature on a routine consent form. It is a process of communication between the patient and surgeon.

Informed consent should include a verbal or written explanation to the patient of the most common possible complications and sequela of surgical procedures. Generally, with reference to complications, surgeons rely on a standard consent form, frequently not unique or specific to the surgical procedure to be performed.

The American Medical Association has noted that forms which serve mainly to satisfy all legal requirements (e.g., "all material risks have been explained to me") may not preclude a patient from asserting that the actual disclosure did not include risks that the patient unfortunately discovered after treatment. Consequently, such consent forms may not prove to be sufficient in a court of law.

In discussing the potential for complications, the severity of potential complications relative to each patient should be considered. For example, osteomyelitis as a complication of great toe implant arthroplasty may have significantly greater impact on a competition ballroom dancer than an individual who is sedentary. Another common example is the patient who is a runner, or otherwise very athletically active, in whom the complication of avascular necrosis following bunionectomy could be much more significant than in a less athletic individual. In discussing complications, reasonable information should be provided to any patient given their individual circumstances. With regard to complications, informed consent disclosure should be tailored to the patient's individual situation thus requiring a combination of good judgment and communication skills.

The likelihood of complications occurring should also be discussed with the patient. For example, a significant nonunion rate is associated with ankle arthrodesis in the patient who smokes. Similarly, elective surgery performed in the diabetic patient, particularly in the presence of neuropathy, vascular disease, or elevated hemoglobin A1c, is associated with a much greater risk of complications. Therefore, the need for patient compliance in overall healthcare as well has postoperative care to reduce the incidence of complications is important to discuss with the patient. Such discussions ideally are documented in the patient's chart. For some procedures, such as tarsal tunnel surgery, excision of a Morton's neuroma, Lapidus procedure, Austin bunionectomy, and ankle arthrodesis, complication rates such as delayed or nonunion are established and should be related to the patient.

Good surgical judgment, together with an integration of patient beliefs and values, is critical in avoiding complications or perceived complications. The specific goals for any surgical procedure should be agreed upon by the patient, family, and surgeon. For example, reduction of a deformity associated with recurring neuropathic ulceration may not require as a goal of the surgery a perfectly functioning or cosmetic result, but rather elimination of pressure. Surgical management of a tarsal coalition may be directed at relief of pain as well as increased ambulatory tolerance, but may not include as a goal restoration of the "normal arch." The concept of limited results, and not a perfect end result, should be accepted by the patient.

Reducing the Risk of Complications

There is no certain manner with which the possibility of complications may be eliminated. Conversely, there are both surgeon and patient factors which can increase the likelihood of a complication associated with surgical intervention. The surgeon should be competent and knowledgeable with procedure to be performed. It is important that the surgeon recognize the limits of his or her professional competence and make appropriate referrals when necessary. The surgeon must not overestimate his or her ability and demonstrate some humility being aware of their individual strengths and weaknesses. Cases should be referred to a colleague when these are beyond his or her capability.

Prior to surgery, the surgeon should ensure that all needed equipment is present and functioning and that the surgeon is familiar with the use of the equipment. This is particularly important in the utilization of new fixation devices which, when mal-applied, can result in an increased risk of complications.

It is important that the surgeon continue to update their individual knowledge to allow patients to benefit from new surgical techniques with improved outcomes and lower complication rates. Thus, continuing professional development and maintenance of surgical competence are important factors in reducing the risks of surgical complications.

Complications and the Noncompliant Patient

Noncompliance is one of the most common causes for treatment failure. It is largely unrecognized, as patients infrequently volunteer that they had failed to comply with the directions of the surgeon. The effects of noncompliance range from trivial to catastrophic and include a variety of behaviors such as failure to take medications prescribed, failure to offload or remain non-weight-bearing, and failure to interdict smoking.

Noncompliance is a common occurrence in the management of the medical/surgical patient. For example, Jowett et al. have demonstrated that noncompliance with bracing is the most common cause of clubfoot relapse following initial correction [15]. Other common examples are the failure of a patient to utilize prophylactic compression stockings to prevent DVT [16] or failure of patient to perform prescribed home physical therapy for the treatment of Achilles tendinosis [17].

Because noncompliance is so common and may result in significant postoperative complications, instructions given to patients for postoperative care should be included in the medical record. The opportunities to do so include the progress notes, the operative note, and the discharge summary. In addition, discharge instructions to the patient should include specifics regarding weight-bearing status, activity level, and other significant factors such as medication use. Compliance with postoperative orders, or the failure to comply with postoperative orders, should be included in follow-up notes. The surgeon should ask about compliance, document the potential effects of noncompliance, and alert the patient to the increased risks of complications as a result of their noncompliance. The patient should be reinstructed regarding their postoperative care when necessary.

When confronted with noncompliance, the surgeon should consider whether the patient understands their problem. An attempt should be made to clarify to the patient the purpose of treatment and have the patient understand the potential effects and consequences of continued therapy noncompliance.

Smoking and Surgical Complications

It is well established that smoking is associated with increased risks of problematic soft tissue healing, increased risk of postoperative infection, increased risk of delayed union and nonunion, and increased risks of thrombosis, platelet adhesions, vasoconstriction, and ischemia [18, 19]. Smoking cessation should be discussed with the patient, and a discussion should be documented. The potential adverse effects of smoking in the perioperative period should also be discussed and documented. Not infrequently, patients demonstrate poor recall of preoperative complication risk discussion and therefore the need for good documentation. In one particular study of foot surgery patients, 11 potential complications were discussed. At which patient recall ranged from zero to a maximum of four complications was discussed. [20]

Summary

Complications may occur following any surgical procedure. Most often, complications are not the result of medical negligence. Complications should be discriminated from failure to cure, from medical error, and from sequela that may occur following any foot or ankle surgical procedure.

References

1. Sokol D, Wilson J. What is a surgical complication? World J Surg. 2008;32:942–4.
2. Thomas JL, Christensen JC, Mendocino RW, Schuberth J, et al. ACFAS scoring scale user guide. J Foot Ankle Surg. 2005;44(5):316–35.
3. Makviva A, Makwana N, Laing P. Correlation of the AOFAS scores with a generic health QUALY score in foot and ankle surgery. Foot Ankle Int. 2007;28(4):494–8.
4. Sink EL, Leunig M, Zaltz I, Gilbert JC, Clohisy J. Reliability of a complication classification system for orthopaedic surgery. Clin Orthop Relat Res. 2012;470(8):2201–6.
5. Sanfillipo JS, Smith S. Complications: what's the standard of care? Clin Obstet Gynecol. 2003;46(1):31–6.
6. Fabri PJ, Zayas-Castrol JL. Human error, not communication and systems, underlies surgical complications. Surgery. 2008;144(4):557–63.

7. Clavien PA, Barkun J, de Oliveira ML, Vauthey JN, Dindi D, Schulick RD, de Santibanes E, et al. The Clavien-Dindo classification of surgical complications: five-year experience. Ann Surg. 2009;250(2):187–96.
8. McKay A, Sutherland FR, Bathe OF, Dixon E. Morbidity and mortality following multivisceral resections in complex hepatic and pancreatic surgery. J Gastrointest Surg. 2008;12:86–90.
9. Permapongkosol S, Link RE, Su LM, Romero FR, et al. Complications of 2,775 urological laparoscopic procedures: 1993–2005. J Urol. 2007;177:580–5.
10. Sundaram CP, Martin GL, Guise A, Bernie J, Bargman V, et al. Complications after a 5-year experience with laparoscopic donor nephrectomy: the Indiana University experience. Surg Endosc. 2007;21:724–8.
11. Wittman AB, Park DM, Hardin BB. How do patients want physicians to handle mistakes? A survey of internal medicine patients in an academic setting. Arch Intern Med. 1996;156(22):2565–9.
12. Nisselle P. Recipe for a writ. Poor rapport+unmet expectation+big bill = a writ. Aust Fam Physician. 1993;22(5):824–7.
13. Vincent C, Young M, Phillips A. Why do people sue doctors? A study of patients and relatives taking legal action. Lancet. 1994;343(8913):1609–13.
14. Beckman HB, Markakis KM, Suchman AL, Frankel RM. The doctor-patient relationship and malpractice. Lessons from plaintiff depositions. Arch Intern Med. 1994;154(12):1365–70.
15. Jowett CR, Morcuenda JA, Ramachandran M. Management of congenital talipes equinovarus using the Ponseti method: a systematic review. J Bone Joint Surg Br. 2011;93(9):1160–4.
16. Bergovist D, Arcelus J, Felicissimo P. Post-discharge compliance to venous thromboembolism prophylaxis in high-risk orthopaedic surgery: results from the ETHOS registry. Thromb Haemost. 2012;107(2):280–7.
17. Knobloch K, Schreibmuellerer O. Eccentric exercises for the management of tendinopathy of the main body of the Achilles tendon with or without the AirHeel™ brace. A randomized controlled trial. A: effects on pain and microcirculation. Disabil Rehabil. 2008;30(20–22):1685–91.
18. Lind J, Kramhøft M, Bødtker S. The influence of smoking on complications after primary amputations of the lower extremity. Clin Orthop. 1991;267:211–7.
19. Silverstein P. Smoking and wound healing. Am J Med. 1992;93(1A):22S–4S.
20. Shurnas P, Coughlin M. Recall of the risks of forefoot surgery after informed consent. Foot Ankle Int. 2003;24(12):904–8.

Part I

Perioperative Complications

2 Venous Thromboembolism Associated with Foot and Ankle Surgery

D. Scot Malay

A vast array of information is available to surgeons to aid in the prevention and management of venous thromboembolism (VTE) [1–4], and readers are encouraged to use these and other sources and to stay abreast of the ever-changing body of knowledge related to these conditions. VTE includes deep vein thrombophlebitis (DVT) and pulmonary embolism (PE), and an appreciation of the clotting cascade can serve as a foundation for understanding clot formation and its prevention and treatment (Fig. 2.1). It is also important for foot and ankle surgeons to maintain a high index of suspicion for VTE, since the condition is prevalent and potentially deadly, and even when it is identified and properly treated, the sequelae of post-thrombotic syndrome (PTS) (Fig. 2.2a–d), which occurs in approximately 30% of VTE patients [5], and chronic pulmonary thromboembolic hypertension (CPTH), which occurs in approximately 4% of PE patients [6], are debilitating. PTS is associated with profound lower extremity edema, chronic stasis dermatitis, and cutaneous ulceration in 5–10% patients that suffer with lower extremity DVT. Still further, it has been estimated that 45,000–75,000 patients in the United States die annually as a result of PE [7], whereas <10% of patients with PE die if timely treatment is administered [8].

VTE develops in response to a mixture of acquired and hereditary exposures that promote hypercoagulability or thrombophilia. Virchow's classic triad of venous stasis, damage to the vein wall, and activation of the clotting cascade serve as the foundation for venous thrombosis. Clots that develop in veins are composed primarily of red and white blood cells combined with platelets and fibrin and are particularly prone to localize in the stagnant blood in the perivalvular segments of the veins of the lower extremity. Venous thrombi that remain fixed in the calf or thigh veins eventually undergo thrombolysis and recanalization, whereas those that break free can migrate with the return of venous blood to the pulmonary arteries where they occlude blood flow to the lungs. Unfortunately, VTE can be difficult to identify, and it can be recurrent. Almost 90% of VTE occur in the lower extremities, and the more proximal the site of VTE in the lower extremity, the greater is the risk of PE. In fact, VTE occurring in the femoral or popliteal veins is associated with a 50% risk of PE if left untreated, whereas the risk of PE is approximately 20–25% for VTE localized to the calf, and, overall, about 15–30% of lower extremity VTE result in PE [9]. PE, in turn, demands compensatory right ventricle inotropism in order to force the blood through the occluded pulmonary artery, which leads to pulmonary artery hypertension and subsequent right heart failure, especially in patients with preexisting cardiac and/or lung disease.

The prevalence of VTE has been estimated to be approximately one million cases per year in the United States [10], and approximately 67% of these cases occur in association with hospitalization, and about half of these patients die as a result of the disease [11]. Risk factors for VTE are present in many hospitalized patients and include comorbidities such as diabetes mellitus, hypertension, hypercholesterolemia, and cigarette smoking, as well as infection, cancer, age >75 years, obesity, and a history of previous VTE [12, 13], surgery, or trauma (Table 2.1) [14]. Following acute myocardial infarction and cerebral vascular accident, VTE is the most common cardiovascular disease [15]. Hereditary conditions, such as protein C and S and antithrombin deficiencies, factor V Leiden, and prothrombin gene mutation, also increase the likelihood of developing VTE.

Diagnosis of Venous Thromboembolism

Clinical Examination

The diagnosis of DVT and/or PE can often be made, or at least strongly suggested, based on the results of the historical review and clinical examination, and combinations of

D. Scot Malay (✉)
Director Podiatric Education and Staff Surgeon, Penn Presbyterian Medical Center, Philadelphia, PA, USA
e-mail: editorjfas@gmail.com

M.S. Lee, J.P. Grossman (eds.), *Complications in Foot and Ankle Surgery*, DOI 10.1007/978-3-319-53686-6_2

Fig. 2.1 The clotting cascade

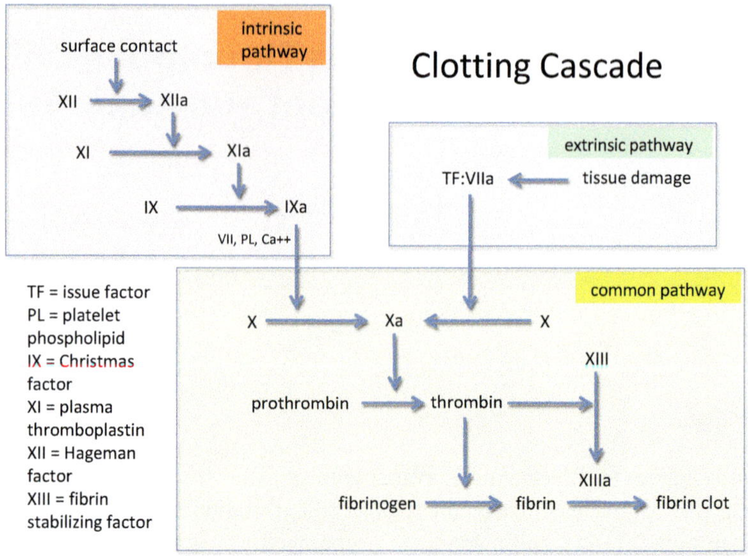

Fig. 2.2 (**a**) Chronic right lateral lesser saphenous venous stasis ulcer in patient with post-thrombotic syndrome. (**b**) Chronic post-thrombotic stasis dermatitis and scarification right lower extremity, lateral view. (**c**) Chronic post-thrombotic stasis dermatitis and scarification right lower extremity, medial view (same patient as viewed in **b**). (**d**) Bilateral postphlebitic stasis dermatitis with post thrombotic syndrome

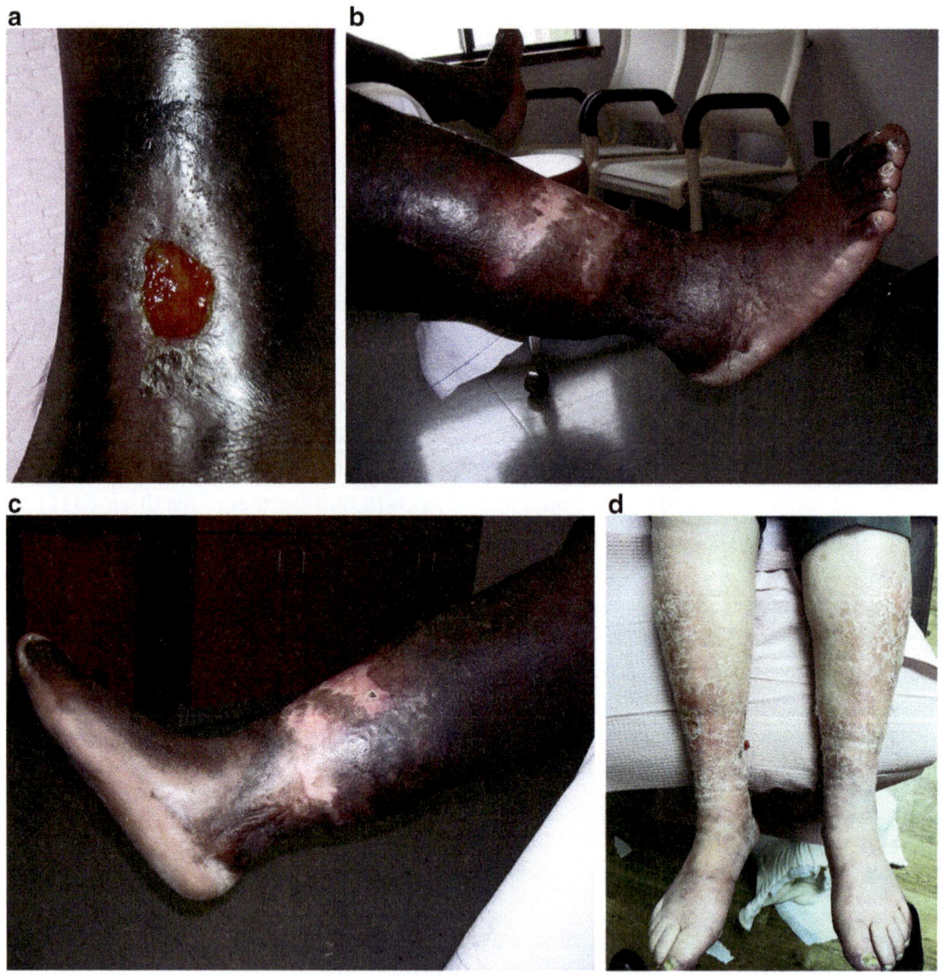

diagnostic criteria have been shown to be more or less suggestive of DVT (Table 2.2) [14, 16]. Clinically, DVT of the lower extremities is commonly associated with pain localized to, and swelling in the extremity distal to, the site of the thrombus. The involved extremity can also be warm, with cutaneous erythema, and regional varicosities may be evident. Homan's sign, which is pain in the calf upon dorsiflexion of the ankle, is commonly thought to be evidence of

Table 2.1 Risk factors for venous thromboembolism

Inherited risk factors	Antithrombin deficiency
	Dysfibrinogenemia
	Elevated levels of factor VIII
	Factor V Leiden mutation
	Hyperhomocysteinemia
	Protein C or S deficiency
	Prothrombin gene mutation
Acquired risk factors	Air travel
	Antiphospholipid syndrome
	Body mass index >30
	Cancer or certain cancer treatments
	Cardiovascular risk factors (smoking, hypertension, hyperlipidemia, diabetes mellitus)
	Heparin-induced thrombocytopenia
	Immobilization[a]
	Indwelling central venous catheter or pacemaker
	Inflammatory bowel disease
	Medical illness (heart failure, chronic obstructive pulmonary disease)
	Myeloproliferative disorder
	Pregnancy, oral contraceptive use, hormone replacement therapy
	Presence of an inferior vena cava filter
	Previous episode of venous thromboembolism
	Surgery[a]
	Trauma[a]

[a]Acquired risk factors related to most, if not all, foot and ankle surgical patients

Table 2.2 The Wells [14, 16] diagnostic criteria suggestive of deep vein thrombosis[a]

Risk factor criteria	Points
Active cancer	1
Recently bedridden >3 days or major surgery within 4 weeks	1
Calf swelling >3 cm compared to contralateral calf measured 10 cm distal to tibial tuberosity	1
Presence of collateral non-varicose superficial veins	1
Entire ipsilateral lower extremity (leg) swollen	1
Ipsilateral tenderness localized to deep venous system	1
Pitting edema greater in the symptomatic lower extremity	1
Paralysis, paresis, or recent immobilization of symptomatic lower extremity	1
History of previously documented DVT	1
Alternative diagnosis to DVT as or more likely	-2

[a]Interpretation: A score ≥ 2 indicates that the probability of DVT is likely, whereas a score < 2 indicates that probability of DVT is unlikely

calf DVT; however, this has been shown to be an unreliable assessment for calf DVT [17]. Multiple thrombosed deep and collateral veins in an extremity can result in a severely edematous, inflamed extremity known as phlegmasia cerulea dolens, which can be limb threatening due to ischemia, and may be associated with prothrombotic disorders such as heparin-induced thrombocytopenia (HIT), myeloproliferative disease, factor V Leiden mutation, polycythemia vera, and paroxysmal nocturnal hemoglobinuria (PNH). As for PE, signs and symptoms include chest pain; tachypnea and dyspnea, along with a sense of impending doom; tachycardia; hyperpyrexia; cough; hemoptysis; syncope; and, frequently, evidence of an associated DVT. Unfortunately, DVT can be clinically silent until the clinical signs of PE become evident.

Diagnostic Laboratory Tests for Venous Thromboembolism

Coagulation Tests

The *partial thromboplastin time* (PTT) is a reliable coagulation screening test, although it may not be sensitive enough to detect subtle coagulopathies. The PTT is also used to monitor heparin anticoagulation therapy, although it is not suitable for monitoring factor VII or platelet factors. The normal range for the PTT is 25–35 s, and it remains normal in von Willebrand's disease, platelet dysfunction, and thrombocytopenia. The PTT is prolonged by defects in clotting factors I, II, V, VIII, IX, X, XI, and XII. The *prothrombin time* (PT) can be used to monitor long-term warfarin anticoagulation therapy. The normal range for the PT is 11–16 s, and it is prolonged with defects in factors I, II, V, VII, and X, as well as in vitamin K deficiency, fat malabsorption (steatorrhea, colitis, jaundice), salicylate or warfarin therapy, and advanced hepatic disease. The *bleeding time* is a simple clinical examination used to assess the overall ability to stop bleeding following a cutaneous prick, and it is particularly sensitive to platelet defects. The normal range (Duke) for the bleeding time is 1–4 minutes, and it is prolonged in thrombocytopenia, abnormal platelet function, and von Willebrand's disease. The *clotting time* is a nonspecific, in vitro screening test used to determine the presence of a major clotting deficiency. The normal range (Lee-White) clotting time is 3–6 min in a capillary tube and 6–17 min in a test tube. The *international normalized ratio* (INR) is a test that was established by the World Health Organization (WHO) and the International Committee on Thrombosis and Hemostasis so that the results of blood clotting tests could be reported by any lab by virtue of the fact that all of the results are standardized with the international sensitivity index for the particular thromboplastin reagent and instrument combination used to perform the test. For warfarin, the usual optimal therapeutic prothrombin time is INR = 2–3.

Platelet Count

The normal range for the *platelet count* is 140,000–340,000/mm^3, and platelets are commonly diminished in pregnancy, leukemia, myelodysplasia, hepatic cirrhosis, aplastic anemia, iron deficiency, vitamin B12 deficiency, HIV/AIDS, Epstein-Barr virus infection, chicken pox, and various toxicities (chemotherapy, alcohol, radiation, other chemicals), hypersplenism, autoimmune diseases, septicemia, idiopathic or thrombotic thrombocytopenic purpura, hemolytic uremia, and disseminated intravascular coagulation. Thrombocytosis, which can predispose to VTE, can be caused by acute hemorrhage and blood loss, surgery, trauma, burn wounds, allergic reactions, cancer, chronic kidney disease, exercise, myocardial infarction, coronary artery bypass, infection, iron deficiency, vitamin deficiency, splenectomy, hemolysis, systemic inflammatory disease (rheumatoid arthritis, inflammatory bowel disease, celiac disease), pancreatitis, and certain medications, including epinephrine, tretinoin, vincristine sulfate, and heparin sodium.

D-Dimer Test

As a result of fibrinolysis, some of the fibrin in a thrombus degrades to form the D-dimer protein, which consists of two cross-linked D fragments of fibrin and which is elevated in the blood in the presence of VTE, rheumatoid arthritis with elevated rheumatoid factor, myeloproliferative disorders, infection, hemorrhage, trauma, and surgery. So, the D-dimer assay is not very specific for VTE, since it is also elevated in several other conditions; nonetheless, when combined with a symptomatic leg and even more so a symptomatic leg and venous Doppler ultrasound imaging of the involved extremity, elevation of the D-dimer can be very specific. The normal value for D-dimer units is ≤250 ng/mL or ≤0.5 mcg/mL fibrinogen equivalent units. As a rule, patient with a low pretest probability of DVT or PE with a negative D-dimer test should undergo further testing, typically imaging evaluation, if VTE is still suspected.

Imaging Studies for Venous Thromboembolism

Duplex Doppler Ultrasound (DDUS)

Duplex Doppler ultrasound (DDUS) imaging of the lower extremity veins is the mainstay diagnostic imaging examination used to identify lower extremity DVT. DDUS is noninvasive, usually readily available and, in comparison to other imaging modalities, relatively inexpensive in terms of the crude cost of the study. Venous DDUS is highly sensitive (95%) and specific (98%) for the diagnosis of DVT in the symptomatic lower extremity, although it is less sensitive in the asymptomatic extremity and in very obese patients [18, 19].

Other Venographic Methods

Contrast, magnetic resonance, and computerized axial tomographic venography can also be used to identify DVT in the lower extremity. The routine use of contrast venography has dwindled over the past 20–30 years, due to the potentially hazardous nature of invasive contrast media (nephrotoxicity), limitations related to inadequate deep vein filling with the contrast dye, and the steady improvement and availability of noninvasive magnetic resonance venography (MRV) and computerized axial tomographic venography (CATV).

Diagnostic Tests for Pulmonary Embolism

When PE is suspected, either with or without a prior diagnosis of DVT, a number of diagnostic laboratory, imaging, and functional tests can be helpful. As previously mentioned above, elevation of the D-dimer units present in the blood can be suggestive of VTE and is most useful in terms of specificity. Hypoxia secondary to diminished pulmonary perfusion related to PE results in an arterial blood gas with a $PaO_2 \leq 80$ mmHg in about 84% of patients with confirmed PE and no previous cardiopulmonary disease [20]. Measured levels of urine prothrombin fragment F1 + 2 can also potentially be used to assess the individual risk of vascular thrombotic complications, including VTE, following total hip arthroplasty and to test for noninvasive detection of sustained coagulation activation [21]. Right heart failure secondary to PE and pulmonary artery hypertension can also lead to elevation of cardiac troponin, as well as elevation of brain natriuretic peptide in patients without renal failure [22]. Radiographic images of the chest might reveal nonspecific signs of atelectasis, consolidation, and pleural effusion, in association with PE; electrocardiography might reveal several findings commonly associated with PE, including the $S_1Q_3T_3$ waveform pattern [23]; and transthoracic as well as transesophageal echocardiography can reveal evidence of right heart failure as a result of PE. The use of a ventilation-perfusion (V-Q) scan, where radiopharmaceutical (a gamma ray emitting xenon or technetium compound) is injected and lung ventilation and perfusion monitored, can be helpful in cases where contrast medium cannot be administered due to allergy or kidney disease or in certain obese or pregnant patients, and it is strongly suggestive of PE when it is abnormal and observed in conjunction with strongly indicative clinical findings. Pulmonary angiography, by means of contrast medium injection or magnetic resonance angiography (MRA), can also be useful, although computerized tomographic pulmonary angiography with contrast, while being expensive and invasive in terms of contrast medium and radiation exposure, has been shown to be more sensitive for PE than VQ scanning [24] and may be more sensitive and more specific than classic contrast pulmonary angiography [25].

Methods of VTE Prophylaxis and Treatment

Patient Education, Mechanical Prophylaxis, and Non-general Anesthesia

Prevention of VTE is a worthwhile and potentially lifesaving endeavor. The basic elements of VTE prophylaxis include patient education, mechanical methods that promote venous blood flow in the extremities, chemoprophylactic measures that inhibit thrombus formation, and variations in anesthesia and fluid management. Nurses [26] and surgeons, as well as house and office staff, can play an important role in teaching patients the basic physiology and warning signs of VTE, both DVT and PE, and this can go a long way in regard to compliance with prophylactic measures and even early diagnosis should a complication develop. As a rule, combined prophylactic modalities decrease significantly the incidence of VTE, in particular DVT [27]. Of course, lower extremity movement, in particular ambulation with active contraction and relaxation of the crural musculature and resultant knee and ankle motion, is an important deterrent to VTE. In fact, most VTE prophylaxis protocols in otherwise healthy individuals are discontinued once regular knee and ankle motions are resumed following foot and ankle surgery. When lower extremity range of motion cannot be implemented, such as when complete bed rest is a required element of treatment or when the extremity is immobilized, then graduated compression stockings (GCS), and intermittent pneumatic compression (IPC) devices on one or both extremities can be employed (Fig. 2.3). A 2010 review of the literature pertaining to the use of GCS revealed that their use reduced the incidence of DVT from 26% to 13% ($p < 0.0001$) in comparison to patients treated without GCS [28]. IPC devices applied to any extremity can also provide beneficial fibrinolytic activity, as evidenced by elevated blood-borne fibrinolytic activity in assays procured from sites distant to the location of the IPC device [29, 30], and this could be particularly useful to foot and ankle surgical patients when both lower extremities have to be in the surgical field [31]. In general, when foot and/or ankle surgery is undertaken on one lower extremity, an IPC device is typically applied to the contralateral lower extremity during the operative procedure and throughout the course of hospitalization.

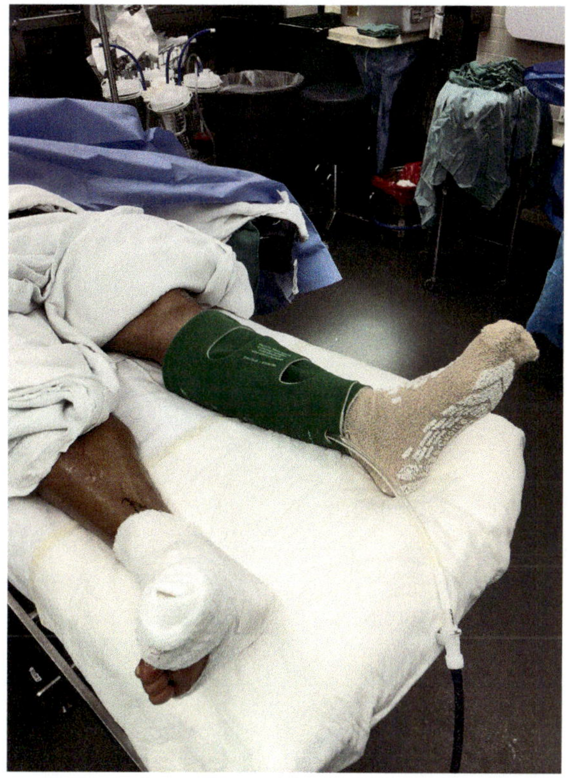

Fig. 2.3 Intermittent pneumatic compression (IPC) device on the left lower extremity of a patient about to undergo right foot surgery

In regard to anesthesia and its potential adverse influence on venous stasis and the development of VTE, it is generally considered favorable to avoid cessation of the calf muscle pump influence on venous return from the lower extremities, and, therefore, avoidance of skeletal muscle paralysis and general anesthesia, when possible, is likely to decrease the risk of DVT [32–35]. In fact, the American Association of Plastic Surgeons has recommended that when possible, the use of non-general anesthesia, such as monitored anesthesia care, local anesthesia with sedation, or neuraxial anesthesia instead of general anesthesia, should be used in order to diminish the risk of VTE [31].

Pharmacological Prophylaxis (Chemoprophylaxis) and Treatment of VTE

Naturally occurring, physiologic anticoagulants such as antithrombin III and activated protein C prevent widespread thrombosis and localize clot formation to sites of vascular injury. The clotting cascade is also balanced by plasmin-mediated fibrinolysis, resulting in the formation of D-dimers and other fibrin degradation products. When the body's intrinsic anticoagulation system requires bolstering to prevent or treat VTE complicating surgery or medical care, a wide range of therapeutic agents are available (Table 2.3), including unfractionated heparin (UFH), which is typically administered subcutaneously (SC) or via intravenous (IV) infusion; low-molecular-weight (fractionated) heparins (LMWHs), which are administered via subcutaneous injection or IV infusion and include agents such as enoxaparin, dalteparin, and tinzaparin; vitamin K antagonists like warfarin, which can be administered orally or via IV infusion; factor Xa inhibitors, which are administered via subcutaneous injection or IV infusion and include agents such as fondaparinux, rivaroxaban, apixaban, and edoxaban; direct thrombin inhibitors like dabigatran, which can be administered orally; and combined factor Xa and thrombin inhibitors like danaparoid, which can be administered via subcutaneous injection or IV infusion. The decision to choose one anticoagulant over another varies by indication and patient-specific factors, and surgeons are always encouraged to use their clinical judgment in order to tailor evidence-based guidelines for VTE prophylaxis or treatment to the particular needs of their individual patients. Useful guidelines for VTE prophylaxis and treatment are available, and readers are encouraged to review these [31, 36–38]. Surgeons are also encouraged to read the clinical pharmacology

Table 2.3 Anticoagulants used for venous thromboembolism prophylaxis and treatment

Category	Agent	Prophylaxis[a, b]	Treatment[a]
Unfractionated heparin (UFH)	Heparin	5000 units SC 2 h preoperative	80 u/kg bolus followed by 18 u/kg/hr IV infusion, or initial IV bolus of 5000, followed by 17,500 u SC twice daily
Low-molecular-weight heparin (LMWH)	Enoxaparin	40 mg SC 2 h preoperative	1.5 mg/kg/day SC once daily or 1 mg/kg SC every 12 h
	Dalteparin	2500 u SC starting 4–8 h after surgery, then 5000 u daily; or 2500 u SC starting 2 h preoperative, then 2500 u SC 4–8 h postoperative on the day of surgery, then 5000 u SC daily; or, 5000 u SC 10–14 h presurgery, then 5000 u SC 4–8 h postoperative on the day of surgery, then 5000 u SC daily	200 u/kg SC daily or 100 u/kg SC every 12 h
	Tinzaparin	50–75 u/kg 2 h preoperative, then 50 u/kg daily for 7–10 days, or 75 u/kg daily postoperative for 7–10 days	175 units/kg SC for 6–7 days
Factor Xa inhibitor	Fondaparinux	2.5 mg SC once daily starting 6–8 h postoperative, for 5–32 days after surgery	5 mg (body weight < 50 kg), 7.5 mg (body weight 50–100 kg), or 10 mg (body weight > 100 kg) SC once daily for 5 days and until a therapeutic oral anticoagulant effect is established
	Rivaroxaban	10 mg orally once daily with or without food	The 15 mg and 20 mg tablets are taken with food, whereas the 10 mg tablets can be taken with or without food. For the treatment of DVT, PE, and reduction in the risk of recurrence of DVT and of PE, 15 mg orally twice daily for the first 21 days for the initial treatment of acute DVT or PE. After the initial treatment period, 20 mg orally once daily with food for the remaining treatment
	Apixaban	2.5 mg orally twice daily	10 mg taken orally twice daily for 7 days, followed by 5 mg taken orally twice daily, for treatment of DVT and PE, or 2.5 mg taken orally twice daily for reduction in the risk of recurrent DVT and PE following initial therapy
	Edoxaban	Not indicated for prophylaxis	60 mg once daily or, if creatinine clearance, 15–50 mL/min or body weight less than or equal to 60 kg or who use certain *P*-glycoprotein inhibitors, 30 mg once daily
Direct thrombin inhibitor	Dabigatran	For patients with creatinine clearance >30 mL/min, 110 mg orally first day, then 220 mg once daily	For patients with creatinine clearance >30 mL/min, 150 mg orally, twice daily after 5–10 days of parenteral anticoagulation and for reduction in the risk of recurrence of DVT and PE for patients with creatinine clearance >30 mL/min, 150 mg orally twice daily after previous treatment
Combined factor Xa, heparinoid thrombin inhibitor	Danaparoid	For nonvascular surgery, if ≤90 kg, 750 u SC 1–4 h preoperative repeated ≥6 h postoperative then 750 u SC twice daily for 7–10 days starting the first postoperative day; and if >90 kg, then 750 u SC 1–4 h preoperative repeated ≥6 h postoperative then 1250 u SC twice daily or 750 u SC three times daily for 7–10 days starting the first postoperative day. In patients with current HIT, body weight ≤ 90 kg, 750 u SC two or three times daily for 7–10 days, following initial IV bolus of 1250 u SC; if >90 kg, then 1250 u SC two or three times daily for 7–10 days after an initial. In patients with past HITT, ≤90 kg, 750 u SC two or three times daily for 7–10 days; and if >90 kg then 1250 u SC two or 750 u SC three times daily for 7–10 days	For a thrombosis <5 days old and weight ≤ 55 kg, 1250–1500 u IV bolus then 400 u/h next 4 h then 300 u/h next 4 h then 150–200 u/h for 5–7 days or maintenance of 1500 u SC twice daily for 4–7 days; if weight 55–90 kg, 2250–2500 u IV bolus then 400 u/h next 4 h then 300 u/h next 4 h then 150–200 u/h for 5–7 days or maintenance of 2000 u SC twice daily for 4–7 days; and if weight > 90 kg, then 3750–2500 u IV bolus then 400 u/h next 4 h then 300 u/h next 4 h then 150–200 u/h for 5–7 days or maintenance of 1750 u SC twice daily for 4–7 days. For thrombosis ≥5 days old and weight ≤ 90 kg, 1250 u IV bolus the 750 u SC two or three times daily; if >90 kg, then 1250 u IV bolus then 750 u SC three times daily or 1250 u SC two or three times daily

(continued)

Table 2.3 (continued)

Category	Agent	Prophylaxis[a, b]	Treatment[a]
Vitamin K antagonist	Warfarin	Warfarin is available as scored tablets of 1, 2, 2.5, 3, 4, 5, 6, 7.5, or 10 mg and as a vial of 5 mg of reconstituted lyophilized powder for injection. Individualized dosing of warfarin is administered orally (or IV) when heparin or heparinoid therapy is already in effect, and it can usually begin (or be resumed if a 5-day overlap, bridging protocol is in effect) on the night of surgery, after which therapy is guided by the INR for at least 10 days and continued up to 4–6 weeks depending on patient-specific factors. Patients that have discontinued their maintenance warfarin therapy preoperatively can typically resume their usual dose beginning the night of surgery or the first postoperative day	After initiation of oral (or IV) administration, aiming for an INR of 2–3, warfarin is usually continued for 3–6 months
Cyclooxygenase inhibitor	Aspirin (acetylsalicylic acid)	325 mg daily for 4–6 weeks, starting the night of surgery, always in combination with physical measures such as GCS and ICD, as well as patient education and avoidance of GA whenever possible	Not indicated for treatment

Abbreviations: *GA* general anesthesia; *GCS* gradient compression stockings; *ICD* intermittent compression device; *IV* intravenous; *SC* subcutaneous, *u* international units

[a]Duration of prophylaxis is usually continued until the involved extremity is mobilized and the duration of treatment is typically 3–6 months post identification of the clot

[b]Prophylaxis entails chemoprophylaxis combined with patient education, mechanical methods, and avoidance of general anesthesia when possible; surgeons and anesthesiologists need to use caution if neuraxial (spinal, epidural) anesthesia is to be used since the risk of spinal or epidural hematoma increases with VTE prophylaxis; and dosage recommendations are based primarily or VTE prophylaxis associated with hip and/or knee surgery or general medical patient care

information contained in the package insert specific to each of these medications in order to review the details related to their proper use for VTE prophylaxis, treatment, and reversal (which is beyond the scope of this text). Surgeons are also encouraged to recruit the medical expertise of other experienced clinicians in the management of acute DVT and/or PE, since the care of such patients can be complicated and requires a wide range of expertise and intervention. Although the primary adverse effect of anticoagulant pharmacological agents is hemorrhage, parenteral administration and patient and surgeon nonadherence to treatment and guidelines are important limitations of their use [39].

Prophylaxis is generally continued until the risk factors are such that VTE is not likely, and this is typically at a time when lower extremity immobilization is discontinued and surgeons need to individualize the duration of prophylaxis based on the needs of each individual patient. The duration of treatment for confirmed DVT and/or PT depends to a large degree on the risk of recurrence. Patients at a high risk for recurrence include those with idiopathic DVT or PE, malignancy, antiphospholipid syndrome, an inferior vena cava filter, obesity, the elderly, and males. As always, the risk of prolonged anticoagulation is hemorrhage.

Anticoagulants that are commonly used for VTE prophylaxis include unfractionated heparin, fractionated heparins such as dalteparin and enoxaparin, the factor Xa inhibitor fondaparinux, and the heparinoid danaparoid, which is particularly useful in patients with a history of heparin-induced thrombocytopenia (HIT). Aspirin can also play a role in prophylaxis [40], although it is not considered to be a sole method of prophylaxis. Warfarin can also be used and is often initiated after surgery using a bridging protocol that also employs heparin or another anticoagulant.

The main goals of treatment for DVT include prevention of PE, postphlebitic syndrome, and recurrent thrombosis. Once VTE is suspected, anticoagulation should be started immediately unless there is a contraindication. In their review of the treatment of VTE, Wells et al. [4] divided therapies into acute (first 5–10 days), long-term (from the end of acute to 3–6 months), and extended (beyond 3–6 months) phases. And, despite the potentially lethal and acutely morbid nature of DVT and PE, they found that low-molecular-weight heparin (LMWH) along with vitamin K antagonists or the use of two oral agents without LMWH, along with ambulation and other physical measures, allows for outpatient management of most cases of DVT and some cases of PE, in the acute phase. Unless there is a specific contraindication, anticoagulation should be initiated as soon as VTE is diagnosed. Beyond the use of LMWH and/or oral therapies combined with physical measures, the use of thrombectomy is reserved for severe VTE threatening limb loss or stroke, and retrievable inferior vena cava (IVC) filters are indicated when anticoagulation is contraindicated. Typically, adequate treatment of DVT and PE entails 3 months of use of anticoagulants, such as single or combinations of LMWH, vitamin K antagonists, or direct factor Xa or factor IIa inhibitors, after which additional therapy used over the long-term and extended phases of VTE is based on the risk of recurrence, cause of the initial thrombus, and the risk of a serious bleeding event over time.

Although prevention of the development of VTE is generally considered a worthwhile aspect of foot and ankle surgery, hemorrhage, particularly bleeding related to methods of anticoagulation and clot prevention, can be problematic and lead to wound as well as systemic complications. Patients with a platelet count <100,000/mm^3; those with active or a history of heparin-induced thrombocytopenia; those taking aspirin, clopidogrel, or nonsteroidal anti-inflammatory drugs; and those with renal or hepatic disease may not be satisfactory candidates for VTE chemoprophylaxis. In such patients, nonpharmacologic methods of prophylaxis, including GCS and ICDs, early active motion with activation of the calf muscle venous pump, and avoidance of general anesthesia if possible are likely to be the mainstays of VTE prophylaxis.

Unfractionated Heparin (UFH) and Low-Molecular-Weight Heparin (LMWH)

Unfractionated heparin (UFH) occurs naturally and is contained in mast cell granules and released via degranulation in response to numerous stimuli, including hypersensitivity and tissue injury, in particular blood vessel disruption. Fractionated heparins (enoxaparin, dalteparin, tinzaparin), which are derived from depolymerization of long-chain polysaccharide heparin, are categorized as low molecular weight and useful as anticoagulants if their molecular weights average ≤ 8000 Daltons. The clotting cascade (Fig. 2.1), via sequential protease activity, amplifies conversion of soluble fibrinogen to insoluble strands of fibrin that combine with platelets to form a thrombus. Antithrombin is a serine protease inhibitor that disrupts the clotting cascade and, as such, serves as the key plasma inhibitor of coagulation. Heparins bind to antithrombin and inhibit factor Xa (activated factor X), thereby impeding the clotting cascade. Interestingly, LMWHs can only bind to and inhibit antithrombin, whereas heparin can bind to antithrombin and inhibit both antithrombin and thrombin. UFH also binds other plasma proteins, whereas LMWH is limited in its binding activity, and as such LMWH is associated with a more consistent dose-response and fewer non-hemorrhagic adverse effects. Heparins can be neutralized by protamine if problematic hemorrhage develops. Moreover, immune-mediated heparin-induced thrombocytopenia (HIT)) can develop in response to administration of heparin, and this can lead to devastating thrombosis. The incidence of HIT in patients that have been heparinized for more than 7 days is approximately 1% [41], and the 30-day incidence of mortality associated with HIT is 16.6% [42].

Factor Xa Inhibitors, Direct Thrombin Inhibitors, and Heparinoids

A number of factor Xa inhibitors can be used for VTE prophylaxis and/or treatment, including fondaparinux, rivaroxaban, apixaban, and edoxaban. Although specific indications may be more broadly defined than just prophylaxis or treatment of DVT and/or PE, all of these agents can potentially be used in the realm of foot and ankle surgery. Fondaparinux is indicated for VTE prevention in patients undergoing hip fracture surgery, hip replacement surgery, knee replacement surgery, and abdominal surgery and for the treatment of acute DVT and/or PE when administered in conjunction with warfarin. Rivaroxaban is indicated to reduce the risk of stroke and systemic embolism in patients with nonvalvular atrial fibrillation, for the treatment of DVT and PE, for the reduction in the risk of recurrence of DVT and of PE, and for the prophylaxis of DVT, which may lead to PE in patients undergoing knee or hip replacement surgery. Apixaban is indicated to reduce the risk of stroke and systemic embolism in patients with nonvalvular atrial fibrillation, for the prophylaxis of DVT, which may lead to PE, in patients who have undergone hip or knee replacement surgery, for the treatment of DVT and PE, and for the reduction in the risk of recurrent DVT and PE following initial therapy. Edoxaban is indicated to reduce the risk of stroke and systemic embolism (SE) in patients with nonvalvular atrial fibrillation and for the treatment of DVT and PE following 5–10 days of initial therapy with a parenteral anticoagulant. The direct thrombin inhibitor dabigatran is indicated to reduce the risk of stroke and systemic embolism in patients with nonvalvular atrial fibrillation, for the treatment of DVT and PE in patients who have been treated with a parenteral anticoagulant for 5–10 days, to reduce the risk of recurrence of DVT and PE in patients who have been previously treated, and for the prophylaxis of DVT and PE in patients who have undergone hip replacement surgery. The combined factor Xa-thrombin inhibitor danaparoid, a heparinoid, is indicated for the treatment of patients with an acute episode of heparin-induced thrombocytopenia (HIT) and for prophylaxis in patients with a history of HIT.

Warfarin

Warfarin remains a very prevalent anticoagulant in the clinical realm, and foot and ankle surgeons routinely encounter patients that use this drug. Warfarin inhibits the synthesis of vitamin K-dependent clotting factors, including factors II, VII, IX, and X, and proteins C and S, which naturally prevent coagulation. Anticoagulation generally occurs within 24 h, and peak antithrombotic effects occur 72–96 h after administration of warfarin. As a rule, the antithrombotic effects of warfarin multiply over time, and regular monitoring of coagulation using the INR or the prothrombin time is required. The pharmacokinetics of warfarin are influenced by a wide range of physiologic conditions (malnutrition, dehydration, old age) and the effects of concomitantly administered medications, in particular certain antibiotics. Generally, the use of warfarin can begin on the night of surgery and guided thereafter by the INR. Patients previously on chronic warfarin therapy prior to their surgery can resume their regular dosage the night of the operation. An INR > 3 warrants cessation of warfarin administration, and 1 mg of vitamin K should be administered orally or SC for an INR >6 in the absence of active hemorrhage, and even higher doses may be used in the presence of bleeding. Fresh frozen plasma can also be administered if active bleeding occurs. Importantly, warfarin should not be administered in conjunction with aspirin or COX-1 inhibiting nonsteroidal anti-inflammatory drugs, although concomitant use of COX-2 inhibitors like celecoxib can be used if needed. For VTE prophylaxis, warfarin should be administered from 10 days to 4–6 weeks, depending on patient-specific factors, whereas, for the treatment of VTE, warfarin is generally administered for 3–6 months, aiming for an INR 2–3.

Aspirin

Historically, aspirin seems to be a prevalent method of VTE prophylaxis in bone and joint surgery, although its efficacy has been questioned by many clinicians due to a limitation of quality evidence. Over the 7–10 day lifespan of a platelet, aspirin (acetylsalicylic acid) irreversibly inactivates cyclooxygenase (COX) by means of acetylation, thereby preventing catalytic oxygenation of arachidonic acid to prostaglandin G2 and the formation of thromboxane A2, a mediator of platelet aggregation and vasoconstriction. Although aspirin is not recommended as a sole option for the prevention of VTE, in patients undergoing elective TKR or who have a contraindication to pharmacologic prophylaxis and undergo a THR or hip fracture surgery, aspirin in conjunction with compression devices as part of a multimodal approach can be acceptable; and existing evidence does not support the hypothesis that aspirin is less likely to cause adverse bleeding events than other anticoagulants [40]. Patients who have given aspirin as postoperative VTE prophylaxis typically receive 325 mg daily for 4–6 weeks, starting the night of surgery, and this is combined with physical measures such as GCS and IPC, as well as patient education and avoidance of general anesthesia when indicated. Surgeons also need to keep in mind that platelet inhibition diminishes the cytoprotective function of prostaglandin in the stomach, thereby predisposing to gastritis, peptic ulcer, and gastrointestinal bleeding, so surgeons employing aspirin for VTE prophylaxis need to take these potential complications into consideration.

Thrombolytic Therapy

Therapeutic thrombolysis, either by means of systemic administration or catheter-directed infusion of the thrombolytic agent, can be used in certain patients, although the risk of bleeding, including intracranial hemorrhage, is higher with thrombolytic therapy than it is with generalized anticoagulation. Two agents, namely, streptokinase (250,000 units infused as a loading does, then 100,000 units/h over the ensuing 24 h) and recombinant tissue plasminogen activator (TPA, 100 mg infused over 2 h), are commonly used for clot lysis. Thrombolysis, in particular catheter-directed infusion aimed at the clot, may diminish the risk of PTS, so it may be a preferred approach in patients with a severe proximal clot or multiple clots, or a previous history of DVT or PTS, and those at risk for limb gangrene but at low risk for hemorrhage [43]. Thrombolytic therapy may also be beneficial for patients with hemodynamically unstable PE with right heart failure.

Pulmonary Embolectomy

In patients with severe PE, who fail to respond favorably to anticoagulation and supportive therapies, including thrombolytic therapy, pulmonary embolectomy may be indicated. The incidence of mortality associated with pulmonary embolectomy is approximately 20% [44].

Inferior Vena Cava (IVC) Filter

There are a number of indications for IVC interruption, including severe PE, thrombosis in the iliac veins or the distal vena cava, inability to adequately anticoagulate or complications related to anticoagulation, and DVT in the presence of preexisting cardiac or pulmonary disease. Alone, an IVC filter is not an adequate therapy for DVT or prevention of PE, so anticoagulation is generally used in conjunction with the filter, if it is not contraindicated. IVC filters can be permanent or retrievable devices, the selection of which is based on the expected duration of use.

Risk Stratification Schemes for VTE Prophylaxis

Long ago, Thomas Bayes pointed out the importance of the baseline probability of a condition (the prevalence of a condition in a specific population) as it relates to the probability of a test being positive for that condition [45]. Since Bayes' famous essay was written, clinical decision rules based on pretest probability have been developed for many diagnostic tests, including those used to identify the presence of

VTE. Such clinical decision rules can be used to classify individuals into high-, medium-, and low-risk categories for the probability of DVT [46–49]. Since the clinical examination of DVT can be unreliable in and of itself, risk stratification of patients based on clinical decision rules that combine clinical and laboratory and imaging tests can increase the accuracy of a diagnosis. In fact, the use of the Wells rules (Table 2.2) [14, 16], combined with the use of the D-dimer test [47], can help surgeons decide when noninvasive imaging of the lower extremity veins is indicated and increases the likelihood of an accurate diagnosis of lower extremity VTE [48]. The Wells criteria [49] for the diagnosis of DVT were determined based on analysis of 1096 outpatients suspected of having DVT. The use of the D-dimer test imparts a negative predictive value (NPV, the probability that the individual does not have the disease of interest if the test result is negative) of 99.1% (95% confidence interval 96.7, 99.9) in patients with a low pretest probability of DVT (a Wells criteria score < 2). In patients with a high pretest probability of DVT (a Wells criteria score ≥ 2), the NPV of the D-dimer test was 89.0% (95% confidence interval 80.7, 94.6).

Overall, it is understood that all patients admitted to the hospital, including those undergoing inpatient or outpatient surgery, are at risk of developing VTE. Of the 38 million hospital discharges in the United States in 2003, 20% were surgical inpatients, and using the American College of Chest Physicians' guidelines for risk stratification [50], it was estimated that 15%, 24%, and 17% were at moderate, high, or very high risk for VTE [51]. Interestingly, PE has been described as the most common cause of preventable hospital death [52–56] and accounts for approximately 150,000–200,000 deaths per year in the United States [57, 58]. Since DVT often precedes PE, its prevention and treatment, once it has been diagnosed, are important aspects of the care of foot and ankle surgical patients, and effective and safe prophylactic measures are available for most high-risk patients [59–62]. Furthermore, numerous evidence-based guidelines have been published for the prevention of VTE in general medical [63, 64] and cancer [65] patients.

VTE Prophylaxis in Hospitalized Patients

One risk stratification scheme that has been found to be useful in the management of a wide range of patients is the Padua Prediction Score, which was developed based on a prospective cohort study that involved 1180 consecutive hospitalized patients who were followed for 90 days following their admission [66]. The Padua Prediction Score was based on the summation of risk factor scores, and a score ≥4 was considered to indicate a high risk for venous thromboembolism (VTE), whereas a score <4 was considered to indicate a low risk for VTE (Table 2.4). Of the patients, 469 (39.7%) were labeled as being at a high risk for thrombosis, and VTE developed in 4 (2.2%) of 186 who received thromboprophylaxis and 31 (11%) of 283 who did not (HR of VTE = 0.13; 95% CI, 0.04–0.40). Furthermore, VTE developed in 2 (0.3%) of 711 low-risk patients (HR of VTE in high-risk patients without prophylaxis as compared with low-risk patients, 32.0; 95% CI, 4.1–251.0), and bleeding occurred in 3 (1.6%) of 186 high-risk patients who had thromboprophylaxis. The authors concluded that their risk assessment model (the Padua Prediction Score) discriminated between medical patients at high and low risk of VTE and that adequate thromboprophylaxis in high-risk patients during hospitalization could result in long-standing (up to 90 days) protection against thromboembolic events with a low risk of bleeding.

Table 2.4 Padua [66] prediction score for VTE risk assessment in hospitalized patients[a]

Risk factor	Score
Active cancer (patients with local or distant metastases and/or in whom chemotherapy or radiotherapy had been performed in the previous 6 months)	3
Previous VTE (excluding superficial vein thrombosis)	3
Reduced mobility (bedrest with bathroom privileges, either due to patient's limitations or on physicians order, for at least 3 days)	3
Known thrombophilia (carrier of defects of antithrombin, protein C or S, factor V Leiden, G20210A prothrombin mutation, antiphospholipid syndrome)	3
Recent (≤1 month) trauma and/or surgery	2
Elderly age (≥70 years)	1
Heart and/or respiratory failure	1
Acute myocardial infarction or ischemic stroke	1
Acute infection and/or rheumatologic disorder	1
Obesity (BMI ≥30)	1
Ongoing hormonal therapy	1

[a]A score ≥ 4 indicates a high risk for venous thromboembolism (VTE), whereas a score < 4 is considered a low risk for VTE

VTE Prophylaxis in Non-orthopedic Surgical and Nonsurgical Patients

Also in 2001, Caprini and colleagues published a risk stratification scheme for VTE in surgical (non-orthopedic) and nonsurgical patients [67], and later in 2010, Caprini and colleagues published a review of VTE risk assessment scoring systems and the results of a validation study of a risk assessment tool for VTE prophylaxis in non-orthopedic surgical patients [68]. In these reports, various risk factors for VTE were categorized and weighted with point values (Table 2.5). In order to determine an individual patient's risk stratum,

Table 2.5 Caprini [67, 68] score risk factors and point values

Risk factor	Score
Age 41–60 years	1
Current swollen leg	1
Varicose veins	1
Obesity (BMI > 25)	1
Minor surgery planned	1
Sepsis (<1 month)	1
Acute myocardial infarction	1
Congestive heart failure (<1 month)	1
Medical patient currently at bed rest	1
History of inflammatory bowel disease	1
History of prior major surgery (<1 month)	1
Abnormal pulmonary function (COPD)	1
Serious lung disease, pneumonia (<1 month)	1
Oral contraceptive or hormone replacement therapy	1
Pregnancy or postpartum (<1 month)	1
History of unexplained stillborn infant, recurrent spontaneous abortion (≥3), premature birth with toxemia or growth-restricted infant	1
Other risk factor	1
Age 61–74 years	2
Central venous catheter	2
Arthroscopic surgery	2
Major surgery (>45 minutes)	2
Malignancy (present or previous)	2
Laparoscopic surgery (>45 minutes)	2
Patient confined to bed (>72 h)	2
Immobilizing plaster cast (<1 month)	2
Age ≥ 75 years	3
Family history of thrombosis (this is most frequently missed risk factor)	3
History of DVT or PE	3
Positive prothrombin 20210A	3
Positive factor V Leiden	3
Positive lupus anticoagulant	3
Elevated serum homocysteine	3
Heparin-induced thrombocytopenia (HIT)	3
Elevated anticardiolipin antibodies	3
Other congenital or acquired thrombophilia (if yes, type should be specified)	3
Stroke (<1 month)	5
Multiple trauma (<1 month)	5
Elective major lower extremity arthroplasty	5
Hip, pelvis, or leg fracture (<1 month)	5
Acute spinal cord injury (paralysis, <1 month)	5

the various risk factor points were added to arrive at the patient's Caprini score. It should be pointed out that the Caprini score, as compared to the Wells criteria (Table 2.2), focuses on risk stratification and not the likelihood of a diagnosis of VTE. Based on prospective risk factor modeling in a large cohort of patients, the Caprini score can be used to determine a patient's risk for VTE, which is used to guide the approach to thrombosis prophylaxis (Table 2.6).

Table 2.6 Recommended prophylaxis for non-orthopedic (not hip or knee arthroplasty) general and abdominal pelvic surgery including gastrointestinal, genitourinary, bariatric, vascular, reconstructive, cardiothoracic, and gynecologic surgery hospitalized surgical patients

VTE risk score[a]	Low risk of bleeding	High risk of bleeding
0 (very low risk)	Early ambulation	Early ambulation
1–2 (low risk)	Intermittent pneumatic compression	Intermittent pneumatic compression
3–4 (moderate risk)	Low-molecular-weight heparin or low-dose unfractionated heparin or intermittent pneumatic compression	Intermittent pneumatic compression
≥5 (high risk)	Low-molecular-weight heparin or low-dose unfractionated heparin and intermittent pneumatic compression	Intermittent pneumatic compression until risk of bleeding diminishes, the chemoprophylaxis

[a]Based on the Caprini score [67, 68]

VTE Prophylaxis in Hip, Knee, and Orthopedic Trauma Surgery

In regard to hip replacement surgery, which carries a high risk of VTE, LMWHs, namely, enoxaparin, tinzaparin, and reviparin, can be used as prophylaxis. These agents behave as separate, noninterchangeable compounds that cannot be therapeutically substituted based upon anti-factor Xa levels, and the choice of LMWH used should be based on clinical experience with each agent [69]. The occurrence of pulmonary embolism and deep venous thrombosis within 30 days after elective primary total hip or knee arthroplasty was more frequent in patients with a body mass index >30 kg/m^2 and in patients with moderate or severe systemic disease resulting in some functional limitation as defined by an American Society of Anesthesiologists (ASA) physical status classification ≥3 [70]. Interestingly, a systematic review of thromboprophylaxis in trauma patients, published in 2013, concluded that there was only weak evidence to recommend the use of DVT prophylaxis for people with severe trauma, that there was some evidence that thromboprophylaxis prevents DVT, and that there was no quality evidence that thromboprophylaxis actually reduced PE or mortality related to trauma [71]. Still further, in a multicenter, non-inferiority design randomized controlled trial, the report for which was published in 2013 [72], the authors concluded that extended prophylaxis for 28 days with aspirin was non-inferior to and as safe as dalteparin for the prevention of VTE after THR in patients who initially received dalteparin for 10 days, and they further speculated that aspirin's low cost and greater convenience could make it a reasonable alternative for extended thromboprophylaxis after THR.

In regard to hip and knee surgery, the American Academy of Orthopaedic Surgeons' expert opinion clinical guideline entitled *Preventing Venous Thromboembolic Disease in Patients Undergoing Elective Hip and Knee Arthroplasty: Evidence-Based Guideline and Evidence Report*, published in 2011 by the American Academy of Orthopaedic Surgeons [73], makes the following ten recommendations for surgeons performing hip or knee arthroplasty:

1. We recommend against routine postoperative duplex ultrasonography screening of patients who undergo elective hip or knee arthroplasty.
2. Patients undergoing elective hip or knee arthroplasty are already at high risk for venous thromboembolism. The practitioner might further assess the risk of venous thromboembolism by determining whether these patients had a previous venous thromboembolism.
3. Patients undergoing elective hip or knee arthroplasty are at risk for bleeding and bleeding-associated complications. In the absence of reliable evidence, it is the opinion of this work group that patients be assessed for known bleeding disorders like hemophilia and for the presence of active liver disease which further increase the risk for bleeding and bleeding-associated complications.
4. We suggest that patients discontinue antiplatelet agents (e.g., aspirin, clopidogrel) before undergoing elective hip or knee arthroplasty.
5. We suggest the use of pharmacologic agents and/or mechanical compressive devices for the prevention of venous thromboembolism in patients undergoing elective hip or knee arthroplasty and who are not at elevated risk beyond that of the surgery itself for venous thromboembolism or bleeding.
6. In the absence of reliable evidence, it is the opinion of this work group that patients undergoing elective hip or knee arthroplasty, and who have also had a previous venous thromboembolism, receive pharmacologic prophylaxis and mechanical compressive devices.
7. In the absence of reliable evidence, it is the opinion of this work group that patients undergoing elective hip or knee arthroplasty, and who also have a known bleeding disorder (e.g., hemophilia) and/or active liver disease, use mechanical compressive devices for preventing venous thromboembolism.
8. In the absence of reliable evidence, it is the opinion of this work group that patients undergo early mobilization following elective hip and knee arthroplasty. Early mobilization is of low cost, minimal risk to the patient, and consistent with current practice.
9. We suggest the use of neuraxial (such as intrathecal, epidural, and spinal) anesthesia for patients undergoing elective hip or knee arthroplasty to help limit blood loss, even though evidence suggests that neuraxial anesthesia does not affect the occurrence of venous thromboembolic disease.
10. Current evidence does not provide clear guidance about whether inferior vena cava (IVC) filters prevent pulmonary embolism in patients undergoing elective hip and knee arthroplasty who also have a contraindication to chemoprophylaxis and/or known residual venous thromboembolic disease. Therefore, we are unable to recommend for or against the use of such filters.

VTE Prophylaxis in Foot and Ankle Surgery

For the purposes of this chapter, foot and ankle surgical patients include any and all inpatients and outpatients managed by surgeons, including patients that undergo surgery localized to the forefoot and toes, mid- and hindfoot, ankle and leg distal to the tibial tuberosity, regardless of whether or not the surgery is undertaken for elective reconstructive interventions, emergent or planned operations, limb salvage or wound care, amputations, and the repair of traumatic injuries. Since immobilization, bed rest, and surgery, as well as trauma, are common elements of many foot and ankle surgical patients, the presence of clinical findings suggestive of DVT in conjunction with just two of these risk factors, according to the Wells criteria [16] (Table 2.2), is highly likely to be associated with the presence of DVT (and possibly PE). Unfortunately for foot and ankle surgeons, in comparison to VTE in association with knee and hip surgery, rigorous study of its association with foot and ankle surgery has not been as thoroughly documented in the peer-reviewed scientific literature. As such, there remains considerable debate as to the routine need for VTE prophylaxis in association with foot and ankle surgery, and definitive methods, in terms of the agents and methods used, dosages, and duration of intervention, have yet to be clearly defined in regard specifically to foot and ankle surgery. Foot and ankle surgeons are encouraged to become familiar with the existing literature, their hospital's institutional protocols, to carefully consider each patient on an individual basis in regard to the risk of developing VTE, and to use the methods that, based on one's experience and understanding of the evidence, prevent the development of VTE. What follows, is a review of the literature related to VTE prophylaxis in foot and ankle surgery.

In a prospective multicenter study published in 1998, Mizel et al. aimed to identify patients with symptomatic thromboembolic disease and to evaluate potential risk factors for VTE in 2733 foot and/or ankle surgery patients [74]. They observed that six (0.22%) patients with clinically significant VTE were identified, four (0.15%) nonfatal pulmonary emboli were identified, and significant risk factor covariates included nonweight bearing and immobilization after surgery. Based on their observations, the investigators concluded that routine prophylaxis for thromboembolic disease after foot and ankle surgery probably was not warranted. Then, in 2002, Solis and Saxby [75] undertook a prospective study to establish the incidence of DVT in patients who had undergone foot and/or ankle surgery, by performing bilateral calf duplex ultrasound examinations at the first postoperative visit. Of 201 consecutive patients, deep calf clots were found in seven (3.5%) patients, but none of these showed progression on follow-up ultrasound or extension proximal to the calf. By the authors' criteria, none of the studied patients required treatment, and they concluded that the rate and progression of DVT after foot and ankle surgery were low and did not require routine prophylaxis. They also noted that risk factors associated with DVT formation were postoperative immobilization, hindfoot surgery, tourniquet use, and advancing age. Also in 2002, Lassen et al. [76] published the results of a prospective, double-blind, placebo-controlled trial to evaluate the efficacy and safety of subcutaneous reviparin (1750 anti-Xa units given once daily during the course of immobilization) in 371 patients who required immobilization in a plaster cast or brace for at least 5 weeks after a leg fracture or rupture of the Achilles tendon, and they performed venography of the injured leg within 1 week after removal of the plaster cast or brace, or earlier if there were symptoms suggesting deep vein thrombosis. They observed that DVT was diagnosed in 17 (9.3%) of the 183 patients randomly assigned to receive reviparin and 35 (18.7%) of 188 patients randomly assigned to receive placebo (odds ratio = 0.45; 95% confidence interval, 0.24–0.82). Most of the thromboses that they observed were distal (14 in the reviparin group and 25 in the placebo group), and there were two (1.1%) cases of PE in the placebo group who also had proximal DVT. There were no differences between the two groups with respect to bleeding or other adverse events. Based on these findings, the authors concluded that DVT was common in persons with leg injury requiring prolonged immobilization and that reviparin given once daily was effective and safe in reducing the risk of VTE.

In 2003, Slaybaugh, Beasley, and Massa [77] published a clinical protocol, a risk assessment tool based on their modification of the previously published Caprini risk stratification tool [67], and prophylaxis and treatment guidelines for DVT and PE that occur in association with foot and ankle surgery. Interestingly, the Slaybaugh, Beasley, and Massey (SBD) risk stratification system for VTE prophylaxis (Tables 2.7 and 2.8) is a system that the authors developed based on their interpretation of the Caprini score as it would, in theory, relate to patients undergoing foot and ankle surgery. Although the SBD foot and ankle risk stratification system has not been validated by means of prospective factor analysis or reliability testing and the precise rationale for their modification of the Caprini risk factor point system was not explicitly defined in the published report, the system has face validity (in this author's opinion).

Table 2.7 SBM[a] venous thromboembolism point system for risk stratification in foot and ankle surgery[b]

Risk factor			Points
Clinical situation		OR time > 105 min	1
		Tourniquet time > 90 min	1
		Rearfoot or ankle sugary	1
		Immobilization in a BK or AK cast >1 week	2
		Medical or surgical patients confined to bed for >72 h	2
		Central venous access	2
		Congestive heart failure	3
		Sever sepsis/infection	3
		Ankle, pilon, or tibial fracture	3
		Multiple trauma	5
		Acute spinal cord injury	5
Medical condition	Clinical status	40–60 years of age	1
		Pregnancy or postpartum	1
		Varicose veins	1
		Obesity defined as >20 pounds > ideal body weight	1
		Diabetes mellitus	1
		Hypertension	1
		Hyperlipidemia	1
		Smoker	1
		Polycystic ovary syndrome	1
		>60 years of age	2
		Oral contraceptive or receiving hormone replacement therapy	2
		Inflammatory bowel disease	2
		Currently treated or history of malignancy	2
		History of deep venous thrombosis or pulmonary embolism	5
	Inherited	Factor V Leiden/activated protein C resistance	3
		Antithrombin III deficiency	3
		Protein S and C deficiency	3
		Dysfibrinogenemia	3
		Homocysteinemia	3
		20210A prothrombin mutation	3
	Acquired	Lupus anticoagulant	3
		Antiphospholipid antibodies	3
		Myeloproliferative disorders	3
		Disorders of plasminogen and plasmin activation	3
		Heparin-induced thrombocytopenia	3
		Hyperviscosity syndromes	3
		Homocysteinemia	3

[a]SBM = Slaybaugh-Beasely-Massa [77]
[b]Risk factor points are added to determine risk stratum, which is used to guide prophylaxis (see Table 2.8)

In a 2006 retrospective analysis of 602 foot and ankle surgical patients from two separate practices, 24 (4% incidence) patients experienced a postoperative VTE complication, the risk factors for which were rheumatoid arthritis, a recent

Table 2.8 SBM[a] pharmacologic venous thromboembolism prophylaxis recommendations by risk stratum for foot and ankle surgery[b]

Patient status and duration of prophylaxis	Risk stratum[c]			
	Low (0–1 risk factor points)	Medium (2 risk factor points)	High (3–4 risk factor points)	Very high (≥5 risk factor points)
Inpatient	No prophylaxis	Beginning first day postoperative and continue throughout hospitalization: enteric coated ASA 325–650 mg orally every 12 h, if ASA contraindicated, then UFH 5000 u SC every 12 h	Beginning first day postoperative and continue throughout hospitalization: enteric coated ASA 325–650 mg orally every 12 h, if ASA contraindicated, then UFH 5000 u SC every 12 h or LMWH SC daily	Beginning preoperative or within 12 h postoperative, UFH 5000 u SC every 8 h, or LMWH SC daily
Outpatient surgery or upon discharge	No prophylaxis	Enteric-coated ASA 325–650 mg orally every 12 h, if ASA contraindicated, then no pharmacologic prophylaxis	Enteric-coated ASA 325–650 mg orally every 12 h or UFH or LMWH preoperative or immediately postoperative, or LMWH beginning the first postoperative day	LMWH SC daily or immediate total or partial weight bearing with ankle range of motion and ASA 325–650 mg orally every 12 h
Duration	No prophylaxis	While hospitalized up to first postoperative visit, then decide whether to extend 7–14 days	While hospitalized up to 7–14 days postoperative, then reassess	While hospitalized up to 10–14 days postoperative, continued while immobilized

Abbreviations: *ASA* acetylsalicylic acid, *LMWH* low-molecular-weight heparin, *SC* subcutaneous, *UFH* unfractionated heparin

[a]SBM = Slaybaugh-Beasely-Massa [77]

[b]Early range of motion and mechanical methods (venous compression stockings and intermittent pressure devices) are recommended in conjunction with pharmacological methods

[c]Risk stratum determined based on the sum of risk factor points described in Table 2.7

history of air travel, previous DVT or PE, and limb immobilization [78]. The authors of that study concluded that the incidence of symptomatic VTE complications could be higher than what had been previously reported (prior to 2006) and that further scientific investigation was needed in order to guide clinical practice.

In a 2007 report of the results of an e-mail-based survey aimed at determining current trends in VTE prophylaxis among 142 American and British foot and ankle surgeons, 27 (19%) of the surgeons indicated that they routinely used VTE prophylaxis in both elective and trauma foot and ankle surgery [79]. The surveyed surgeons in that report indicated that the most common situation in which VTE prophylaxis was used involved postoperative immobilization of the lower extremity, or when postoperative non-weight-bearing ambulation was employed. The respondents also indicated that the most common reasons for not using VTE prophylaxis on a routine basis were the known low incidence of VTE following foot and ankle surgery and the lack of published evidence indicating that it was beneficial. The investigators concluded that further clinical research was required in order to adequately guide practice.

In 2008, Wukich and Waters [80] reviewed a cohort of 1000 patients that had been treated over a 1.5-year period, and identified 4 (0.4%) cases of DVT and 3 (0.3%) cases of nonfatal PE. They also observed that the patients who developed DVT had ≥2 identifiable risk factors. Based on the <1% incidence of VTE following foot and ankle surgery, Wukich and Waters concluded that routine prophylaxis in association with foot and ankle surgery was not supported by their evidence.

In a 2010 survey focusing on VTE prophylaxis practices in elective foot and ankle surgery amongst 159 members of the British Orthopaedic Foot and Ankle Society (BOFAS), 84 (53%) respondents, accounting for 33,500 foot and ankle operations per annum, estimated the incidence of DVT, PE and fatal PE to be 0.6%, 0.1% and 0.02, respectively [81]. Furthermore, and despite recognized biases, they concluded that 10,000 patients would have to be treated (number needed to treat) in order to prevent a single fatal PE and, based on their observations, they questioned guidelines that called for routine VTE chemoprophylaxis in elective foot and ankle surgery.

In a retrospective cohort study of English National Health Service patients, published in 2011, symptomatic VTE, PE, and mortality within 90 days following fixation of an ankle fracture (45,949 patients), first metatarsal osteotomy (33,626 patients), hindfoot fusion (7033 patients), and total ankle replacement (TAR, 1633 patients), observed over a 42-month period, revealed the following incidences of DVT, PE, and mortality, respectively: after fixation of an ankle fracture—0.12%, 0.17% and 0.37%; after first metatarsal osteotomy—0.01%, 0.02% and 0.04%; after hindfoot fusion—0.03%, 0.11% and 0.11%; and after TAR—0, 0.06%, and 0. The risk factors that were significantly associated with VTE were older age and multiple comorbidities following ankle fracture repair [82]. Based on these national data, the investigators concluded that VTE, PE, and death following foot and ankle surgery were extremely rare, and although the fracture subset was at a higher risk, there was no evidence that VTE prophylaxis reduced the risk and, for most patients, prophylaxis was not required.

In a review of the incidence of VTE and PE following surgical repair of acute Achilles tendon rupture in 88 patients who underwent surgery without VTE prophylaxis, 5 (5.7%) cases of VTE and 1 (1.1%) case of PE were identified [83]. Based on their retrospective observations, the authors recommended routine VTE prophylaxis for patients undergoing acute repair of a ruptured Achilles tendon.

Using the 2007–2009 National Trauma Data Bank, Shibuya et al. [84] showed that the incidence of VTE and PE associated with foot and ankle trauma was 0.28% and 0.21%, respectively. They also observed that older age (DVT, odds ratio [OR] 1.02, 95% confidence interval [CI] 1.01–1.03; PE, OR 1.02, 95% CI 1.01–1.03), obesity (DVT, OR 2.35, 95% CI 1.33–4.14; PE, OR 3.06, 95% CI 1.68–5.59), and higher injury severity score (DVT, OR 1.22, 95% CI 1.16–1.28; PE, OR 1.21, 95% CI 1.14–1.29) were statistically and clinically significant risk factors for DVT and PE following foot and ankle trauma. Based on the observed low incidence of DVT and/or PE, the authors concluded that routine pharmacologic thromboprophylaxis might be contraindicated in foot and ankle trauma, and clinicians were encouraged to undertake careful, individualized assessment of the risk factors associated with DVT/PE in order to decide when chemoprophylaxis was indicated.

In a retrospective study that focussed on the incidence of symptomatic VTE complications observed in a consecutive series of 2654 patients that underwent elective foot and ankle surgery, of whom 1078 (40.62%) received 75 mg aspirin as VTE prophylaxis between 2003 and 2006 and 1576 (59.38%) patients received no form of chemical thromboprophylaxis between 2007 and 2010, the overall incidence of VTE was 0.42% (DVT, 0.27%; PE, 0.15%) and 27 (1.01%) patients were lost to follow-up [85] Assuming that those lost to follow up developed VTE, the overall incidence of VTE was 1.43%. Based on this worst-case scenario incidence of VTE of 1.43%, the authors concluded that routine VTE chemoprophylaxis was not indicated for foot and ankle surgery unless the patient was categorized at high risk for VTE.

Interestingly, in regard to major lower extremity amputation, the authors of a systematic review concluded that there was insufficient evidence to make any meaningful conclusions regarding VTE prophylaxis [86].

In a comparison of 130 patients that underwent foot and/or ankle surgery and treated with a below-the-knee cast for 4 weeks and non-weight-bearing ambulation for up to 6 weeks to 88 patients that underwent hallux surgery and treated without a cast or non-weight bearing, none of whom were administered any form of VTE prophylaxis, and all of whom underwent venous compression ultrasonography between 2 and 6 weeks postoperative; the overall incidence of VTE was 5.09% and that of PE was 0.9% [87]. Since none of the cases of VTE or PE in this particular study occurred in the hallux surgery group, the incidence of VTE or PE was 8.46% in the cast/non-weight-bearing group. Interestingly, 90.9% of patients in the VTE group had a total risk factor score of ≥5, and 73.7% of patients in the non-VTE group had a total risk factor score of ≥5, and the mean time to the diagnosis of VTE was 33.1 days. Based on their findings, the investigators recommended that VTE prophylaxis be routinely used for patients that undergo foot and/or ankle surgery requiring the use of a short-leg cast and non-weight bearing and that it should be carried out until weight bearing is resumed either with or without immobilization or until immobilization is discontinued whether with or without non-weight bearing, between 28 and 42 days following the surgery.

Even though it is generally known that the incidence of venous thromboembolism (VTE) is lower following foot and ankle surgery, in comparison to hip or knee surgery, it is important to consider the potential complications secondary to VTE, including pulmonary embolism (PE), in comparison to the costs, risks, and effectiveness of venous thromboembolism (VTE) prophylaxis. An e-mail-based survey of 100 active American Orthopaedic Foot and Ankle Society (AOFAS) committee members (80% of which responded) inquired as to the use, type, and duration of VTE prophylaxis following elective ankle fusion surgery in three different clinical scenarios, including a 50-year-old female with no risk factors, a 50-year-old female with a history of PE, and a 35-year-old female on birth control pills [88]. In response to the first scenario, 45 (57%) of the respondents said that no prophylaxis was required, and in response to the second scenario, 78 (97.5%) said that prophylaxis was required, whereas in response to the third scenario, 49 (61.3%) said that they would employ some form of prophylaxis. Among the respondents, the most common forms of prophylaxis were aspirin, 49% (24/49), and LMWH, 47% (23/49); and the recommended duration of VTE prophylaxis ranged from 1 day to more than 6 weeks. These investigators concluded that wide variation existed in regard to VTE following foot and ankle surgery, and further research was needed in order to more precisely define guidelines for VTE following foot and ankle surgery.

As noted earlier, in comparison to VTE in association with knee and hip surgery, rigorous study of its association with foot and ankle surgery has not been as thoroughly documented in the peer-reviewed scientific literature. As such, there is considerable debate as to the routine need for VTE in association with foot and ankle surgery, and definitive methods, in terms of the agents and methods used, dosages, and duration of intervention, have yet to be clearly determined. In still another systematic review of English language literature, up to 2012, the overall incidence of symptomatic VTE associated with foot and ankle surgery was ≤0.55%, and there was an increased incidence in foot and ankle trauma patients with the highest incidence reported in tendo-Achilles surgery [89]. In that review, moreover, the reported risk factors included previous history of VTE, immobilization, high BMI, age, comorbidities, contraceptive pill, and air travel, and there was a cumulative effect resulting in higher risk when two or more risk factors are present.

Finally, in an analysis of 200 consecutive patients treated with plaster cast immobilization for ankle fracture, wherein oral anticoagulant therapy was administered for prevention of venous thromboembolism in those patients that were deemed to be at high risk for thrombosis, only one (0.5%) patient developed a DVT [90]. Based on this observation, they concluded that oral anticoagulation prophylaxis was suitable for ambulatory trauma patients temporarily immobilized for the nonsurgical treatment of an ankle fracture.

Since 2008, ten reports [78, 80–85, 87, 88, 90], describing results based on 211,067 foot and ankle surgical patients, observed the incidence of DVT to range from 0.01% to 8.46%, the incidence of PE to range from 0.02% to 0.9%, and the incidence of mortality to be 0.02–0.37% (the incidence of mortality based on observations in 88,241 patients). Of note, the highest incidences of DVT were 8.46% and 5.7%, observed in patients that were immobilized in a below-the-knee cast for 4–6 weeks non-weight bearing [87] and those that underwent acute surgical repair of Achilles tendon rupture, respectively. It is also interesting to note that 61.3% of orthopedic surgeons responding to a survey indicated that they would use VTE prophylaxis in a 35-year-old female on birth control pills who was undergoing elective ankle arthrodesis and that aspirin was the chemoprophylaxis of choice in 49% of these surgeons [88]. Unfortunately, further research is required in order for surgeons to be able to know for sure whether or not routine VTE prophylaxis is truly beneficial in foot and ankle surgery. In fact, in their position statement approved July 9, 2013 [91], the American Orthopaedic Foot and Ankle Society said "There is currently insufficient data for the American Orthopaedic Foot & Ankle Society (AOFAS) to recommend for or against routine VTED [venous thromboembolic disease] prophylaxis for patients undergoing foot and ankle surgery. Further research in this field is necessary and is encouraged." Still further, in their clinical consensus statement [92], the American College of Foot and Ankle Surgeons claimed "The decision to prescribe chemical prophylaxis during nonoperative or operative management of foot and ankle disorders should be based on each patient's unique risk benefit-analysis. This involves weighing the risks and consequences of bleeding against those of developing VTED. Exactly what constitutes sufficient risk to warrant chemical prophylaxis is not clear. Factors associated with the greatest risk include a personal history of VTED, active or recent cancer, a hypercoagulable state, and prolonged lower extremity immobilization." As such, surgeons are encouraged to pursue VTE prophylaxis based on the recommendations that they believe are meaningful, in conjunction with their own experience and knowledge of their individual patient's needs.

In conclusion, VTE is prevalent in surgical patients, and it can result in substantial morbidity as well as mortality. There are well-established risk assessment models that can be used to stratify the risk of VTE in hospitalized patients and others that focus on patients undergoing total hip or total knee arthroplasty. And even though there have been numerous peer-reviewed publications that focus on VTE in association with foot and ankle surgery, to date, a specific foot and ankle surgical VTE risk assessment model has not been validated. As such, foot and ankle surgeons are in the position of having to extrapolate the information in general medical and hip and knee VTE prophylaxis guidelines and combine this with their knowledge of their individual patient's needs in order to determine how to minimize the risk of VTE.

References

1. McKinsey JF, Aleander J, Byer A, Cherr GS, Gewertz BL, Lawrence PF, Nelson PR. Diseases of the vascular system. In: Lawrence PF, editor. Essentials of General Surgery. 5th ed. Philadelphia: Lippincott Williams & Wilkins; 2013. p. 472–9.
2. Goldhaber SZ. Deep venous thrombosis and pulmonary thromboembolism. In: Kassper DL, Hauser SL, Jameson JL, Fauci AS, Longo DL, Loscalzo J, editors. Harrison's Principles of Internal Medicine. 19th ed. New York: McGraw-Hill Education; 2015. Chapt. 300.
3. Asuka Ozaki A, Bartholomew JR. Venous thromboembolism (deep venous thrombosis & pulmonary embolism). Cleveland Clinic Center for Continuing Education, OH, 2012 (http://www.clevelandclinicmeded.com/medicalpubs/diseasemanagement/cardiology/venous-thromboembolism/, last visited 1 Aug 2016).
4. Philip S, Wells PS, Forgie MA, Rodger MA. Review: treatment of venous thromboembolism. JAMA. 2014;311(7):717–28. doi:10.1001/jama.2014.65.
5. Kahn SR. How I treat postthrombotic syndrome. Blood. 2009;114:4624–31.
6. Pengo V, Lensing AW, Prins MH, Marchiori A, Davidson BL, Tiozzo F, Albanese P, Biasiolo A, Pegoraro C, Iliceto S, Prandoni P, Thromboembolic Pulmonary Hypertension Study Group. Incidence of chronic thromboembolic pulmonary hypertension after pulmonary embolism. N Engl J Med. 2004;350(22):2257–64.
7. Heit JA. Venous thromboembolism: disease burden, outcomes and risk factors. J Thromb Haemost. 2005;3(8):1611–7.
8. Carson JL, Kelley MA, Duff A, Weg JG, Fulkerson WJ, Palevsky HI, Schwartz JS, Thompson BT, Popovich Jr J, Hobbins TE, et al. The clinical course of pulmonary embolism. N Engl J Med. 1992;326(19):1240–5.
9. Kucher N. Clinical practice. Deep-vein thrombosis of the upper extremities. N Engl J Med. 2011;364:861–9.
10. Anderson Jr FA, Wheeler HB, Goldberg RJ, Hosmer DW, Patwardhan NA, Jovanovic B, Forcier A, Dalen JE. A population-based perspective of the hospital incidence and case-fatality rates of deep vein thrombosis and pulmonary embolism. The Worcester DVT Study. Arch Intern Med. 1991;151(5):933–8.
11. Heit JA, O'Fallon WM, Petterson TM, Lohse CM, Silverstein MD, Mohr DN, Melton III. LJ. Relative impact of risk factors for deep vein thrombosis and pulmonary embolism: a population-based study. Arch Intern Med. 2002;162(11):1245–8.
12. Ageno W, Becattini C, Brighton T, Selby R, Kamphuisen PW. Cardiovascular risk factors and venous thromboembolism: a meta-analysis. Circulation. 2008;117(1):93–102.

13. Alikhan R, Cohen AT, Combe S, Samama MM, Desjardins L, Eldor A, Janbon C, Leizorovicz A, Olsson CG, Turpie AG, MEDENOX Study. Risk factors for venous thromboembolism in hospitalized patients with acute medical illness: analysis of the MEDENOX study. Arch Intern Med. 2004;164(9):963–8.
14. Wells PS, Anderson DR, Ginsberg J. Assessment of deep vein thrombosis or pulmonary embolism by the combined use of clinical model and noninvasive diagnostic tests. Semin Thromb Hemost. 2000;26(6):643–56.
15. Goldhaber SZ. Pulmonary embolism thrombolysis: a clarion call for international collaboration. J Am Coll Cardiol. 1992;19(2):246–7.
16. Wells PS, Anderson DR, Bormanis J, Guy F, Mitchell M, Gray L, Clement C, Robinson KS, Lewandowski B. Value of assessment of pretest probability of deep-vein thrombosis in clinical management. Lancet. 1997;350(9094):1795–8.
17. Levi M, Hart W, Büller HR. Physical examination—the significance of Homan's sign. Ned Tijdschr Geneeskd. 1999;143(37):1861–3.
18. Lensing AW, Prandoni P, Brandjes D, Huisman PM, Vigo M, Tomasella G, Krekt J, Wouter Ten Cate J, Huisman MV, Büller HR. Detection of deep-vein thrombosis by real-time B-mode ultrasonography. N Engl J Med. 1989;320(6):342–5.
19. Mattos MA, Londrey GL, Leutz DW, Hodgson KJ, Ramsey DE, Barkmeier LD, Stauffer ES, Spadone DP, Sumner DS. Color-flow duplex scanning for the surveillance and diagnosis of acute deep venous thrombosis. J Vasc Surg. 1992;15(2):366–75.
20. Stein PD, Terrin ML, Hales CA, Palevsky HI, Saltzman HA, Thompson BT, Weg JG. Clinical, laboratory, roentgenographic, and electrocardiographic findings in patients with acute pulmonary embolism and no pre-existing cardiac or pulmonary disease. Chest. 1991;100(3):598–603.
21. Borris LC, Breindahl M, Ryge C, Sommer HM, Lassen MR. uF1 + 2 study group. Prothrombin fragment 1 + 2 in urine as an indicator of sustained coagulation activation after total hip arthroplasty. Thromb Res. 2007;121(3):369–76.
22. Vuilleumier N, Simona A, Méan M, Limacher A, Lescuyer P, Gerstel E, Bounameaux H, Aujesky D, Righini M. Comparison of cardiac and non-cardiac biomarkers for risk stratification in elderly patients with non-massive pulmonary embolism. PLoS One. 2016;11(5):e0155973. doi:10.1371/journal.pone.0155973.
23. Sreeram N, Cheriex EC, Smeets JL, Gorgels AP, Wellens HJ. Value of the 12-lead electrocardiogram at hospital admission in the diagnosis of pulmonary embolism. Am J Cardiol. 1994;73(4):298–303.
24. Anderson DR, Kahn SR, Rodger MA, Ovacs MJ, Morris T, Hirsch A, Lang E, Stiell I, Kovacs G, Dreyer J, Dennie C, Cartier Y, Barnes D, Burton E, Pleasance S, Skedgel C, O'Rouke K, Wells PS. Computed tomographic pulmonary angiography vs ventilation-perfusion lung scanning in patients with suspected pulmonary embolism: a randomized controlled trial. JAMA. 2007;298(23):2743–53.
25. Blum A, Bellou A, Guillemin F, Douek P, Laprévote-Heully MC, Wahl D, GENEPI study group. Performance of magnetic resonance angiography in suspected acute pulmonary embolism. Thromb Haemost. 2005;93(3):503–11.
26. Tietze M, Gurley J. VTE prevention: development of an institutional protocol and the nurse's role. Medsurg Nurs. 2014;23(5):331–3. 342
27. Kakkos SK, Caprini JA, Geroulakos G, Nicolaides AN, Stansby GP, Reddy DJ. Combined intermittent pneumatic leg compression and pharmacological prophylaxis for prevention of venous thromboembolism in high-risk patients. Cochrane Database Syst Rev. 2008;4:CD005258.
28. Sachdeva A, Dalton M, Amaragiri SV, Lees T. Elastic compression stockings for prevention of deep vein thrombosis. Cochrane Database Syst Rev. 2010;7:CD001484. doi:10.1002/14651858.CD001484.pub2.
29. Comerota AJ, Chouhan V, Harada RN, Sun L, Hosking J, Veermansunemi R, Comerota Jr AJ, Schlappy D, Rao AK. The fibrinolytic effects of intermittent pneumatic compression: mechanism of enhanced fibrinolysis. Ann Surg. 1997;226:306–13. discussion 313
30. Knight MT, Dawson R. Effect of intermittent compression of the arms on deep venous thrombosis in the legs. Lancet. 1976;2:1265–8.
31. Pannucci CJ, MacDonald JK, Ariyan S, Gutowski KA, Kerrigan CL, Kim JY, Chung KC. Benefits and risks of prophylaxis for deep venous thrombosis and pulmonary embolus in plastic surgery: a systematic review and meta-analysis of controlled trials and consensus conference. Plast Reconstr Surg. 2016;137(2):709–30. doi:10.1097/01.prs.0000475790.54231.28.
32. Swanson E. The case against chemoprophylaxis for venous thromboembolism prevention and the rationale for SAFE anesthesia. Plast Reconstr Surg Glob Open. 2014;2:e160.
33. Bitar G, Mullis W, Jacobs W, Matthews D, Beasley M, Smith K, Watterson P, Getz S, Capizzi P, Eaves III. F. Safety and efficacy of office based surgery with monitored anesthesia care/sedation in 4778 consecutive plastic surgery procedures. Plast Reconstr Surg. 2003;111:150–6. discussion 157
34. Ersek RA. General anesthesia gases are a common denominator in cases of thromboembolism. Aesthet Surg J. 2009;29:340–1.
35. Hafezi F, Naghibzadeh B, Nouhi AH, Salimi A, Naghibzadeh G, Mousavi SJ. Epidural anesthesia as a thromboembolic prophylaxis modality in plastic surgery. Aesthet Surg J. 2011;31:821–4.
36. Scottish Intercollegiate Guidelines Network (SIGN). Prevention and management of venous thromboembolism. A national clinical guideline. Edinburgh (UK): Scottish Intercollegiate Guidelines Network (SIGN); 2010. p. 101. (SIGN publication; no. 122)
37. Jobin S, Kalliainen L, Adebayo L, Agarwal Z, Card R, Christie B, Haland T, Hartmark M, Johnson P, Kang M, Lindvall B, Mohsin S, Morton C. Institute for Clinical Systems Improvement. Venous Thromboembolism Prophylaxis. http://bit.ly/VTEProphy1112. Updated November 2012.
38. Hospital for Special Surgery Quality Assurance Committee Final Report DVT/PE prophylaxis (https://www.hss.edu/conditions_dvt-pe-prophylaxis.asp, last visited August 13, 2016).
39. Frostick S. Pharmacological thromboprophylaxis and total hip or knee replacement. Br J Nurs. 2016;25(1):45–53. doi:10.12968/bjon.2016.25.1.45.
40. Stewart DW, Freshour JE. Aspirin for the prophylaxis of venous thromboembolic events in orthopedic surgery patients. A comparison of the AAOS and ACCP Guidelines with review of the evidence. Ann Pharmacother. 2013;47(1):63–74.
41. Chong BH. Heparin-induced thrombocytopenia. J Thromb Haemost. 2003;1(7):1471–8. Review
42. Baroletti S, Piovella C, Fanikos J, Labreche M, Lin J, Goldhaber SZ. Heparin-induced thrombocytopenia (HIT): clinical and economic outcomes. Thromb Haemost. 2008;100(6):1130–5.
43. Kearon C, Akl EA, Comerota AJ, Prandoni P, Bounameaux H, Goldhaber SZ, Nelson ME, Wells PS, Gould MK, Dentali F, Crowther M, Kahn SR, American College of Chest Physicians. Antithrombotic therapy for VTE disease: antithrombotic therapy and prevention of thrombosis, 9th ed: American College of Chest Physicians Evidence-Based Clinical Practice Guidelines. Chest. 2012;141:e419S–94S.
44. Stein PD, Alnas M, Beemath A, Patel NR. Outcome of pulmonary embolectomy. Am J Cardiol. 2007;99(3):421–3.
45. Bayes T. An essay towards solving a problem in the doctrine of chances [Offprint title: "A method of calculating the exact probability of all conclusions founded on induction."]. Philos Trans R Soc Lond. 1764;53:370–418.
46. Sandler DA, Martin JF, Duncan JS, Blake GM, Ward P, Ramsay LE, Lamont AC, Ross B, Sherriff S, Walton L. Diagnosis of deep-vein thrombosis: Comparison of clinical evaluation, ultrasound, plethysmography, and venoscan with X-ray venogram. Lancet. 1984;2(8405):716–9.

47. Wells PS, Anderson DR, Rodger M, Forgie M, Kearon C, Dreyer J, Kovacs G, Mitchell M, Lewandowski B, Kovacs MJ. Evaluation of D-dimer in the diagnosis of suspected deep-vein thrombosis. N Engl J Med. 2003;349(13):1227–35.
48. Tamariz LJ, Eng J, Segal JB, Krishnan JA, Bolger DT, Streiff MB, Jenckes MW, Bass EB. Usefulness of clinical prediction rules for the diagnosis of venous thromboembolism: a systematic review. Am J Med. 2004;117(9):676–84.
49. Wells PS, Owen C, Doucette S, Fergusson D, Tran H. Does this patient have deep vein thrombosis? JAMA. 2006;295(2):199–207.
50. Guidelines and Expert Panel Reports: Antithrombotic Therapy for VTE Disease, published February 2016 (http://www.chestnet.org/Guidelines-and-Resources/Guidelines-and-Consensus-Statements/Antithrombotic-Guidelines-9th-Ed, last visited 15 May 2016).
51. Anderson Jr FA, Zayaruzny M, Heit JA, Fidan D, Cohen AT. Estimated annual numbers of US acute-care hospital patients at risk for venous thromboembolism. Am J Hematol. 2007;82:777.
52. Lindblad B, Eriksson A, Bergqvist D. Autopsy-verified pulmonary embolism in a surgical department: analysis of the period from 1951 to 1988. Br J Surg. 1991;78:849.
53. Stein PD, Henry JW. Prevalence of acute pulmonary embolism among patients in a general hospital and at autopsy. Chest. 1995;108:978.
54. White RH, Zhou H, Romano PS. Incidence of symptomatic venous thromboembolism after different elective or urgent surgical procedures. Thromb Haemost. 2003;90:446.
55. Sandler DA, Martin JF. Autopsy proven pulmonary embolism in hospital patients: are we detecting enough deep vein thrombosis? J R Soc Med. 1989;82:203.
56. Martino MA, Borges E, Williamson E, Siegfried S, Cantor AB, Lancaster J, Roberts WS, Hoffman MS. Pulmonary embolism after major abdominal surgery in gynecologic oncology. Obstet Gynecol. 2006;107:666.
57. Dismuke SE, Wagner EH. Pulmonary embolism as a cause of death. The changing mortality in hospitalized patients. JAMA. 1986;255:2039.
58. Horlander KT, Mannino DM, Leeper KV. Pulmonary embolism mortality in the United States, 1979–1998: an analysis using multiple-cause mortality data. Arch Intern Med. 2003;163:1711.
59. Clagett GP, Reisch JS. Prevention of venous thromboembolism in general surgical patients. Results of meta-analysis. Ann Surg. 1988;208:227.
60. Collins R, Scrimgeour A, Yusuf S, Peto R. Reduction in fatal pulmonary embolism and venous thrombosis by perioperative administration of subcutaneous heparin. Overview of results of randomized trials in general, orthopedic, and urologic surgery. N Engl J Med. 1988;318:1162.
61. Leizorovicz A, Haugh MC, Chapuis FR, Samama MM, Boissel JP. Low molecular weight heparin in prevention of perioperative thrombosis. BMJ. 1992;305:913.
62. Nurmohamed MT, Rosendaal FR, Büller HR, Dekker E, Hommes DW, Vandenbroucke JP, Briët E. Low-molecular-weight heparin versus standard heparin in general and orthopaedic surgery: a meta-analysis. Lancet. 1992;340:152.
63. Geerts WH, Pineo GF, Heit JA, Bergqvist D, Lassen MR, Colwell CW, Ray JG. Prevention of venous thromboembolism: the Seventh ACCP Conference on Antithrombotic and Thrombolytic Therapy. Chest. 2004;126:338S.
64. Geerts WH, Bergqvist D, Pineo GF, Heit JA, Samama CM, Lassen MR, Colwell CW, American College of Chest Physicians. Prevention of venous thromboembolism: American College of Chest Physicians Evidence-Based Clinical Practice Guidelines (8th Edition). Chest. 2008;133:381S.
65. Lyman GH, Khorana AA, Falanga A, Clarke-Pearson D, Flowers C, Jahanzeb M, Kakkar A, Kuderer NM, Levine MN, Liebman H, Mendelson D, Raskob G, Somerfield MR, Thodiyil P, Trent D, Francis CW, American Society of Clinical Oncology. American Society of Clinical Oncology guideline: recommendations for venous thromboembolism prophylaxis and treatment in patients with cancer. J Clin Oncol. 2007;25:5490–505.
66. Barbar S, Noventa F, Rossetto V, Ferrari A, Brandolin B, Perlati M, De Bon E, Tormene D, Pagnan A, Prandoni P. A risk assessment model for the identification of hospitalized medical patients at risk for venous thromboembolism: the Padua Prediction Score. J Thromb Haemost. 2010;8(11):2450–7. doi:10.1111/j.1538-7836.2010.04044.x.
67. Caprini JA, Arcelus JI, Reyna JJ. Effective risk stratification of surgical and nonsurgical patients for venous thromboembolic disease. Semin Hematol. 2001;38(2 Suppl 5):12–9.
68. Caprini JA. Risk assessment as a guide for the prevention of the many faces of venous thromboembolism. Am J Surg. 2010;199(1 Suppl):S3–10. doi:10.1016/j.amjsurg.2009.10.006.
69. Lassen MR, Backs S, Borris LC, Kaltoft-Sørenson M, Coff-Ganes H, Jeppesen E. Deep-vein thrombosis prophylaxis in orthopedic surgery: hip surgery. Semin Thromb Hemost. 1999;25(Suppl 3):79–82.
70. Mantilla CB, Horlocker TT, Schroeder DR, Berry DJ, Brown DL. Risk factors for clinically relevant pulmonary embolism and deep venous thrombosis in patients undergoing primary hip or knee arthroplasty. Anesthesiology. 2003;99:552–60.
71. Barrera LM, Perel P, Ker K, Cirocchi R, Farinella E, Morales Uribe CH. Thromboprophylaxis for trauma patients. Cochrane Database Syst Rev. 2013;3:CD008303.
72. Anderson DR, Dunbar MJ, Bohm ER, Belzile E, Kahn SR, Zukor D, Fisher W, Gofton W, Gross P, Pelet S, Crowther M, MacDonald S, Kim P, Pleasance S, Davis N, Andreou P, Wells P, Kovacs M, Rodger MA, Ramsay T, Carrier M, Vendittoli PA. Aspirin versus low-molecular-weight heparin for extended venous thromboembolism prophylaxis after total hip arthroplasty: a randomized trial. Ann Intern Med. 2013;158(11):800–6. doi:10.7326/0003-4819-158-11-201306040-00004.
73. Preventing Venous Thromboembolic Disease in Patients Undergoing Elective Hip and Knee Arthroplasty: Evidence-based Guideline and Evidence Report, published in 2011 by the American Academy of Orthopaedic Surgeons. http://www.aaos.org/search/?srchtext=Preventing+Venous+Thromboembolic, last accessed 8 Aug 2016.
74. Mizel MS, Temple HT, Michelson JD, Alvarez RG, Clanton TO, Frey CC, Gegenheimer AP, Hurwitz SR, Lutter LD, Mankey MG, Mann RA, Miller RA, Richardson EG, Schon LC, Thompson FM, Yodlowski ML. Thromboembolism after foot and ankle surgery. A multicenter study. Clin Orthop Relat Res. 1998;348:180–5.
75. Solis G, Saxby T. Incidence of DVT following surgery of the foot and ankle. Foot Ankle Int. 2002;23(5):411–4.
76. Lassen MR, Borris LC, Nakov RL. Use of the low-molecular-weight heparin reviparin to prevent deep-vein thrombosis after leg injury requiring immobilization. N Engl J Med. 2002; 347(10):726–30.
77. Slaybaugh RS, Beasley BD, Massa EG. Deep venous thrombosis risk assessment, incidence, and prophylaxis in foot and ankle surgery. Clin Podiatr Med Surg. 2003;20(2):269–89.
78. Hanslow SS, Grujic L, Slater HK, Chen D. Thromboembolic disease after foot and ankle surgery. Foot Ankle Int. 2006;27(9):693–5.
79. Gadgil A, Thomas RH. Current trends in thromboprophylaxis in surgery of the foot and ankle. Foot Ankle Int. 2007;28(10):1069–73.
80. Wukich DK, Waters DH. Thromboembolism following foot and ankle surgery: a case series and literature review. J Foot Ankle Surg. 2008;47(3):243–9. doi:10.1053/j.jfas.2008.02.003.
81. Hamilton PD, Hariharan K, Robinson AH. Thromboprophylaxis in elective foot and ankle patients--current practice in the United Kingdom. Foot Ankle Surg. 2011;17(2):89–93. doi:10.1016/j.fas.2011.02.004.
82. Jameson SS, Augustine A, James P, Serrano-Pedraza I, Oliver K, Townshend D, Reed MR. Venous thromboembolic events follow-

ing foot and ankle surgery in the English National Health Service. J Bone Joint Surg (Br). 2011;93(4):490–7. doi:10.1302/0301-620X.93B4.25731.
83. Saragas NP, Ferrao PN. The incidence of venous thromboembolism in patients undergoing surgery for acute Achilles tendon ruptures. J Foot Ankle Surg. 2011;17(4):263–5. doi:10.1016/j.fas.2010.12.002.
84. Shibuya N, Frost CH, Campbell JD, Davis ML, Jupiter DC. Incidence of acute deep vein thrombosis and pulmonary embolism in foot and ankle trauma: analysis of the National Trauma Data Bank. J Foot Ankle Surg. 2012;51(1):63–8. doi:10.1053/j.jfas.2011.10.017.
85. Griffiths JT, Matthews L, Pearce CJ, Calder JD. Incidence of venous thromboembolism in elective foot and ankle surgery with and without aspirin prophylaxis. J Bone Joint Surg (Br). 2012;94(2):210–4. doi:10.1302/0301-620X.94B2.27579.
86. Robertson L, Roche A. Primary prophylaxis for venous thromboembolism in people undergoing major amputation of the lower extremity. Cochrane Database Syst Rev. 2013;12:CD010525.
87. Saragas NP, Ferrao PN, Saragas E, Jacobson BF. The impact of risk assessment on the implementation of venous thromboembolism prophylaxis in foot and ankle surgery. Foot Ankle Surg. 2014;20(2):85–9. doi:10.1016/j.fas.2013.11.002.
88. Shah K, Thevendran G, Younger A, Pinney SJ. Deep-vein thrombosis prophylaxis in foot and ankle surgery: what is the current state of practice? Foot Ankle Spec. 2015;8(2):101–6. doi:10.1177/1938640014546858.
89. Mangwani J, Sheikh N, Cichero M, Williamson D. What is the evidence for chemical thromboprophylaxis in foot and ankle surgery? Systematic review of the English literature. Foot (Edinb). 2015;25(3):173–8. doi:10.1016/j.foot.2014.07.007.
90. Haque S, Davies MB. Oral thromboprophylaxis in patients with ankle fractures immobilized in a below the knee cast. Foot Ankle Surg. 2015;21(4):266–8. doi:10.1016/j.fas.2015.02.002.
91. Position Statement: The Use of VTED Prophylaxis in Foot and Ankle Surgery. The American Orthopaedic Foot and Ankle Society (http://www.aofas.org/search/pages/results.aspx?k=position%20statement%20VTED, last visited August 6, 2016).
92. Fleischer AE, Abicht BP, Baker JR, Boffeli TJ, Jupiter DS, Schade VL. American College of Foot and Ankle Surgeons' clinical consensus statement: risk, prevention, and diagnosis of venous thromboembolism disease in foot and ankle surgery and injuries requiring immobilization. J Foot Ankle Surg. 2015;54:497–507.

Complication Management: Nonunions

3

Alan Catanzariti and Kyle Moore

Introduction

The concern related to complications can consume a substantial amount of healthcare providers' time and thought. In surgical disciplines, seemingly minor complications can invoke major frustration and anxiety for both the practitioner and patient. At the core of the near-constant impetus to improve surgical technologies and techniques are the quality of patient care and the goal of reducing complications. The successful management of surgical complications requires a thorough understanding of the pathology in question and the aptitude to instill confidence in the patient regarding the practitioner's ability to deliver effective treatment. Surgeons can manage their fears of complications and begin to better understand the subtle nuances that are unique to successful complication management by developing a comprehensive knowledge base. Nonunion is a complex surgical complication that results in an absence of healing across two opposing bony surfaces. Various anatomic locations in the lower extremities have been identified as having relatively high propensities for nonunion. Nonunion of tibial shaft fractures can occur in 10–60% of cases [1–4]. Hindfoot and ankle arthrodeses are associated with a nonunion rate of approximately 10%, although rates ranging from 6–33% have also been reported for triple arthrodesis [5–8]. The first metatarsophalangeal joint (first MTP) and first tarsometatarsal joint (first TMT) arthrodeses have nonunion rates below 10% [9–14]. Surgical nonunion is not uncommon in the foot and ankle. Thus, surgeons should have a relatively high index of suspicion, particularly in situations in which there is a predisposition to nonunion.

This chapter will focus on the complex facets that are integral to nonunion management in the foot and ankle with a special emphasis on nonunion in elective surgical patients, i.e., those individuals who have undergone previous osteotomy and/or arthrodesis for the purpose of surgical reconstruction and have developed a nonunion. Despite the focus on nonunion in elective surgical patients, the general principles and management techniques discussed can also be applied to the treatment of nonunions with traumatic etiology.

Nonunion is a chronic condition that is capable of causing significant pain, deformity, and instability in lower extremities. Nonunion can arise when a bone sustains injury in the form of a fracture, osteotomy, or resection for joint arthrodesis. Osteotomies, arthrodesis procedures, and fractures are considered to have progressed to nonunion when the biologic mechanisms of bone healing cease to function appropriately [15]. A plethora of time lines and variability in the descriptions of nonunion exist, and surveys have revealed significant inconsistencies regarding the definition of the onset of nonunion [16]. Previous reports have described nonunion as a fracture that is unable to heal within 6–8 months of observation [17–19]. Currently, the Federal Drug Administration (FDA) characterizes nonunion as "established when a minimum of 9 months has elapsed since injury, and the fracture site shows no visibly progressive signs of healing for a minimum of 3 months" [15, 20]. For the purpose of this discussion, we describe nonunion as a multifactorial disease state that is rooted in the body's inability to heal two opposing bony surfaces. Ultimately, these cases necessitate interventions from external sources, either via surgical or nonsurgical means, to facilitate osseous union. Although a preset time frame of 9 months might be helpful in certain situations, we by no means feel that it is necessary to delay treatment until this time frame has passed.

In their 1976 report, Weber and Cech classified fracture nonunion by correlating radiographic findings with biologic healing efforts [21]. These authors subdivided nonunion types into hypertrophic, oligotrophic, and atrophic. Hypertrophic nonunions promote callus formation, maintain sufficient vascularity and biologic activity for healing, and normally only require improved stability to facilitate union.

A. Catanzariti (✉) • K. Moore
West Penn Hospital, The Foot and Ankle Institute, 4800 Friendship Avenue, North Tower, 1st Floor, Pittsburgh, PA 15524, USA
e-mail: acatanzariti@faiwp.com; kmoore6@wpahs.org

M.S. Lee, J.P. Grossman (eds.), *Complications in Foot and Ankle Surgery*, DOI 10.1007/978-3-319-53686-6_3

Oligotrophic nonunions exhibit only a minute amount of callus radiographically, and although they do not completely lack biologic activity, they are much less active than desired. Finally, atrophic nonunions are considered to be nearly devoid of biologic activity and are deemed nonviable. This classification system is based on radiological appraisals and has limited value for prognosis and treatment due to the advent of advanced imaging.

Furthermore, it is not possible to discuss nonunion without also establishing a framework for defining delayed union. Unfortunately, the differentiation of delayed union and nonunion can be nebulous. For the purpose of this discussion, we define delayed union as a prolonged time to bone healing compared to the average, "normal" course. The same factors that predispose a patient to nonunion can certainly contribute to delayed union. However, the absence of biologic activity that is encountered in nonunion does not exist to the same degree in delayed union.

Basic Science of Bone Healing

The bony skeleton is the structural framework that serves as the attachment sites of the body's various ligaments, muscles, and tendons. This framework affords protection to some of the most vital organs in the human body and is a storehouse for physiologically crucial nutrient deposits [22]. The bone is one of the few tissues in the human body with full regenerative capacity that is also capable of healing without scar formation [22–24].

Despite its perceived rigidity, the bone has the ability to withstand substantial deformation under tensile, torsional, and compressive stresses. When external forces exceed a bone's capacity to deform, a fracture occurs. Purposeful "fractures" can occur in the forms of osteotomy or joint resection for arthrodesis, and surgeons can capitalize on the regenerative capacity of the bone to provide reconstructive correction.

Almost instantaneously after a traumatic insult occurs, the involved segments of the damaged bone undergo a reparative process via a highly regulated series of events [22–26]. The initial induction and inflammatory phases promote the recruitment of phagocytic cell lines, bone-forming pluripotent mesenchymal cells, and growth factors. The swelling that occurs around the site soon after injury facilitates physiologic splinting of the opposing surfaces. The adjacent bone margins then begin to unite by one of the two distinct healing models that are commonly referred as primary (direct) and secondary (indirect) healing.

The large majority of osseous injuries (which are frequently treated nonoperatively) undergo secondary healing. This healing is characterized by the presence of exuberant bony callus, initial widening of fracture gap due to resorption of the damaged ends, and an overall lack of stable fixation [22, 23, 27]. Within 2–3 weeks of the injury, the fracture site is partially stabilized and gradually bridged by soft, cartilaginous callus [23]. The newly formed collagenous substrate subsequently undergoes ossification that results in a stable bony segment.

In contrast, for the majority of elective surgical reconstructions that involve osteotomy or arthrodesis, primary osseous repair is typically the desired method of healing. This repair is characterized by an absence of callus around the site and a lack of widening of the fracture line. There are a few critical prerequisites to achieving this outcome that has been described by Danis as *soudure autogene* or the autologous weld [28]. First, close anatomic reduction of the adjoining segments and direct contact of the surfaces should be obtained. In regions in which direct bone-to-bone contact is not present, the gaps must be limited to approximately 1 mm of space between the segments [15, 29, 30]. Secondly, stable fixation that is capable of resisting deforming forces and facilitating adequate compression across the fracture site must be delivered. When these criteria are met, the opposing damaged surfaces are recanalized via new Haversian systems instead of being resorbed [31]. Cutting cones will facilitate the ingrowth of new vasculature and the delivery of bone-forming cells and thereby lead to the development of a functionally "bridged" bony segment. Following the union of the damaged segments, the newly formed bone will begin a remodeling phase according to Wolff's law [32].

Etiology of Nonunion

Successful bone healing requires the orchestration of numerous complex mechanisms and factors. At the most basic level, the bone must have adequate vascularity, have sufficient contact with the opposing surface, and be provided with stability around the surgical site to facilitate union. A patient can be predisposed to nonunion when a deviation exists at any level of the elaborate bone healing cascade or when the basic factors of vascularity, surface contact, and stability are lacking. To successfully manage nonunion, surgeons must determine the etiology behind the occurrence and then provide intervention directed at the areas of deficiency. Ultimately, therapeutic interventions for management of nonunion should be directed toward improving the mechanical and biological environment at the nonunion site.

The factors that contribute to nonunion can be subdivided into local factors and host factors (Table 3.1). Local factors can be considered to be any abnormalities that occur at the nonunion site and are frequently correlated with technical error. For example, excessive periosteal stripping or thermal necrosis at the surgical site during bony resection can lead to an avascular local environment, and there is an established

Table 3.1 Summary of factors associated with impaired bone healing

Local factors	Host factors
Infection	Tobacco use
Insufficient fixation	Vitamin D deficiency/insufficiency
Poor reduction/gapping	Thyroid dysfunction
Malalignment	Parathyroid dysfunction
Poor site preparation/debridement	Diabetes mellitus
Thermal necrosis	Premature weight bearing
Soft tissue interposition	Malnutrition
Soft tissue/periosteal stripping	Arterial insufficiency
	Pharmaceuticals (NSAIDs, steroids)

relationship between local soft tissue injury and an increased incidence of nonunion [33–35]. Moreover, inadequate bone surface contact or malalignment can create gaps that cannot be bridged by normal physiologic processes. Malalignment can also generate abnormal stress across the arthrodesis or osteotomy site during the phases of healing. Poor surgical site preparation due to insufficient removal of the joint cartilage, inadequate penetration of the subchondral plate, or interposed soft tissues can serve as a direct barrier to bony bridging in arthrodesis procedures. Furthermore, inadequate or inappropriate fixation that fails to stabilize the arthrodesis or osteotomy site can lead to excessive surgical site motion. Although micromotion at the bone-to-bone interface has been shown to positively affect healing, gross instability due to insufficient fixation can be detrimental to achieving successful union [23, 36–40].

While not solely a technical error, surgical site infection can be a local factor that also contributes to nonunion. Infection of the local soft tissues can lead to necrosis and a dysvascular environment. Overt bacterial infection of the bone weakens its structural integrity and can cause failure of the fixation construct that leads to instability of the surgical site. Diseased fibrous tissue and interposed necrotic bone segments can be barriers to the ingrowth of healthy vascular channels and can inhibit the delivery of growth factors.

There are numerous preexisting medical conditions that are capable of contributing to the incidence of surgical nonunion. While not directly affecting the surgical site in the same manner as the previously described local factors, certain medical conditions can have adverse effects on the bone healing cascade. For the purpose of this discussion, the authors refer to these patient conditions as host factors. One host factor that is often cited as a cause of nonunion is tobacco use [15, 41–44]. Nicotine has been shown to uncouple the tightly regulated angiogenesis and osteogenesis pathways that are formed during normal bone healing [45]. Prolonged use of tobacco leads to a reduced oxygen-carrying capacity and results in generalized tissue hypoxia. The proliferation and activity of bone-forming osteoblasts are significantly diminished in subjects exposed to nicotine [46–48]. Moreover, the overall bone mineral density of smokers can be significantly less than that of individuals who do not use tobacco products, and this difference is further exacerbated in elderly and postmenopausal patients [49–52]. These combined effects lead to an increase risk of nonunion in smokers that has been reported to be 2–16-fold higher in hindfoot arthrodesis and to a significant increase in overall complications such as wound dehiscence and infection [43, 44, 52].

Endocrine and metabolic irregularities have also been shown to contribute to nonunion. Specifically, vitamin D deficiency, diabetes mellitus, parathyroid disease, thyroid dysfunction, hypogonadism, and malnutrition can have significant implications in the bone healing cascade [53–55]. One specific report of nonunion patients by Brinker and colleagues showed that 31 of 37 (84%) individuals who met their screening criteria suffered underlying metabolic or endocrine abnormalities [55].

The prolonged use of pharmaceuticals, such as nonsteroidal anti-inflammatory drugs (NSAIDs), chemotherapy agents, anticoagulants, antibiotics, and advanced biologic antirheumatic drugs, has been hypothesized to contribute to nonunion [24, 56–70]. Although no absolute agreement exists regarding the roles of medications in elective foot and ankle surgical nonunion, causal links between diminished bone healing and certain pharmacological regimens have been reported in both clinical and laboratory models [24, 56–70]. For example, Jeffcoach and colleagues found a significant increase in complications in patients receiving NSAIDs after suffering traumatic long bone fracture [63]. Various animal model studies have shown significant implications of NSAID use on bone healing due to abnormalities in prostaglandin production at the fracture site [24, 64–67]. The long-term use of corticosteroids can predispose patients to osteopenia by inhibiting osteoblastogenesis and has been cited as one of the most common causes of secondary osteoporosis [24, 61, 62]. The cytotoxic and antiproliferative properties of chemotherapeutic drugs have been shown to inhibit healing in arthrodesis subjects [59, 60]. Furthermore, antibiotics, specifically fluoroquinolones, have been alleged to adversely affect bone healing by altering endochondral ossification and inducing chondrocyte death [68–70].

Patient Evaluation

To formulate a comprehensive treatment plan for a nonunion patient, one must begin by obtaining a thorough history and physical examination. Details of the initial surgery, including time lines before and after the intervention, the pathology that leads to the original operation, previous treatments, and other complications throughout the treatment course, should be reviewed. A complete analysis of the patient's past medical and social histories is essential. Particular emphasis should be placed on comorbidities that are known to adversely affect bone healing, such as diabetes mellitus, peripheral vascular disease, vitamin D deficiency, thyroid dysfunction, malabsorption syndromes, autoimmune disease, and tobacco use. Pharmaceuticals linked to aberrations in bone metabolism, such as immunosuppressive agents, NSAIDs, and high-potency steroids, should also be noted.

A thorough appraisal of the previous clinical, surgical, and inpatient hospital records should be conducted prior to revision surgery. Obtaining a complete copy of the patient's external records is particularly important if complications, such as surgical site infections, wound healing issues, or venous thrombotic events, transpired during the postoperative course. Patients should understand the importance of such records and be encouraged to bring reports and film copies of diagnostic imaging when available.

Furthermore, in-depth understandings of the patient's current pain, disability status, and future treatment goals should be acquired. For example, a patient might seem to be a surgical candidate from an objective standpoint. However, certain medical or social issues might limit or preclude the option of additional surgery. A patient might be unable to proceed with further surgical intervention due to an inability to withdraw from social responsibilities or due to concurrent medical conditions. The provider might be relegated to employing nonoperative care in lieu of surgical therapy. These situations are best elucidated early in the planned treatment course.

Physical examination of the involved lower limb requires a comparison to the contralateral extremity. Disparities of temperature, edema, and erythema should be noted. Inspection of the soft tissue envelope for signs of open lesions, drainage, or skin atrophy should also be performed. Baseline neuromotor and vascular statuses as assessed by palpation of pulses, capillary refill times, and manual muscle testing should be examined and documented.

The suspected or confirmed nonunion site(s) should be palpated for tenderness, and manual stress should be applied to assess apparent gross instability. The ranges of motion of the contiguous joints of the nonunion should be evaluated for crepitation or limitation. Close attention should be given to the presence of tenderness, malalignment, diminished range of motion, and additional signs of degenerative changes at these neighboring joints. Such findings may be useful guides for future treatment. For example, when malalignment exists at a nonunion site, secondary angulation through compensation might occur at the adjacent joints. Such situations can arise when a severe varus deformity exists at a tibiotalar arthrodesis nonunion. Long-standing compensatory eversion at the subtalar joint (STJ) to achieve a plantigrade foot can result in arthrosis that might require realignment arthrodesis during the ankle revision. Revision of the tibiotalar arthrodesis without addressing the subsequent STJ deformity can create a continued source of pain even if ankle union is achieved.

Laboratory testing can be beneficial when evaluating and formulating a treatment plan for a nonunion patient. Updated chemistry and hematology (CMP, CBC) panels should be obtained and reviewed for all patients, especially when a surgical intervention is planned. When a patient's nutritional status is in question, evaluations of the albumin, prealbumin, total lymphocyte count, and transferrin levels can be useful to ascertain the healing potential [71, 72]. Furthermore, due to the roles that vitamin D and calcium abnormalities play in nonunion, blood levels should be obtained for the majority of patients undergoing treatment. Vitamin D levels below 20 ng/mL typically warrant repletion therapy in the majority of cases [73–75].

In situations in which an underlying infectious etiology of the nonunion is suspected, acute phase reactant testing, including erythrocyte sedimentation rate (ESR) and C-reactive protein (CRP) tests, can be helpful aids for diagnosis. Acute phase reactants have high sensitivity and specificity in the diagnosis of osteomyelitis [76, 77]. A 2013 report by Stucken et al. compared the utilities of ESR and CRP in the diagnosis of infection in nonunion patients. The authors determined that the combination of ESR and CRP is a significantly accurate predictor of infection in such cases [78]. If suspicions of infection are accompanied by increases in CRP and ESR values, a biopsy of the nonunion site for gram staining, culture and sensitivity, and histologic review should be performed.

Numerous imaging modalities are available to evaluate foot and ankle nonunion including radiographs, radionucleotide scans, linear and computerized tomography (CT scanning), and magnetic resonance imaging (MRI). Depending on the specific nature of a nonunion, one or a combination of these techniques can be employed for evaluation, treatment guidance, and progress monitoring.

Plain film radiographs have become a mainstay tool in the assessment of bone healing after fracture, osteotomy, and arthrodesis. Bone union or arthrodesis is traditionally deemed to have occurred when orthogonal X-rays show trabecular bridging across three of four cortices, and patient complaints of pain and swelling have begun to subside [79, 80] (Fig. 3.1). Standard radiographs have proven to be a particularly valuable tool in the assessment of nonunion. Findings on serial radiographs frequently serve as the first indication that union is delayed or has failed to occur following surgery.

Serial X-rays should be evaluated in a chronological manner. Multiplane projections consisting of the dorsoplantar (DP) and oblique (MO) foot and anteroposterior (AP) and mortise ankle and lateral foot and ankle should be assessed for healing, bone quality, and residual or recurrent deformity. Additional specialized alignment radiographs, such as Saltzman and Harris-Beath views, can be useful to better assess the relationship of the foot/ankle to the lower leg [81, 82] (Fig. 3.2). Disuse osteopenia, sclerosis, bone callus, and progression of radiolucent lines at the suspected nonunion site should be noted and quantified. The presence of hardware loosening, breakage, and/or migration is indicative of excessive surgical site motion and warrants further investigation. The concern about an infectious component should also be heightened when sinus tracks or radiograph signs of infection are present [83, 84].

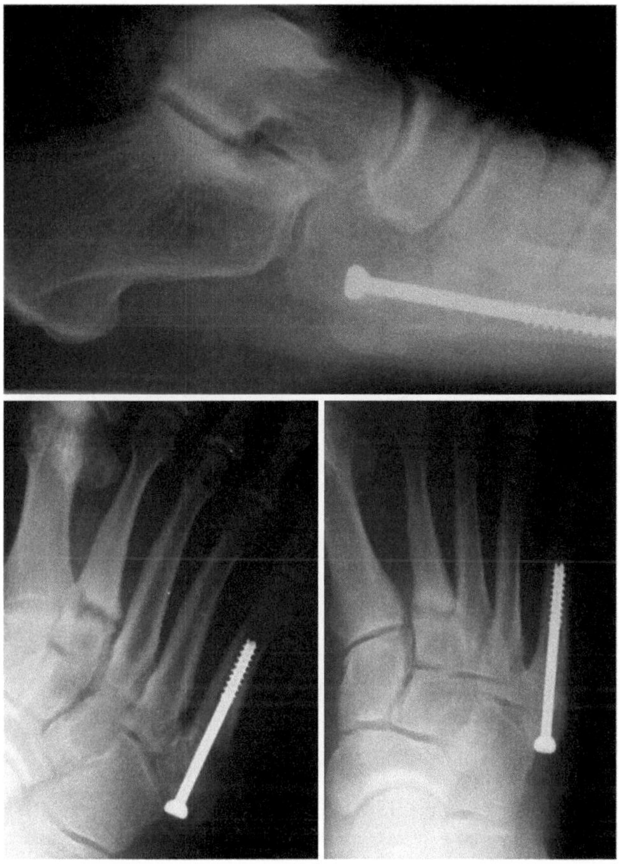

Fig. 3.1 AP, oblique and lateral radiographs demonstrating bridging across 3 of 4 cortices

Despite the role of plain film X-rays, two-dimensional X-rays cannot adequately or thoroughly discern bony union in all cases. Visualizing trabeculation across an arthrodesis or osteotomy site can be difficult when internal fixation, a bone graft, or bone graft substitute has been utilized. Patients complaining of continued postoperative pain and swelling even after apparent radiographic union has occurred often warrant further investigation beyond standard X-rays. In such instances, three-dimensional imaging modalities, such as CT scanning, have proven to be exceedingly useful. Hindfoot joints exhibit a nonplanar orientation, and the significant superimposition that is present throughout the midfoot can make standard radiographs appear equivocal when evaluating nonunion. The nonplanar and compact natures of these joints can be better evaluated with helical CT scans than with standard films (Fig. 3.3). A 2006 report by Coughlin prospectively compared standard radiographs to CT scans in the evaluation of union in hindfoot arthrodesis. The study reported a significant difference in the reliabilities of the detection of true bone union between CT scans and radiographs [85]. The evaluation of CT scans allows radiologists and surgeons to quantify the percentage of fusion mass, which is difficult with plain radiographs in most instances (Fig. 3.4). It is recommended that a measurement of 50% or more bridging at an arthrodesis site be achieved before it is considered a successful union [86]. Furthermore, a thorough analysis of the adjacent joints can be performed when CT scanning is used for nonunion. When adjacent arthritis is present, the decision to incorporate these joints into the fusion mass during revision surgery might be considered.

If the viability, vascularity, or suspected infection of the nonunion site or adjacent bone is in question, MRI and bone scintigraphy scans have been demonstrated to be useful [87–90]. The sensitivity of MRI in the detection of avascular necrosis (AVN) in the foot and ankle is nearly 100% [87, 91].

Fig. 3.2 (**a**) Bilateral calcaneal axial radiographs (**b**) Bilateral hindfoot alignment radiographs

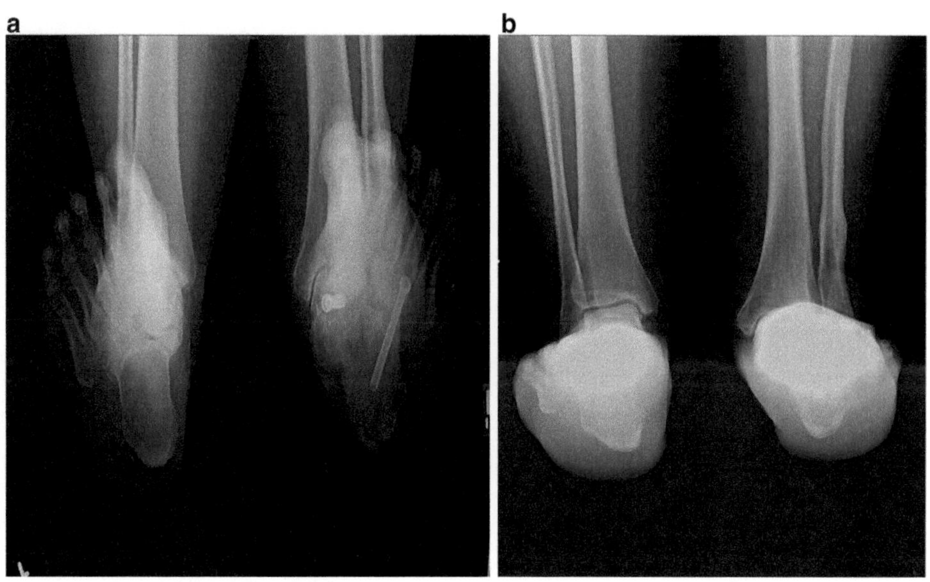

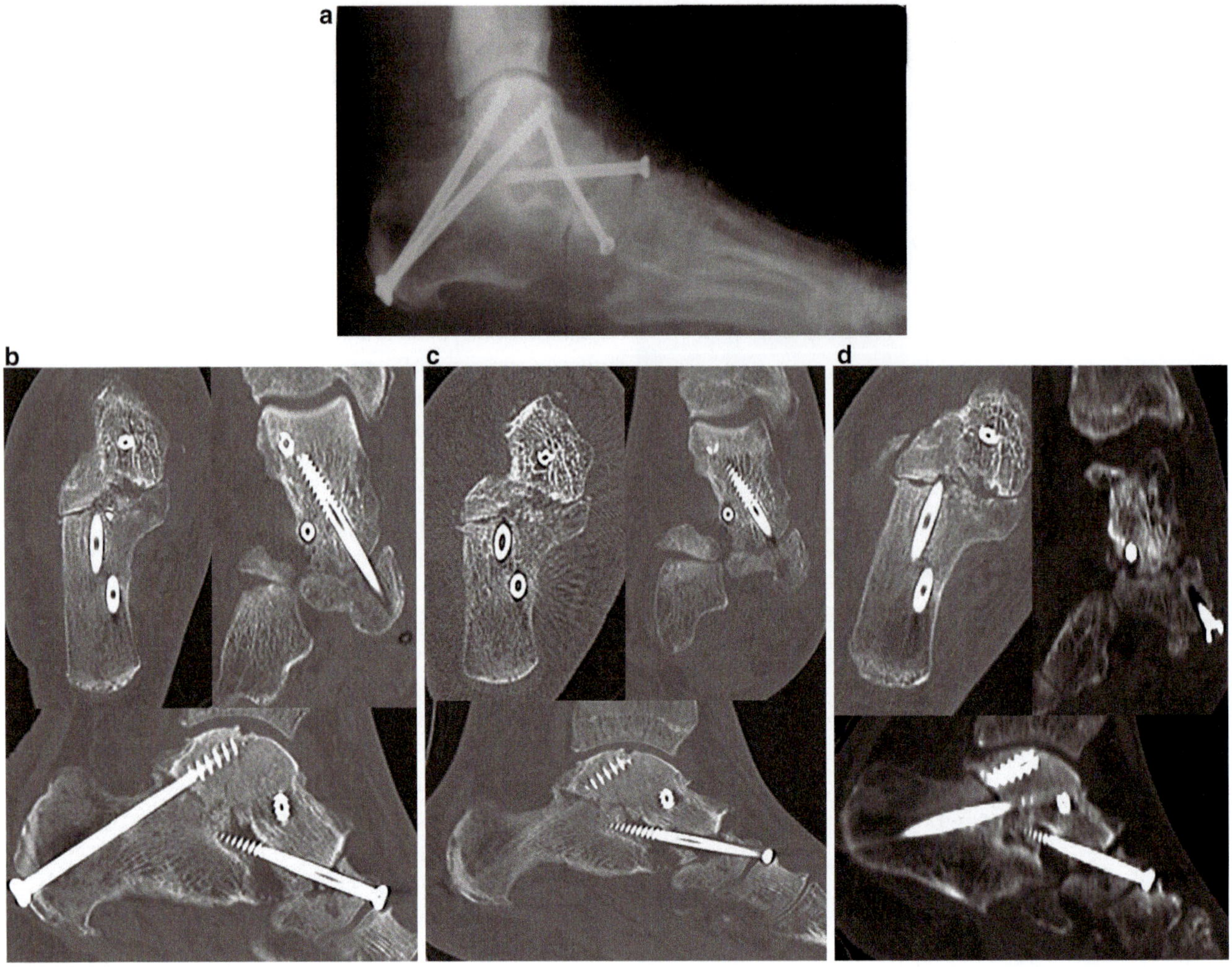

Fig. 3.3 (**a**) Lateral radiograph with fractured screw (inferior-medial to superior-lateral) across talonavicular joint 6-months following selected hindfoot arthrodesis for end-stage adult acquired flatfoot. This view fails to demonstrate evidence of joint consolidation. (**b**) 3-months status post axial and lateral CT scans showing absence of consolidation at both the talonavicular and subtalar joints. (**c**) 6-months status post CT scan with continued absence of consolidation. (**d**) 9-months status post CT scan clearly demonstrating nonunion following an extended course of immobilization, nonweightbearing and electrical stimulation

Fig. 3.4 CT scan demonstrating near complete consolidation after subtalar joint arthrodesis

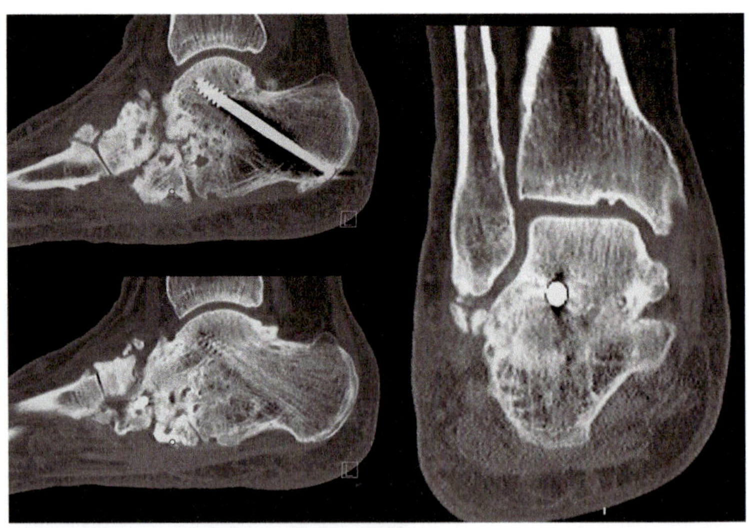

Adjacent articular surfaces remote to the site of nonunion can also be thoroughly assessed for degenerative changes, which can help to guide future surgical planning. However, the use of MRI after surgical reconstruction can be problematic due to artifacts and scatter if ferromagnetic implants have been utilized. In such circumstances, nuclear bone scintigraphy scans (technicium-99m MDP) have been shown to adequately detect both unifocal and multifocal AVNs at acceptable rates and are not hindered by retained hardware. Furthermore, white blood cell-labeled nuclear scans (indium-111) can be utilized in conjunction with traditional scanning techniques to detect underlying infection at the nonunion site. Combining Tc-99m MDP and indium-111 scans increases the accuracy, specificity, and sensitivity of the diagnoses of concomitant bone infections in nonunion patients to greater than 90% [87, 92].

In patients for whom a suspicion of underlying osteopenia or osteoporosis is present, bone densitometry scanning can be a valuable tool. The healthcare community recommends bone density testing (via dual-energy X-ray absorptiometry (DEXA)) for postmenopausal women at the age of 65 and for male and female patients with risk factors such as tobacco use, alcoholism, chronic steroid use, and endocrine disorders that contribute to osteoporosis prior to age 65 [93–95]. When a bone mass deficiency is present in a nonunion patient, the patient might benefit from the utilization of additional orthobiologics or fixation methods, such as locked plating constructs and/or external fixation, which have proven successful in the osteoporotic/osteopenic bone.

Nonunion Management/Treatment Strategies

Treatment strategies should obviously be focused on healing the nonunion. However, nonunions in the foot and ankle are often associated with malunions and deformities. Additionally, the joints in close proximity might be stiff, malaligned, and painful due to compensation, particularly in cases of long-standing nonunions. Therefore, one should employ a global approach that accounts for the entire foot, ankle, and lower leg. The ultimate goal is a well-aligned, painless, and functional foot and ankle. Obtaining this goal can be challenging and is certainly not possible for every patient. Nonetheless, some degree of pain relief and improved function should be expected. The surgeon needs to develop a treatment plan and then determine a realistic prognosis, and the plan and prognosis should be thoroughly communicated to the patient. Patients should understand that the treatment process will be long and cumbersome and will often require multiple surgical sessions. While some nonunions heal rather easily, others require a long period of time to heal.

Patient goals typically include pain relief and normal function. The primary goals for the surgeon include union, normal architecture/alignment, resolution of symptoms, and functionality. The goals must be kept realistic and attainable. Obviously, these goals will vary based on the patient's unique situation and circumstances. Factors such as medical history, prior surgery, anatomic site, compliance, etc. will directly affect the patient's prognosis and should be the starting point of any discussion between the patient and surgeon. The surgeon should provide reasonable options and associated outcomes based on his/her experience and the current literature. Furthermore, the surgeon and patient should agree on the definition of an acceptable outcome. The patient's motivation, disability, social problems, litigation issues, mental status, and desires should be considered before a revision is undertaken.

Revision surgery to address nonunion often requires much thought, thorough planning, patient education, patient optimization, appropriate technology and resources, extended convalescence, advanced imaging, further surgery, and long-term follow-up. Patients should have clear understandings of their problems. Surgical consultation and informed consent should provide clarity and understanding regarding each patient's unique situation. This process might require several visits and various types of educational media for the patient to thoroughly comprehend his or her situation and develop realistic expectations. Such patients and their families should understand the uncertainties associated with nonunion healing, the extended course of treatment, and that multiple surgical interventions might be required.

Appropriate consultation with other services is important prior to surgery. Any issues that might adversely affect patient outcomes should be addressed by the appropriate specialist before surgical intervention.

If preoperative noninvasive lower limb arterial studies demonstrate poor perfusion, a vascular surgery consultation is recommended. These tests might indicate that the proposed surgery might not heal. A vascular intervention can be performed to increase arterial perfusion or might indicate that the patient is not a surgical candidate.

If incision placement is necessary in an area that is predisposed to dehiscence or if soft tissue deficits are anticipated following realignment, a plastic surgery consultation is recommended. A plastic surgeon might suggest an optimal site for incision placement or perform soft tissue reconstruction concomitantly during revision for the nonunion.

Unfortunately, patients with long-standing nonunions might be dependent on oral narcotics. Referral to pain management is helpful both during the course of treatment and ultimately for the detoxification and weaning of the patient off of all narcotic medications [96–98].

Obtaining a preoperative physical therapy consultation is particularly important in situations in which premature weight bearing was a contributing factor to nonunion. A physical therapist can provide gait training that accounts for the postoperative activity expectations and the use of assistive or adaptive devices. Furthermore, such training provides an opportunity for the patient to develop a relationship with a physical therapist who will work with him or her following surgery. Rehabilitation will be necessary following surgery for independent transfer and ambulation. Ultimately, physical therapy will be necessary to address the strengths and ranges of motion of the surrounding joints.

A nutritionist consultation should be considered for patients who are malnourished or obese. It has been clearly established that poor dietary intakes of proteins, particularly albumin, and vitamins can contribute to delayed union or nonunion. Furthermore, a nutritionist can help a severely obese patient reduce his or her weight. Obesity obviously makes the offloading of the surgical site technically very difficult [53, 99–101].

Endocrinology consultations are beneficial for patients with diabetes, particularly those patients with elevated HgA1c levels. Hoogwerf et al. have demonstrated a linear relationship between the incidence of complications and elevated HgA1c levels in patients with diabetes mellitus [102].

Therefore, tight glucose control should be a part of patient optimization when diabetes mellitus is present. Furthermore, in a 2007 report by Brinker et al., the investigators strongly recommended endocrinology referrals for patients with nonunion when technical errors have been excluded [55], i.e., the patient's failure to heal was not caused by underutilization of fixation, fixation failure, or infection. Endocrinology can isolate the metabolic deficiency that contributed to the nonunion and treat the abnormality to optimize the patient throughout their treatment course. These treatments can include the repletion of low vitamin D levels, thyroid hormone, and the optimization of blood glucose.

Depression is not uncommon in patients with chronic medical conditions; thus, patients with nonunions often exhibit signs of clinical depression. Referral to their primary care physician or psychiatrist might be beneficial [103–106].

Although the majority of revision procedures to address nonunion can be performed in one surgical setting, there are situations in which multiple surgeries are required. Factors that influence this decision include prior operative procedures, fixation that necessitates removal, the fixation that will be utilized for the revision, the necessity of harvesting an autogenous bone graft, and the times anticipated for the various parts of the surgery. It is important to anticipate technical difficulties and unforeseen challenges that might develop during surgery. Unfortunately, technical difficulties occur even under ideal circumstances and with the best of plans. Maintaining a surgical schedule that provides a margin to accommodate these unanticipated problems is recommended.

Procedures as simple as removing hardware can be rather difficult even when the appropriate instrumentation and image intensification are available. Such procedures can require a significant amount of time and effort that might be better utilized to address other, more important aspects of the procedure. Therefore, it might be better to stage the surgery so that the fixation can be removed during the initial surgical session and debridement, realignment, fixation, etc. can be performed in the next surgical session. Additionally, if intramedullary nails, large diameter screws, or other types of devices with large diameters are removed, the patient can be permitted a period of time to allow these bony deficits to fill in or consolidate. These processes can be expedited via the use of adjuvant nonsurgical therapies, such as pulsed electromagnetic field and ultrasonic therapies. The goal is to improve bone quality, which might enhance the effectiveness of the fixation that will be used in subsequent procedures.

In situations in which osteomyelitis is suspected, staged procedures are recommended. Although preoperative advanced imaging is helpful in the diagnosis of osteomyelitis, a definitive diagnosis can only be made with bone cultures and biopsy. Because infection will adversely affect bony union, it is imperative that the organisms are identified and appropriate antibiotics are administered if osteomyelitis is present. The primary surgical session can be used to obtain a bone biopsy and cultures to rule out or treat osteomyelitis. Additionally, hardware can also be removed during this initial surgical session.

Staging provides time for the patients to contemplate their upcoming procedures and develop a thorough understanding of their situation. Staging also provides an opportunity to address metabolic deficiencies or issues such as elevated HgA1c or hypovitaminosis D. Additionally, staging can provide time for a patient to implement smoking cessation program if necessary.

Lastly, the staging of procedures gives the surgeon an opportunity to ascertain the patient's ability to comply and to determine whether there are socioeconomic, psychological, family, or other factors that require attention.

Deformity Assessment

Deformity is invariably associated with nonunion in the foot and ankle. In addition to addressing nonunion, surgeries must also address any existing deformity (Fig. 3.5). Deformity, whether secondary to inadequate reduction during the index procedure or due to gradual development following a failed union, must be completely reduced. One of the major surgical goals is to obtain complete realignment. Any residual deformity will result in stress or an unevenly distributed axial load on the nonunion site and increase the risk of failure following revision. Residual deformities can further result in compensatory gaits that predispose surrounding joints to degenerative processes. Thus, deformity assessments must be thorough and comprehensive. Evaluations should include clinical examination, radiographs, and advanced imaging.

Clinical examination should include both static and dynamic assessments. Frontal, transverse, and sagittal plane deformities should be evaluated in both open and closed kinetic chains. Open kinetic chain evaluations of both the nonunion site and the surrounding joints are important.

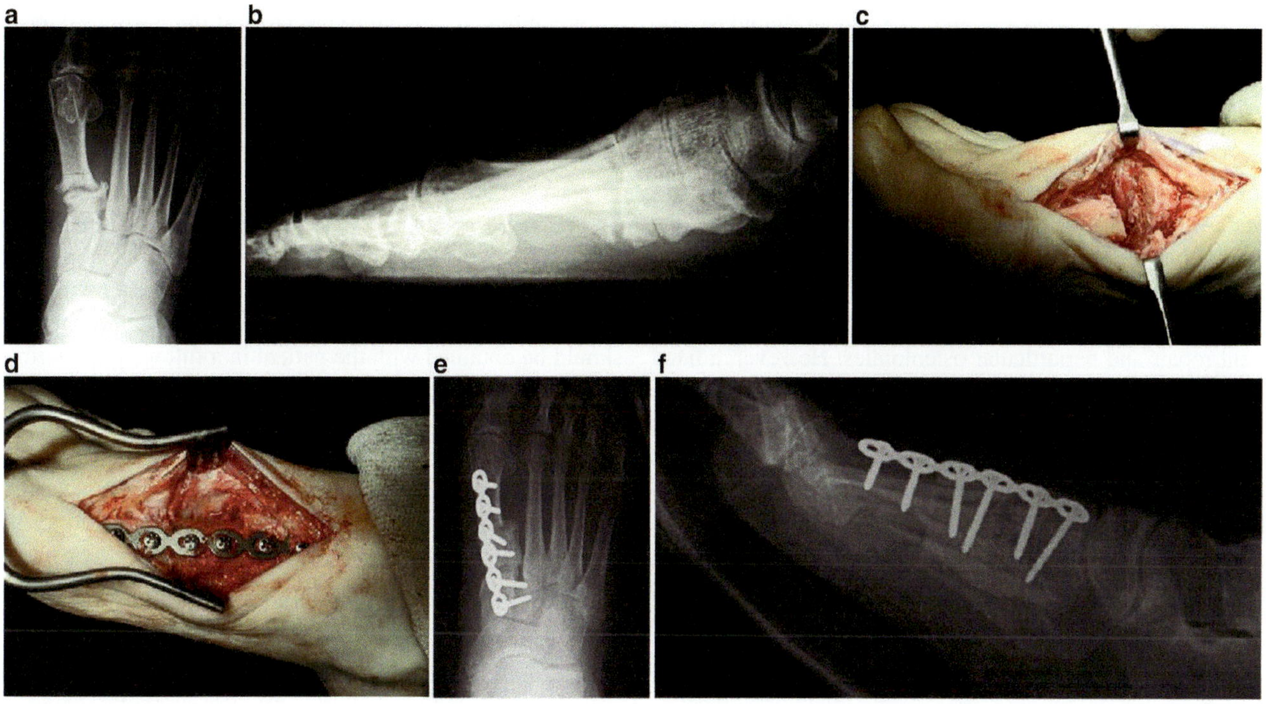

Fig. 3.5 (**a**) AP radiograph showing nonunion following a first metatarsal base osteotomy for hallux valgus reconstruction resulting in severe shortening. (**b**) Lateral radiograph demonstrating significant first ray elevation. (**c**) Skeletal deficit following resection of the nonunion. (**d**) Defect filled with a structural autogenous bone graft and secured with plate fixation. (**e, f**) AP and lateral radiographs demonstrating restoration of length and sagittal plane realignment

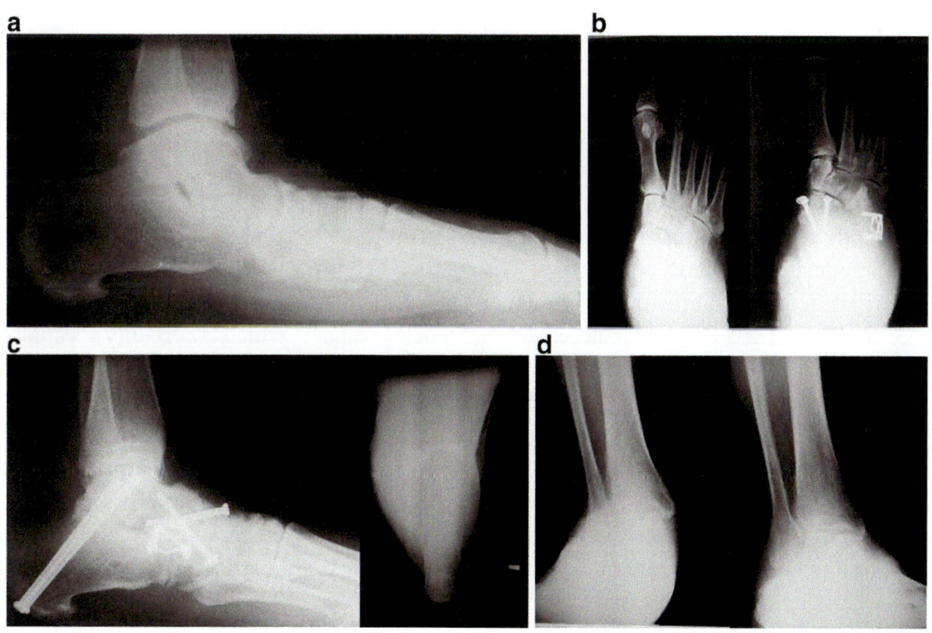

Fig. 3.6 (**a**) Lateral radiograph of late-stage adult-acquired flat foot with significant angular deformity. (**b**) Preoperative and postoperative radiograph following triple arthrodesis. Note the undercorrection of transverse plane deformity with inadequate talar head coverage by the navicular. (**c**) 6-months status post lateral and axial radiographs demonstrating nonunion. (**d**) AP radiograph of the ankle showing valgus deformity

Compensatory deformities can often develop in adjacent joints. A long-standing nonunion of the subtalar joint (STJ) following arthrodesis for stage III adult-acquired flatfoot with residual valgus deformity might develop ankle valgus (Fig. 3.6). Revision surgery of the STJ nonunion should also address the ankle valgus to obtain complete realignment. Furthermore, one must ascertain whether the ankle valgus is fixed or reducible. An attempt should be made to passively manipulate the deformity into realignment. This determination can be made during open kinetic chain assessment. Closed kinetic chain or weight-bearing assessment is also very important. The level of deformity and the areas of compensation can be determined. The patient should be able to place the foot and ankle into a corrected position during weight bearing. If this cannot be accomplished, then the deformity is fixed. If the patient cannot place the ankle joint into a position that parallels the subtalar deformity at the nonunion site, the joint deformity is fixed and requires correction. If the patient can achieve the corrected position, the joint deformity might resolve with realignment of the nonunion. Reducible valgus deformities of the ankle can be managed with joint-sparing procedures, such as deltoid ligament repair and periarticular osteotomies. However, a fixed deformity might require ankle arthrodesis or total ankle replacement to obtain complete realignment. Another example is the compensatory forefoot supinatus/varus that develops due to an ankle or hindfoot nonunion in valgus deformity. The supinatus/varus might require correction during surgical management of the nonunion. Such deformities will be exposed and magnified following ankle or hindfoot realignment. A fixed supinatus/varus requires surgery. However, a reducible deformity might resolve without intervention following ankle or hindfoot realignment [107].

Plain radiographs are an important part of deformity assessment because they can fully characterize all other deformities associated with the nonunion. Radiographs can be used to evaluate length, angulation, rotation, and translation. It is occasionally important to obtain weight-bearing radiographs of the contralateral extremity as well as the involved extremity. Stress radiology can be helpful in the evaluation of the competence of the collateral ligaments of the ankle.

Shortening is not uncommon with nonunion. One must ascertain the degree of shortening that is acceptable from a functional standpoint. It is important to anticipate the quantity of bony resection that will be necessary to develop a healthy cancellous substrate at the nonunion site. This quantity will have implications in terms of the type and size of bone graft that will be required. Furthermore, this quantity will also influence the type of fixation that is necessary and whether adjacent joints will need to be included in the arthrodesis.

Angular deformities, particularly in the frontal and sagittal planes, can be thoroughly reviewed with plain radiographs. Nonunion following STJ or ankle joint arthrodesis can often be associated with a severe frontal plane deformity. Plain radiographs will demonstrate the extent of the deformity so that plans can be made for realignment during revision surgery of the nonunion. Templates can be helpful when planning realignments for frontal plane deformities. One can determine whether complete realignment is possible based on the extent of the deformity. There are situations in which a complete reduction of a severe deformity can place a compromised soft tissue envelope at risk for wound problems. In such situations, one must accept incomplete realignment or consider shortening the bony segment. Otherwise, one should prepare for possible soft tissue reconstruction.

Nonunions following arthrodeses of the tarsometatarsal, midfoot, and midtarsal articulations are often associated with sagittal plane deformities. Axial loads will invariably result in dorsiflexion deformities. Plain radiographs will demonstrate the degree of deformity so that the surgeon can plan accordingly.

Therefore, plain radiographs are very important for planning deformity corrections during revision nonunion surgeries. These evaluations should be comprehensive, and all appropriate views should be obtained. Radiographs should be obtained with the patient in a full weight-bearing position and should be performed bilaterally, particularly when significant deformities involving the hindfoot and ankle are present.

Although advanced imaging can be quite helpful in the evaluation of nonunion, such imaging has limited utility in terms of deformity assessment. CT scans can be helpful in evaluations of transverse plane deformities, particularly rotational and translational problems. These deformities can be clinically and radiographically difficult to evaluate. A CT scan can provide information regarding the magnitude and direction of the deformity, particularly in cases involving the STJ and ankle joints.

Principles and Techniques for Revision Surgeries of Nonunions

Full-thickness incisions down to the bone should be utilized in virtually all cases. Undermining should be avoided or kept to a minimum to facilitate retraction. The goal is to avoid disrupting the blood supply at the incision site. However, one must be cognizant of the vital structures located in a particular area, particularly nerves and tendons, to avoid damaging them. In situations involving severe deformities that require significant realignment, incisions should be placed opposite the tension side of the soft tissue envelope. Such location might be in areas that are remote from the original incision, which is certainly acceptable. Otherwise, placing an incision on the tension side of the soft tissue envelope can result in wound problems.

Thorough dissection and evacuation of scar tissue is important because it will permit direct access to the nonunion site, which is essential for adequate debridement and joint preparation. Additionally, the removal of scar tissue that contributes to joint contracture allows for manipulation so that alignment can be restored.

The nonunion must be identified and thoroughly evacuated. All devitalized and necrotic tissue should be completely removed. Joint access is very important, and having appropriate instrumentation to facilitate access is helpful. Various types of distracters are available to provide and maintain access to the nonunion site. Following debridement, the host tissue can be prepared with a combination of fenestration and fish scaling. Depending on the specific anatomic site, sharp drill bits should be advanced under constant irrigation into the deep subchondral tissues to create vascular channels. The goal is for blood to enter the nonunion site and deliver cells, bone marrow, growth factors, etc. Following fenestration, the host tissue should be further developed into a healthy cancellous substrate via the use of small, sharp osteotomes. This procedure should be performed aggressively, but care should be taken to preserve the cortical and subchondral bone at the perimeter of the nonunion site so that the structural integrity is maintained. This structural integrity of perimeter bone will be important to facilitate realignment and support a stiff fixation construct. Although many such cases will involve bone grafts or bone graft substitutes, bone grafts cannot manifest biologic activity without an adequate blood supply. Therefore, meticulous attention to preparation of host tissues is important for enhancing union.

The primary goal of fixation is to provide a stable construct that eliminates motion. Motion during healing impedes the consolidation of bony surfaces and the incorporation of bone grafts. Although a firm surgical plan is required in these cases, one must respond to intraoperative findings and developments that require alternative forms of fixation. The surgeon should plan for "alternative" forms of fixation and have these devices readily available. As these revision nonunion cases evolve, adaptability is critically important to achieving the primary goal of stability.

The choice of fixation is often affected by factors such as osteopenia, the location of the nonunion, proximity to surrounding joints, previous fixation, patient compliance, the amount of bone loss following debridement, the patient's ability to tolerate non-weight bearing, the surgeon's technical acumen with specific techniques and devices, and industry/technical support. Situations involving severe osteopenia or bone loss might require super constructs or the sacrifice of nearby joints (Fig. 3.7).

Recent advances in technology have provided many excellent options for fixation. Screws should purchase cortices or compact subchondral bone whenever possible. Locking plate technology is an excellent option for patients with osteopenia or poor quality bone (Fig. 3.8). Alternatively, supplemental external fixators that neutralize the nonunion site are a reasonable option in this same patient population (Fig. 3.9).

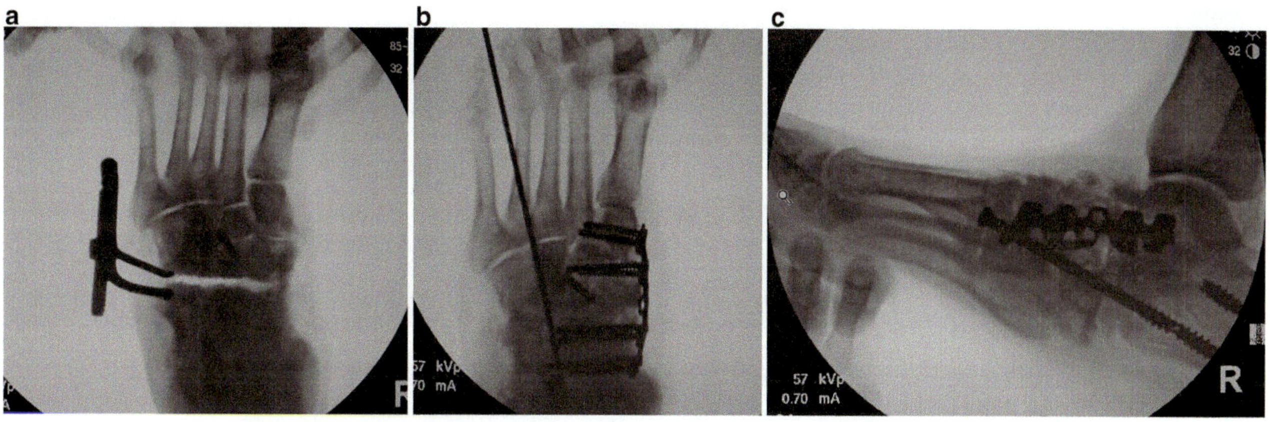

Fig. 3.7 (a) Intraoperative AP image following debridement of midtarsal nonunion. (b, c) Revision of nonunion showing super-construct fixation with a locking plate that extends distally to include the medial cuneiform

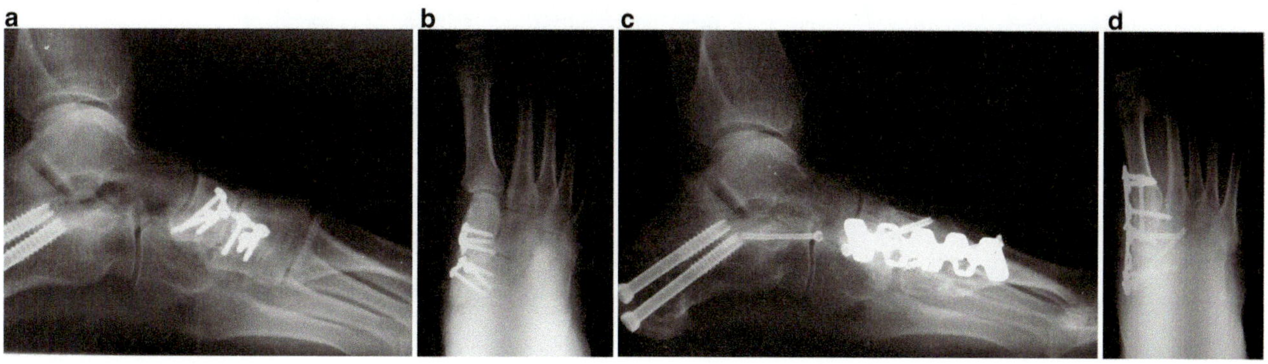

Fig. 3.8 (a, b) Nonunion following naviculocuneiform arthrodesis. (c, d) Revision with locking plate that extends distally to the 1st tarsometatarsal articulation which was included in the fusion mass

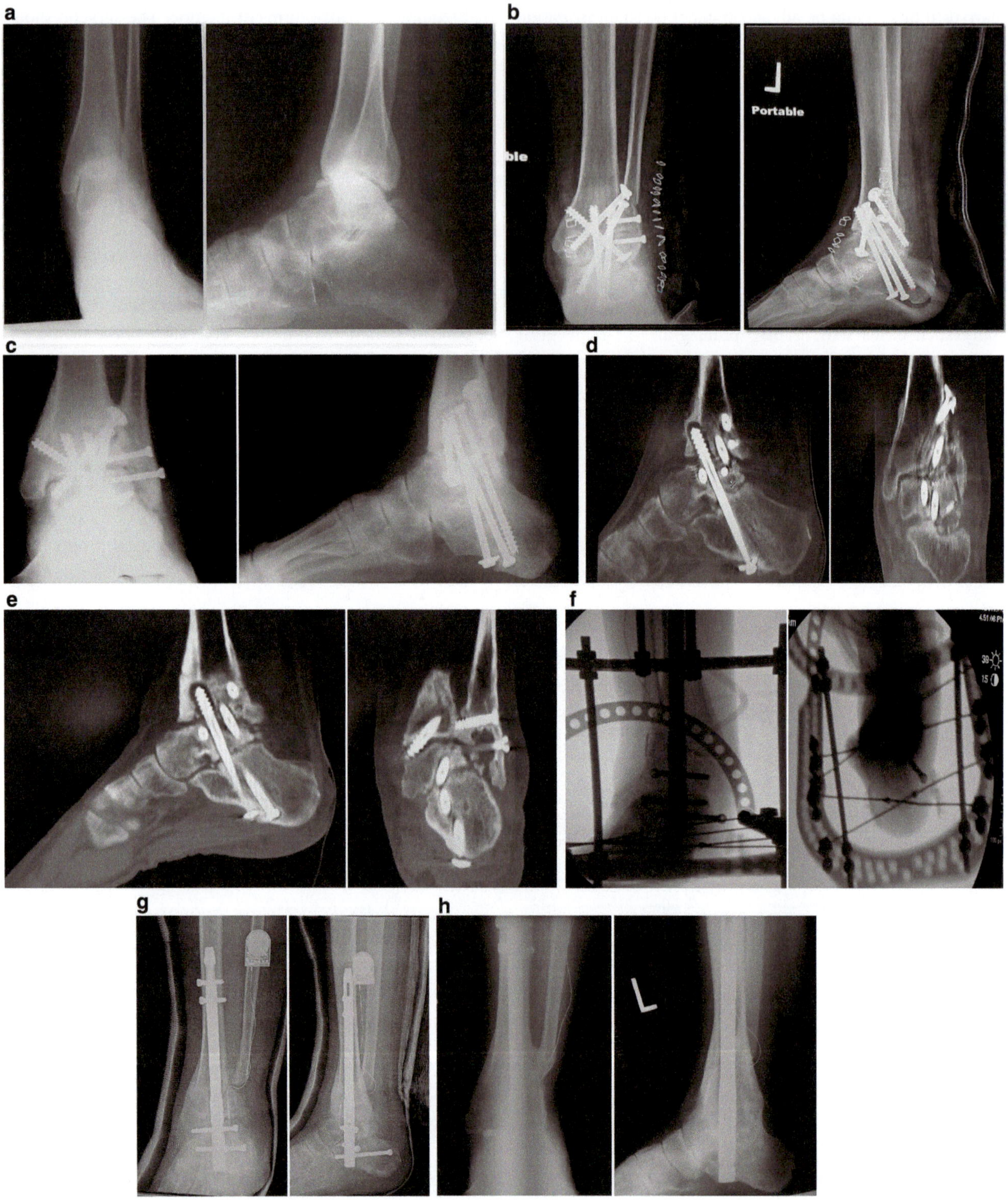

Fig. 3.9 (**a**) AP and lateral radiograph demonstrating severe ankle and subtalar arthritis (**b–e**) Plain film radiographs and serial CT scans demonstrating no consolidation across arthrodesis sites (**f**, **g**) Revision tibiotalocalcaneal arthrodesis with intramedullary nail, external fixation and implantable bone growth stimulator (**h**) AP and lateral radiograph demonstrating consolidation of revision tibiotalocalcaneal arthrodesis

Surgical Revision Techniques: Specific Anatomic Sites

First Metatarsophalangeal (MTP) Joint

The incidence of nonunion following the first MTP arthrodesis is relatively low. The incidences are higher in patients with hallux rigidus who develop subsequent end-stage arthrosis and patients with posttraumatic arthritis than in patients with diagnoses of hallux valgus. End-stage arthrosis, whether secondary to hallux rigidus or posttraumatic arthritis, is often associated with a thicker subchondral plate that can be sclerotic and avascular. These patients have a higher predisposition to nonunion than patients with hallux valgus. Therefore, joint preparation must be thorough and adequate such that the subchondral plates are penetrated and methodically broken to enhance blood flow. Some of the reaming systems used for joint debridement might be inadequate in these cases or should be supplemented with drilling techniques and fish scaling rather than used alone.

Patients who have undergone a distal first metatarsal osteotomy for hallux rigidus are also at risk for avascular necrosis (AVN). Advanced imaging to evaluate or rule out AVN can be helpful in this group of patients. One can then plan for appropriate debridement techniques and the use of bone grafts or orthobiologics to augment arthrodesis.

Positioning the hallux in plantar flexion will result in a significant axial load during the propulsive phase of the gait. These patients can develop nonunion, particularly if they begin weight bearing prior to the complete consolidation of the arthrodesis site. One of the reasons that the first MTP arthrodesis has such a low incidence of nonunion is that the hallux is typically positioned in dorsiflexion which offloads the arthrodesis site during weight bearing.

Revision surgery should be based on the reasons for nonunion. Regardless of the factors involved, revision should include thorough debridement and joint preparation, autogenous cancellous bone and/or orthobiologics, appropriate positioning, and a stable fixation construct. A structural bone graft is rarely necessary, and some shortening is certainly acceptable in this situation. The calcaneus or distal tibial metaphysis provides regional sources of autogenous cancellous bone. The authors typically use 6-mm or 8-mm trephines in a percutaneous manner to harvest the bone for first MTP nonunion revisions. Fixation constructs should extend to cortical bone remote from the arthrodesis site via either long screws or a long plate (Fig. 3.10). Although the authors typically permit immediate weight bearing following first MTP arthrodesis, a 6-week period of non-weight bearing is recommended following revision for nonunion.

Tarsometatarsal (TMT) Joint(s)

The first TMT arthrodesis (the modified Lapidus procedure) is a common procedure for hallux valgus reconstruction. Additionally, this joint is often included when global TMT arthrodesis is performed for posttraumatic arthritis and deformity. Nonunions of the TMT joints and all of the midfoot articulations are vertically oriented nonunions that have some shear component in which the osseous segments slide past each other when subjected to axial load. Nonunion of the first TMT joint is often associated with first ray elevation secondary to axial loading. Additionally, shortening is not uncommon with this particular nonunion, particularly in long-standing cases (Fig. 3.11). Therefore, revision goals should include union, sagittal plane realignment, and restoration of length. A structural bone graft might be necessary when shortening is significant (Figs. 3.12 and 3.13). However, the majority of these cases do not require a structural bone graft, particularly when sagittal and transverse realignments are easily achieved. Debridement of nonviable bone and scar tissue, the development of a healthy host environment, autogenous cancellous bone grafts, the use of orthobiologics, and stable fixation are often sufficient to address nonunion of the first TMT joint. Locking plate technology lends itself well to this situation.

Arthrodesis of the lesser TMT joints (second and third) might be required for posttraumatic arthritis or deformity involving the TMT complex. Nonunion of the lesser TMT joints might develop following global arthrodesis (joints 1–3). Fortunately, nonunion following lesser TMT arthrodesis is rarely associated with malalignment. Revision typically requires thorough debridement, host preparation, bone grafting/orthobiologics, and stable fixation.

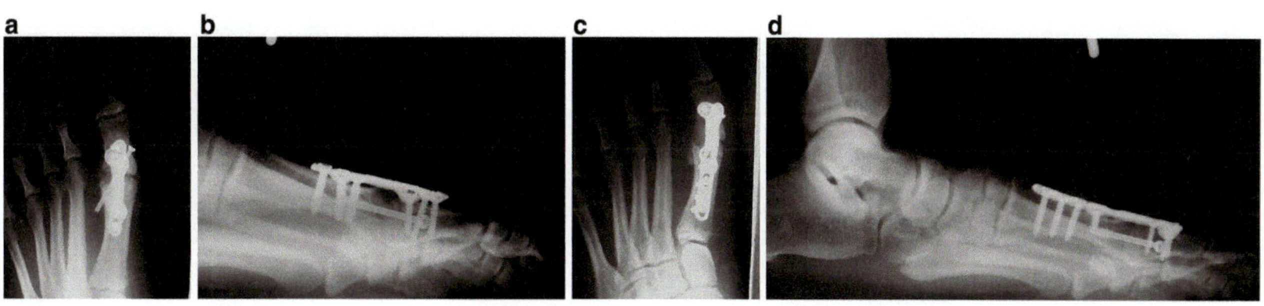

Fig. 3.10 (**a**, **b**) Nonunion status post 1st MPJ arthrodesis (**c**, **d**) Revision with a long locking plate that extends far beyond the arthrodesis site. The goals are to engage quality cortical bone and disperse axial loading over a relatively large implant

Tritarsal Complex

Nonunion is not uncommon following isolated, selected, or triple arthrodeses. Revision surgery should address not only the nonunion but also other associated problems.

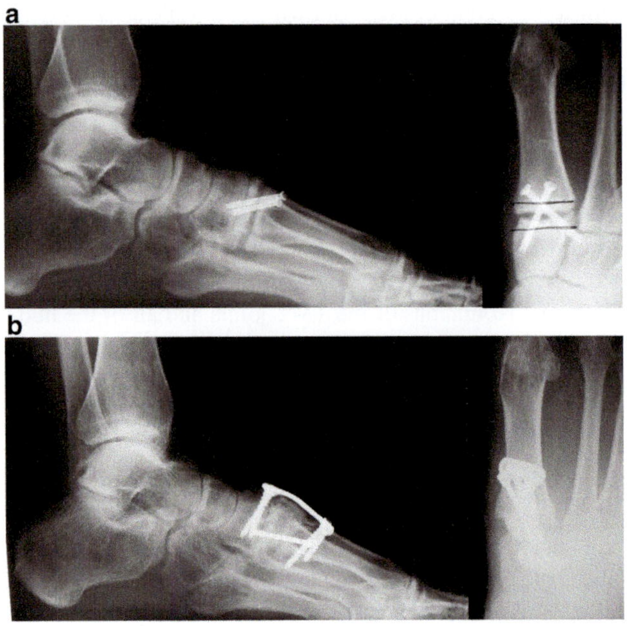

Fig. 3.11 (**a**) First ray shortening and elevation following 1st tarsometatarsal arthrodesis. (**b**) Revision with autogenous structural bone graft and plate. Note restoration of length and sagittal plane alignment

These might include undercorrection, malunion, ankle valgus or varus with associated collateral ligament attenuation, medical column instability not recognized during the initial surgery, soft tissue contractures that were not adequately released during the initial surgery, and unrecognized suprastructural issues. The goals of revision surgery are union, restoration of a plantigrade foot, and the preservation of function. Preoperative considerations should include specialized radiographs to evaluate alignment, appropriate advanced imaging, and patient optimization. Intraoperative goals include the development of a healthy cancellous substrate at the nonunion site and realignment. Specialized technology, appropriate instrumentation, bone grafts, orthobiologics, and image intensification help to accomplish these goals. In addition to revision of the nonunion, procedures should include osteotomies, the release of soft tissue contractures, superconstructs, and extended arthrodesis to include other joints whenever necessary.

Nonunion following isolated arthrodesis of the STJ can be surgically managed with isolated revision of the STJ or conversion into a triple arthrodesis. The highest incidence of nonunion following STJ arthrodesis occurs in patients with posttraumatic arthritis following calcaneal fractures. The authors prefer isolated revision of the STJ nonunion in the absence of malalignment and when degenerative changes are absent from the talonavicular (TNJ) and calcaneocuboid (CCJ) joints. This judgment is often based on

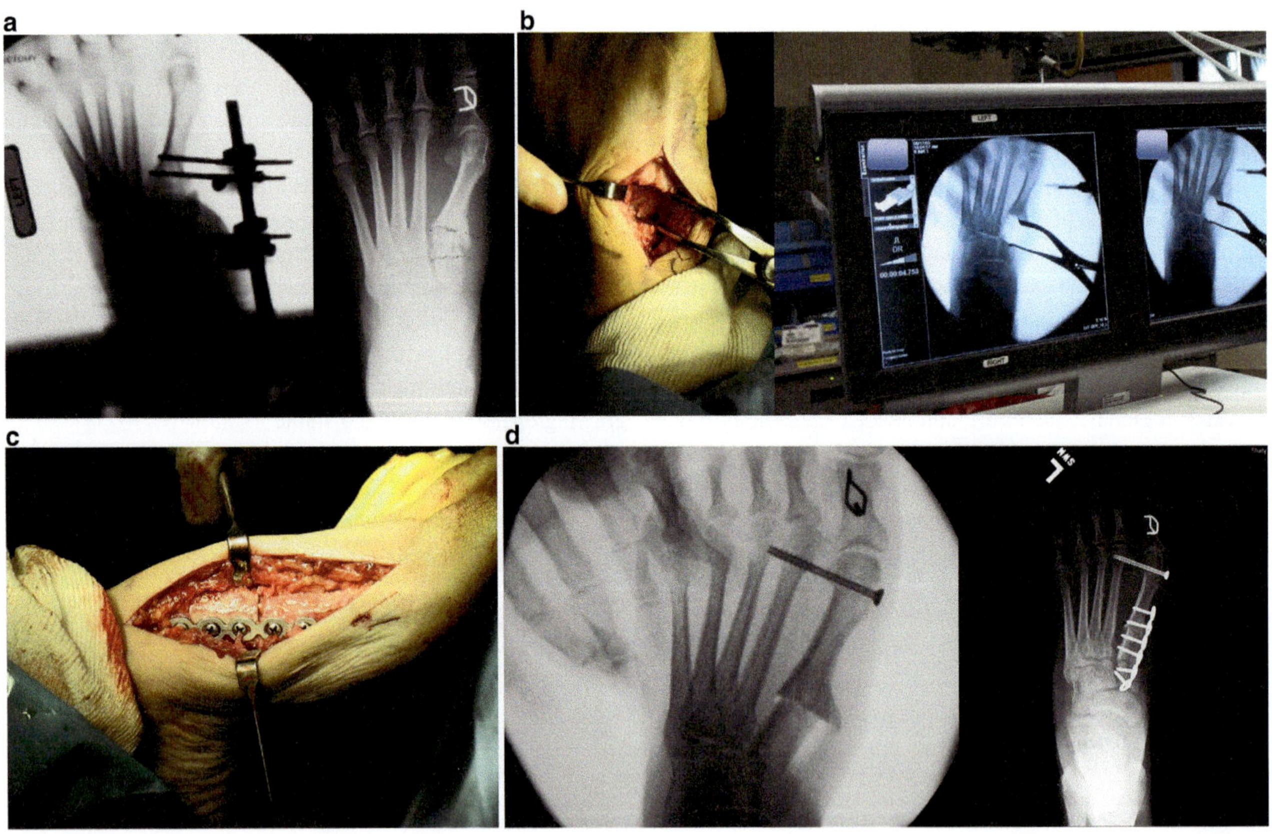

Fig. 3.12 (**a**) Status post 1st tarsometatarsal nonunion with significant shortening. (**b**) Skeletal defect following debridement. (**c**) Structural autogenous bone graft with plate fixation. (**d**) Restoration of length and alignment

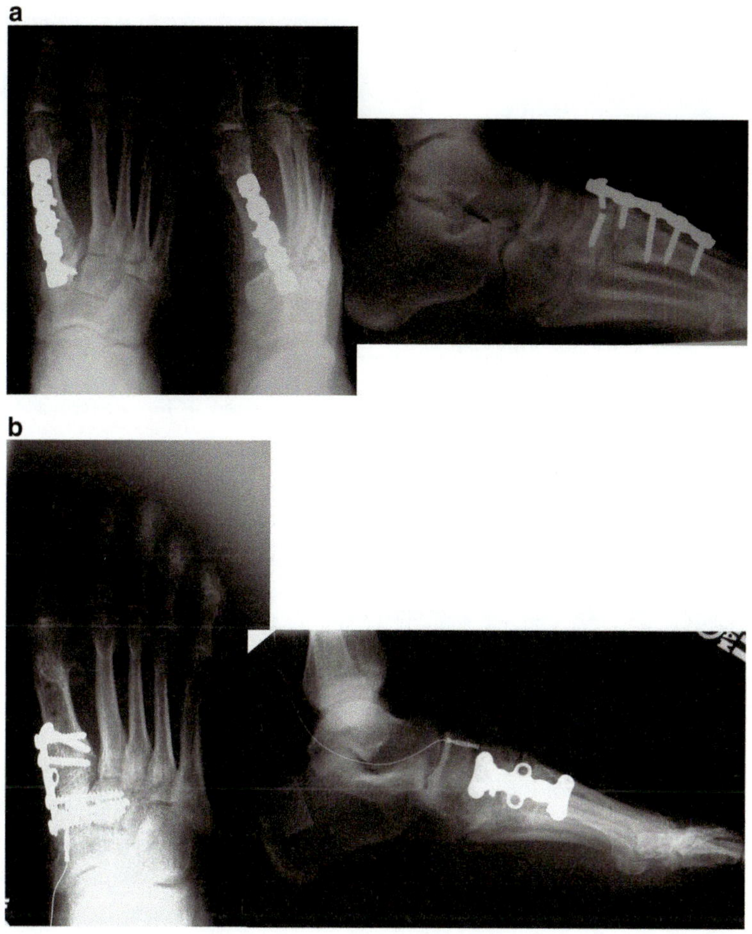

Fig. 3.13 (**a**) Nonunion following 1st tarsometatarsal joint arthrodesis (**b**) Revision 1st TMT arthrodesis with structural graft, locking plate, implantable bone growth stimulator

clinical assessment and preoperative imaging. The fixation construct typically includes large diameter compression screws (Fig. 3.14). The authors prefer multiple screws that engage the cortices or subchondral areas. However, when malalignment is present or there are factors that will adversely affect the fixation construct, we prefer to convert the STJ nonunion into a triple arthrodesis (Fig. 3.15). This procedure enhances the stiffness of the entire tritarsal complex following fixation and provides multiple options for fixation.

The rate of nonunion following TNJ arthrodesis has been reported to be relatively high [108, 109]. Isolated revision is difficult even when the alignment is good. The authors invariably convert nonunions of the TNJ into triple arthrodeses (Fig. 3.16). CCJ arthrodesis enhances the compression of the TNJ and allows easier realignment when deformity is present. Additionally, incorporation of the STJ into the fusion mass adds further stiffness to the entire construct. Complete elimination of all tritarsal motion will enhance the possibility of union during revision TNJ surgery. Our fixation construct of the talonavicular joint typically includes lateral compression screws and a medial locking plate. However, we have also used multiple compression screws that are strategically placed to deliver even compression throughout the arthrodesis site (Fig. 3.18d and e).

Selected arthrodesis for stage III or IV adult-acquired flatfoot has become a common procedure. Although the incidence of nonunion has not been reported, the authors have observed a higher rate relative to triple arthrodesis, particularly at the TN joint [110]. Our preference is to convert nonunions of either the STJ or TNJ into triple arthrodeses (Fig. 3.17).

Nonunion of any or all of the tritarsal joints is possible following triple arthrodesis (Fig. 3.18). The principles of addressing nonunion remain the same. Debridement, joint preparation, realignment, bone graft/orthobiologics, and enhanced fixation are required. A static neutralization external fixator is occasionally used to augment the internal fixation construct if osteopenia is severe or there are concerns about premature weight bearing.

Ankle Joint

Nonunion following ankle arthrodesis is most common in patients who have developed posttraumatic arthritis following pilon and Weber C fractures [111]. Ankle nonunions involve large, transversely oriented adjacent surfaces with

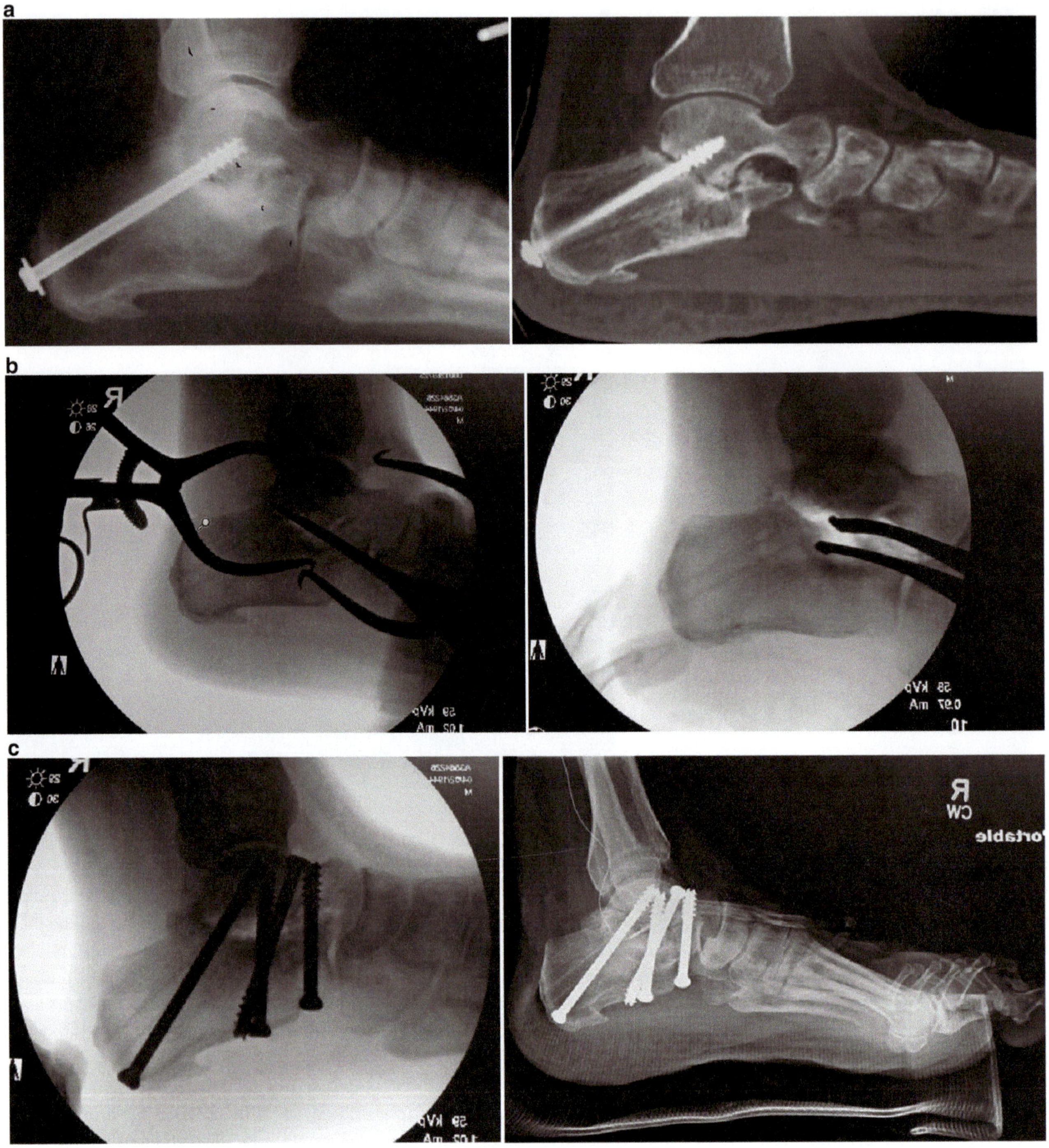

Fig. 3.14 (a) Nonunion status post isolated subtalar joint arthrodesis. (b) Intraoperative image-intensification confirming nonunion location. Distraction provides access to allow adequate debridement and preparation. (c) Fixation construct using compression screws engaging cortical and compact subchondral bone to enhance screw purchase and construct stiffness. Note electrical bone growth stimulator

good bony apposition that are generally stable to axial compression and should proceed to union. The revision of ankle joint nonunion depends on the original surgical approach and fixation. The majority of surgical approaches are either anterior or lateral, and we recommend using the same approach for revision. However, in cases in which a poor soft tissue envelope places the patient at risk for wound problems, an alternative approach should be considered (Fig. 3.19). A posterior approach is a reasonable alternative in these situations.

Debridement of ankle nonunion resulting in substantial bone loss can be difficult to manage. One must determine if

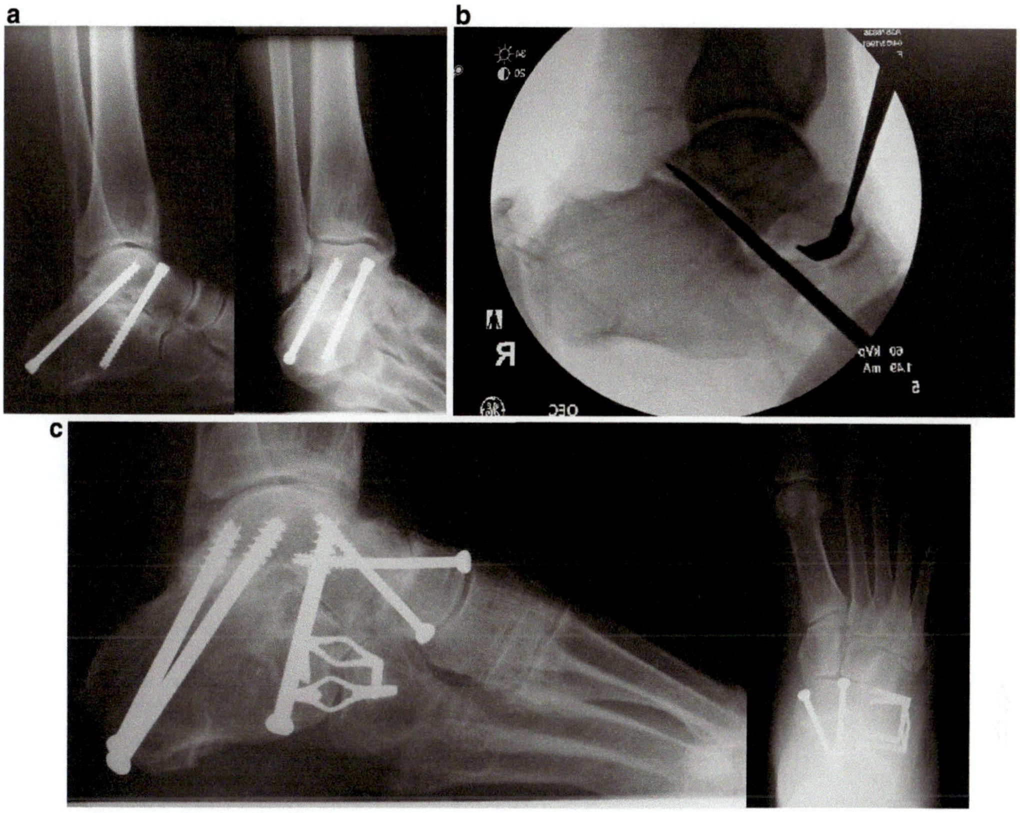

Fig. 3.15 (**a**) Nonunion following subtalar joint arthrodesis. (**b**) Intraoperative identification of nonunion. (**c**) Conversion into triple arthrodesis

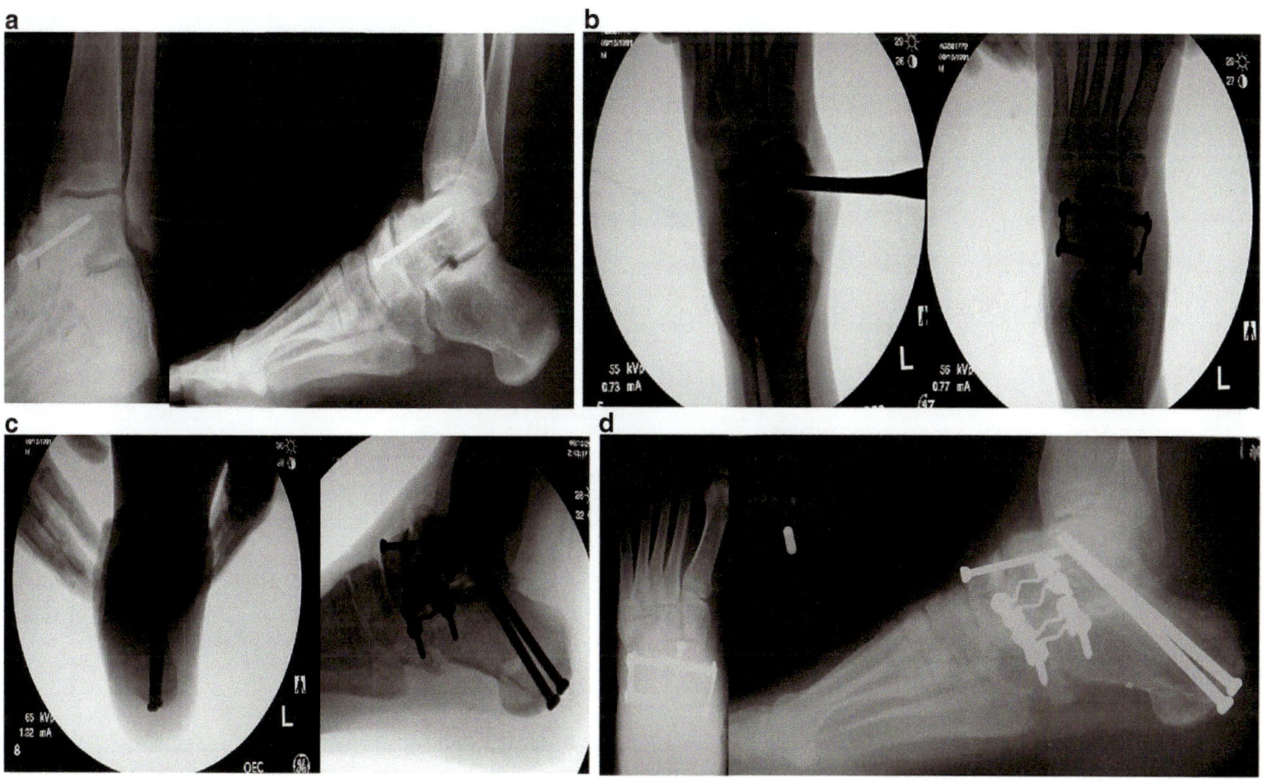

Fig. 3.16 (**a**) Nonunion following talonavicular arthrodesis. (**b**) Intraoperative identification of nonunion and conversion into a triple arthrodesis. Fixation accomplished with a combination of screws and locking plates. (**c**) Intraoperative images of final construct. (**d**) 3-months status post surgery

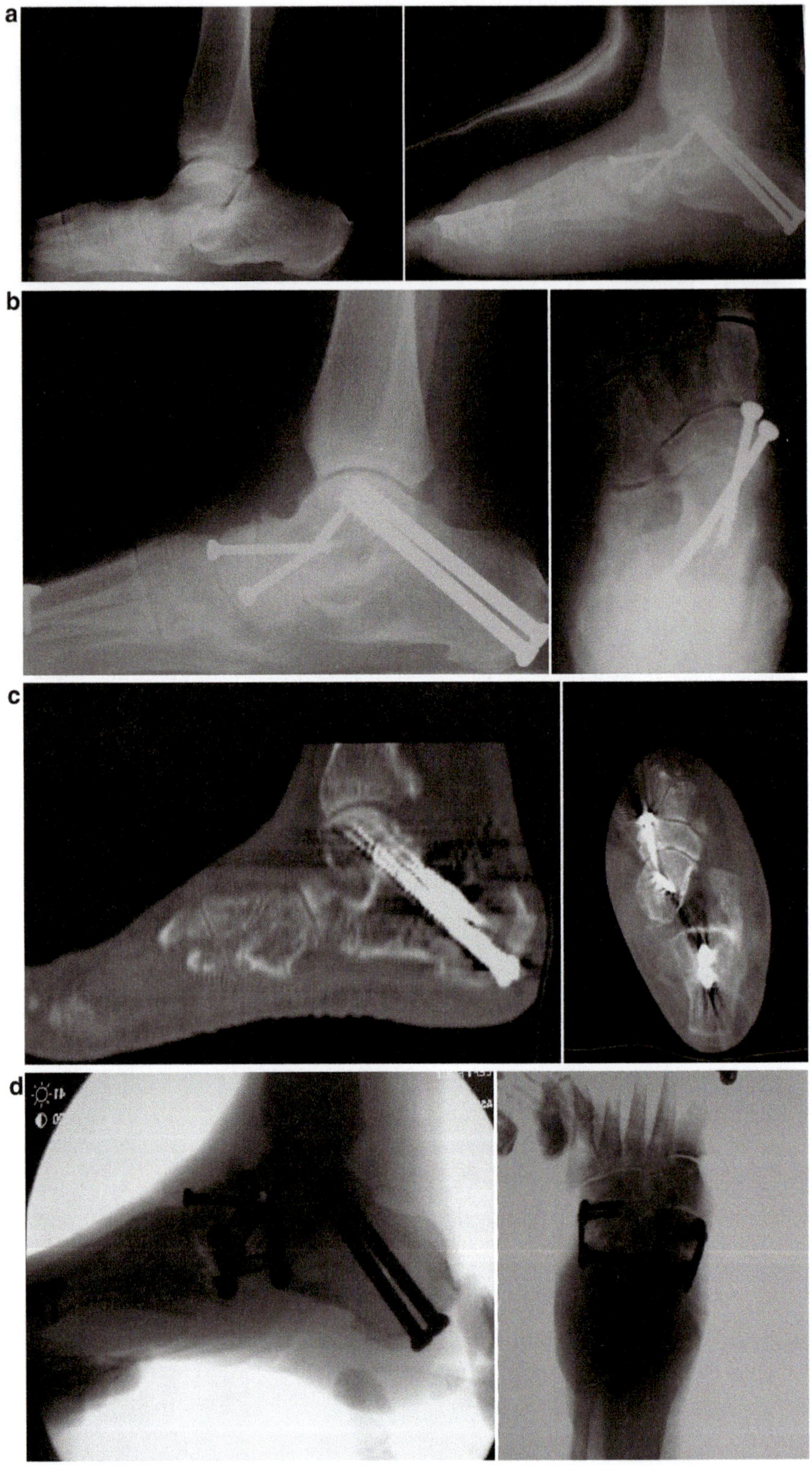

Fig. 3.17 (**a**, **b**) Status post selected hindfoot arthrodesis for end-stage adult acquired flatfoot. Implants traversing the talonavicular joint are short and located along the medial aspect of the joint with virtually no lateral compression. (**c**) CT scan confirms absence of consolidation at the talonavicular joint. (**d**) Conversion into triple arthrodesis. Fixation with screws and locking plates

there will be adequate bone to support an isolated revision of the ankle nonunion following debridement. Obtaining a solid fixation construct without sacrificing the STJ can be challenging with extensive bony debridement, particularly during a second or third revision. Alternatives include tibiotalocalcaneal or tibiocalcaneal arthrodeses (Fig. 3.20).

Although some shortening can be tolerated, excessive shortening can result in significant gait disturbances and

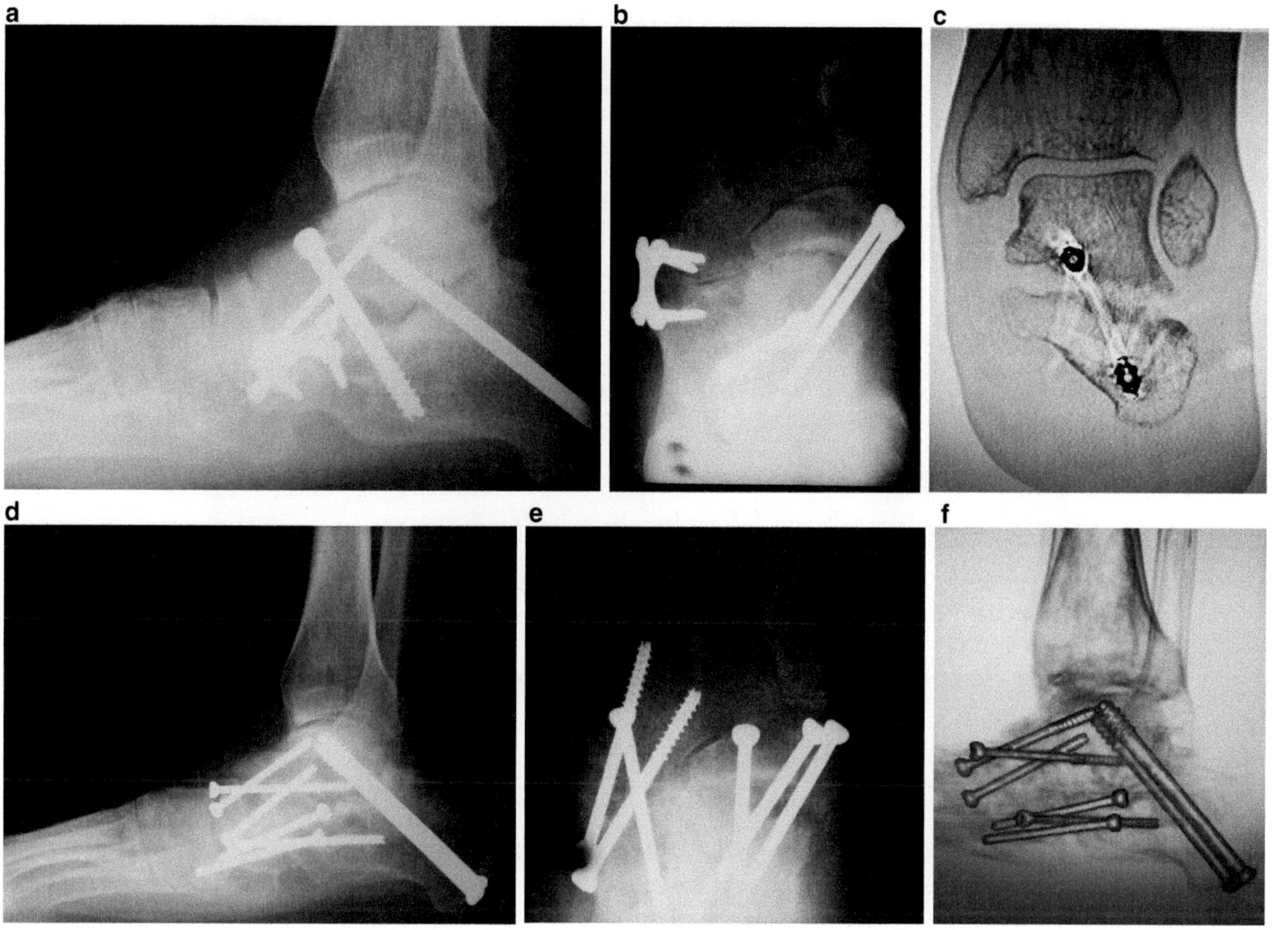

Fig. 3.18 (**a**, **b**) Radiographs demonstrating nonunion of all tritarsal joints following triple arthrodesis. (**c**) CT scan confirmation of nonunion. (**d**, **e**) Status post revisional triple arthrodesis. Note 2-point fixation of all tritarsal joints. (**f**) CT scan confirmation of consolidation

compensatory issues in the suprastructural skeleton. Additionally, acute shortening of the ankle can result in complications such as venous congestion, wound bunching with subsequent breakdown, edema, and tissue necrosis. Autogenous bone grafts or engineered bone might be considered in these cases [112]). Another option is a large segmental allograft, which has no limits in volume. However, large allografts do not always completely incorporate and can be predisposed to fracture. Distraction osteogenesis of the tibia is another option for maintaining length. The advantages of this technique include early weight bearing, stimulation of regional blood flow, and management of large defects (up to 10 cm.). This technique requires technical expertise and patient compliance [113].

The anatomy of the ankle lends itself well to multiple fixation options following nonunion revision. Screws, plates (standard and locking), intramedullary devices, and external fixators provide a range of good options for securing a stiff construct to support revision surgery.

Postoperative Management

Biologic responses are influenced by load and stability. Revisional nonunion surgeries invariably require extended periods of immobilization and non-weight bearing. Physical therapy consultations that provide instructions for non-weight bearing are recommended, especially if the patient is unable to comply prior to surgery. Devices such as knee walkers, wheelchairs, etc. can be helpful for these patients. Patients who lack family support are good candidates for placement into subacute nursing facilities. Deep venous thrombosis prophylaxis is recommended and dictated by risk factors. Patients should resume preoperative supplementation if indicated for any previously diagnosed deficiencies. The use of electrical stimulation or ultrasound might be considered to augment healing following surgery. Progress to union should be monitored with serial radiographs and advanced imaging. The authors typically confirm consolidation with CT scans prior to weight bearing.

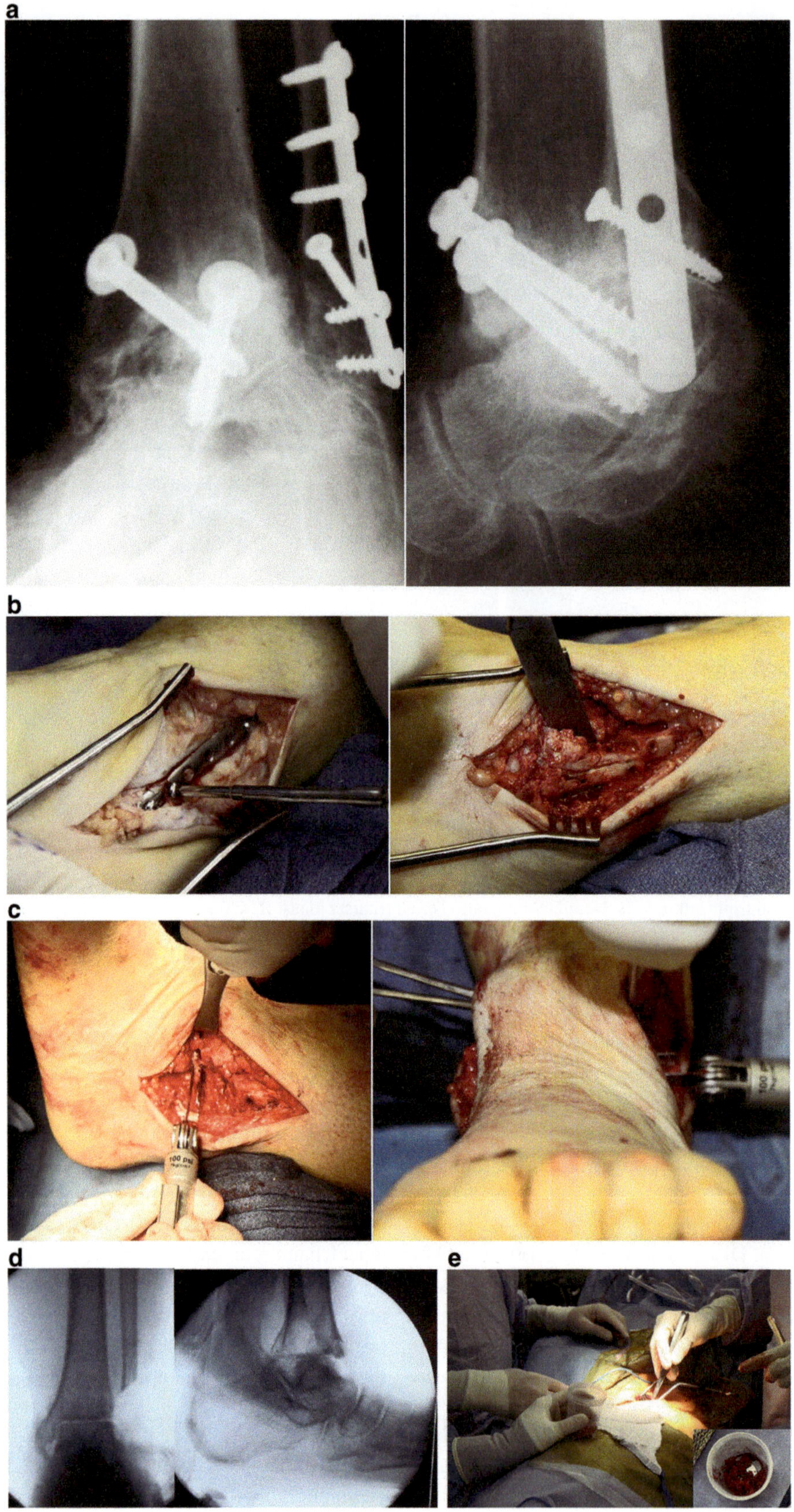

Fig. 3.19 (**a**) Nonunion status post ankle arthrodesis through anterior approach. (**b**) Revision through lateral approach. Removal of hardware and osteotomy of fibula. (**c**) Resection of nonunion. (**d**) Intraoperative images following debridement. (**e**) Harvest of cancellous bone graft from ipsilateral iliac crest. (**f**) Drilling of subchondral plate and packing of bone graft. Note fixation construct using screws that engage cortices and subchondral bone. (**g**) 3-months status post radiographs demonstrating consolidation. (**h**) CT scan confirmation of consolidation

f g h

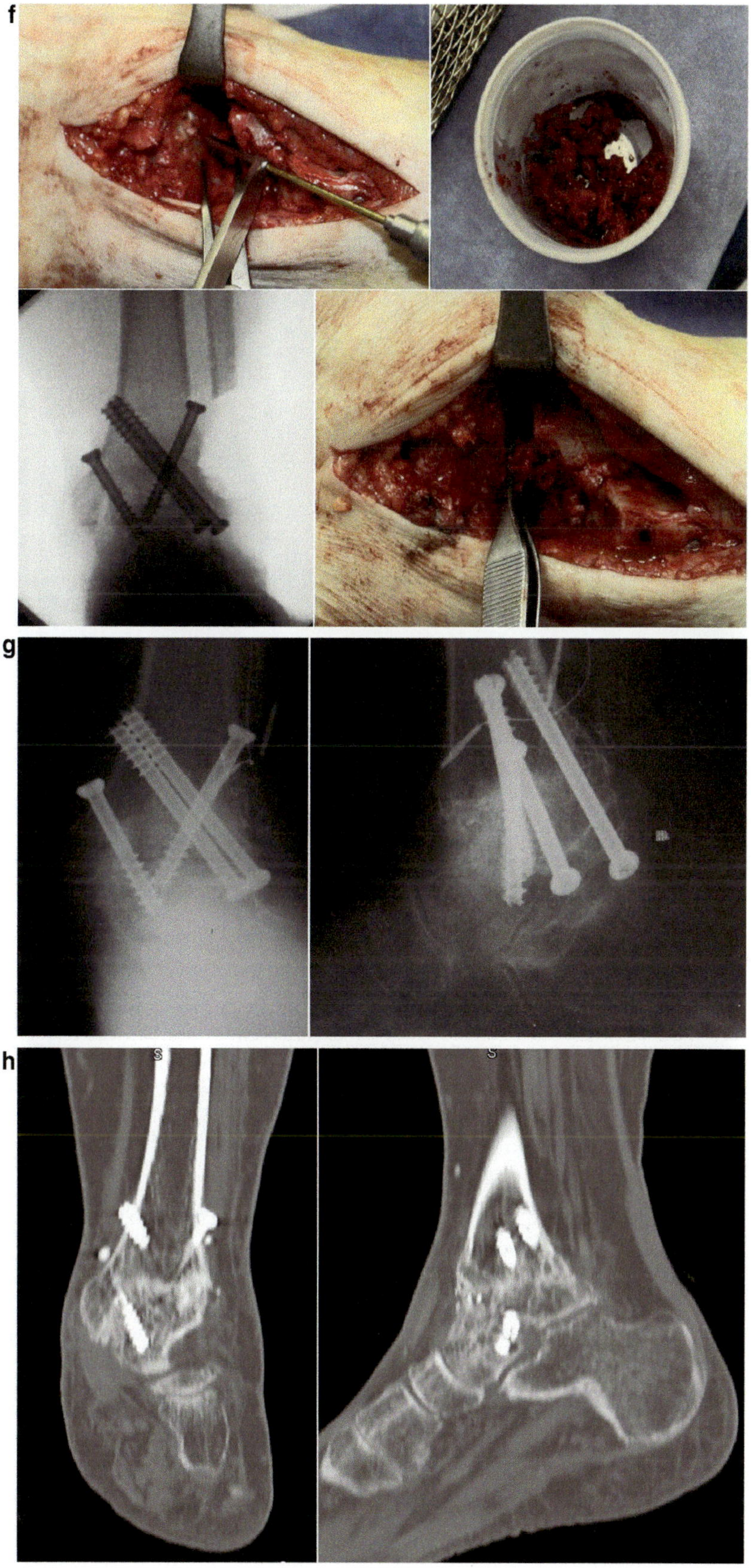

Fig. 3.19 (continued)

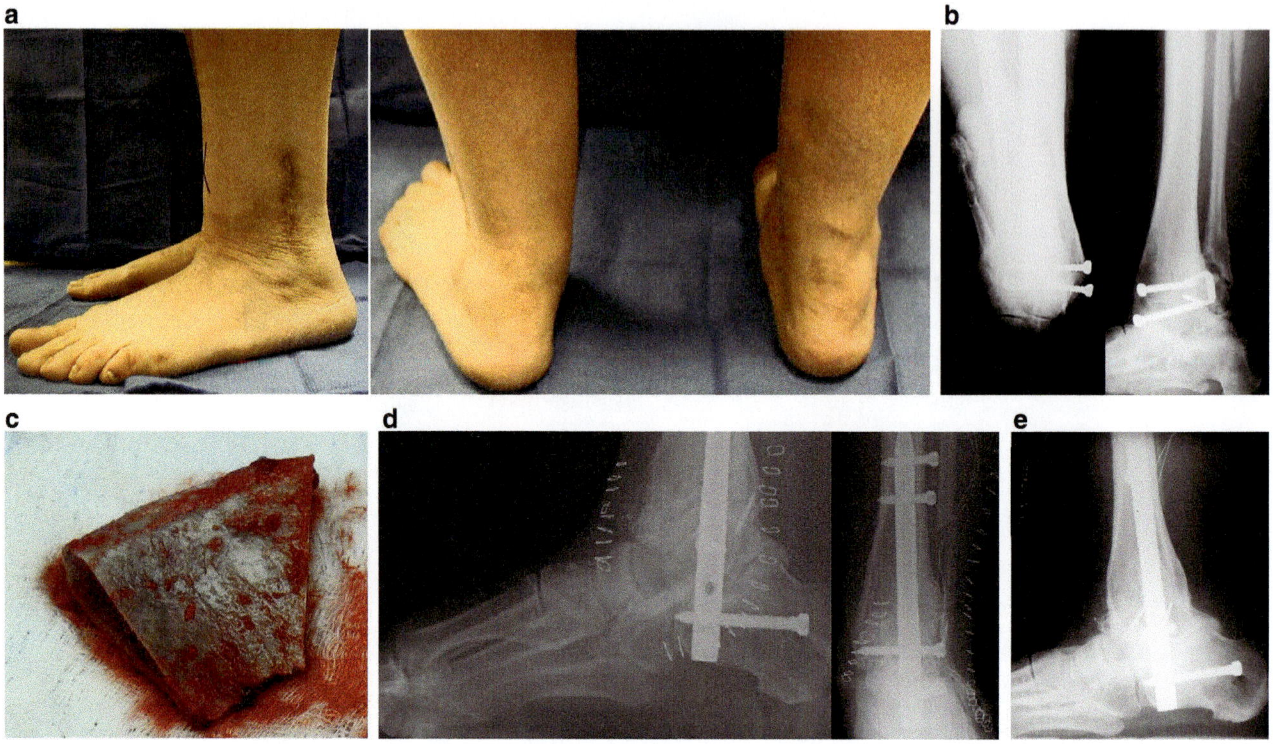

Fig. 3.20 (**a**) Nonunion following ankle arthrodesis with residual valgus deformity (**b**) Radiographs demonstrating nonunion. (**c**) Structural graft harvested from iliac crest. (**d**) Conversion into tibiotalocalcaneal arthrodesis with intramedullary nail. (**e**) One-year status post surgery demonstrating union

Conclusion

Surgical nonunion is a complex condition encountered by foot and ankle surgeons. The successful management of nonunions requires an understanding of bone healing, an awareness of medical conditions that contribute to abnormalities of bone metabolism, knowledge of technical issues that predispose patients to nonunion, and a thorough comprehension of fixation principles. Many cases benefit from a multidisciplinary team approach, and recruiting the assistance of other medical/surgical specialists and allied health professionals is encouraged to achieve successful outcomes.

References

1. Riemer BL, DiChristina DG, Cooper A, et al. Nonreamed nailing of tibial diaphyseal fractures in blunt polytrauma patients. J Orthop Trauma. 1995;9:66–75.
2. Caudle RJ, Stern PJ. Severe open fractures of the tibia. J Bone Joint Surg Am. 1987;69(6):801–7.
3. Sanders R, Jersinovich I, Anglen J, DiPasquale T, Herscovici Jr D. The treatment of open tibial shaft fractures using an interlocked intramedullary nail without reaming. J Orthop Trauma. 1994;8:504–10.
4. Govender S, Csimma C, Genant HK, et al. Recombinant human bone morphogenetic protein-2 for treatment of open tibial fractures: a prospective, controlled, randomized study of four hundred and fifty patients. J Bone Joint Surg Am. 2002;84-A(12):2123–34.
5. Sangeorzan BJ, Smith D, Veith R, et al. Triple arthrodesis using internal fixation in treatment of adult foot disorders. Clin Orthop Relat Res. 1993;294:299–307.
6. Wukich DK, Bowen JR. A long-term study of triple arthrodesis for correction of pes cavovarus in Charcot-Marie-Tooth disease. J Pediatr Orthop. 1989;9(4):433–7.
7. Saltzman CL, Fehrle MJ, Cooper RR, et al. Triple arthrodesis: twenty-five and forty-four-year average follow-up of the same patients. J Bone Joint Surg Am. 1999;81-A(10):1391–402.
8. Maskill MP, Loveland JD, Mendicino RW, Saltrick K, Catanzariti AR. Triple arthrodesis for the adult acquired flatfoot deformity. Clin Podiatr Med Surg. 2007;24:765–78.
9. Goucher NR, Coughlin MJ. Hallux metatarsophalangeal joint arthrodesis using dome-shaped reamers and dorsal plate fixation: a prospective study. Foot Ankle Int. 2006;27(11):869–76.
10. Doty J, Coughlin M, Hirose C, et al. Hallux metatarsophalangeal joint arthrodesis with a hybrid locking plate and a plantar neutralization screw: a prospective study. Foot Ankle Int. 2013;34(11):1535–40.
11. Roukis TS. Nonunion after arthrodesis of the first metatarsal-phalangeal joint: a systematic review. J Foot Ankle Surg. 2011;50(6):710–3.
12. Catanzariti AR, Mendicino RW, Lee MS, Gallina MR. The modified Lapidus arthrodesis: a retrospective analysis. J Foot Ankle Surg. 1999;38(5):322–32.
13. Donnenwerth MP, Borkosky SL, Abicht BP, et al. Rate of nonunion after first metatarsal-cuneiform arthrodesis using joint curettage and two crossed compression screw fixation: a systematic review. J Foot Ankle Surg. 2011;50(6):707–9.

14. Thompson IM, Bohay DR, Anderson JG. Fusion rate of first tarsometatarsal arthrodesis in the modified Lapidus procedure and flatfoot reconstruction. Foot Ankle Int. 2005;26(9):698–703.
15. Brinker MR. Nonunions: evaluation and treatment. In: Browner BD, Levine AM, Jupiter JB, Trafton PG, editors. Skeletal trauma: basic science, management, and reconstruction. 3rd ed. Philadelphia, PA: W.B. Saunders; 2002. p. 507–604.
16. Bhandari M, Guyatt GH, Swiontkowski MF, et al. A lack of consensus in the assessment of fracture healing among orthopaedic surgeons. J Orthop Trauma. 2002;16(8):562–6.
17. Muller ME, Allgower M, Schneider R, Willenegger H. Manual of Internal Fixation: Techniques Recommended by the AO group. 2nd ed. Berlin: Springer Verlag; 1979.
18. Lack WD, Starman JS, Seymour R, et al. Any cortical bridging predicts healing of tibial shaft fractures. J Bone Joint Surg Am. 2014;96(13):1066–72.
19. Nicoll EA. Fractures of the tibial shaft: a survey of 705 cases. J Bone Joint Surg (Br). 1964;46:373–87.
20. Bishop JA, Palanca AA, Bellino MJ, et al. Assessment of compromised fracture healing. J Am Acad Orthop Surg. 2012; 20(5):273–82.
21. Weber BG, Čech O. Pseudarthrosis: pathophysiology, biomechanics, therapy, results. New York: Grune & Stratton; 1976. Print
22. Mandracchia VJ, Nelson SC, Barp EA. Current concepts of bone healing. Clin Podiatr Med Surg. 2001;18(1):55–77.
23. McKibbin B. The biology of fracture healing in long bones. J Bone Joint Surg (Br). 1978;60(2):150–62.
24. Pountos I, Georgouli T, Blokhuis TJ, et al. Pharmacological agents and impairment of fracture healing: what is the evidence? Injury. 2008;39(4):384–94.
25. Lindholm R, Lindholm S, Liukko P, et al. The mast cell as a component of callus in healing fractures. J Bone Joint Surg (Br). 1969;51(1):148–55.
26. Ham AW. A histological study of the early phases of bone repair. J Bone Joint Surg Am. 1930;12(4):827–44.
27. Charnley J. The closed treatment of closed fractures. 3rd ed. Edinburgh and London: E & S Livingstone Ltd; 1975.
28. Danis soudure autogene-Danis R. Théorie et pratique de l'ostéosynthèse. Paris: Masson; 1949.
29. Schenk R, Willenegger H. Zur Histologie der primären Knochenheilung: Modifikationen und grenzender Spaltheilung in Abhängigkeit von der Defektgrösse. Unfallheilkunde. 1977;81: 219–27.
30. Augat P, Margevicius K, Simon J, et al. Local tissue properties in bone healing: influence of size and stability of the osteotomy gap. J Orthop Res. 1998;16(4):475–81.
31. Schenk R, Willenegger H. Morphological findings in primary fracture healing. Symp Bioi Hung. 1967;7:75.
32. Wolff J. The law of bone remodeling [translated from the 1892 original, Das Gesetz der Transformation der Knochen, by P. Maquet and R. Furlong]. Berlin: Springer Verlag; 1986.
33. Chatziyiannakis AA, Verettas DA, Raptis VK, et al. Nonunion of tibial fractures treated with external fixation. Contributing factors studied in 71 fractures. Acta Orthop Scand Suppl. 1997;275: 77–9.
34. Hak DJ, Fitzpatrick D, Bishop JA, et al. Delayed union and nonunions: epidemiology, clinical issues, and financial aspects. Injury. 2014;45(suppl 2):S3–7.
35. Trueta J. Studies of the development and decay of the human frame. London: William Heinemann Ltd.; 1968.
36. Perren SM. Physical and biological aspects of fractures healing with special reference to internal fixation. Clin Orthop Relat Res. 1979;138:175–96.
37. Perren SM. Evolution of internal fixation of long bone fractures. The scientific basis of biological internal fixation: choosing a new balance between stability and biology. J Bone Joint Surg (Br). 2002;84(8):1093–110.
38. Hak DJ, Toker S, Yi C, et al. The influence of fracture fixation biomechanics on fracture healing. Orthopedics. 2010;33(10):752–5.
39. Bassett CA, Herrmann I. Influence of oxygen concentration and mechanical factors on differentiation of connective tissue in vitro. Nature. 1961;190:460–1.
40. Fukada E, Yasuda I. On the piezoelectric effect of bone. J Phys Soc Jpn. 1957;12(10):1158–62.
41. Haverstock BD, Mandracchia VJ. Cigarette smoking and bone healing: implications in foot and ankle surgery. J Foot Ankle Surg. 1998;37(1):69–74.
42. Sherwin MA, Gastwirth CM. Detrimental effects of cigarette smoking on lower extremity wound healing. J Foot Surg. 1990; 29(1):84–7.
43. Cobb TK, Gabrielsen TA, Campbell II DC, et al. Cigarette smoking and nonunion after ankle arthrodesis. Foot Ankle Int. 1994;15(2):64–7.
44. Ishikawa SN, Murphy GA, Richardson EG. The effect of cigarette smoking on hindfoot fusions. Foot Ankle Int. 2002;23(11): 996–8.
45. Ma L, Zheng LW, Sham MH, et al. Uncoupled angiogenesis and osteogenesis in nicotine-compromised bone healing. J Bone Miner Res. 2010;25(6):1305–13.
46. Zheng LW, Ma L, Cheung LK. Changes in blood perfusion and bone healing induced by nicotine during distraction osteogenesis. Bone. 2008;43(2):355–61.
47. Ma L, Sham MH, Zheng LW, et al. Influence of low-dose nicotine on bone healing. J Trauma. 2011;70(6):117–21.
48. Ma L, Zwahlen RA, Zheng LW, et al. Influence of nicotine on the biologic activity of rabbit osteoblasts. Clin Oral Implants Res. 2011;22(3):338–42.
49. Lee S, do Yoon H, Kim KN, et al. Association between urine cotinine levels and bone mineral density in lumbar spine and femoral neck among adult males. Spine. 2014;39(4):311–7.
50. Daniell HW. Osteoporosis of the slender smoker. Vertebral compression fractures and loss of metacarpal cortex in relation to postmenopausal cigarette smoking and lack of obesity. Arch Intern Med. 1976;136(3):298–304.
51. Law MR, Hacksaw AK. A meta-analysis of cigarette smoking, bone mineral density and risk of hip fracture: recognition of a major effect. BMJ. 1997;315(7112):841–6.
52. Scolaro JA, Schenker ML, Yannascoli S, et al. Cigarette smoking increases complications following fracture: a systematic review. J Bone Joint Surg Am. 2014;96(8):674–81.
53. Day SM, DeHeer DH. Reversal of the detrimental effects of chronic protein malnutrition on long bone fracture healing. J Orthop Trauma. 2001;15(1):47–53.
54. Simpson AH, Mills L, Noble B. The role of growth factors and related agents in accelerating fracture healing. J Bone Joint Surg (Br). 2006;88(6):701–5.
55. Brinker MR, O'Conner DP, Monla YT, et al. Metabolic and endocrine abnormalities in patients with nonunions. J Orthop Trauma. 2007;21(8):557–70.
56. Friedlaender GE, Tross RB, Doganis AC, et al. Effects of chemotherapeutic agents on bone. Short-term methotrexate and doxorubicin (adriamycin) treatment in a rat model. J Bone Joint Surg Am. 1984;66(4):602–7.
57. Gravel CA, Le TT, Chapman MW. Effect of neoadjuvant chemotherapy on distraction osteogenesis in the goat model. Clin Orthop Relat Res. 2003;412:213–24.
58. Hausman MR, Schaffler MB, Majeska RJ. Prevention of fracture healing in rats by an inhibitor of angiogenesis. Bone. 2001; 29(6):560–4.
59. Hazan EJ, Hornicek FJ, Tomford W, et al. The effect of adjuvant chemotherapy on osteoarticular allografts. Clin Orthop Relat Res. 2001;385:176–81.
60. Tortolani PJ, Park AE, Louis-Ugbo J, et al. The effects of doxorubicin (Adriamycin) on spinal fusion: an experimental model of

posterolateral lumbar spinal arthrodesis. Spine J. 2004;4(6): 669–74.
61. O'Brien CA, Jia D, Plotkin LI, et al. Glucocorticoids act directly on osteoblasts and osteocytes to induce their apoptosis and reduce bone formation and strength. Endocrinology. 2004;145(4): 1835–41.
62. Weinstein RS, Jilka RL, Parfitt AM, et al. Inhibition of osteoblastogenesis and promotion of apoptosis of osteoblasts and osteocytes by glucocorticoids. Potential mechanisms of their deleterious effects on bone. J Clin Invest. 1998;102(2):274–82.
63. Jeffcoach DR, Sams VG, Lawson CM, et al. Nonsteroidal anti-inflammatory drugs' impact on nonunion and infection rates in long-bone fractures. J Trauma Acute Care Surg. 2014;76(3): 779–83.
64. Endo K, Sairyo K, Komatsubara S, et al. Cyclooxygenase-2 inhibitor delays fracture healing in rats. Acta Orthop. 2005; 76(4):470–4.
65. Gerstenfeld LC, Thiede M, Seibert K, et al. Differential inhibition of fracture healing by non-selective and cyclooxygenase-2 selective non-steroidal anti-inflammatory drugs. J Orthop Res. 2003;21(4):670–5.
66. Giordano V, Giordano M, Knackfuss IG, et al. Effect of tenoxicam on fracture healing in rat tibiae. Injury. 2003;34(2):85–94.
67. Sudmann E, Bang G. Indomethacin-induced inhibition of haversian remodeling in rabbits. Acta Orthop Scand. 1979;50(6 pt 1):621–7.
68. Huddleston PM, Steckelberg JM, Hanssen AD, et al. Ciprofloxacin inhibition of experimental fracture healing. J Bone Joint Surg Am. 2000;82(2):161–73.
69. Mont MA, Mathur SK, Frondoza CG, Hungerford DS. The effects of ciprofloxacin on human chondrocytes in cell culture. Infection. 1996;24(2):151–5.
70. Perry AC, Prpa B, Rouse MS, et al. Levofloxacin and trovafloxacin inhibition of experimental fracture-healing. Clin Orthop Relat Res. 2003;414:95–100.
71. Seltzer MH, Fletcher HS, Slocum BA, et al. Instant nutritional assessment in the intensive care unit. J Parenter Enter Nutr. 1981;5(1):70–2.
72. Cross MB, Yi PH, Thomas CF, et al. Evaluation of malnutrition in orthopaedic surgery. J Am Acad Orthop Surg. 2014;22(3):193–9.
73. Holick MF. Vitamin D deficiency. N Engl J Med. 2007;357(3): 266–81.
74. Dawson-Hughes B, Heaney RP, Holick MF, et al. Estimates of optimal vitamin D status. Osteoporos Int. 2005;16(7):713–6.
75. Malabanan A, Veronikis IE, Holick MF. Redefining vitamin D insufficiency. Lancet. 1998;351(9105):805–6.
76. Rabjohn L, Roberts K, Troiano M, et al. Diagnostic and prognostic value of erythrocyte sedimentation rate in contiguous osteomyelitis of the foot and ankle. J Foot Ankle Surg. 2007;46(4):230–7.
77. Fleischer AE, Didyk AA, Woods JB, et al. Combined clinical and laboratory testing improves diagnostic accuracy for osteomyelitis in the diabetic foot. J Foot Ankle Surg. 2009;48(1):39–46.
78. Stucken C, Olszewski DC, Creevy WR, et al. Preoperative diagnosis of infection in patients with nonunions. J Bone Joint Surg Am. 2013;95(15):1409–12.
79. Sarmiento A, Sobol PA, Sew Hoy AL, et al. Prefabricated functional braces for the treatment of fractures of the tibial diaphysis. J Bone Joint Surg Am. 1984;66(9):1328–39.
80. Whelan DB, Bhandari M, McKee MD, et al. Interobserver and intraobserver variation in the assessment of the healing of tibial fractures after intramedullary fixation. J Bone Joint Surg (Br). 2002;84(1):15–8.
81. Lamm BM, Mendicino RW, Catanzariti AR, Hillstrom HJ. Static rearfoot alignment: a comparison of clinical and radiographic measures. J Am Podiatr Med Assoc. 2005;95(1):26–33.
82. Mendicino RW, Catanzariti AR, John S, Child B, Lamm BM. Long leg calcaneal axial and hindfoot alignment radiographic views for frontal plane assessment. J Am Podiatr Med Assoc. 2008;98(1):75–8.
83. Lew DP, Waldvogel FA. Osteomyelitis. Lancet. 2004;364(9431): 369–79.
84. Cierny III G, Mader JT, Penninck JJ. A clinical staging system for adult osteomyelitis. Clin Orthop Relat Res. 2003;414:7–24.
85. Coughlin MJ, Grimes JS, Traughber PD, et al. Comparison of radiographs and CT scans in the prospective evaluation of the fusion of hindfoot arthrodesis. Foot Ankle Int. 2006;27(10): 780–7.
86. Jones C, Coughlin M, Shurnas P. Prospective CT scan evaluation of hindfoot non-unions treated with revision surgery and low-intensity ultrasound stimulation. Foot Ankle Int. 2006;27(4):229–35.
87. Buchan CA, Pearce DH, Lau J, et al. Imaging of postoperative avascular necrosis of the ankle and foot. Semin Musculoskelet Radiol. 2012;16(3):192–204.
88. Solicito V, Jacobs AM, Oloff LM, Soave R, Bernstein A. The use of radionucleotide bone and joint imaging in arthritic and related diseases. J Foot Surg. 1984;23(2):173–82.
89. Visser HJ, Jacobs AM, Oloff L, Drago JJ. The use of differential scintigraphy in the clinical diagnosis of osseous and soft tissue changes affecting the diabetic foot. J Foot Surg. 1984;23(1):74–85.
90. Jacobs AM, Klein S, Oloff L, Tuccio MJ. Radionuclide evaluation of complications after metatarsal osteotomy and implant arthroplasty of the foot. J Foot Surg. 1984;23(1):86–96.
91. Mont MA, Ulrich SD, Seyler TM, et al. Bone scanning of limited value for diagnosis of symptomatic oligofocal and multifocal osteonecrosis. J Rheumatol. 2008;35(8):1629–34.
92. Palestro CJ, Love C, Bhargava KK. Labeled leukocyte imaging: current status and future directions. QJ Nucl Med Mol Imaging. 2009;53(1):105–23.
93. Baim S, Binkley N, Bilezikian JP, et al. Official positions of the international society for clinical densitometry and executive summary of the 2007 ISCD position development conference. J Clin Densitom. 2008;11(1):75–91.
94. Kanis JA. Diagnosis of osteoporosis and assessment of fracture risk. Lancet. 2002;359(9321):1929–36.
95. Watts NB, Bilezikian JP, Camacho PM, et al. American association of clinical endocrinologists medical guidelines for clinical practice for the diagnosis and treatment of postmenopausal osteoporosis. Endocr Pract. 2010;16(suppl 3):1–37.
96. Goldman B. Use and abuse of opioid analgesics in chronic pain. Can Fam Physician. 1993;39:571–6.
97. Savage SR. Opioid use in the management of chronic pain. Med Clin North Am. 1999;83:761–86.
98. Tennant Jr FS, Rawson RA. Outpatient treatment of prescription opioid dependence: comparison of two methods. Arch Intern Med. 1982;142:1845–7.
99. Einhorn TA, Levine B, Michel P. Nutrition and bone. Orthop Clin North Am. 1990;21:43–50.
100. Guarniero R, de Barros Filho TE, Tannuri U, et al. Study of fracture healing in protein malnutrition. Rev Paul Med. 1992; 110:63–8.
101. Pollak D, Floman Y, Simkin A, et al. The effect of protein malnutrition and nutritional support on the mechanical properties of fracture healing in the injured rat. J Parenter Enter Nutr. 1986;10:564–7.
102. Hoofwerf BJ, Sferra J, Donley BG. Diabetes mellitus—overview. Foot Ankle Clin. 2006;11(4):703–15.
103. Dworkin SF, Von Korff M, LeResche L. Multiple pains and psychiatric distrurbance: an epidemiologic investigation. Arch Gen Psychiatry. 1990;47:239–44.
104. Katon W. The impact of major depression on chronic medical illness. Gen Hosp Psychiatry. 1996;18:215–9.

105. Katon W, Sullivan MD. Depression and chronic medical illness. J Clin Psychiatry. 1990;51:3–11.
106. Krishan KR, France RD. Chronic pain and depression. South Med J. 1987;80:558–61.
107. Evans EL, Catanzariti AR. Forefoot supinatus. Clin Podiatr Med Surg. 2014;31:405–13.
108. Mann RA, Beaman DN. Double arthrodesis in the adult. Clin Orthop Relat Res. 1999;356:74–80.
109. Granata JD, Berlet GC, Ghotge R, et al. Talonavicular joint fixation: A biomechanical comparison of locking compression plates and lag screws. Foot Ankle Spec. 2014;7:20–31.
110. Catanzariti AR, Adeleke AT. Double arthrodesis through a medial approach for end-stage adult-acquired flatfoot. Clin Podiatr Med Surg. 2014;31(3):435–49.
111. Frey C, Halikus NM, Vu-Rose T, et al. A review of ankle arthrodesis: predisposing factors to nonunion. Foot Ankle Int. 1994;15(11):581–97.
112. Stock U, Vacanti J. Tissue engineering: current state and prospects. Annu Rev Med. 2001;52:443–51.
113. Kanellopoulos A, Soucacos P. Management of nonunion with distraction osteogenesis. Injury. 2006;37(Suppl 1):S51–5.

Management of Incision Complications

4

Meagan M. Jennings, Alan Sue, and Nicholas Todd

As surgeons, our incision is one of the most important steps during the surgical procedure. Not only does it allow us access to the anatomy below, but it is a representation to the patient of our work. Although much of incision healing is based on patient factors such as underlying medical comorbidities and a patient's collagen, we as surgeons can optimize many factors of incision wound healing. Taking care not to skive our incision, minimizing tension with retraction, ensuring adequate return of vascularity, and appropriate hemostasis are a few examples of ways we can contribute to optimal incision healing. However, when incisions have complications and do not heal optimally, we, too, are responsible again for managing the wound and optimizing its healing potential.

Skin and wound healing is a regulated process of cellular and molecular mechanism. An incision made through the skin or wounds from an injury results in a loss of the normal physiological function. The body responds to this insult by both regeneration and repair. Regeneration involves replacing or substitution of the tissue, while repair results in scar and fibrotic formation. The majority of wound healing processes in surgery focus on repair as scar and fibrosis are formed after an incision is made. The goal of wound healing in surgery is to minimize scar formation and implement techniques to facilitate or promote wound healing. This chapter will focus on these various techniques, but in order to fully understand the repair or regenerative process of wounds or incision(s), we must focus on the physiology and histology of wound healing.

M.M. Jennings (✉) • A. Sue • N. Todd
Orthopedics and Podiatry, Palo Alto Foundation Medical Group, Mountain View, CA 94040, USA
e-mail: mmjfootankle@gmail.com

Histology and Physiology

The layered histology of the skin includes three main layers: epidermis, dermis, and hypodermis. The epidermis has five layers from superficial to deep: stratum corneum, stratum luciduim, stratum granulosum, stratum spinosum, and stratum basale. Keratinocytes make up the majority of the epidermis and are generated in the stratum basale layer. During wound healing, the keratinocytes are responsible for the epidermal growth by replicating and pushing older cells to the surface. These older cells that are pushed to the surface take on a more flattened appearance resulting in stratified squamous keratinized epithelium and are replenished every 48 h. The epidermal layer stratum basale projects and communicates with the dermal layer through "rete ridges." The epidermis also contains hair follicles, sebaceous glands, eccrine sweat glands, and apocrine glands. The rete ridges and sebaceous glands contain epithelial stem cells that are able to generate into basal keratinocytes and are essential to the wound epithelial regeneration process. When physical abrasions such as burns affect the deeper layers and destroy the epithelial stem cells, this results in a decrease in production of keratinocytes and improper healing and eventual scarring.

The dermal layer is the layer deep to the epidermis. The dermis is made up of two layers: superficial or papillary dermis and deeper layer or reticular dermis. The dermal layer functions to provide blood supply to the skin and contains the dermal appendages such as apocrine glands, eccrine glands, and hair follicles. Damage to the dermis with extension to the reticular dermal layer most likely results in scarring.

The epidermis and dermis play an important role in the histological process of wound healing. The physiological process involved in wound healing can be separated into four overlapping phases:

M.S. Lee, J.P. Grossman (eds.), *Complications in Foot and Ankle Surgery*, DOI 10.1007/978-3-319-53686-6_4

1. Hemostasis
2. Inflammation
3. Proliferation/repair
4. Maturation/remodeling

Hemostasis is the first stage of physiological wound healing. This phase occurs immediately after injury to the soft tissue has occurred and lasts for some hours. During the hemostasis phase, the body initiates inflammation, which causes recruitment of cells and factors to assist in the healing process. The insult to the epidermal layer provides initial removal of antigens and microorganisms. This process then promotes the clotting cascade to promote initial hemostasis and causes the release of cytokines and hormones to set off the next phase of healing. Concurrently the body initiates a short period of platelet-induced vasoconstriction, which fills the gap with clot material comprised of growth factors and cytokines. The clot also consists of fibrin molecules which serve as a scaffold or bridge for migration of leukocytes, keratinocytes, growth factors, etc. After the short period of vasoconstriction, the body responds with a period of vasodilation. The platelet cells cause the leukocytes to release chemotactic and growth factors to initiate the inflammatory response and collagen synthesis and assist in the reepithelialization process.

Inflammation is the second stage of physiological wound healing. As described in the previous section, during the coagulation period, the inflammatory phase becomes active. The inflammatory phase is divided into two main phases: The initial phase involves recruitment of neutrophils during the first 24 h, and the later phase includes appearance and maturation of monocytes. The initial phase involving the neutrophils lasts for about 3–5 days. Neutrophils are of vital importance as they undergo a phagocytotic process destroying bacteria and degrading necrotic tissue. The neutrophils also play a part in recruitment of other cells during the inflammatory process. After 3 days, macrophages enter the zone of injury and begin to eliminate pathogens and cell debris. They (macrophages) are also involved in secretion of cytokines to promote the next stage of wound healing and possess immunologic functions, angiogenesis, tissue formation, and wound contracture. The inflammatory phase is vital in the tissue regeneration/repair process and has been shown the inhibition of this phase results in chronic wound, delayed healing, and long-term scarring. The factors that could inhibit this process would include high bacterial load, trauma, foreign material, etc.

Proliferation/repair phase occurs 3–10 days after the injury. The main focus of the proliferation phase is by filling in the wound defect, formation of granulation tissue, and to reinstate the vascular network. After the inflammatory process has debrided the wound of necrotic and bacterial tissue, the influx of keratinocytes layers to fill the deficit occurs. The stem cells from the apocrine and follicles differentiate into keratinocytes, which repopulate and migrate over the edge of the wound bridging the deficit. When the keratinocytes encounter the extracellular matrix, they lay down a new basement membrane and subsequently lay down layers on top of the previous epithelial layer filling the deficit. These cells migrate and replicate until they come into physical contact from the other side which then stops the replicating process. Angiogenesis or repair of the vascular network begins as vessels bud from arterial vessels surrounding the wound. Growth factors are responsible for the early phase of angiogenesis as they bind to specific receptors causing destruction of the basement membrane allowing cells to enter the wound and repair the vascular network. The last step of the proliferation phase is formation of granulation tissue. Granulation tissue is composed of fibroblasts, granulocytes, macrophages, and collagen bundles. The key component during the formation of granulation tissue is characterized by the fibroblasts. The fibroblasts' main function is to generate or produce collagen and extracellular matrix substances. This function generates the provisional wound matrix in which cell organization takes place.

Remodeling is the last phase of wound healing which occurs from day 21 to 1 year. The granulation tissue formation ceases through the apoptosis of the cell. During the remodeling stage, the components of the extracellular matrix undergo a transformation specifically the collagen type III. During the remodeling process, the collagen type III is replaced by the stronger collagen type I. With the incorporation of the collagen type I, the strength of the wound dramatically increases. Thus, it is wise to inform patients that scar remodeling occurs for up to a year.

Surgical Wounds

Surgical incisions are considered acute wounds if they heal in the expected time frame and without complications. The major goal in caring for surgical patients is prevention of complications such as surgical site infections (SSIs) and wound healing failure by way of careful monitoring and appropriate interventions. Interventions include reducing modifiable risk factors associated with healing complications and providing systemic support to facilitate healing. Factors impeding wound healing include excessive bleeding, hematoma/seroma, allergic reactions, infection or increased bioburden, dehiscence, tissue necrosis, mechanical factors and tension, excessive granulation tissue, systemic conditions (i.e., diabetes mellitus, obesity, malnutrition), external agents (i.e., tobacco, drugs), and hypertrophic scar formation. It is important to consider all of these things before, during, and after surgery to maximize healing potential.

Bleeding Complications

Surgical complications from bleeding may occur as an acute bleed during surgery, immediate postoperative bleeding in the first few hours postoperatively, or late postoperative bleeding several days after surgery. For all of these issues, there are intrinsic and extrinsic factors that need to be considered. It is important for the surgeon to understand the physiology behind bleeding vessels and address them appropriately both as a clinician and a technician. As a clinician, one should consider the patient and any medical disorders or medications that may affect the clotting cascade, which is twofold: platelet mediated and fibrin mediated. The details of these two mechanisms will not be discussed here. For surgeons using epinephrine at the surgical site for better visualization, masked bleeding can be unveiled when the epinephrine wears off. This can cause hyperemia and excessive swelling and hematoma formation. Tourniquet use can also have similar consequences if the tourniquet is not deflated prior to wound closure. Thus, all potential areas of bleeding should be explored prior to wound closure to avoid these complications.

When acute intraoperative bleeding is present, it is typically due to transecting or partial vessel injury. The surgeon must achieve hemostasis via cautery, and/or ligatures should be used to tie off both segments of the transected vessel. Arterial injury should be addressed almost always by repairing the vessel with sutures or tying off the artery with ligatures. Cautery for arterial injury is often not adequate due to the nature of the vessel and its function.

Hematoma/seroma formation can cause increased tension on a wound site and incision. It can also serve as a nutrition source for microbes. An increase in the incidence of hematomas is mostly due to the clinical use of anticoagulants as well as the now recommended prophylactic standards for the prevention of deep vein thrombosis (DVT). When a hematoma or seroma occurs, intervention is required. Aspiration of the hematoma or seroma should be performed via needle aspiration if there is incomplete coagulation of the fluid collection. However, if a fluid collection has coagulated and cannot be needle aspirated, removing a suture or staple can be performed and manual expression used to remove the fluid collection or coagulation (Figs. 4.1 and 4.2).

Allergic reactions can be type I anaphylaxis or type IV contact sensitivity. Reactions can occur to any substance or medication used during the surgical procedure. Thus, it is imperative to obtain an accurate history of your surgical patient to minimize potential reactions. Local anesthetics, skin preparation agents, topical antibiotics, and adhesives are among some of the most common offenders.

Local anesthetics are injected often preemptively for intraoperative analgesia and to reduce the amount of general anesthetics required. Local anesthetics fall into one of the two major groups: ester- or amide-type anesthetics. The esters cross-react with para-aminobenzoic acid (PABA) esters and other related compounds and thus have been associated with a higher incidence of allergic reactions. The amide anesthetics which include lidocaine, bupivacaine, etidocaine, and prilocaine are most commonly used in foot and ankle surgery. There have been much fewer incidences of allergic reactions to these drugs.

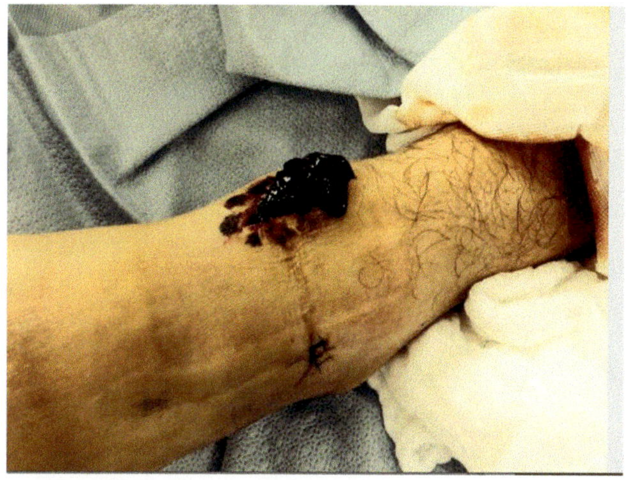

Fig. 4.1 A 34-year-old male presented to the clinic with chronic ankle pain from numerous inversion ankle injuries. Radiographs revealed a large osseous fragment (figure) over the anterior medial aspect of the ankle. After several months of conservative therapy, it was decided that the patient would undergo arthroscopic debridement of the ankle and removal of loose body. The ankle was debrided arthroscopically, but it was decided during the surgery to remove the fragment via medial ankle arthrotomy. The fragment was removed, and patient was instructed to be non-weight bearing. He presented to the clinic 1 week later ambulating on the affected extremity. A hematoma was present over the medial aspect of the ankle. There was minimal erythema/edema over the hematoma. It was decided to treat in a conservative fashion. For 1 week, he was placed in a posterior splint and instructed to place warm compresses over the dressings. At 1 week, there was increased erythema/edema, and patient was taken to the OR for incision and drainage (Fig. 4.2). Deep cultures were positive for *E. coli*. One month following surgery, patient was healed with casting and 2 weeks of oral antibiotics

Skin preparation agents such as povidone-iodine have been shown to cause an acute contact dermatitis in sensitized patients. The iodophor compound slowly releases the iodine. The contact dermatitis consisting of vesicle formation and weeping may develop in the area of the surgical incision and thus predispose the patient to a secondary infection. Treatment typically consists of application of wet dressing and topical steroids. If severe, systemic steroids may be required to treat the adverse reaction. Chlorhexidine gluconate tends to cause little skin irritation and has a very weak sensitizing potential while providing a prolonged bactericidal effect.

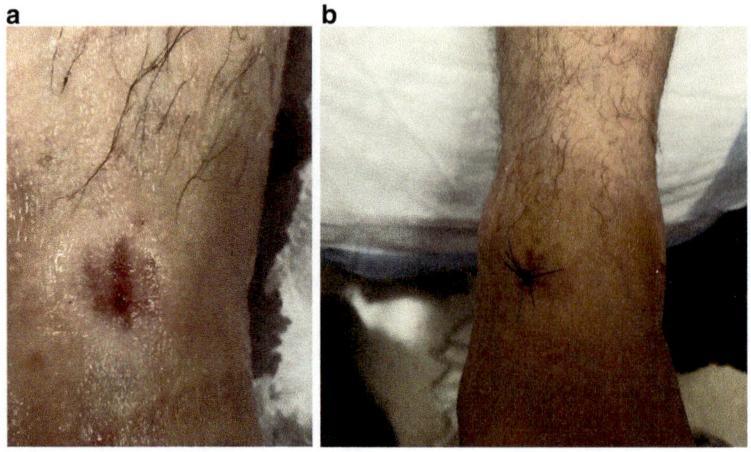

Fig. 4.2 Seroma. A 61-year-old male underwent arthroscopic ankle stabilization. Against medical advice, patient took off his splint and began ambulating. At his 2-week postoperative appointment, he developed a small seroma (**a**) over the medial portal. Treatment included Betadine dressing with posterior splint for 1 week. One week following his Betadine dressing, there was still small amount of fluid originating from the seroma. The surrounding area had no erythema/edema or purulence. The seroma was treated by placement of full-thickness 3-0 nylon sutures without any debridement (**b**). The patient was placed in a cast, and this was changed on a weekly basis (total of 3 weeks). The incision healed and the sutures removed. The patient started his physical therapy regimen and has had no further complications

Topical antibiotics can produce contact sensitivity. The most common sensitizer is neomycin which causes sensitivity reaction in 6–8% of patients. Bacitracin is often found in many over-the-counter products with neomycin, but alone, it does not appear to be a potent sensitizer. When examining patients with a contact dermatitis, one may mistake it for an infection. It is important to look for vesicle formation and involvement of the skin up to the incision. Typically, a dressing reaction or tape reaction will not involve the incision.

Adhesive allergy can cause severe reaction in many patients. Reactions can include rapid severe blistering or more chronic erythema with skin irritation. It is best to avoid adhesives all together including steri-strips and adhesive products such as Mastisol and Benzoin tincture and hold bandages in place with elastic wraps instead (Fig. 4.3).

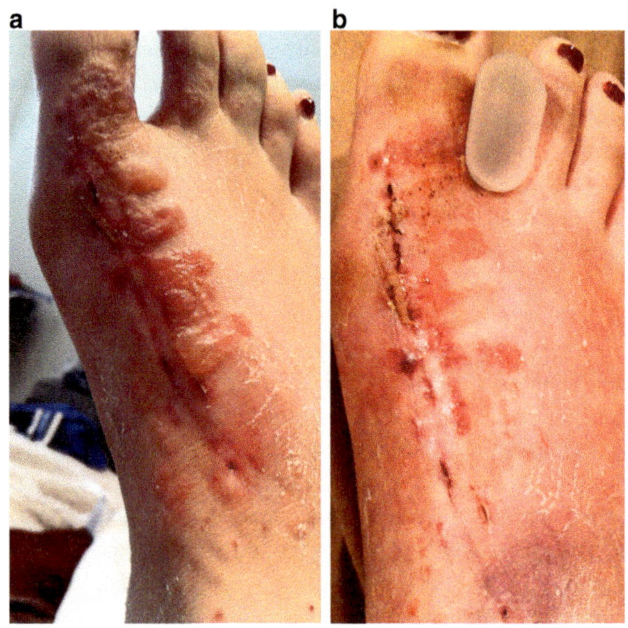

Fig. 4.3 (**a**) and (**b**) Allergic reaction to Steri-Strip adhesive after bunion surgery. Patient was treated with topical corticosteroids and dry dressings for seepage until symptoms resolved in about 7 days

Surgical site infections (SSIs) are a serious impediment to surgical incision healing. According to the Centers for Disease Control (CDC), approximately 300,000 are reported each year and have associated costs both economically and in terms of mortality and morbidity [1]. SSIs occur within 30 days of surgery or within 1 year if an implant is used and the infection involves that site. SSIs are classified into superficial and deep. *Superficial incision infection* involves only the skin and subcutaneous tissue at the incision. *Deep incision infection* involves the deep tissues including the muscle and fascia (Fig. 4.4). Factors have been identified for both categories of infection in multiple studies. Superficial infections are most commonly seen in patients with previous operations, prolonged duration of surgery, low albumin, and chronic obstructive pulmonary disease, whereas deep infections have been most common in patients with low albumin and previous operations.

The most common pathogen in SSI per CDC is *Staphylococcus aureus*, which accounts for 30% of infections. This is followed by coagulase-negative *Staphylococcus* at 13.7%, *Enterococcus* spp. at 11.2%, *E. col* at 9.6%, and *Pseudomonas aeruginosa* at 5.6% [2]. It is important to identify the pathogen if possible in treating an SSI in order to administer appropriate antibiotic therapy. It is also important to choose the appropriate prophylactic antibiotic and administer it consistently with the Surgical Infection Prevention

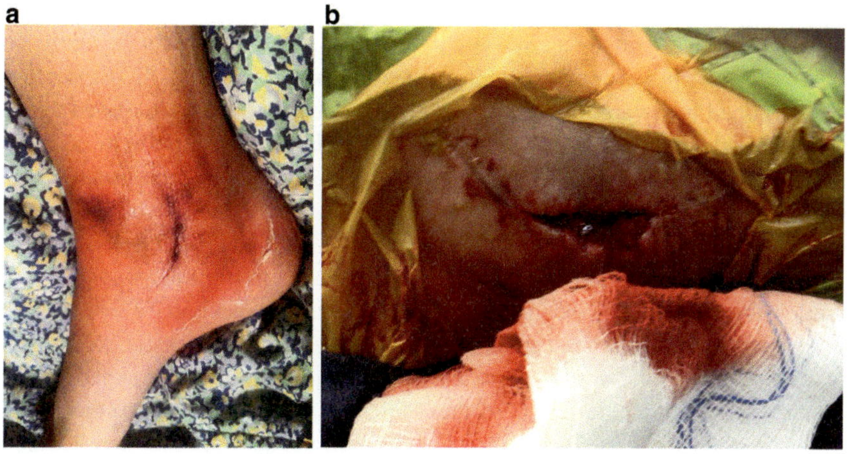

Fig. 4.4 A 27-year-old female sustained Weber C ankle fracture. The first image (**a**) shows the patient 3 weeks following surgery when patient presented with increased pain and edema on the medial incision. There was a small area of incision dehiscence and clinical signs of infection. Patient started on IV antibiotics, and after 48 h of minimal improvement, patient was taken to the operating room. (**b**) Patient had two sequential debridements in the operating room 48 h apart. Hardware was retained until union was achieved as confirmed with CT. Upon union, the hardware was removed and a wound VAC was placed. Patient healed over the next 4 weeks via secondary intention

Collaborative and the Surgical Care Improvement Project to minimize the surgical wound infection and bacterial load at the surgical site prior to incision.

The guidelines currently state antibiotic administration should be within 60 min prior to injection or incision. The typical prophylactic antibiotic choice in orthopedic surgery is 1 g IV cephalexin and 2 g IV if over 80 kg. In patients with a known allergy to cephalosporins, either 600 or 900 mg of clindamycin can be administered. In patients with previous methicillin-resistant *Staphylococcus aureus* (MRSA) or sensitivity to clindamycin, 1 g IV vancomycin should be administered over 60 min prior to surgical incision. Intraoperatively, antibiotic should be readministered in any surgical case lasting over 3 h.

Risk factors for SSI can be broken into *intrinsic* and *extrinsic*, and several studies have identified both [3–6]. Intrinsic risks are inherent to the patient such as systemic disease, whereas extrinsic risks are due to surgeon, technique, and perioperative issues such as greater blood loss, hypothermia, use of blood products, and surgery time over 2 h.

Understanding which risk factors we can mediate and minimize will help decrease the incidence of SSIs and subsequent incision morbidity. Thus, thorough patient evaluation is vital and proper patient selection important.

Wound dehiscence is almost always related to another complicating issue with the most common being hematoma, wound infection, or premature suture removal. Healing may be affected by wound tension, external trauma, underlying medical comorbidities, and external factors such as smoking. Issues such as hematoma aspiration and early suture removal for infection drainage or hematoma/seroma aspiration can also lead to wound failure (Fig. 4.5).

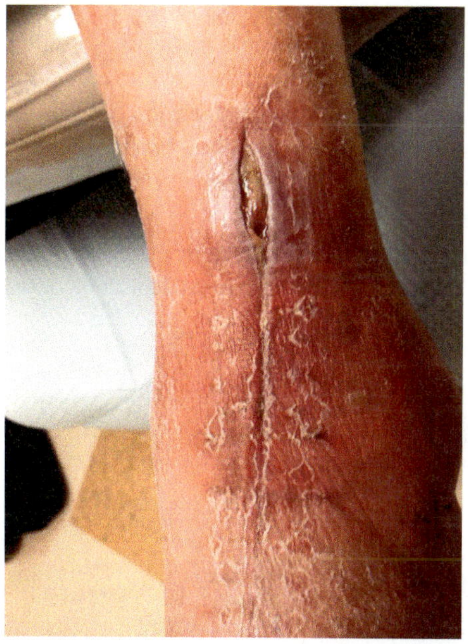

Fig. 4.5 Anterior ankle incision with proximal wound dehiscence. Note fibrotic tissue in the wound. This required serial debridement and local wound care and went on to heal by secondary intention

Management of the dehisced wound depends on the cause. Typically, wound dehiscence can be treated by local wound care and allowing healing by secondary intention. However, some surgeons may choose to be more aggressive depending on the state of the wound, the patient, and the type of surgery that was performed. If a soft tissue procedure was performed and a superficial wound dehiscence is now present, often with local debridement in the office and ongoing wound care, the wound will heal. Often, one must limit motion of the affected area as well to minimize wound disruption.

It is important to minimize excessive fibrous tissue formation along the edges of the incision. This can often require serial, weekly debridements in the office. If a wound dehiscence occurs over an area with retained hardware, typically, it is in the patient's best interest to address these surgically due to the underlying risk of infection and sequelae of contamination of exposed hardware.

A wound that opens and is recognized within 24 h may be able to be repaired primarily unless there is nonviable material at the base or margins of the incision. The wound should be closed under aseptic technique using the least traumatic suture material (e.g., monofilament nylon). The use of prophylactic antibiotics is controversial and is left to the surgeon's discretion.

Necrosis of a wound is almost always the result of another complication such as hematoma/seroma, increased tension, infection, or inadequate vascularity. Any of these complications can cause full-thickness tissue loss and require further intervention and repair. When using tissue flaps, necrosis can occur if the dimensions of the flap are not appropriate (i.e., flaps should be no more than three times the width of its base 3:1 length-to-base ratio). Inadvertent cutting, cautery use, or ligation of arterial feeders can also compromise tissue blood flow and viability. Wound tension can lead to ischemia and subsequent necrosis as well. Tobacco use may cause tissue hypoxemia and lead to tissue necrosis. When necrosis occurs, early debridement should be performed only if there is evidence of infection; otherwise, the necrosis should be allowed to fully demarcate prior to debridement (Fig. 4.6).

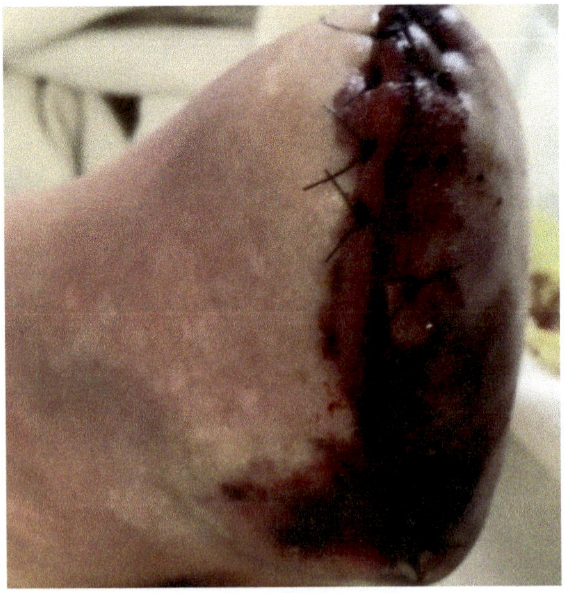

Fig. 4.6 Necrosis along the transmetatarsal amputation incision indicated by the black dusky skin. Patient was followed closely with incision checks every 4–5 days. No debridements were performed. Sutures were removed after 4 weeks and necrosis resolved without further intervention

Tension can cause both wound dehiscence and necrosis of tissue. It may account for early postoperative pain and lead to scar widening. If suture closure was excessively tight, one may develop "railroad track" scarring. It is necessary during wound closure to take appropriate measures to correct for excessive tension. There are various surgical techniques that can be used. One technique is creating a relaxing incision parallel to the primary incision approximately 2–3 cm from the wound edge. The initial wound is closed, and the secondary wound is then fully undermined and closed. This is a tension-sharing method. A second technique is to perform tissue expansion. This may be done with formal tissue expanders or other plastic surgery techniques that will not be discussed here. A third acceptable method of tension reduction is partial closure of the wound. This technique creates both primary wound healing with the approximated part of the wound and secondary wound healing of the defect (Fig. 4.7).

Excessive granulation tissue is an excessive overgrowth of "proud flesh." It consists of an overgrowth of fibroblasts and endothelial cells. This tissue often bleeds easily and is prone to infection due to its friable nature. It most often is present in wounds allowed to heal by secondary intention. If granulation tissue extends above the skin surface in a primarily closed incision, it prevents reepithelialization, and without its removal, the wound will not heal. This tissue can be removed in an anesthetized wound by curettage and hemostasis with cautery, or silver nitrate can be used to treat the tissue and does not require anesthesia.

Incision Closure

There are numerous techniques and materials available for closing surgical incisions. Guidelines state that the type of suture material used does not matter as long as the primary repair is anatomic and perfused [7]. Typically, a layered closure is used; however, the choice of suture technique depends on the type and anatomic location of the wound, the skin thickness, and degree of tension. In foot and ankle surgery, absorbable sutures are used to close tissues deeper than the epidermis and to provide tissue support, relieve skin tension, and reduce wound dead space [8]. Current evidence indicates that external or internal retention sutures do not prevent dehiscence and that dehiscence is more likely associated with other factors such as trauma and wound contamination. Staples can be used to close the epidermis with no increase in infection [8].

Removal of sutures or staples typically is performed within 10–14 days of their placement. Sutures left in too long can lead to suture scar marks and local tissue reaction. However, sutures removed prematurely can lead to wound

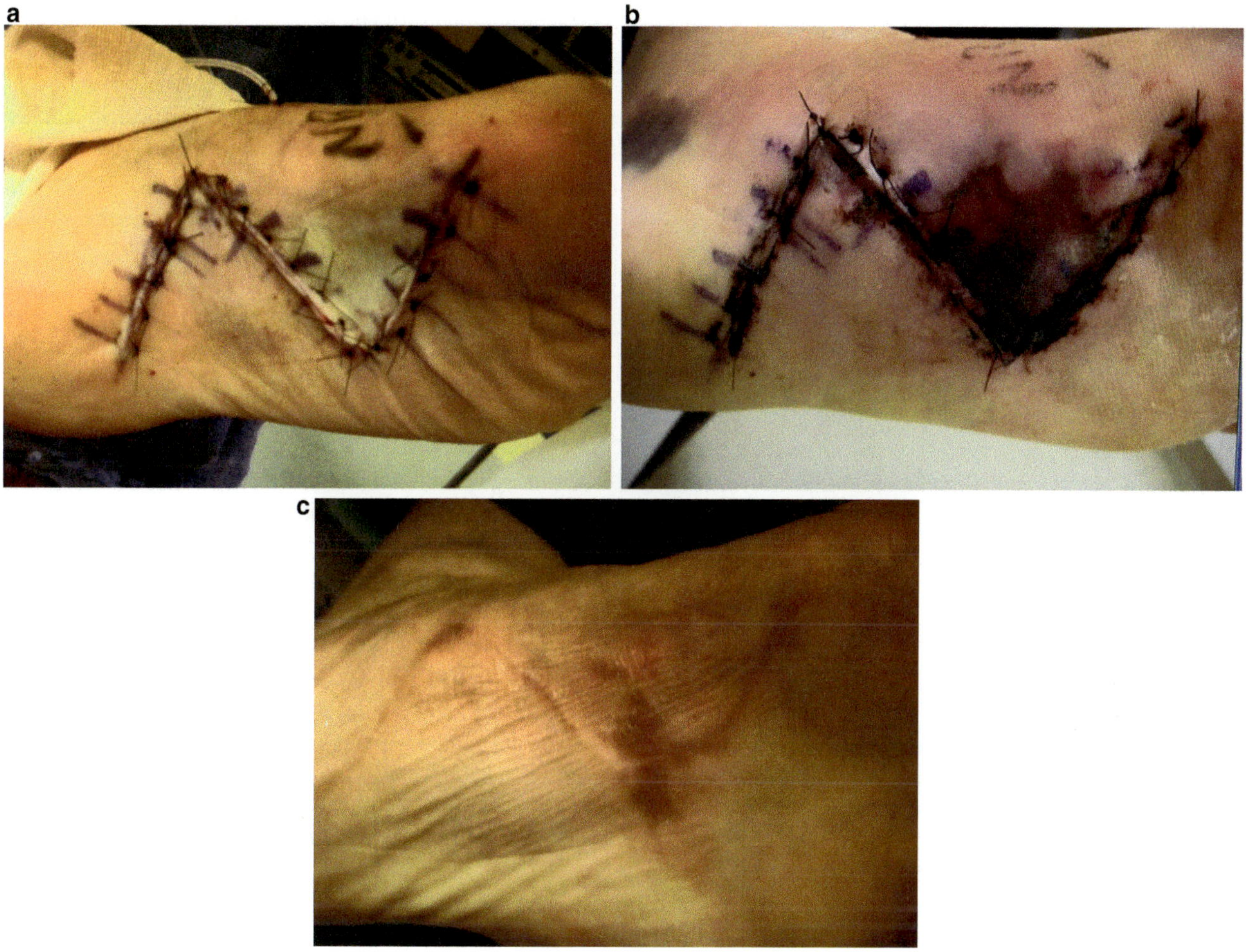

Fig. 4.7 Tension along the closure indicated by blanching of the skin (**a**) often times can lead to necrosis of tissue (**b**). This went on to heal without debridement (**c**)

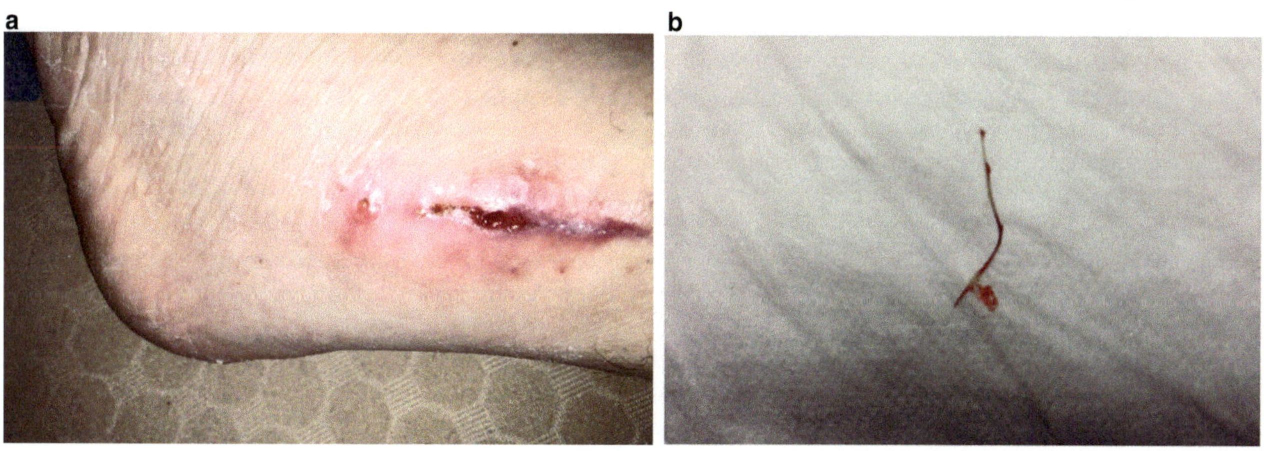

Fig. 4.8 (**a**) Suture abscess with distal wound dehiscence on an ORIF fibula with retained Vicryl suture. Suture abscess was debrided and Vicryl suture removed (**b**). Local wound care allowed healing without further complication

opening. Absorbable suture reactions do occur. In these instances, when the suture is causing a small abscess or inflammatory reaction, it is best to remove the suture to facilitate wound healing (Fig. 4.8).

Tissue adhesives can also be used to facilitate incision closure. A Cochrane review of eight randomized trials including 630 patients compared adhesive to suture used for incision closure and identified no difference in rates of dehiscence or infection [9]. However, adhesives are not recommended for use with complex lacerations, wounds with increased tension, or incision edges that are difficult to approximate. Adhesives slough off 5–10 days after application and thus may not be ideal for foot and ankle surgery where most incisions require maintenance of closure material for 10–14 days.

Adhesive tapes, also known as Steri-Strips, are reinforced microporous surgical adhesive tapes that can serve as an adjunct to wound closure. However, if a patient has skin sensitivity to adhesives, these should be avoided due to potential excessive inflammatory reaction, which then can lead to incision breakdown. Steri-Strips alone typically cannot suffice for wound closure; however, in certain instances, they can replace skin sutures and supplement subcuticular running suture closure.

Systemic Conditions

Numerous systemic conditions and medications can affect surgical outcomes and tissue healing. Medications that affect wound healing include glucocorticoids, chemotherapeutic agents, cyclosporine, penicillamine, metronidazole, and B-aminopropionitrile. Circulatory conditions that most likely will affect wound healing include diabetes, coronary insufficiency, congestive heart failure, and hypertension. Pulmonary disease may decrease oxygen saturation. Immunosuppression and chronic disease can predispose patient to secondary infection, and coagulopathies predispose patients to hematoma formation which can lead to further wound healing issues.

Hyperglycemia is defined as whole blood glucose level greater than 200 mg/dl and is associated with diminished wound strength and significant reduction in the phagocytic ability of neutrophils in 48 h postoperatively. Tight glycemic control with blood glucose levels from 80–180 mg/dl is optimal for patient wound healing [10]. Consistent careful monitoring and glucose control are important well into the postoperative period.

Obesity is a growing concern and is an independent predictor of SSI [11]. Increased body mass index and subcutaneous fat are significantly associated surgery-related complications including wound infection [11–12]. Regardless of surgical procedure, the incidence of postsurgical wound complications in patients who are obese compared to normal weight is high with reported rates of 15 to 22% [13]. In patients with obesity, perfusion and oxygenation of the surgical wound are more likely to be compromised. Intraoperative measures such as increased perioperative FiO2 and systemic warming to maintain normothermia are important. The standard dose of prophylactic antibiotics should be doubled if a patient's weight is over 220 lb or BMI is greater than 35.

Incision Care

To optimize incision healing, topical incision care should follow some basic principles:

- Incisions should be kept dry without prolonged moisture exposure including topical antibiotics.
- Original postoperative dressing should be maintained for 48–72 h.

Dressings provide initial protection, exudate absorption, and thermal insulation for acute wounds. Use of topical antibiotics on closed surgical incisions is not supported by current evidence and is not recommended by recent guidelines [10, 14]. In a comparison trial of no ointment, paraffin, and mupirocin ointment on excised and sutured skin lesions ($n = 562$ wounds), there was no difference reported in wound infection rate and significantly fewer scar complications in the patients treated without any ointment [15].

Hypertrophic Scarring and Keloids

Hypertrophic scars are thickened and raised scar tissue at the incision site. Often times they are symptomatic. They differ from keloids in that they do not extend beyond the margins of the wound. The greatest predictor of hypertrophic scarring is a patient history of similar scars with other surgical procedures.

Widened scars however are a result of increased tension force, and more than 80% of widening occurs in the first 6 months postoperatively [16]. Suturing techniques can sometimes help prevent this by using buried suture that will retain its tensile strength as long as possible. Prevention is the best treatment for this type of scar. Typically, more active people tend to be at higher risk to scar widening due to long-term stresses and collagen remodeling at greater levels. It is important to inform patients that scars may widen for a full year after surgery.

With hypertrophic scarring, it is important to recognize this complication early and initiate treatment typically with high-potency topical steroids or intralesional steroid injections. Both should decrease symptoms and help flatten the scar; however, the scar will always be wide and irregular texture. Thus, it is important to counsel patients on this risk preoperatively.

Keloids are excessive scar that exceeds its margins and the original site of trauma or surgery. These are often painful scars and occur most commonly in blacks and people of Mediterranean descent. Treatment of keloids is difficult. Steroid injections can be tried and allow acceptable containment of the keloid for some patients, but in many, there is insignificant impact on the keloid. Surgical excision often puts the patient at high risk for development of another keloid and one that is larger than the original keloid. Sutures may act as a catalyst for keloid formation. Carbon dioxide laser treatment of keloids has shown some success, although varied.

Conclusion: Managing Incision Complications

When a patient presents postoperatively with signs of incision breakdown or delayed healing, it is important to be aggressive in management. Initially, examining the wound is an imperative first step. Questions the surgeon should ask him or herself include:

- What is the extent of incision breakdown (i.e., superficial, deep, suture reaction)?
- What are the clinical signs surrounding the incision—erythema, edema, serous drainage, purulent drainage, warmth, and fibrotic tissue?
- Is a culture necessary, and will it improve and better guide treatment?
- How can I better manage this patient systemically?
- Do I need to consult another specialist to optimize this patient for healing?

Debridement of nonviable tissue including any foreign body such as suture should be performed upon initial presentation of incision breakdown. Typically, if the incision is void of any clinical signs of infection, culture typically is not necessary. However, if subsequent visits with the patient reveal increasing signs of erythema, serous or purulent drainage, and nonviable tissue, wound culture should be performed to help guide antibiosis. With superficial wounds, continue serial wound debridements typically weekly or more often as necessary. Immobilization of the limb and minimizing motion at the area of the incision will also facilitate healing. Optimizing comorbidities such as strict blood glucose control is imperative for patient wound healing. With positive cultures, it can be beneficial to consult infectious disease especially if the wound appears to have deep extension and possible tracking to the bone. Typically, if weekly visits are not showing decreased surface area over a period of 3 to 4 weeks, it may be wise to consider surgical excision of the dehisced portion of the wound with primary closure in a clean wound.

Incisional complications can vary in degree of morbidity for the patient. It is important as the surgeon that you are proactive in managing these complications. From aspirating a hematoma to wound excision with delayed primary closure to addressing the hypertrophic scar, your patient has enlisted you as the expert in caring for them.

Incision Complication Case Examples

Case #1 Bunion incision complication—a 62-year-old male underwent bunion surgery, fell, and had displacement of the capital fragment at 2 weeks post-op. Patient was taken back to the operating room and revision surgery was performed. After revision and suture removal, patient returned 2.5 weeks later with incision area appearing as in image (a). Debridement in the operating room was performed and culture taken positive for *Serratia marcescens*. Antibiotics started and wound VAC placement with granular wound bed (b). Extensor hallucis longus tendon noted in wound. With VAC removal, wound and tendon showed necrosis (c). Plastic surgery consulted and vascular flap created for wound coverage with excision of EHL (d–f). Final appearance of the foot at 16 weeks post-graft coverage (g).

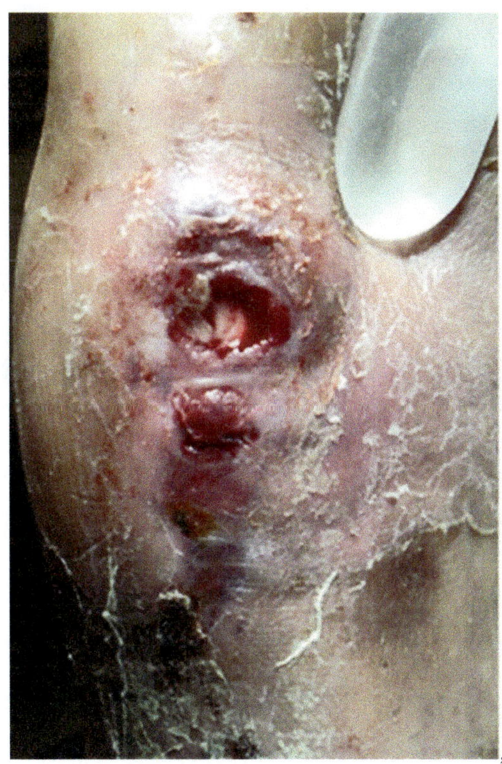

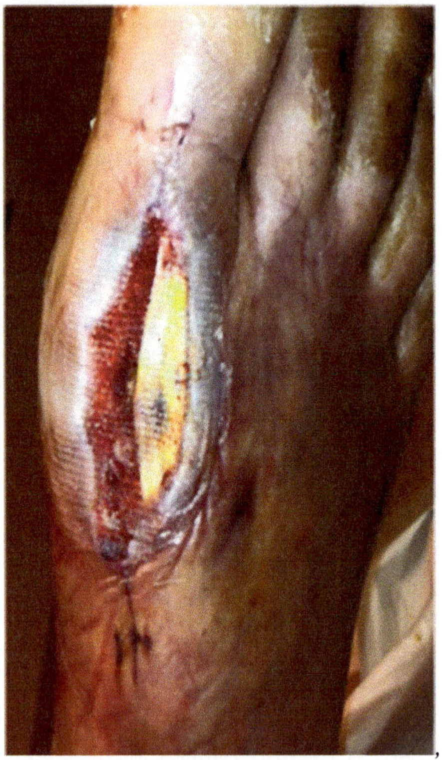
,

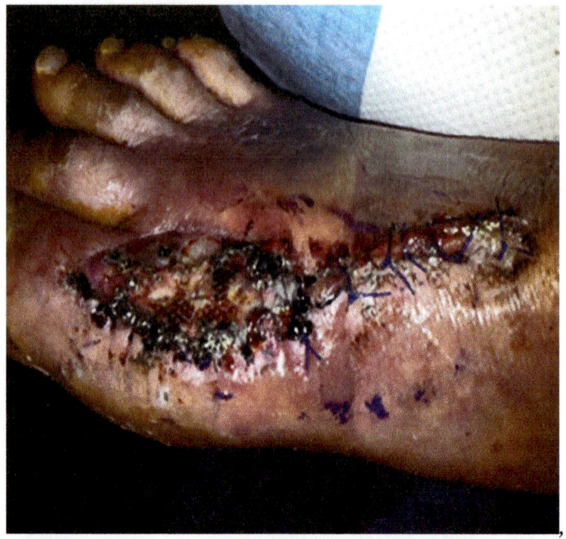
,

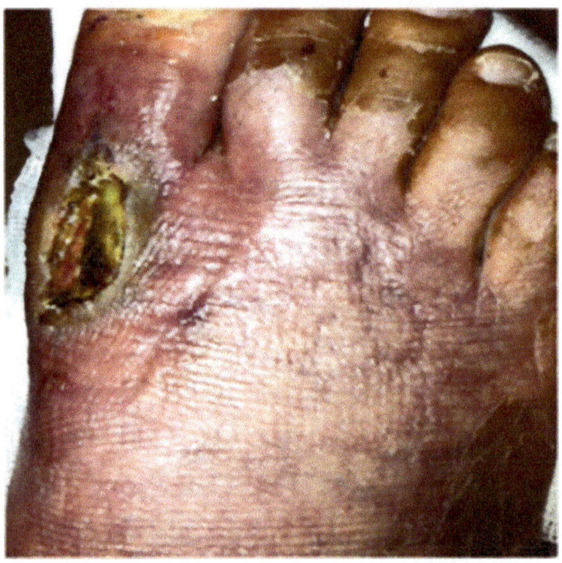

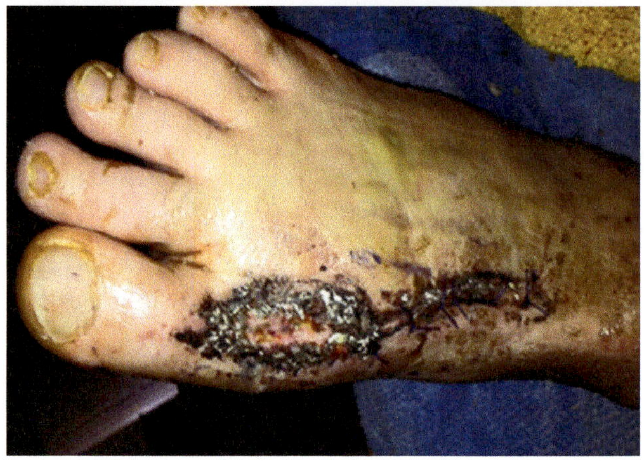

Case #2 This is a 56-year-old female with history of multiple unsuccessful foot surgeries where reconstructive surgery was attempted after calcaneal fracture and subtalar joint arthrodesis. These procedures ended up failing, and an extensive interposition graft of the calcaneus malunion with Achilles reconstruction and fixation was performed to restore the rearfoot. The patient then was noncompliant with her postoperative follow-up due to her living situation.

Here the patient's incision 3 weeks post-op from interposition graft of the calcaneal malunion with Achilles reconstruction shows dehiscence of the wound due to patient noncompliance on a lateral extensile incision type. The wound does not probe to the bone but shows ecchymotic changes with incisional blistering. The wound was extensively debrided, and wound cultures were taken. The area was then cleaned with Hibiclens and then placed in a short leg non-weight-bearing cast for 1 week with wound checks and light debridements weekly after that. Patient went on to heal without further issue.

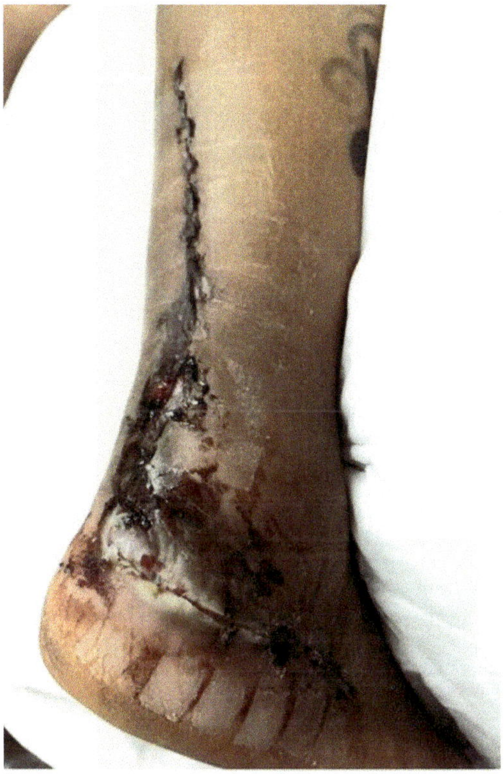

Case #3 A 19-year-old female treated at an outside facility with arthroplasty of the fourth digit. She presented with wound dehiscence and underlying infection (A). She was immediately taken to the operating room for incision and drainage

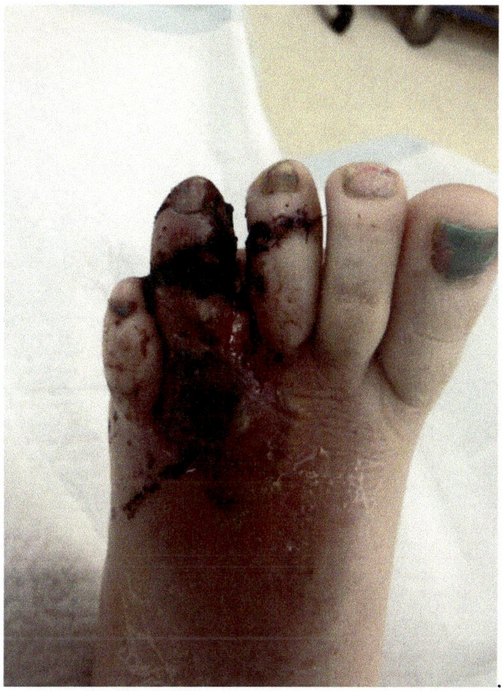

(B) Debridement was taken down to the level of the extensor tendon

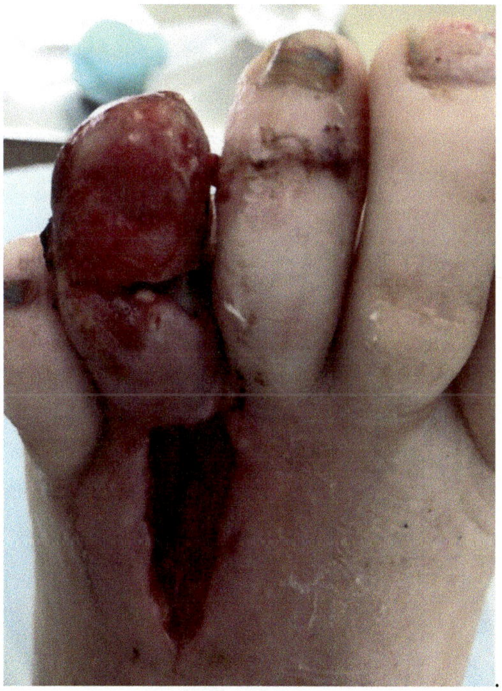

Extreme care was taken to ensure that vascular supply was not disrupted. (C and D) After four operative debridements and IV antibiotics, patient was started on negative pressure therapy

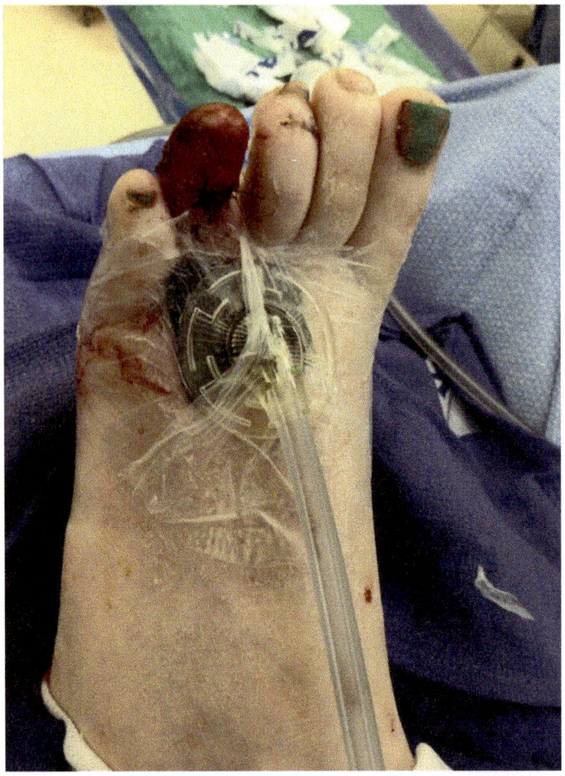

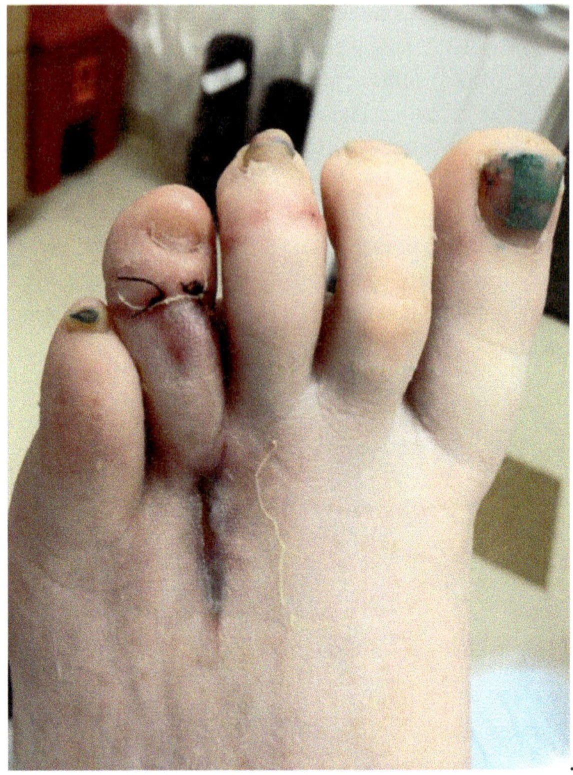

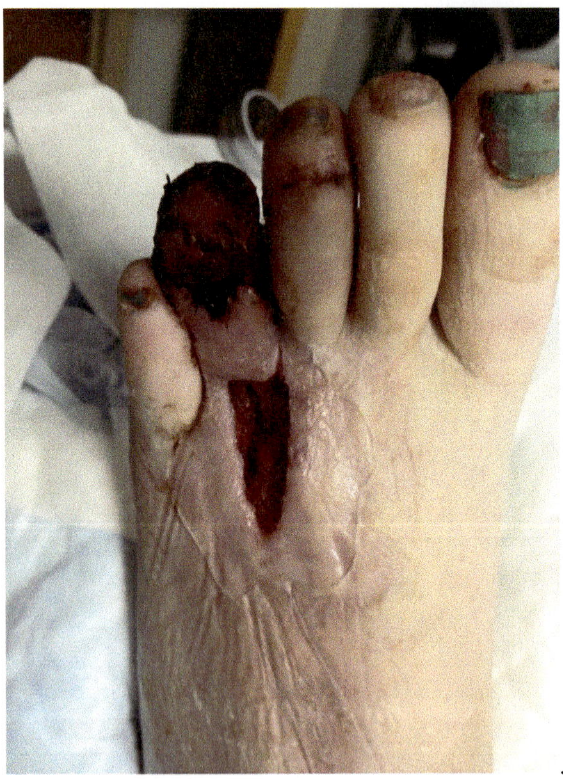

(E) Six weeks following initial treatment, patient is shown with healed wound. The digit was functional and patient was able to return to college

References

1. Anderson DJ, et al. Strategies to prevent surgical site infections in acute care hospitals. Infect Control Hosp Epidemiol. 2008;29:S51.
2. Hidron AI, et al. NHSN annual update: antimicrobial-resistant pathogens associated with healthcare-associated infections: annual summary of data reported to the National Healthcare Safety Network at the Centers for Disease Control and Prevention, 2006-2007. Infect Control Hosp Epidemiol. 2008;29:996–1011.
3. Barie PS. Surgical site infections: epidemiology and prevention. Surg Infect. 2002;3:59.
4. Haridas M, Malangoni MA. Predictive factors for surgical site infection in general surgery. Surgery. 2008;144:496.
5. Kompatscher P, et al. Comparison of the incidence and predicted risk of surgical site infection after breast reconstruction. Anesth Plast Surg. 2003;27(4):308.
6. Malone DL, et al. Surgical site infections: reanalysis of risk factors. J Surg Res. 2002;103(1):89.
7. Franz MG, et al. Optimizing healing of the acute wound by minimizing complications. Curr Probl Surg. 2007;44:679.
8. Hollander JE. Wound closure options. In: Singer AJ, Hollander JE, editors. Lacerations and acute wounds: an evidence-based guide. Philadelphia: FA Davis; 2003.
9. Coulthard P et al. Tissue adhesive for closure of surgical incisions. Cochrane Database Syst Rev. 2002; (3):CD004287.
10. Harrington G, et al. Surgical-site infection rates and risk factor analysis in coronary artery bypass graft surgery. Infect Control Hosp Epidemiol. 2004;25:472.
11. Tsukada K, et al. Body fat accumulation and postoperative complications after abdominal surgery. Am Surg. 2004;70:347.
12. Patel VP, et al. Factors associated with prolonged wound drainage after primary total hip and knee arthroplasty. J Bone Joint Surg Am. 2007;89:33.

13. Franz MG, et al. Guidelines to aid healing of acute wounds by decreasing impediments of healing. Wound Repair Regen. 2008; 16:723.
14. Leaper D, et al. Prevention and treatment of surgical site infections: summary of NICE guidance. BMJ. 2008;337:a1924.
15. Dixon AJ, et al. Randomized clinical trial of the effect of applying ointment to surgical wounds before occlusive dressing. Br J Surg. 2006;93:937.
16. Sommerlad BC, Creasey JM. The stretched Scar: a clinical and histological study. Br J Plast Surg. 1978;31:34–45.

5 Surgical Infections

Michelle Butterworth and Trevor Payne

Introduction

The risk of postoperative infection after foot and ankle surgery has been reported as low as 0.5% and as high as 6.5% [1] and tends to be higher than other parts of the body [2]. Infection prevention, timely recognition of infection, and choosing the most prudent course of treatment are critical and can make the difference between a salvageable outcome versus undesirable results including major reconstruction, amputation, loss of function and quality of life, significantly increased healthcare costs, and even death.

Prevention

Patient Selection

The foundation of a successful outcome in elective surgery is proper patient selection, particularly in procedures with a higher risk of infection such as repair of open fracture, use of external fixation, or prosthetic joint implantation [2, 3]. When considering surgical intervention, special attention should be directed to intrinsic risk factors. These include factors such as advanced age or poor nutrition status; use of tobacco or recreational drugs; concurrent remote infections or history of previous infections; inflammatory conditions such as crystalline arthropathies and rheumatoid arthritis; immunocompromised states including diabetes mellitus, HIV, and immunosuppressant therapies; and other comorbidities which may impair healing such as peripheral arterial disease, peripheral neuropathy, and Charcot neuroarthropathy. Many of these risk factors may be modified by optimization of the underlying condition such as blood glucose control in diabetic patients and smoking cessation.

M. Butterworth (✉)
Pee Dee Foot Center, Kingstree, SC 29556, USA
e-mail: mbutter@ftc-i.net

T. Payne
Augusta Foot and Ankle, Evans, GA 30809, USA

Glucose Control in Diabetes Mellitus

Risk stratification and early recognition is especially important in diabetic patients, who often present with special surgical considerations in combination with a higher overall risk of developing postoperative infections [4–7]. In 2010, Wukich et al. conducted a 1000-patient retrospective review which demonstrated that the presence of diabetes-related peripheral vascular disease, peripheral neuropathy, Charcot neuroarthropathy, or a history of diabetic ulcers was associated with a tenfold increase in incidence of postoperative infection, including a fivefold increase in the incidence of severe complicated infections which ultimately required hospitalization, when compared to both nondiabetic patients and diabetic patients who had none of these complications [4]. As diabetic management advances, more emphasis is being placed upon HgA1C levels, which provide a better long-term snapshot of patients' glucose levels and treatment adherence. Jupiter et al. demonstrated a significant relationship between HgA1C greater than 7.0% and increased incidence of postoperative infection risk—a correlation which steepened when HgA1C surpassed 7.3% [8]. Humphers et al. reported a 1.59 relative risk increase of postoperative infection following foot and ankle surgery, for every 1% increase of HgA1C above 7.0% [9].

To mitigate these risks, tight glucose control should be an essential prerequisite for elective surgeries, as glucose levels of even 150–175 ml/dl have been shown to negate the inherent immunity needed to prevent infection [10]. Of course, non-elective emergent cases warrant surgical treatment regardless of the patient's glucose compliance. The risks of uncontrolled diabetes and the strategy of reducing infection risk through tight glucose control should be explained to the patient. This patient education regarding long-term implementation of structured diabetic control, particularly through diet and exercise, cannot be underestimated as it can profoundly affect the surgical outcome.

M.S. Lee, J.P. Grossman (eds.), *Complications in Foot and Ankle Surgery*, DOI 10.1007/978-3-319-53686-6_5

Smoking Cessation

Several recent studies have shown the detrimental effects that smoking can have on postsurgical infections [11–16]. Specifically, current smokers have a greater than fourfold increased risk of infection, compared to patients who have never smoked. Even former smokers who quit smoking an average of 17 years prior to intervention demonstrated a nearly twofold increased risk of complications compared to those who had never smoked [17] . Fortunately, smoking cessation at least 4 weeks prior to surgery has been shown to decrease the risk of postoperative infections, through a proposed mechanism of reversing the impairment of the immune response to peripheral tissues [18]. In order to maximize compliance, patients should be educated about the benefits of preoperative smoking cessation on immunological response and surgical outcome. Research shows that smokers are typically unaware of the significant negative risks that smoking can have on surgical outcomes and are inclined to quit with adequate instruction [19].

Prophylactic Antibiotics

Many healthcare systems have adopted preoperative prophylactic antibiotic protocols supplied by the Surgical Care Improvement Project (SCIP) or The Joint Commission, while other institutions have devised their own individual mandates and protocols. The American College of Foot and Ankle Surgeons recently published a commentary noting the lack of compelling evidence to demonstrate the benefit of prophylactic antibiotics for foot and ankle surgery and the need for future high-level evidence to legitimize their use [20]. Based on available research from multiple other specialties, the consensus panel devised the following recommendations:

- Prophylactic antibiotics are appropriate in surgery involving bone, hardware and prosthetic joints, and any prolonged surgical cases. The use of antibiotics in soft tissue procedures is according to surgeon preference on a case-by-case basis.
- Prophylactic antibiotics should be used in patient populations with inherent increased risk (i.e., diabetics, immunocompromised patients), regardless of the type of surgical procedure.
- When used, prophylactic antibiotics should be narrow in spectrum and cover only the most commonly identified organism in postoperative infections, *Staphylococcus aureus*. Neither routine, preoperative nasal swabbing for MRSA colonization nor prophylactic MRSA coverage for positive nasal colonization was recommended.
- When administered, prophylactic antibiotics should be given 60 min before surgery (before tourniquet inflation) and discontinued within 24 h of the operation.

For first-line prophylactic agent, the Infectious Diseases Society of America recommends cefazolin 2 g (3 g for patients over 120 kg). For patients with a beta-lactam allergy, clindamycin 900 mg or vancomycin 15 mg/kg can be substituted [21].

Surgical Site Preparation

Lowering the exogenous bacterial load via proper preparation of the surgical site is another way in which the surgeon can reduce the risk of infection. Presurgical disinfectant preparations have many forms, with the two main categories being povidone-iodine and chlorhexidine—both of which have been shown to be more efficacious in an alcohol-based form [22, 23]. Several studies have shown that chlorhexidine is superior in decreasing bacterial burden and is the best choice [23–26]. Furthermore, Keblish et al. showed that application of the solution with bristled brush compared to a soft sponge technique yielded higher rates of skin decontamination [27]. In addition to presurgical scrubs with high yield decontaminates, Ng et al. showed the efficacy of 4% chlorhexidine foot baths 20 min prior to the normal presurgical prophylactic scrub technique [28]. This method could be useful especially in patients with high-risk infection potential. In addition, sterile gown and glove technique, as well as shaving of hair in the surgical field, are standards of care.

Surgeons should also take care to minimize the risk of postoperative infections arising from locations other than the surgical site. For example, incentive spirometry, deep breathing exercises, directed coughing, and early ambulation should be used to prevent postoperative pulmonary illnesses such as atelectasis and pneumonia [29]. In addition, Foley catheters should be used only when indicated and only for as long as necessary, to reduce the risk of catheter-associated urinary tract infections [30, 31]. Other factors, such as length of surgery, length of hospital stay, and hypothermia, should be considered and reduced whenever possible [32–34].

Evaluation

Triage of Systemic Infections

Postoperative fever can be an indicator for systemic infection. The timing of fever in the postoperative phase can give insight to the causative factor. Fever within the first 24 h is typically a result of postanesthetic overshoot or atelectasis. Fever within the first 24–48 h may be caused by thrombophlebitis and pulmonary embolism, or it may just be benign. Fever developing within 3–4 days postoperatively may be due to a urinary tract infection or a wound infection.

Systemic inflammatory response syndrome or "SIRS" is a clinical indicator of a systemic inflammatory state which can reflect a variety of underlying conditions including, but not limited to, systemic infection. Patients with positive SIRS criteria (listed below), or systemic signs and symptoms such as nausea, vomiting, abdominal pain, diarrhea, fever, chills, and night sweats, may be suffering from systemic infection and therefore need rapid antibacterial, supportive, and potential surgical interventions. A complete set of vital signs (with complete blood count when it is available) is essential in screening for SIRS, which is classified by two or more of the following:

- Body temperature <36°C (96.8°F) or >38°C (100.4°F)
- Heart rate >90 beats per minute
- Tachypnea of >20 breaths per minute or $PaCO^2$ < 4.3 kPa (32 mmHg)
- White blood cell count <4000 cells/mm^3 (4 × 10^9 cells/L) or >12,000 cells/mm^3 (12 × 10^9 cells/L) or the presence of greater than 10% immature granulocytes

Though it would not be within the scope of a foot and ankle surgeon to manage this spectrum of conditions alone, it is important to be familiar with the definitions, pathogenesis, and course of the systemic infectious syndromes ranging from SIRS to septic shock. Sepsis is defined by positive SIRS criteria plus the presence of a known or suspected source of infection. Severe sepsis is defined by sepsis plus the presence of at least one sign of end-organ dysfunction (oliguria or other signs of acute kidney injury, altered mental status, increased liver enzyme abnormalities, metabolic acidosis, or respiratory distress). Septic shock is defined by sepsis plus the presence of hypotension (systolic blood pressure of <90 mmHg or a >40 mmHg decrease from patient's baseline) which does not resolve with initial attempts at fluid resuscitation. Any of these clinical presentations should trigger early and aggressive treatment by a well-qualified multidisciplinary team who is familiar with the management of sepsis and critically ill patients, which typically includes hospital admission and parenteral empiric antibiotic therapy as well as fluids and blood pressure support where indicated.

History and Physical Exam

In the absence of signs for systemic infection, the initial postoperative visit should begin with consideration of the patient's medical history and risk factors, as well as the course of events since the operation was performed. In situations where a patient presents to a physician other than the one who performed the surgery, medical records should be acquired in order to properly evaluate the patient for possible complications specific to both the patient and the intervention they received. Suspicion of infection and consideration of broad-spectrum antimicrobial treatments should have a lower threshold if the history contains patient risk factors such as poorly controlled diabetes, smoking, or high-risk procedures such as open fracture fixation [3, 35, 36].

Patient history should include ascertaining the timing of infectious symptom onset. Acute postoperative infections occur any time within the first 4 weeks of surgical intervention, most often presenting within the first 2 weeks [37]. Patients who are ultimately diagnosed with infection may complain of worsening rather than improving symptoms or of a "double-peak" effect, whereby symptoms initially improve but then regress into a worsening state. An exception to this timeline are infections caused by *Streptococcus pyogenes* (group A β-hemolytic streptococcus) or *Clostridium perfringens*, rare but debilitating organisms which arise as early as 24–36 h after introduction and present with a more rapid course, with manifestations including erythema, bacteremia, and necrotizing fasciitis. Due to scarcity of this type of infection, suspicions should be tempered by considering indications for infection and worsening symptoms over a rapid period of time soon after surgery [37].

Alternatively, chronic postsurgical infections persist beyond initial management attempts or present several weeks after the intervention—up to 1 year if hardware is present [38]. For these patients, historical information about prior interventions including debridements, aspirations, washouts, and culture results must be evaluated and weighed against the evolving clinical presentation [39].

On examination, the local cardinal signs of infection including increased pain (dolar), redness (rubor), swelling (tumor), heat (calor), and loss of function (function lasso) are often the first clues that an infection is present; however, they can also be normal postoperative findings. Although these findings can be present in both a postoperative infection and the normal healing process, the intensity of these findings are often greater in the presence of infection and can be used as a differentiating factor (Fig. 5.1). An intimate understanding of normal foot and ankle anatomy and a thorough physical evaluation, including dermatological, vascular, neurological, and musculoskeletal components, are therefore necessary to differentiate infection from normal postoperative features as early as possible. Exam findings which should raise suspicion of infection include purulent drainage expressed from a wound or surgical site, malodor, induration, fluctuance, erythema which extends beyond 5 cm from the surgical site, sinus tract formation, cessation of healing, and continued or increased pain [40, 41] (Fig. 5.2). Special consideration should be given if there is suspicion of joint infection. Pain out of proportion upon motion of the affected joint is 100% sensitive for septic arthritis and should be correlated with other findings including the classic signs of inflammation, axial load pain, and evidence of joint effusion [42].

Laboratory Studies

When the history and physical findings are suspicious for infection, it is helpful to order laboratory studies for further evaluation, including a complete blood count with differential and inflammatory markers such as erythrocyte sedimentation rate (ESR) and C-reactive protein (CRP). This data can be helpful in demonstrating a heightened inflammatory state and can be trended over time to gauge responsiveness to the selected treatment. However, these are nonspecific markers of inflammation which can occur in the setting of infection or as a natural response to trauma and surgery itself. In the absence of obvious signs of infection such as a draining sinus tract, an increased white blood cell (WBC) count combined with an increased ESR and CRP has shown 100% sensitivity but 24% specificity for detecting the presence of infection [43]. While an abnormal WBC count (outside the range of 4–10 × 10^3 leucocytes/ul) indicates an ongoing acute inflammatory response in the body, an increased immature granulocyte percentage can be more indicative of bacterial infection in particular. ESR represents greater migration of erythrocytes in the blood and changes in fibrinogen in response to inflammation. When it is elevated above its normal baseline level of less than 20 mm/hr, it has been shown to be highly sensitive for osteomyelitis but much less sensitive for infection in general [44, 45]. Therefore, a single increased postoperative WBC count or ESR value has poor diagnostic and prognostic value by itself and should be clinically correlated with history and physical findings, as well as trends over time [46].

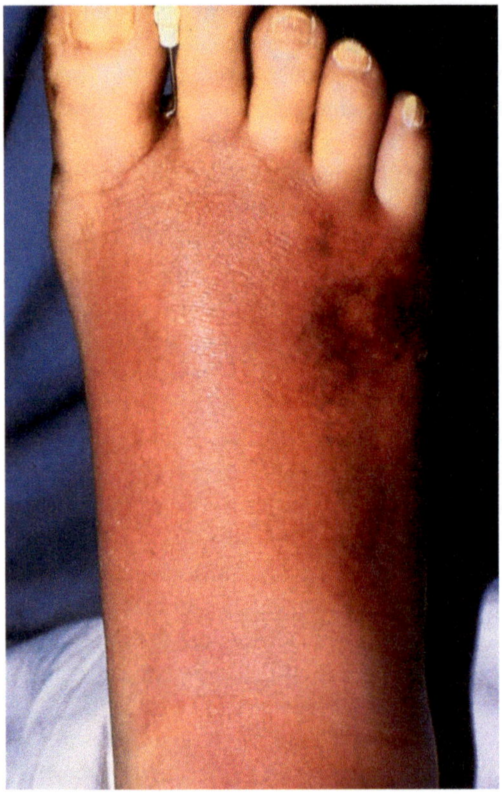

Fig. 5.1 Clinical presentation 3 days post-op. Notice the significant intensity and extent of the erythema and edema. There is no drainage, but with these cardinal signs of infection, one should be concerned about a deep abscess

CRP is produced by the liver during times of acute inflammation and does not normally occur in the body. It is indicative of some acute inflammatory change at any increase above 0.6 mg/dl. Under normal circumstances, CRP levels can be expected to rise and equilibrate at 24–72 h after surgical intervention, followed by a gradual but consistent decrease with resolution to normal levels after 7 days. When correlated with other signs and symptoms, infection should

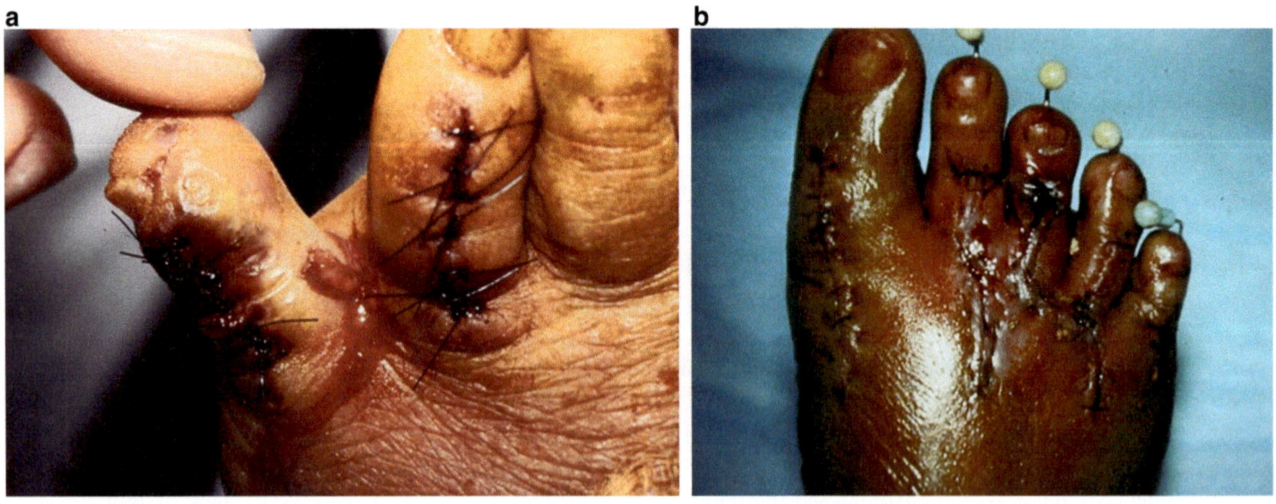

Fig. 5.2 (**a**) Purulent drainage from the interdigital space post hammertoe repair. This requires incision and drainage for adequate decompression. (**b**) Postoperative infection with notable erythema and edema. There is also the start of wound dehiscence and incisional serous drainage. Patient will need to be monitored closely for deep infection. If no response to antibiotic therapy, incision and drainage may be warranted

be suspected when CRP continues to increase after this time frame or undergoes a "second rise" to levels of 100 mg/mL or above, after the initial decrease [47]. The location of surgical intervention can also have an impact on the postsurgical CRP value. For example, Neumaier showed that the average CRP levels at 2 days after open reduction and internal fixation (ORIF) of femoral fractures was 136 mg/L, compared to 46 mg/L at 2 days after ORIF of ankle fractures [48]. While the initial increase was proportional to the amount of injury and amount of subsequent dissection performed, levels which remained higher than 100 mg/L after 4 days were associated with infection in both groups [49]. Proper utilization of CRP as a correlation to postoperative infection has shown a sensitivity of 85–92% and specificity of 86–93% [48, 50]. In pediatric patients, Laporta et al. showed that CRP levels over 11 mg/DL at 48 h had a sensitivity of 87% and specificity of 89% for postoperative infection [51].

Other infectious markers, such as CD64, TNF-α, and IL-6, have been proposed and are being studied, but require further research before recommendations can be made regarding their diagnostic or prognostic clinical use [52–55]. Procalcitonin has shown some promise as a diagnostic marker for sepsis and severe sepsis in critically ill postsurgical ICU patients who are unable to communicate their history and symptoms [53]. However, there is not enough evidence to support its utilization in foot and ankle postoperative infections.

Other laboratory values such a metabolic panel, albumin, and pre-albumin, while not helpful in the diagnosis of infection, provide an overall look at the patient's general health and nutritional status and, therefore, may be indirectly prognostic of a patient's ability to ward off and recover from infection. Finally, studies such as blood lactate levels [56] are important prognostic markers in the management of sepsis.

Imaging Studies

Imaging techniques can be very helpful in evaluating infection. There are many imaging techniques available including plain radiographs, ultrasonography, various types of scintigraphy, CT scans, and magnetic resonance imaging (MRI). The important thing to remember is that the imaging study alone is just an aid and should not be relied upon to make the diagnosis of infection. The physician must utilize a combination of imaging studies, laboratory values, and clinical evaluation to make an accurate diagnosis and devise a proper treatment plan.

At the first suspicion of infection, plain radiographs should be ordered to look for early signs of hardware failure, migration of hardware or prostheses, changes in bone density and joint space margins, or other alarm signs such as gas in the tissues, which can result from aggressive infectious

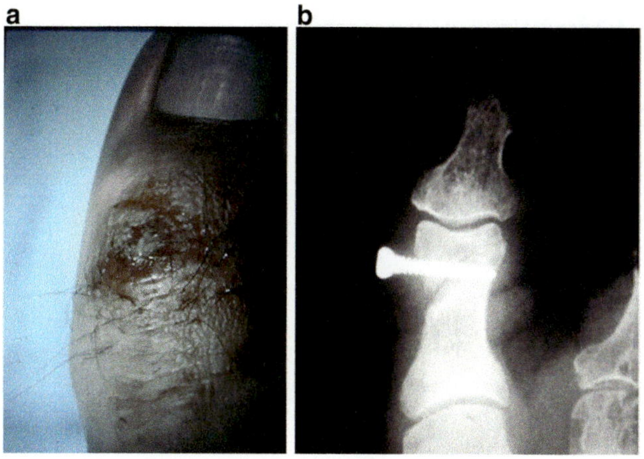

Fig. 5.3 (**a**) Clinical presentation 3 weeks post-op Akin osteotomy. Notice localized edema and discoloration around the location of the screw head. (**b**) Obvious loosening of the screw and failure of the internal fixation. Infection is part of the differential diagnosis

agents including *Clostridia* species [57] (Fig. 5.3). Although their specificity and sensitivity are low during the acute phase of infection versus normal postoperative changes, they should be the first imaging study obtained to evaluate possible infection. They can act as a baseline for comparison and are useful for serial evaluations of changes over time. The classic radiographic findings of osteomyelitis are well known and include soft tissue swelling, periosteal reaction, cortical erosion, and osteolysis and destruction (Fig. 5.4). The radiographic manifestations of osteomyelitis, however, appear after the destruction of bone and may take up to 4 weeks for the osseous changes to actually be visualized on plain films. Because of this delay, plain film radiographs should not be relied upon for the diagnosis of osteomyelitis [58].

Ultrasonography is a viable option for the detection of fluid collections including abscesses and joint effusions as small as 1–2 mL and is particularly useful for guiding procedures in real time, such as needle aspiration of a fluid collection for fluid culture sampling [59]. Limitations include inability to assess bone stock as sound waves are not able to penetrate the hard outer cortical layer [60, 61].

Advanced imaging selections should be based on the type and location of the suspected infection and other related factors. For example, computed tomography (CT) provides some detail about bone quality and integrity, by detecting erosions, sclerosis, and other bony abnormalities [62]. To investigate suspected septic arthritis, however, MRI should be selected as it is superior in both sensitivity (100%) and specificity (75%) [63] and can better evaluate septic arthritis by analyzing soft tissue in addition to pertinent osseous structures. Imaging features which may suggest septic arthritis include evidence of joint effusion, chondral destruction, adjacent decreased bone density, soft tissue inflammation, or abscesses.

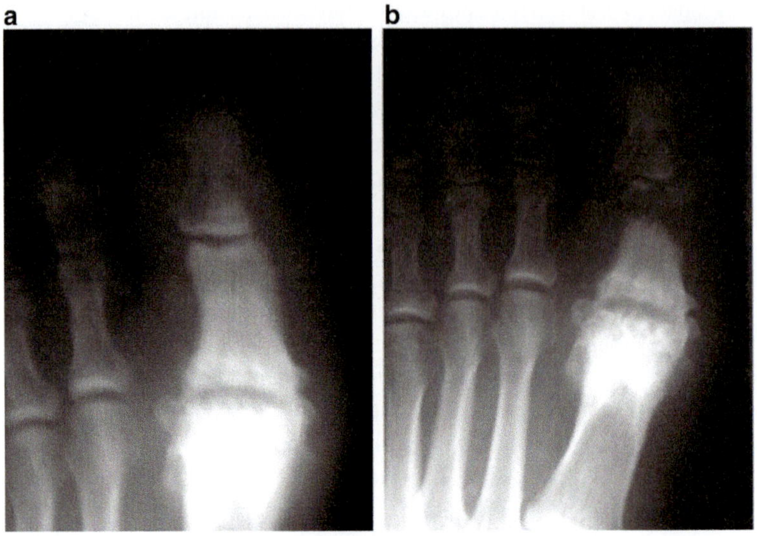

Fig. 5.4 (**a**) Osteolysis with obvious cortical destruction of the hallux. Findings are consistent with osteomyelitis. (**b**) Two weeks later significant osseous destruction is noted with rapid continuance and extension of the osteomyelitis. The distal portion of the proximal phalanx is practically absent

These advanced imaging techniques are very useful for evaluating inflammatory changes when there is no hardware; but when hardware is present, artifact effects significantly reduce their utility [64]. For suspected prosthetic joint infections, advanced imaging is not recommended due to lack of visualization, low specificity for infection, and high cost. An exception is titanium hardware, which permits better visualization of soft tissue in the same viewing field when evaluated by MRI, although some artifact effects will still be present [65] (Fig. 5.5).

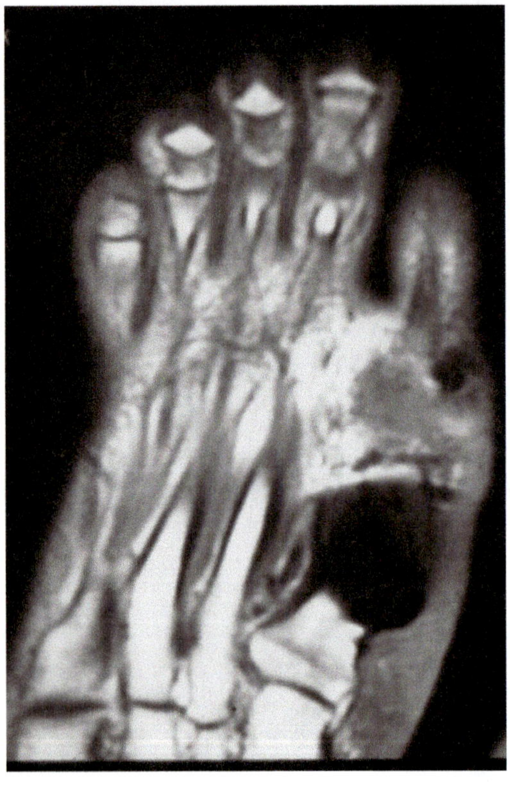

Fig. 5.5 Decreased signal intensity on this MRI represents artifact secondary to the titanium screws utilized. This is the typical void made by internal fixation and will obscure the surrounding anatomic area

Scintigraphy or bone scans are very common imaging modalities utilized in evaluating infections, but they are not reliable during the acute phase of the postoperative course. There are many different scintigraphy modalities available. The technetium (^{99m}Tc MDP) study is the most basic and common bone scan but is the least specific for infection. In an attempt to increase the specificity for infection, white blood cell-labeled bone scans of various kinds have been developed, but still have limitations. They are all markers of metabolic activity so are very sensitive to any inflammatory process, including infection and normal postoperative healing. Although bone scans are sensitive, they are nonspecific for infection and should have limited use postoperatively since they can both produce false-positive results and misguide the physician's treatment plan (Fig. 5.6). Palestro et al. compared the sensitivity and specificity of three different types of bone scans for their accuracy in diagnosing osteomyelitis. The ^{99m}Tc MDP scan had a specificity of only 27%, while the indium-labeled white blood cell scan (^{111}In-WBC) had the same specificity as the monoclonal antigranulocyte antibody (Moab) in vivo white blood cell-labeled scan, but was still only 67% specific [66]. Although WBC-labeled bone scans are more specific than technetium scans, their use in the acute postoperative phase is still limited, and they are more useful in detecting chronic or late-presenting infections. Recent evidence has suggested that bone scans combining ^{111}In-WBC and ^{99m}Tc-sulfur colloid single-photon emission computed tomography (SPECT) could diagnose prosthetic joint infections with a reported accuracy of 95–97%; however, further testing is needed to determine how to utilize this modality in a cost-effective way [67].

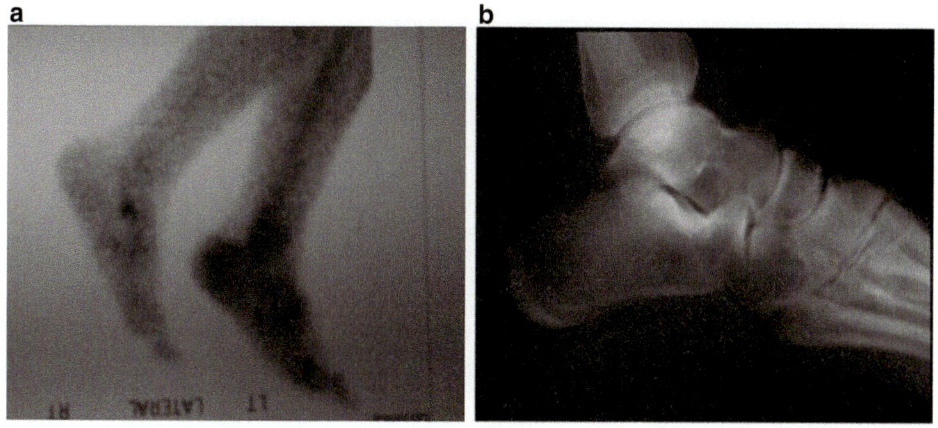

Fig. 5.6 (**a**) Patient is status post heel surgery with a wound dehiscence. This technetium bone scan was read as positive for osteomyelitis of the calcaneus. This is a false-positive result confirming the high sensitivity but low specificity for diagnosing infection. (**b**) A plain film radiograph and clinical exam of the same patient reveal a superficial, healthy plantar ulceration with no probing to bone, no clinical signs of infection, and no radiographic evidence of osteomyelitis

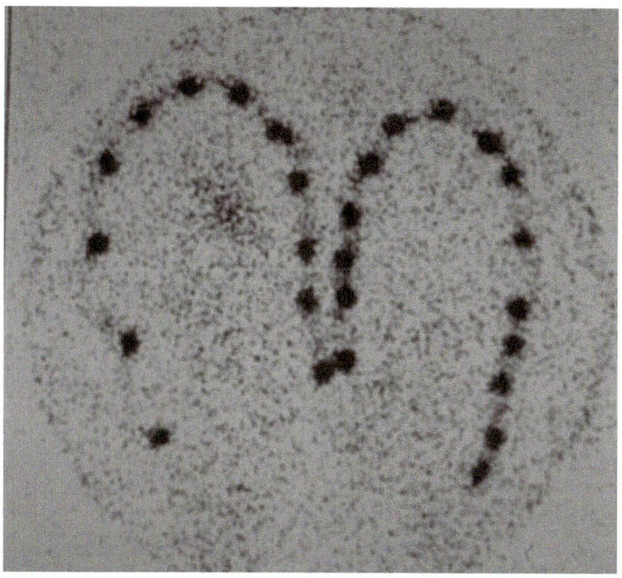

Fig. 5.7 This is an indium white blood cell-labeled scan. It was read as positive for osteomyelitis; however, it is very difficult to visualize the anatomic structures and differentiate soft tissues from osseous structures

The other drawback of bone scans in evaluating infections is the inability to readily distinguish structures individually. Results are often generalized to a large relative area around the infection, due to superimposed focal uptake in all tissue layers such as bone, tissue, and joint areas. Anatomic structures are poorly visualized making evaluation difficult (Fig. 5.7).

MRI has been described as the imaging modality of choice for the evaluation of postoperative infection. It offers superior visualization of anatomic structures and can differentiate between soft tissue and osseous infection (Fig. 5.8). It can also be utilized for preoperative planning to determine the extent of infection and the level of debridement needed. Additionally, it can be utilized to look for other sources of infection, such as a deep abscess, if the patient is not responding adequately to the treatment protocol. Finally, it can also be utilized to monitor an infection and the response to treatment (Fig. 5.9). A meta-analysis was performed over a 40-year time frame comparing MRI with plain radiographs, bone scans, and white blood cell-labeled studies for diagnosing osteomyelitis. They concluded that MRI was a strong test to aid in both confirming and excluding osteomyelitis of the foot and that a positive MRI results in an 84% chance of having the diagnosis of osteomyelitis and other exam findings such as substantial wound depth and probing to bone cinch the diagnosis. They also stated that the use of technetium bone scanning in the diagnosis of osteomyelitis of the foot should be limited and the lack of adequate specificity creates many false-positive results [68] (Fig. 5.10). Another study added the probe to bone test and compared it with radiographs, bone scans, white blood cell-labeled scans, and MRI for the diagnosis of osteomyelitis. The probe to bone test was actually more specific than any imaging modality, and MRI was the second most specific test. Radiographs and white blood cell-labeled scans were equal in specificity, and bone scans were the least specific [69].

Microbiology Studies

Microbiology studies such as gram stains, cultures, and sensitivities are an exceptionally important part of the diagnostic process and should be used to guide antibiotic selections whenever possible. Ideally, cultures should be taken prior to administration of antibiotics to reduce the risk of a false-negative result. However, in life-threatening situations such as suspected sepsis, or when cultures cannot be taken in a timely fashion, antibiotic treatment should not be delayed for the sake of acquiring more accurate cultures. In such cases, treatment should be administered, with cultures at the earliest opportunity.

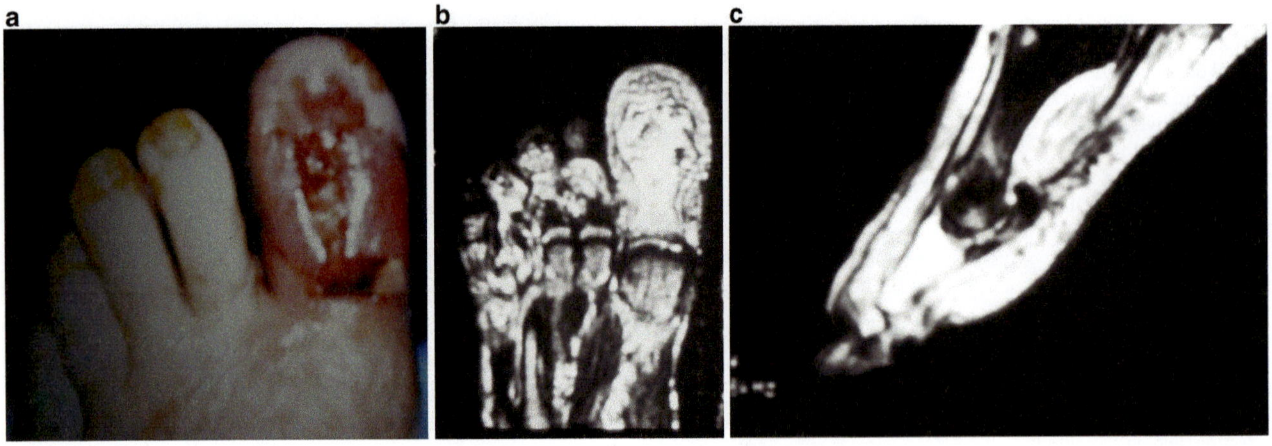

Fig. 5.8 (**a**) Patient is status post phenol and alcohol procedure with persistent erythema, edema, and drainage. (**b**) and (**c**) These T2-weighted magnetic resonance images show increased signal intensity of the entire hallux consistent with osteomyelitis. MRI provides great anatomic visualization and unfortunately shows that the infection has extended through the soft tissue boundaries invading bone

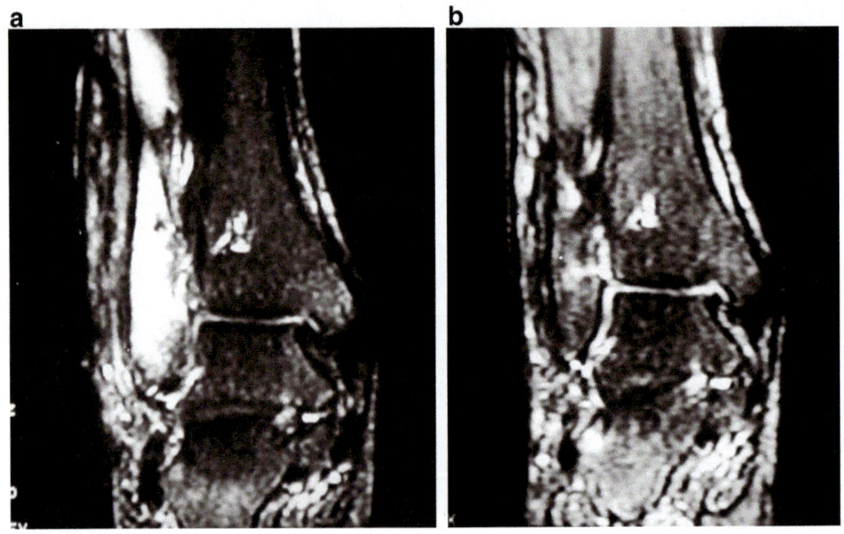

Fig. 5.9 (**a**) Patient had an open fibula fracture resulting in osteomyelitis evidenced by the increased signal intensity. (**b**) After 6 weeks of intravenous antibiotics, this MRI shows successful treatment and eradication of the infection

When obtaining wound cultures, it is important to understand that superficial ulcerations and tissues are poor specimens which are contaminated with normal skin flora and are not recommended for attempting to identify pathogens responsible for deeper infections [70]. Whenever possible, deep wound cultures should be taken as they are more reliable for the accurate detection of offending pathogens [71]. If possible, augmentation of deep cultures with both purulent fluid cultures and deep tissue specimens can enhance the accuracy and precision of the resulting pathogenic profile [72]. Prior to deep culture acquisition, contamination should be prevented by reducing the superficial bacterial load overlying the infection site, via sterile water or normal saline lavage, debridement, and scrubbing with an iodine or chlorhexidine alcohol-based cleanser.

When bone infection is suspected, bone biopsy and cultures are predictive of responsiveness to targeted antibiotics [70] and should always be obtained when accessible or exposed through surgical site dehiscence. If a bone culture is not accessible, consider obtaining deep sinus tract cultures, as this has been shown to correlate well with potential osseous infections when properly executed and when the swab probes to bone [71].

When bacteremia or sepsis is suspected, due to abnormal vital signs or the presence of systemic symptoms such as nausea or vomiting and chills, blood cultures should be obtained as quickly as possible [64, 73]. March et al. have shown that a full antibacterial susceptibility panel can be produced within 120 min when taken from positive blood culture samples [74]. Blood cultures should be procured from two separate venous sites with 20 min in between, to avoid false-negative results, as patients with even severe sepsis can demonstrate rare or discontinuous bacteria in circulation at any one time.

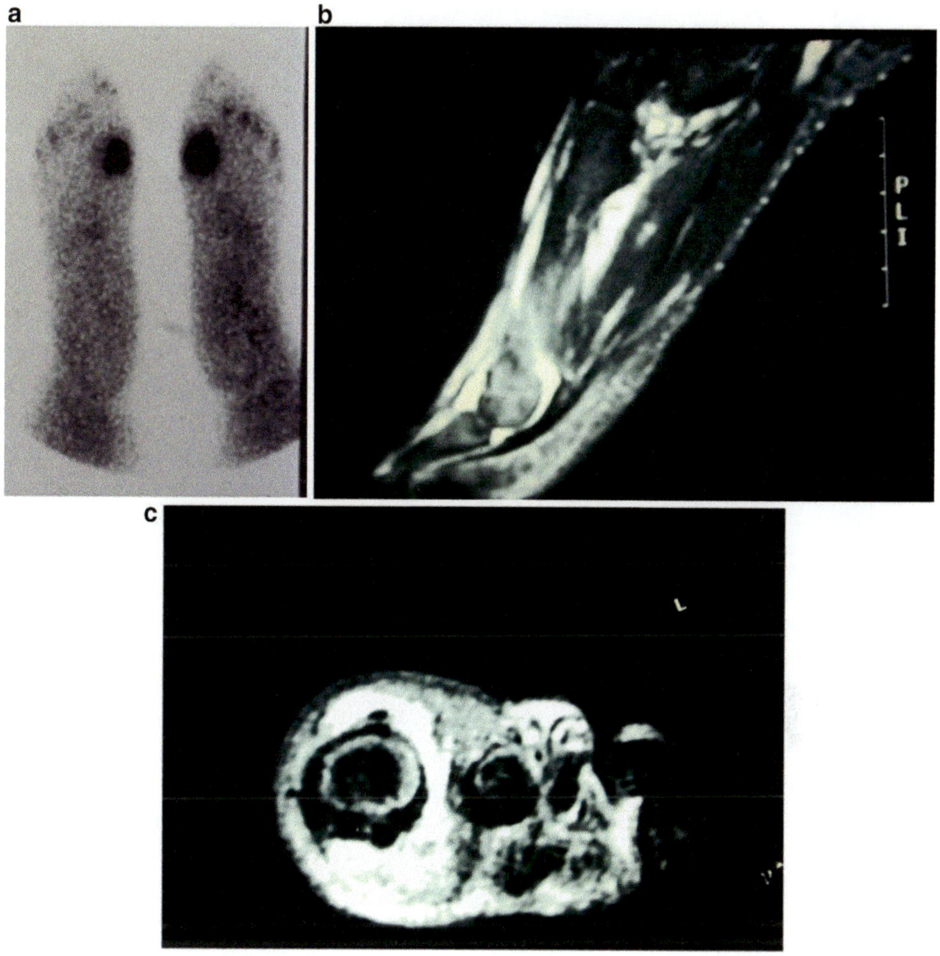

Fig. 5.10 (**a**) Patient is status post 4 weeks bilateral bunionectomy. She presented with localized erythema and edema and increased pain. This technetium bone scan was read as positive for osteomyelitis. (**b**) and (**c**) An MRI was performed on the same patient showing an increased signal intensity of the soft tissues surrounding the first metatarsophalangeal joint but no extension into the bone. This proves that the bone scan was a false-positive result and should not be utilized in the postoperative phase

Ideally, multiple culture samples should be taken from any tissues with suspected infection and with two or more cultures positive for the same species being highly indicative that infection is present and the identified pathogen is responsible [57]. Depending on the type of suspected infection, this may include sterilely acquired aspirate of any fluid collection, direct fluid sampling from a sinus tract to its terminal recess, tissue specimens from surgical debridement, and blood cultures. When hardware infection is suspected, it is recommended that five to six cultures be taken to adequately represent the infected area about the hardware.

The most common organisms responsible for postoperative infections are gram-positive agents including *Staphylococci* and *Streptococci* species, followed by the gram-negative organisms such as *Escherichia coli.* Postsurgical tissue infected with colonized *Staphylococcus* becomes intensely erythematous, edematous, and tender. Abscesses may then form consisting of either a thick, creamy, yellow purulence commonly seen with *S. aureus* or a white-colored purulence if *S. epidermidis* is present. The gas-forming gram-positive species, *Clostridium perfringens*, is a less common but potentially devastating organism which can cause gas gangrene or necrotizing fasciitis and should therefore be treated with extreme prudence. In rare cases, necrotizing fasciitis can also be caused by particularly virulent strains of *Streptococcus pyogenes* or *Staphylococcus aureus* (Fig. 5.11). Gram-positive cocci remain the most common bacteria associated with postoperative osteomyelitis [75]. *S. aureus, S. epidermidis*, and *Streptococcal* species account for up to 73% of the osteomyelitis following musculoskeletal surgery [76].

When prostheses or other hardware is involved, biofilms can present other unique challenges. Biofilms are formed when bacteria colonize implanted synthetic material, bind host fibrinogen and fibronectin, and produce barriers of protein complexes. These biofilm barriers impair both antibiotics and components of the host immune system and therefore complicate management of the infection [77, 78]. In prosthetic joint infections, the most common biofilm-producing agents include staphylococcal species such as *S. aureus* and *S. epidermidis* [79.

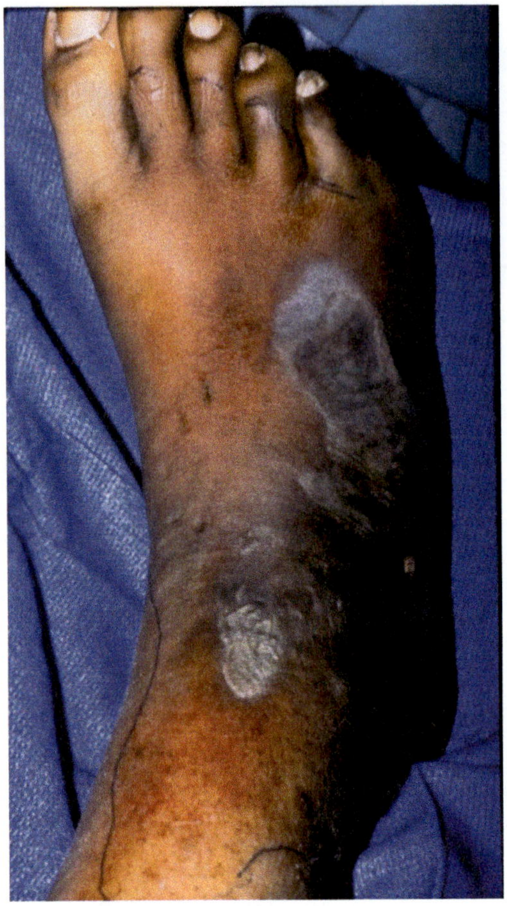

Fig. 5.11 Patient with severe infection, necrotizing fasciitis, and status post lateral ankle surgery

Arthrocentesis and Joint Fluid Analysis

Arthrocentesis is a critically important diagnostic procedure which is used to analyze and culture the joint space fluid in cases of suspected septic arthritis [80, 81]. Many physicians are hesitant to proceed with arthrocentesis due to the possibility of iatrogenic contamination or "seeding the joint," but the evidence shows that this is not a common occurrence. In a retrospective study by Geirsson et al., incidence of iatrogenic infection during joint fluid aspiration was only 0.037% [82]. Relative contraindications include anticoagulation or overlying infection, but this should be weighed against the indication of the procedure for diagnosing septic arthritis. The aspiration should be done in an aseptic manner and may be facilitated by ultrasound guidance. The collected fluid sample should be sent for gram stain, cytology, crystal analysis under polarized light, and culture with sensitivities. The Infectious Diseases Society of America recommends that antibiotics be stopped 2 weeks before the recovery of joint fluid whenever possible, in order to maximize the chances of a positive culture [40]. In cases where this is not feasible, Von Essen et al. showed that blood agar bottles can be utilized in place of traditional agar plates to grow aspirated samples with high dependability. This method was able to more accurately isolate organisms in patients receiving antibiotic therapy, compared to samples which had previously yielded negative results using conventional methods [83].

A typical septic joint will have a turbid appearance and a WBC count >50,000 mm^{-3}. It does however need to be correlated with other elements of the patient's presentation. Van der Bruggen et al. showed that a synovial fluid sample containing a WBC >9000/μl, in combination with an elevated ESR and CRP, had a 100% positive predictive value and 98% accuracy for detecting prosthetic joint infection [67]. Recently, molecular testing has become more commonplace in the diagnosis of acute infection. A wide array of PCR techniques have been developed for rapid diagnosis of pathological presence. However, simply having the DNA of pathologies in a sample can still result from contamination. At this time, PCR is recommended for those cases when infection is highly suspected but cultures have produced a negative result. The PCR should be calibrated to include staphylococcal and streptococcal species as well as any other common organisms found in a regional antibiogram.

A different profile of pathogens should be considered when septic arthritis is suspected. While MSSA is still the most common causative organism present in over one-third of reported cases, and up to 70% of pediatric cases [39, 84–86], there has been a recent increase in the proportion of cases caused by MRSA, such that it is now attributed to approximately 25% of all cases [39, 84, 86]. Other causative agents in order of frequency include *Streptococcus* species and gram-negative cocci such as *Escherichia coli*, *Proteus mirabilis*, *Klebsiella*, and *Enterobacter*, which are involved in about 20% of septic arthritis cases [64]. Additionally, anaerobic and biofilm-forming microorganisms should be considered when hardware or prostheses are present [87].

Types of Infections

Surgical site infections are classified by the level of tissue that they affect and include superficial incisional, deep incisional, and organ/space infections [38]. Superficial incisional infections involve only the skin and subcutaneous structures and are diagnosed within 30 days of the initial surgical intervention by the presence of any one of the following criteria: (1) purulent drainage from the surgical site; (2) microorganisms aseptically obtained from the superficial incisional site; (3) clinical findings of erythema, pain, or edema at the incision site and a positive culture after intentional opening of the incision site by a surgeon; and (4) clinical diagnosis by a surgeon or physician based on experience.

Deep incisional infections involve deeper layers of the incision, such as muscle and facial layers, and present up to

1 year after surgical placement of implanted devices or hardware or within 30 days of most other types of surgery. The findings associated with this infection are the same as for superficial incisional infections, with addition of clinical signs of abscess formation, imaging results that suggest deep involvement, or spontaneous dehiscence of the incision.

Organ/space infections involve deep intra-compartmental tissues and structures which were surgically manipulated at the time of the intervention. In the realm of foot and ankle surgery, some examples include joint infections, osteomyelitis, and orthopedic hardware or prosthesis infections. Like deep incisional infections, organ/space infections also present up to 1 year after surgical placement of implanted devices or hardware, or within 30 days of most other types of surgery [38].

Management

Initial Approach

Suspicion of infection should prompt the surgeon to consider appropriate antibiotic and surgical management options and hospital admission options for serious infections requiring parenteral administration or interdisciplinary approaches. Antibiotic selections will be discussed, as will surgical considerations for special circumstances such as osteomyelitis, hardware infections, and septic arthritis. Patients should be informed about the nature and expected course of their infection, risks and benefits of available management options including any expected patient responsibilities, and the possibility that multiple-staged interventions may be necessary to achieve full resolution.

Antibiotic Management

According to the Infectious Diseases Society of America's guidelines on surgical site infections, a patient presenting after a clean orthopedic procedure with a temperature >38.5°C, heart rate >110 bpm, or erythema extending beyond the wound margins for >5 cm should be started on a short course of intravenous antibiotic therapy targeted against *Staphylococcus aureus* and *Staphylococcus epidermidis*. A first-generation cephalosporin or any agent which is effective against methicillin-susceptible *Staphylococcus aureus* (*MSSA*) is acceptable [41].

Coverage for methicillin-resistant *Staphylococcus aureus* (*MRSA*) is not routinely recommended and should only be utilized when specific risk factors are present—these include positive nasal colonization for MRSA, a prior MRSA infection, recent hospitalization, or recent antibiotic treatment [88, 89]. When indicated, coverage for MRSA can be achieved with vancomycin, daptomycin, linezolid, or ceftaroline. The addition of piperacillin-tazobactam, a carbapenem, or ceftriaxone and metronidazole may sometimes be warranted to cover for gram-negative and anaerobic infections, such as in cases where the surgical wound has been complicated by exposure to the exogenous environment or contaminated bodily fluids [41]. The addition of these antibiotics may also be preferable for immunocompromised patients, including those with diabetes mellitus, in order to provide broader coverage until culture and sensitivity results have been obtained.

Septic arthritis is an exception to many of these general guidelines. While there are conflicting guidelines on this topic, it is the author's belief that septic arthritis should be initially treated with broad-spectrum antibiotics to cover both MRSA and gram-negative agents, due to the higher prevalence of these organisms in joint infections as previously discussed.

When biofilms are likely, such as in the presence of hardware or prostheses, the minimum inhibitory concentration (MIC) may be increased by factors of 10–1000. This is due to antagonism of antibiotic mechanisms by biofilm proteins, rather than a lack of penetration as is commonly believed [90]. Such cases may require prolonged use of oral antimicrobial agents and combination therapy in order to achieve long-term suppression of biofilm-producing organisms [40]. Additionally, agents such as rifampin may be used as an adjunct, resulting in biofilm penetration and superior bactericidal effects against staphylococcal species when used with agents such as cephalosporins, linezolid, daptomycin, and vancomycin [91].

As culture results become available, the antimicrobial regimen should be adapted as needed to target the identified pathogens. Responsiveness to the selected treatment regimen should be gauged by frequent reevaluations of the patient's clinical course, as well as trends in WBC count/differential and inflammatory markers. Antibiotics are continued until there has been satisfactory resolution of the clinical signs of infection, imaging studies do not show any further evidence of soft tissue or osseous infection, and laboratory values are within an acceptable range. This can be several weeks for soft tissue infections and up to 6 weeks for osteomyelitis. For high-risk patients or those who do not respond to initial treatments as expected, it is recommended that the treatment team include an infectious disease specialist moving forward.

Surgical Management

Abscess formation, osteomyelitis, and infected retained hardware should be part of the differential diagnosis if the patient has not responded adequately to antibiotic therapy and/or local wound care measures when treating a postoperative

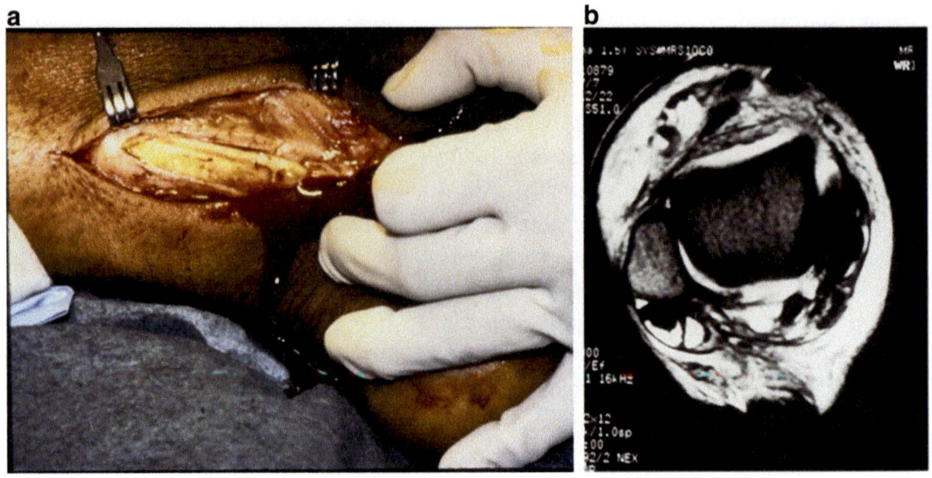

Fig. 5.12 (**a**) Incision of the peroneal tendon sheath expressed significant purulent drainage. (**b**) MRI with increased signal intensity confirming infection along the peroneal tendon sheath

infection. The surgeon should perform any necessary laboratory studies and imaging to help aid in a working diagnosis and plan on surgical intervention.

Management of Abscesses and Soft Tissue Infections

When a postoperative abscess or deep soft tissue infection is present, incision and drainage is necessary. Complete release of tension and expression of all drainage is crucial. The incision should continue until the wound has been adequately decompressed. Infections often track along tendon sheaths so special attention should be made to inspect these structures and ensure satisfactory drainage (Fig. 5.12). While multiple debridements are usually needed to contain infection, the initial procedure should include decompression, acquisition of deep tissue cultures, and debridement of all necrotic and nonviable tissue, leaving only healthy tissue with viable borders. It is recommended to leave vital structures such as neurovascular tissue whenever possible, due to its important role in future healing.

In order to adequately reduce the bacterial burden in the tissues, copious lavage with several liters of normal saline should be performed twice, once prior to taking deep cultures and again after debridement prior to concluding the procedure. The quantity of the solution is more important than the type of solution for irrigation. Antibiotic-impregnated irrigation is not necessary and has little advantage over normal saline solution because the antibiotic is not in contact with the soft tissues for any sufficient amount of time. The irrigation solution should also be delivered under high pressure providing mechanical debridement of the site. This is best accomplished with a Pulsed Lavage apparatus, but if unavailable an 18-gauge needle and 20–50 cc syringe can be utilized.

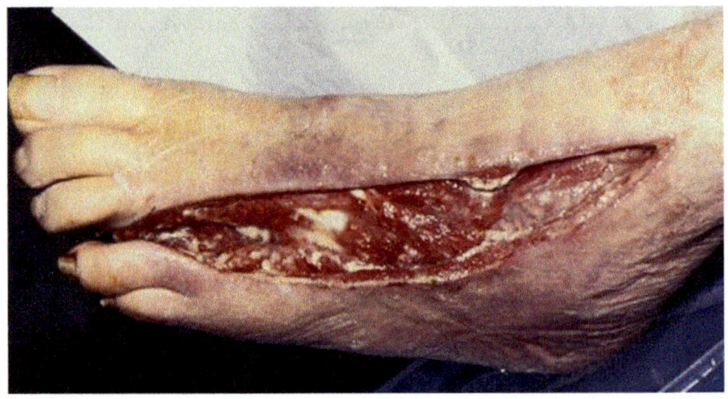

Fig. 5.13 Patient is status post 5 days incision and drainage of abscess following neuroma excision. The wound now displays healthy, red granulation tissue, no drainage, and resolved cellulitis and is now ready for delayed primary closure

Any foreign material must be removed, and an open passage must remain in the wound to allow for continued drainage and resolution of the infection. The wound is usually packed open with gauze-type material, and daily dressing changes and wound care are performed. Once the wound appearance is satisfactory, it may be closed by delayed primary repair or allowed to close through secondary intention. The wound should show no signs of necrosis, purulence, or erythema prior to closure (Fig. 5.13). Mild edema and serous-type drainage secondary to the inflammatory process are acceptable for wound closure.

Management of Osteomyelitis

When the infection has progressed beyond the soft tissue level and osseous involvement has occurred, debridement of necrotic and nonviable bone is mandated. Debridement of bone should be carried out until there is evidence of healthy, bleeding osseous surfaces (Fig. 5.14). Simpson et al. recommends excision of bone with a 5 mm clear border to ensure

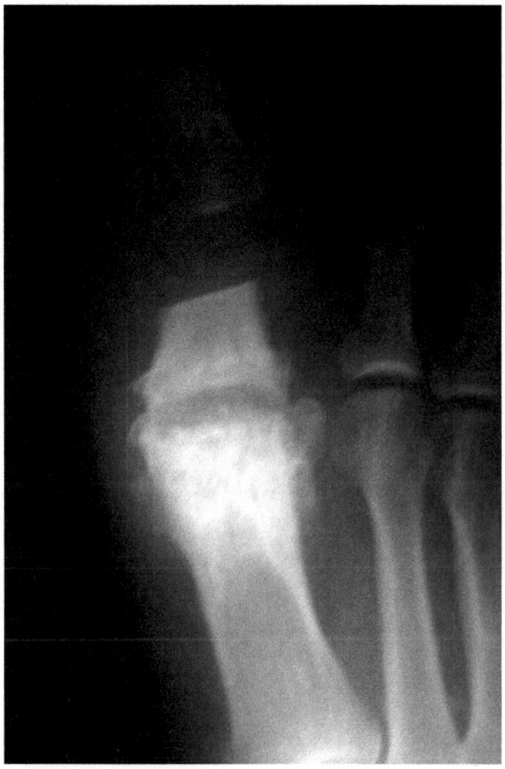

Fig. 5.14 Radiograph displaying successful resection of osteomyelitis of the proximal phalanx of the hallux. Well-delineated osseous border remains with no further evidence of cortical erosion or osteolysis

eradication of the osteomyelitis and minimize the risk of recurrence [92]. The bone should also be explored for a medullary or subperiosteal abscess. The periosteal tissue can be incised, any medullary abscess drained, and any areas of devitalized or detached bone excised. Failure to remove any areas of infection or necrotic tissue may result in a delayed response or poor outcome. It may take several debridements to adequately resect all infected and nonviable bone.

When large portions of bone are removed due to infection, parenteral antibiotic treatment can be augmented with antibiotic-impregnated cement beads or spacers such as polymethyl methacrylate, placed within the tissue and bone void in between debridement margins (Fig. 5.15). The incorporated antibiotic should be heat liable, such as tobramycin and vancomycin. After confirmation that the wound has been cleared of infection, a late-staged fusion with autogenous bone graft and spanning internal fixation is a viable option [93]. Alternatively, if the patient is unable to undergo a harvest procedure, several allografts can be used. In this case, auto-populating the allograft with bone marrow aspirate from the calcaneus or distal tibia can increase the healing potential and help avoid a nonunion, especially in cases involving large-spanning defects.

Management of Hardware Infections

When hardware is involved, infection at any point prior to osseous union may contribute to morbidity and negatively affect long-term function. The question of whether to remove or retain hardware should depend on the integrity of the contiguous bone, the hardware function, and the time frame of the infection (Fig. 5.16). For acute infections occurring within 6 weeks of the primary procedure, where hardware is stabilizing a healing fracture, fusion, or osteotomy site which has not yet incorporated, it is recommended to temporarily retain the hardware. There is relative confidence that the infection can be managed and suppressed with parenteral antibiotics and aggressive serial debridements as needed [2, 3, 57, 94–96]. Once the bone has fully healed, as evidenced by callus crossbridging and pain-free weight-bearing, it is recommended that hardware be removed, as retention beyond this point has been linked to a very high rate of recurrent infections [94, 97–99].

In cases involving gross instability of the bony interphase or gapping osteomyelitis, hardware should be removed and the site secured with external fixation whenever possible [97]. At this point, treatment should focus on the eradication of infection, with the goal of reconstructive salvage at a later point.

Management of Septic Arthritis

Septic arthritis is characterized by bacterial infection within the joint space, leading to joint effusion which increases intra-articular pressure. When intra-articular pressure surpasses local arterial pressures, the cartilage becomes underperfused, resulting in cell death and subsequent synovium breakdown [64, 100, 101]. Postoperative joint infections are serious complications which can be life-altering due to their ability to destroy normal joint anatomy and function and life-threatening due to the potential of conversion to systemic infection. Inpatient mortality rates associated with septic joints can reach 15%, with increased chances of deleterious outcomes correlated to a delay in either diagnosis or treatment [102–104]. Therefore, detection and management of septic arthritis require keen clinical judgment and rapid deployment of appropriate management strategies.

Postoperative septic arthritis can be caused by iatrogenic contamination during the surgical procedure [100] which usually occurs through a break in sterile technique or by transfer of bacteria from superficial tissues into the joint space during an otherwise sterile procedure. Alternatively, it can be caused by contiguous spread from a nearby infection or hematogenous spread from a remote infection, due to a lack of a basement membrane at the cartilage-joint interface [73].

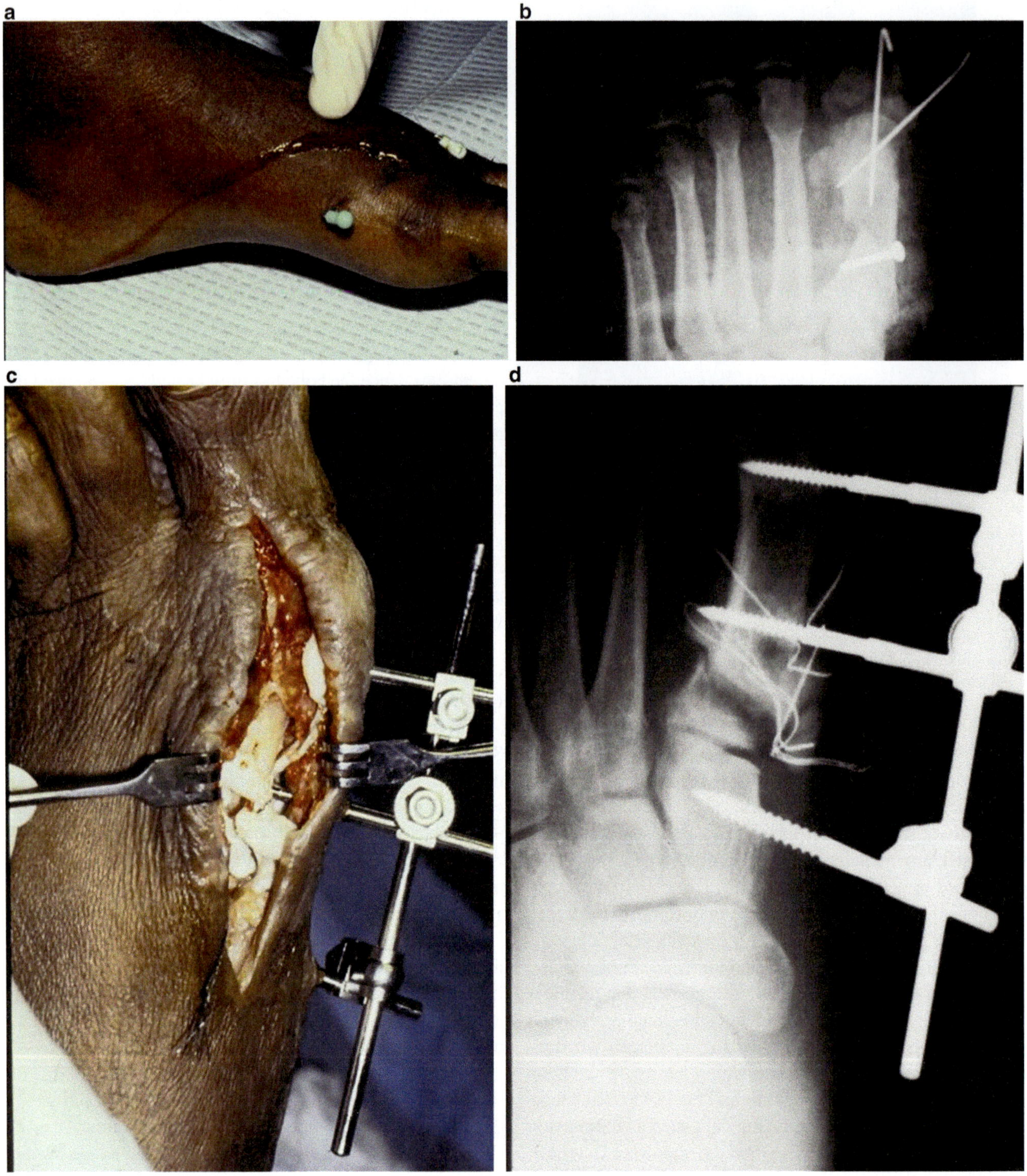

Fig. 5.15 (**a**) and (**b**) Patient status post bunionectomy with purulent drainage, unstable fixation, and obvious extensive infection. (**c**) and (**d**) Incision and drainage was performed, and all nonviable tissue and unstable internal fixation was removed. The wound was packed with antibiotic-impregnated PMMA beads, and osseous structure and integrity was maintained with external fixation

When septic arthritis is suspected, an arthrocentesis should be performed to confirm the diagnosis and identify the pathogen, as previously discussed. Prompt intervention should be undertaken with a three-pronged approach: administration of parenteral antibiotics, evacuation of purulent material, and debridement of nonviable tissue (Fig. 5.17). In the ankle joint, arthroscopic lavage should be performed with at least three liters of normal saline. Other joints, however, are best

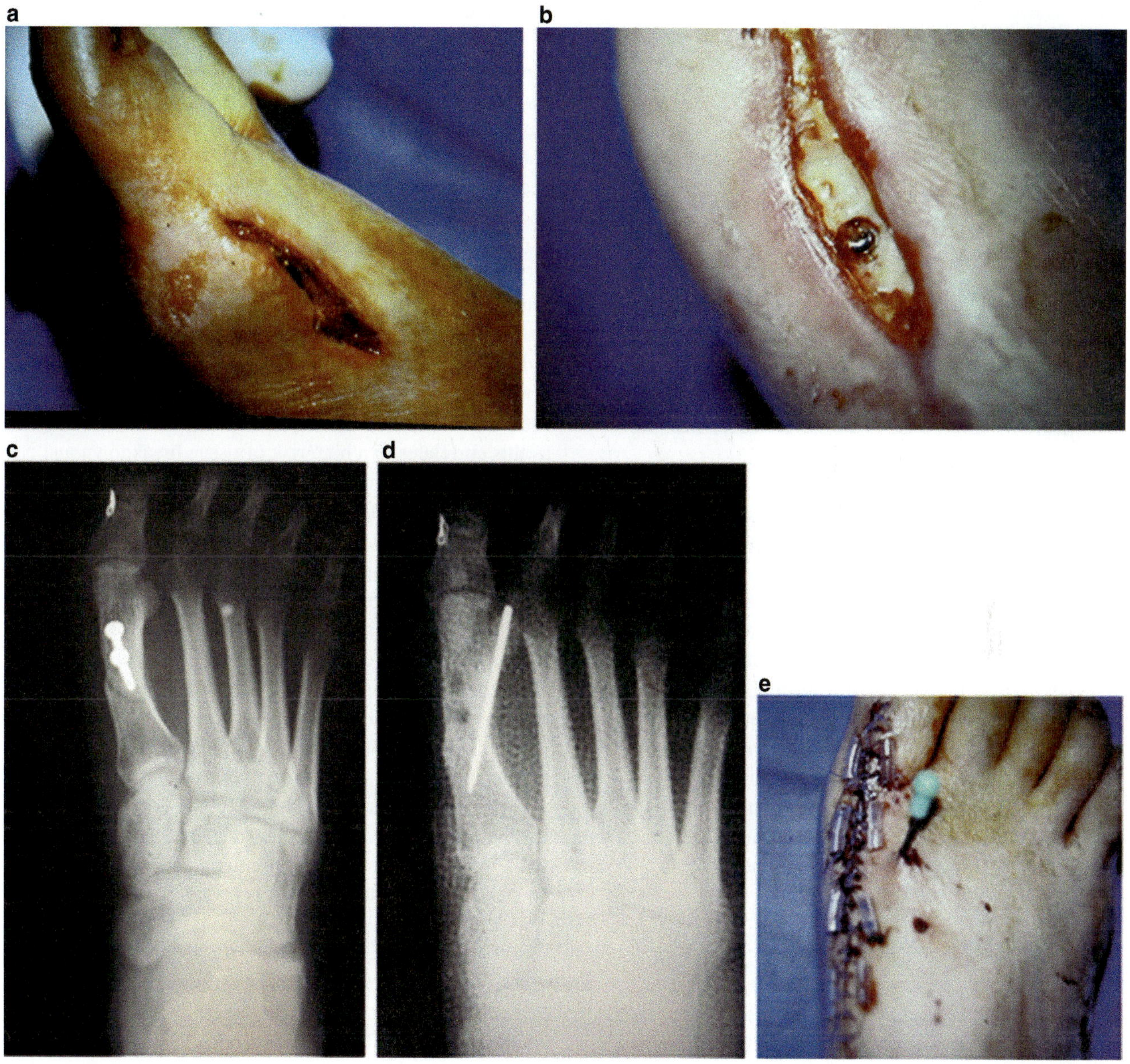

Fig. 5.16 (**a**) and (**b**) Patient had wound dehiscence 3 weeks status post bunionectomy. Oral antibiotics and local wound care were performed. The internal fixation (screw head) can be visualized in the wound. Fixation was maintained initially but then became loose and unstable over the ensuing weeks. (**c**)and (**d**) Patient was taken to the OR 6 weeks after the initial surgery. The screws were removed, and a percutaneous K-wire was placed to aid in stability until complete osseous union was achieved. (**e**) The wound was excised, and delayed primary closure was obtained with reduction of tension along the wound edges

evaluated utilizing an open method. When attempted arthroscopically, complications which warrant immediate conversion to open debridement include concurrent observed articular damage and osteomyelitis [105]. Furthermore, aspiration is not recommended as a primary means of treatment for post-surgical septic arthritis, as visualization and inspection of the joint surfaces is strongly encouraged in order to evaluate and debride any damaged cartilage and surrounding soft tissue.

Management of Prosthetic Joint Infections

Management of septic joints becomes more complicated when a prosthesis is involved. For patients with suspected prosthetic joint infection (PJI), it is critical to take a team-based approach, using the services and expertise of surgeons, infectious disease specialists, radiologists, and plastic surgeons, in order to obtain optimal outcomes.

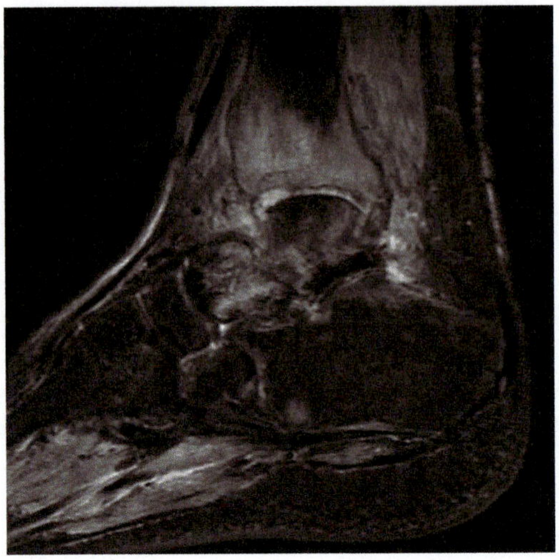

Fig. 5.17 Septic arthritis of the ankle on MRI. Infection occurred after hardware removal following talocalcaneal arthrodesis. Noted osseous changes of the tibia and talus as well as increased signal intensity in the tibiotalar joint

Open surgical debridement is the standard of care and should ideally include 3–6 culture samples. These cultures should be taken directly around multiple periprosthetic tissue sites and from the prosthetic itself to ensure optimal comparison to presurgical arthrocentesis results. The least invasive method for addressing PJI is debridement, antibiotics, and implant retention (DAIR), which is a reasonable strategy in patients who present with a fixed implant without migration or sinus tract, within 30 days of initial implantation and less than 3 weeks from onset of symptoms [40].

More aggressive treatment consists of single- or double-stage revisions. Single-stage revisions are best suited to cases in which there is good bone stock, adequate soft tissue coverage, and a pathogenic organism which has been identified preoperatively and is susceptible to orally bioavailable antibiotics. In addition, the exchanged implant should contain antibiotic-impregnated bone cement. In contrast, a two-stage revision is indicated in circumstances where there is poor soft tissue coverage or there are resistant organisms, in which no prior two-stage revision has been attempted, reimplantation of new prosthetic over a prolonged period of time is viable, and there is a functionally good outcome anticipated [40].

In some patients, permanent resection of the joint area is indicated. This is reasonable in patients who are nonambulatory, with poor soft tissue coverage and pathogens which are highly resistant to antibacterial therapy. Patients who are unable to proceed with the obligatory multiple surgical exchange, or those who have previously failed an attempted two-stage revision, are also better suited to this strategy due to a high risk of reinfection [40].

Continued Wound Management

Sometimes, adequate debridement will result in a significant wound defect in which deep tissues are open to the outside environment. These wounds, as with any infections, should not be closed primarily but allowed to drain during the initial healing process, with regular dressing changes to promote declaration of viable tissues. If enough soft tissue is present at the resolution of infection, delayed primary closure can be utilized to ultimately cover the wound and reduce the risk of reinfection. This is preferable to delayed secondary intention closure methods, in which the superficial skin is left open indefinitely while healing occurs from the wound margins inward. However, delayed primary closure should not be used when it would cause high tension at the wound margins, as this correlates to a high risk of tissue breakdown and can lead to recurrent infection. Instead, if there is not enough native tissue to close the defect, negative-pressure wound care therapy should be employed to provide coverage of the wound site and promote new, healthy granular tissue. After suitable granulation tissue has formed, definitive coverage with a split-thickness skin graft is recommended [106–110]. In addition to these considerations, large defects can result in vascular compromise and may require a pedicle free flap with intact and independent blood supply. Amputation can unfortunately, ultimately result but should be a last resort after other strategies have failed.

Once definitive surgical intervention has been completed, antibiotics are typically continued over the ensuing weeks until infectious signs and symptoms including erythema, edema, drainage, and pain have subsided. The patient should also be monitored for signs of infection recurrence. This should include trending of vital signs and laboratory values, which should show a steady normalization of any previously evident inflammatory changes (such as increased WBC count, ESR, and CRP), repeat imaging studies as necessary, and reevaluation of the postoperative sight. Patients should have increased range of motion with reduced pain, over a time frame of days to weeks. Early physical therapy can provide better postoperative outcomes, and the patient should slowly progress back to normal function.

Conclusion

Postoperative infections pose a variety of challenges to the foot and ankle surgeon. With a proactive approach of careful patient selection, modification of risk factors such as blood glucose control and smoking cessation, and implementation of presurgical protocols, these incidences can be minimized. Successful management of this complication is hinged on the practitioner's ability to identify the infection quickly, using appropriate laboratory, imaging, and culturing modalities.

Multimodal management strategies, including multispecialty teams, timely antibiotic implementation, and surgical intervention, are paramount to a favorable outcome.

References

1. Butterworth P, Gilheany MF. Postoperative infection rates in foot and ankle surgery: a clinical audit of Australian podiatric surgeons, January to December 2007. Aust Health Rev. 2010;34(2):180–5.
2. Berkes M, Obremskey WT, Southeast Fracture Consortium. Maintenance of hardware after early postoperative infection following fracture internal fixation. J Bone Joint Surg Am. 2010;92(4):823–8.
3. Zalavras CG, Christensen T. Infection following operative treatment of ankle fractures. Clin Orthop Relat Res. 2009;467:1715–20.
4. Wukich DK, Lowery NJ. Postoperative infection rates in foot and ankle surgery: a comparison of patients with and without diabetes mellitus. J Bone Joint Surg Am. 2010;92(2):287–95.
5. Wukich DK, McMillen RL. Surgical site infections after foot and ankle surgery: a comparison of patients with and without diabetes. Diabetes Care. 2011;34(10):2211–3.
6. Wukich DK, Crim BE. Neuropathy and poorly controlled diabetes increase the rate of surgical site infection after foot and ankle surgery. J Bone Joint Surg Am. 2014;96(10):832–9.
7. Wukich DK, Joseph A. Outcomes of ankle fractures in patients with uncomplicated versus complicated diabetes. Foot Ankle Int. 2011;32(2):120–30.
8. Jupiter DC, Humphers JM. Trends in postoperative infection rates and their relationship to glycosylated hemoglobin levels in diabetic patients undergoing foot and ankle surgery. J Foot Ankle Surg. 2014;53(3):307–11.
9. Humphers JM, Shibuya N. The impact of glycosylated hemoglobin and diabetes mellitus on wound-healing complications and infection after foot and ankle surgery. J Am Podiatr Med Assoc. 2014;104(4):320–9.
10. Furnary AP, Wu Y. Eliminating the diabetic disadvantage: the portland diabetic project. Semin Thorac Cardiovasc Surg. 2006; 18(4):302–8.
11. Haskins IN, Amdur R. The effect of smoking on bariatric surgical outcomes. Surg Endosc. 2014;28(11):3074–80.
12. Durand F, Berthelot P. Smoking is a risk factor of organ/space surgical site infection in orthopaedic surgery with implant materials. Int Orthop. 2013;37(4):723–7.
13. Duchman KR, Gao Y. The effect of smoking on short-term complications following total hip and knee arthroplasty. J Bone Joint Surg Am. 2015;97(13):1049–58.
14. Jain RK, Shukla R. Epidemiology and risk factors for surgical site infections in patients requiring orthopedic surgery. Eur J Orthop Surg Traumatol. 2015;25(2):251–4.
15. Bydon M, Macki M, De la Garza-Ramos R. Smoking as an independent predictor of reoperation after lumbar laminectomy: a study of 500 cases. J Neurosurg Spine. 2015;22(3):288–93.
16. Sørensen LT. Wound healing and infection in surgery. The clinical impact of smoking and smoking cessation: a systematic review and meta-analysis. Arch Surg. 2012;147(4):373–83.
17. Bettin CC, Gower K. Cigarette smoking increases complication rate in forefoot surgery. Foot Ankle Int. 2015;36(5):488–93.
18. Sørensen LT, Toft B. Smoking attenuates wound inflammation and proliferation while smoking cessation restores inflammation but not proliferation. Wound Repair Regen. 2010;18(2):186–92.
19. Webb AR, Robertson N. Smokers know little of their increased surgical risks and may quit on surgical advice. ANZ J Surg. 2013;83(10):753–7.
20. Dayton P, DeVries JG. American college of foot and ankle surgeons' clinical consensus statement: perioperative prophylactic antibiotic use in clean elective foot surgery. J Foot Ankle Surg. 2015; 54(2):273–9.
21. Bratzler DW, Dellinger EP, Olsen KM, Perl TM, Auwaerter PG, Bolon MK, Fish DN, Napolitano LM, Sawyer RG, Slain D, Steinberg JP, Weinstein RA, American Society of Health-System Pharmacists (ASHP), Infectious Diseases Society of America (IDSA), Surgical Infection Society (SIS), Society for Healthcare Epidemiology of America (SHEA). Clinical practice guidelines for antimicrobial prophylaxis in surgery. Surg Infect. 2013;14(1):73–156.
22. Bibbo C, Patel DV. Chlorhexidine provides superior skin decontamination in foot and ankle surgery. Clin Orthop Relat Res. 2005;438:204–8.
23. Yammine K, Harvey A. Efficacy of preparation solutions and cleansing techniques on contamination of the skin in foot and ankle surgery: A systematic review and meta-analysis. Bone Joint J. 2013;95-B(4):498–503.
24. Scowcroft T. A critical review of the literature regarding the use of povidone iodine chlorhexidine gluconate for preoperative surgical skin preparation. J Perioper Pract. 2012;22(3):95–9.
25. Dumville JC, McFarlane E. Preoperative skin antiseptics for preventing surgical wound infections after clean surgery. Cochrane Database Syst Rev. 2015;2015:CD003949.
26. Ostrander RV, Botte MJ. Efficacy of surgical preparation solutions in foot and ankle surgery. J Bone Joint Surg Am. 2005;87(5): 980–5.
27. Keblish DJ. Preoperative skin preparation of the foot and ankle: bristles and alcohol are better. J Bone Joint Surg Am. 2005;87(5): 986–92.
28. Ng AB, Adeyemo FO. Preoperative footbaths reduce bacterial colonization of the foot. Foot Ankle Int. 2009;30(9):860–4.
29. Restrepo RD, Wettstein R. Incentive spirometry: 2011. Respir Care. 2011;56(10):1600–4.
30. Nicolle LE. Catheter-related urinary tract infection. Drugs Aging. 2005;22(8):627–39.
31. Ángeles-Garay U, Morales-Márquez LI, Sandoval-Balanzarios MA, Velázquez-García JA, Maldonado-Torres L, Méndez-Cano AF. Risk factors related to surgical site infection in elective surgery. Cir Cir. 2014;82(1):48–62.
32. Kalish JA, Farber F, Sf C. Factors associated with surgical site infection after lower extremity bypass in the Society for Vascular Surgery (SVS) Vascular Quality Initiative (VQI). J Vasc Surg. 2014;60(5):1238–46.
33. Seamon MJ, Jessica W. The effects of intraoperative hypothermia on surgical site infection: an analysis of 524 trauma laparotomies. Ann Surg. 2012;255(4):789–95.
34. Mazzeffi M, Zivot J. In-hospital mortality after cardiac surgery: patient characteristics, timing, and association with postoperative length of intensive care unit and hospital stay. Ann Thorac Surg. 2014;97(4):1220–5.
35. Gustilo RB, Anderson JT. Prevention of infection in the treatment of one thousand and twenty-five open fractures of long bones: retrospective and prospective analyses. J Bone Joint Surg Am. 1976;58(4):453–8.
36. Castillo RC, Bosse MJ, Group L S. Impact of smoking on fracture healing and risk of complications in limb-threatening open tibia fractures. J Orthop Trauma. 2005;19(3):151–7.
37. Dellinger EP. Surgical site infections. In: Jong EC, Stevens DL, editors. Netter's infectious diseases. Philadelphia: Elsevier; 2012. p. 295–8.
38. Mangram AJ, Horan TC. Guideline for prevention of surgical site infection, 1999. Centers for Disease Control and Prevention (CDC) hospital infection control practices advisory committee. Am J Infect Control. 1999;27(2):97–132. 97-132

39. Dubost JJ, Couderc M. Three-decade trends in the distribution of organisms causing septic arthritis in native joints: single-center study of 374 cases. Joint Bone Spine. 2014;81(5):438–40.
40. Osmon DR, Berbari EF, America ID. Executive summary: diagnosis and management of prosthetic joint infection: clinical practice guidelines by the Infectious Diseases Society of America. Clin Infect Dis. 2013;56(1):1–10.
41. Stevens DL, Bisno AL. Practice guidelines for the diagnosis and management of skin and soft tissue infections: 2014 update by the Infectious Diseases Society of America. Clin Infect Dis. 2014;59(2):e10–52.
42. Carpenter CR, Schuur JD. Evidence-based diagnostics: adult septic arthritis. Acad Emerg Med. 2011;18(8):781–96.
43. Li SF, Cassidy C. Diagnostic utility of laboratory tests in septic arthritis. Emerg Med J. 2007;24(2):75–7.
44. Lipsky B. Bone of contention: diagnosing diabetic foot osteomyelitis. Clin Infect Dis. 2008;47(4):528–30.
45. Karr J. The diagnosis of osteomyelitis in diabetes using erythrocyte sedimentation rate. J Am Podiatr Med Assoc. 2002;92(5):314.
46. Caird MS, Flynn JM. Factors distinguishing septic arthritis from transient synovitis of the hip in children. A prospective study. J Bone Joint Surg Am. 2006;88(6):1251–7.
47. Kang BU, Lee S-H. Surgical site infection in spinal surgery: detection and management based on. J Neurosurg Spine. 2010;13(2):158–64.
48. Neumaier M, Scherer MA. C-reactive protein levels for early detection of postoperative infection after fracture surgery in 787 patients. Acta Orthop. 2008;79(3):428–32.
49. Santonocito C, De Loecker L. C-reactive protein kinetics after major surgery. Anesth Analg. 2014;119(3):624–9.
50. Nunes BK, Lacerda RA. Systematic review and meta-analysis of the predictive value of C-reactive protein in postoperative infections. Rev Esc Enferm USP. 2011;45(6):1488–94.
51. Laporta Baez Y, Palomero R. C-reactive protein in the diagnosis of postoperative infection in pediatric. J Pediatr Surg. 2011; 46(9):1726–31.
52. Hartley JC, Harris KA. Molecular techniques for diagnosing prosthetic joint infections. J Antimicrob Chemother. 2014;69(Suppl 1):i21–4.
53. Saeed K. Diagnostics in prosthetic joint infections. J Antimicrob Chemother. 2014;69(Suppl 1):11–9.
54. Patel R, Osmon DR. The diagnosis of prosthetic joint infection: current techniques and emerging technologies. Clin Orthop Relat Res. 2005; 437:55–8.
55. Trampuz A, Osmon DR. Molecular and antibiofilm approaches to prosthetic joint infection. Clin Orthop Relat Res. 2003; 414: 69–88.
56. Mikkelsen ME, Miltiades AN. Serum lactate is associated with mortality in severe sepsis independent of organ failure and shock. Crit Care Med. 2009;37(5):1670–7.
57. Trebse R, Pisot V. Treatment of infected retained implants. J Bone Joint Surg Br. 2005;87(2):249–56.
58. Buckholz JM. The surgical management of osteomyelitis: with special reference to a surgical classification. J Foot Ankle Surg. 1985;26(Suppl):S17.
59. Maher MM, Gervais DA. The inaccessible or undrainable abscess: how to drain it. Radiographics. 2004;24(3):717–35.
60. Tien YC, Chih HW. Clinical application of ultrasonography for detection of septic arthritis in children. Kaohsiung J Med Sci. 1999;15(9):542–9.
61. Zieger MM, Dorr V. Ultrasonography of hip joint effusions. Skelet Radiol. 1987;16(8):607–11.
62. Seltzer S. Value of computed tomography in planning medical and surgical treatment of chronic osteomyelitis. J Comput Assist Tomogr. 1984;8(3):482–7.
63. Christian S, Kraas J. Musculoskeletal infections. Semin Roentgenol. 2007;42(2):92–101.
64. García-Arias M, Balsa A. Septic arthritis. Best Pract Res Clin Rheumatol. 2011;25(3):407–21.
65. Ahmad FU, Sidani C. Postoperative magnetic resonance imaging artifact with cobalt-chromium versus titanium spinal instrumentation: presented at the 2013 Joint Spine Section Meeting. Clinical article. J Neurosurg Spine. 2013;19(5):629–36.
66. Palestro C, Caprioli R, Love C, et al. Rapid diagnosis of pedal osteomyelitis in diabetics with a technetium-99 m-labeled monoclonal antigranulocyte antibody. J Foot Ankle Surg. 2003;42(1):2–8.
67. van der Bruggen W, Bleeker-Rovers CP. PET and SPECT in osteomyelitis and prosthetic bone and joint infections: a systematic review. Semin Nucl Med. 2010;40(1):3–15.
68. Kapoor A, Page S, LaValley M, et al. Magnetic resonance imaging for diagnosing foot osteomyelitis; a meta-analysis. Arch Intern Med. 2007;167(2):125–32.
69. Jeffcoate WJ, Lipsky BA. Controversies in diagnosing and managing osteomyelitis of the foot in diabetes. Clin Infect Dis. 2004;39(2):115–22.
70. Senneville E, Lombart A. Outcome of diabetic foot osteomyelitis treated nonsurgically: a retrospective cohort study. Diabetes Care. 2008;31(4):637–42.
71. Bernard L, Uçkay I. Two consecutive deep sinus tract cultures predict the pathogen of osteomyelitis. Int J Infect Dis. 2010; 14(5):e390–3.
72. Malone M, Bowling FL. Deep wound cultures correlate well with bone biopsy culture in diabetic foot. Diabetes Metab Res Rev. 2013;29(7):546–50.
73. Goldenberg D. Septic arthritis. Lancet. 1998;351(9097):197–202.
74. March GA, García-Loygorri MC. A new approach to determine the susceptibility of bacteria to antibiotics directly from positive blood culture bottles in two hours. J Microbiol Methods. 2015;109:49–55.
75. Lavery LA, Sariaya M, Ashry H, Harkless LB. Microbiology of osteomyelitis in diabetic foot infections. J Foot Ankle Surg. 1995;34:61–4.
76. Ericson C, Lingren L, Lindberg L. Cloxacillin in the prophylaxis of post-operative infections of the hip. J Bone Joint Surg Am. 1973;55:808–13.
77. Trampuz A, Zimmerli W. Prosthetic joint infections: update in diagnosis and treatment. Swiss Med Wkly. 2005;135(17–18):243–51.
78. Richards JJ, Melander C. Controlling bacterial biofilms. ChemBioChem. 2009;10(14):2287–94.
79. Aparna MS, Yadav S. Biofilms: microbes and disease. Braz J Infect Dis. 2008;12(6):526–30.
80. Ernst AA, Weiss SJ. Usefulness of CRP and ESR in predicting septic joints. South Med J. 2010;103(6):522–6.
81. Mathews CJ, Kingsley G. Management of septic arthritis: a systematic review. Ann Rheum Dis. 2007;66(4):440–5.
82. Geirsson AJ, Statkevicius S. Septic arthritis in Iceland 1990–2002: increasing incidence due to iatrogenic infections. Ann Rheum Dis. 2008;67(5):638–43.
83. von Essen R, Holtta A. Improved method of isolating bacteria from joint fluids by the use of blood culture bottles. Ann Rheum Dis. 1986;45(6):454–7.
84. Frazee BW, Fee C. How common is MRSA in adult septic arthritis? Ann Emerg Med. 2009;54(5):695–700.
85. Dubost JJ, Soubrier M. No changes in the distribution of organisms responsible for septic arthritis over a 20 year period. Ann Rheum Dis. 2002;61(3):267–9.
86. Ross J. Septic arthritis. Infect Dis Clin N Am. 2005;19(4):799–817.
87. Brook I. Microbiology and management of joint and bone infections due to anaerobic bacteria. J Orthop Sci. 2008;13(2):160–9.

88. Gurusamy KS, Koti R. Antibiotic prophylaxis for the prevention of methicillin-resistant *Staphylococcus aureus* (MRSA) related complications in surgical patients. Cochrane Database Syst Rev. 2013;19(8):23959704.
89. Klevens RM, Morrison MA, Investigators AB. Invasive methicillin-resistant *Staphylococcus aureus* infections in the United States. JAMA. 2007;298(15):1763–71.
90. Jacqueline C, Caillon J. Impact of bacterial biofilm on the treatment of prosthetic joint infections. J Antimicrob Chemother. 2014;69(Suppl 1):i37–40.
91. Saginur R, StDenis M. Multiple combination bactericidal testing of staphylococcal biofilms from implant-associated infections. Antimicrob Agents Chemother. 2006;50(1):55–61.
92. Simpson A, Deakin M, Latham J. Chronic osteomyelitis. The effect of the extent of surgical resection on infection-free survival. J Bone Joint Surg Br. 2001;83-B:403–7.
93. Stapleton JJ, Rodriguez RH, Jeffries LC, Zgonis T. Salvage of the first ray with concomitant septic and gouty arthritis by use of a bone block joint distraction arthrodesis and external fixation. Clin Podiatr Med Surg. 2008;25:755–62.
94. Lall RR, Wong AP. Evidence-based management of deep wound infection after spinal instrumentation. J Clin Neurosci. 2015;22(2): 238–42.
95. Marschall B, Obremskey WT. Maintenance of hardware after early postoperative infection following fracture internal fixation. J Bone Joint Surg. 2010;92:823–8.
96. Marsh JL, Saltzman CL. Ankle fractures. In: Heckman JD, Bucholz RW, editors. Rockwood and green's fractures in adults, vol. 2. Philadelphia, PA: Lippincott; 2005. p. 2148–247.
97. Rightmire E, Zurakowski D. Acute infections after fracture repair: management with hardware in place. Clin Orthop Relat Res. 2008;466(2):466–72.
98. Hedequist D, Haugen A. Failure of attempted implant retention in spinal deformity delayed surgical site infections. Spine. 2009; 34(1):60–4.
99. Maruo K, Berven SH. Outcome and treatment of postoperative spine surgical site infections: predictors of treatment success and failure. J Orthop Sci. 2014;19(3):398–404.
100. Morgan DS, Fisher D. An 18 year clinical review of septic arthritis from tropical Australia. Epidemiol Infect. 1996;117(3):423–8.
101. Kaandorp CJ, Van Schaardenburg S. Risk factors for septic arthritis in patients with joint disease. A prospective study. Arthritis Rheum. 1995;38(12):1819–25.
102. Gupta MN, Sturrock RD. A prospective 2-year study of 75 patients with adult-onset septic arthritis. Rheumatology. 2001;40(1): 24–30.
103. Söderquist B, Jones I. Bacterial or crystal-associated arthritis? Discriminating ability of serum inflammatory markers. Scand J Infect Dis. 1998;30(6):591–6.
104. Coakley G, Mathews C, British Society for Rheumatology Standards, Guidelines and Audit Working Group BSR & BHPR, BOA, RCGP and BSAC guidelines for management of the hot swollen joint in adults. Rheumatology. 2006;45(8):1039–41.
105. Shirtliff ME, Mader JT. Acute septic arthritis. Clin Microbiol Rev. 2002;15(4):527–44.
106. Richter D, Hahn MP. Arthrodesis of the infected ankle and subtalar joint: technique, indications and results of 45 consecutive cases. J Trauma. 1999;47(6):1072–8.
107. Pelham FR, Kubiak EN. Topical negative pressure in the treatment of infected wounds with exposed orthopaedic implants. J Wound Care. 2006;15(3):111–6.
108. Patzakis MJ, Zalavras CG. Chronic posttraumatic osteomyelitis and infected nonunion of the tibia: current management concepts. J Am Acad Orthop Surg. 2005;13:417–27.
109. Attinger C, Cooper P. Soft tissue reconstruction for Calcaneal fractures or osteomyelitis. Orthop Clin North Am. 2001;32(1): 135–70.
110. Mullner T, Mrkonjic L. The use of negative pressure to promote the healing of tissue defects: A clinical trial using the vacuum sealing technique. Br J Plast Surg. 1997;50(3):194–9.

Suggested Reading

111. Allareddy V, Das A. Prevalence, predictors, and outcomes of methicillin-resistant *Staphylococcus aureus* infections in patients undergoing major surgical procedures in the United States: a population-based study. Am J Surg. 2015;210(1):59–67.
112. Costerton JW, Stewart PS. Bacterial biofilms: a common cause of persistent infections. Science. 1999;284(5418):1318–22.
113. Gomes F, Teixeira P. Evaluation of antimicrobial activity of certain combinations of antibiotics against in vitro *Staphylococcus epidermidis* biofilms. Indian J Med Res. 2012;135(4):542–7.
114. Kaandorp CJ, Dinant HJ. Incidence and sources of native and prosthetic joint infection: a community based prospective survey. Ann Rheum Dis. 1997;56(8):470–5.
115. Kodumuri P, Geutjens G. Time delay between diagnosis and arthroscopic lavage in septic arthritis. Does it matter? Int Orthop. 2012;36(8):1727–31.
116. Ross JJ, Davidson L. Methicillin-resistant *Staphylococcus aureus* septic arthritis: an emerging clinical syndrome. Rheumatology. 2005;44(9):1197–8.
117. Saleh-Mghir A, Muller-Serieys C. Adjunctive rifampin is crucial to optimizing daptomycin efficacy against rabbit prosthetic joint infection due to methicillin-resistant *Staphylococcus aureus*. Antimicrob Agents Chemother. 2011;55(10):4589–93.
118. Stutz G, Kuster MS. Arthroscopic management of septic arthritis: stages of infection and results. Knee Surg Sports Traumatol Arthrosc. 2000;8(5):270–4.
119. Trampuz A, Hanssen AD. Synovial fluid leukocyte count and differential for the diagnosis of prosthetic knee infection. Am J Med. 2004;117(8):556–62.
120. Zimmerli W, Trampuz A. Prosthetic-joint infections. N Engl J Med. 2004;351(16):1645–54.

Complications Associated with Comorbid Conditions

6

Gage M. Caudell and Mindi Feilmeier

Introduction

Complications after surgery are unfortunately unavoidable. Fortunately, most complications are mild, but in a few, they can have a high mortality. Foot and ankle surgical procedures commonly have a higher risk of surgical site infection in comparison to other orthopedic surgical sites because of the colonization of bacteria [1]. There is evidence that after proper aseptic technique of the foot, a significant amount of bacteria can still be found [1]. When combining these risk factors with a patient's comorbidities, the risk of complications can increase significantly. This chapter will help the foot and ankle surgeon recognize potential risks involving patients with comorbidities.

This chapter will break down comorbid conditions into systemic and autoimmune diseases, chronic infectious disorders, and substance abuse. Many patients undergoing foot and ankle surgery will have multiple comorbid conditions, leading to more risk of complications.

Diabetes

Patients with diabetes are well known to the foot and ankle surgeon. A significant amount of time and effort has been dedicated to efforts to determine the pathomechanics of diabetes in relation to surgery. Even though there is more research to do, the data we have supports that patients with diabetes have a much higher risk of complications, including surgical site infection, in comparison to nondiabetics.

G.M. Caudell (✉)
Fort Wayne Orthopedics, 7601 West Jefferson Blvd, Fort Wayne, IN 46804, USA

M. Feilmeier
School- Des Moines University, College of Podiatric Medicine and Surgery, 3200 Grand Ave, Des Moines, IA 50312, USA
e-mail: Mindi.Feilmeier@dmu.edu

Patients with diabetes whose blood glucose levels regularly average above 200 mg/dl have a higher risk of surgical site infection [2]. In one study looking at cardiac surgery patients, they were able to control other comorbid conditions and concluded that blood glucose levels above 200 mg/dl had a significant risk of infection compared to patients with blood glucose levels below [2]. It is well known that poorly controlled diabetes leads to decreased phagocytosis and bactericidal activity of neutrophils. It has been shown that the threshold of proper neutrophil function is a blood glucose of less than 200 mg/dl [3].

There has been little research looking at surgical site infection in patients who have undergone foot and ankle surgery. One retrospective study looking at 1000 patients showed 2.8% of nondiabetic patients undergoing foot and ankle surgery developed infection compared to 13.2% in patients with diabetes [4]. Also in that study, the author concluded neuropathy as a factor in patients with diabetes developing an infection [4]. This finding is consistent with other research. Patients who do not have neuropathy likely do not have any more risk of infection than a nondiabetic patient [5].

It is our opinion that these patients also have other factors that are difficult to stratify. Oftentimes these patients are noncompliant with taking their medications, thus leading them down a path that includes neuropathy and other comorbid conditions associated with diabetes. If these patients are not compliant with managing their diabetes, one may question their ability to be compliant with instructions after surgery.

Renal Disease

Renal disease is a condition that is often times associated with other comorbidities, such as diabetes, malnutrition, congestive heart failure, anemia, and coronary artery disease. These patients are inherently at risk of complications because they do not properly excrete toxins within the body, often times leading to an impaired immune response. Patients with renal disease are at significant risk of developing renal osteodystrophy, especially in those who are on dialysis.

M.S. Lee, J.P. Grossman (eds.), *Complications in Foot and Ankle Surgery*, DOI 10.1007/978-3-319-53686-6_6

Renal osteodystrophy, also known as chronic kidney disease-mineral and bone disorder (CKD-MBD), causes malabsorption of calcium and phosphorous which leads to thinning of the bone and an increased risk of fracture [6]. It is known that patients with renal disease often times develop calcification of their arteries [7]. Because of this, the risk of wound healing complications significantly rises and makes it challenging for the foot and ankle or orthopedic surgeon to be able to properly manage these musculoskeletal problems in these patients [7]. Other potential causes of increased mortality and morbidity are elevated plasma homocysteine, enhanced coagulability, excess arterial calcification, and endothelial dysfunction [8].

Review of the literature demonstrates no available research looking at foot and ankle surgery and patients with chronic kidney disease. There is research looking at total knee and hip arthroplasty and chronic renal disease. All of these studies are consistent with an increased risk of morbidity/mortality [9]. In a study looking at more than 500 patients with chronic renal disease undergoing elective total joint procedures, there was found to be a significant increase in morbidity after surgery [10].

Current recommendations state that patients who are undergoing elective surgery and have chronic renal disease should receive hemodialysis the day before in order to minimize the adverse effects of fluid and electrolyte abnormalities [11]. The surgeon should weigh the risk of surgery when evaluating these patients.

Obesity

One in five Americans are clinically obese [12]. Obesity is defined as a person with a BMI greater than or equal to 30. It has been reported that obesity will continue to significantly rise over the next 15 years [12]. Most surgeons would conclude that obese patients have a higher risk of complications. This idea, however, is not very well supported in the literature. It is thought that because obese patients have larger amounts of adipose tissue, there is a risk of loss of adherence of the skin to the underlying subcutaneous tissue and this could lead to an increased risk of wound dehiscence and risk of infection [13]. Most obese patients have other comorbid conditions such as diabetes, congestive heart failure, and coronary artery disease. It is because of these additional comorbid conditions that obese patients may have a higher risk of surgical complications.

There are few studies evaluating obesity and foot and ankle surgery. Most studies have looked at obesity and ankle fractures. Many have concluded that obese patients have a higher risk of a more severe fracture [14, 15]. One study compared patients with a BMI less than 30 and a BMI above or equal to 30 and determined that obese patients do not have a higher risk of infection or development of nonunions [15]. Therefore, the current literature does not necessarily support obesity alone as a risk factor for increased surgical complications.

Malnutrition

Patients with protein and vitamin deficiencies are known to have increased risk of surgical complications [16]. It is believed that 50% of hospital patients are malnourished [16, 17]. Key laboratory markers include serum albumin, total lymphocyte count, and transferrin. Transferrin assists in decreasing inflammation as well as in impeding bacterial survival [18]. It has been shown that a transferrin of <226 mg/dL increases the rate of wound complications [19]. Lymphocytes are key to the body's humoral and cell-mediated immunity. A decrease in total lymphocyte count below 1500/mm^3 (1.5…109/L) increases the rate of infection [19]. Protein deficiency interferes with wound healing and humoral and cell-mediated immunity, thus lowering the host resistance and increasing risk of surgical site infection [20]. Serum albumin is one of the key markers used in assessment of nutritional status. Serum albumin of <3.5 g/dL indicates a nutritional deficiency and an increased risk of complications [16, 19]. Albumin, even though a good nutritional marker, also has limitations. It has a long half-life; therefore, it can take time to see the effects of any changes in diet [21]. Prealbumin is a better marker in identifying acute changes in protein because it reaches its peak at 2 days [21]. When evaluating the malnourished patient, a combination of all these markers should be utilized, and a proper consultation with a dietitian should be considered.

Osteoporosis

It is well know that osteoporosis leads to an increased incidence of fractures [22]. It is not well known if osteoporosis increases the risk of surgical complications [22]. Osteoporosis leads to thinning of the cortex and weakening of the bone. After surgical fixation of fractures or in patients undergoing elective orthopedic procedures such as osteotomies and arthrodesis, there is concern that there may be failure of fixation due to the compromised bone. There have been many biomechanical studies showing evidence that screw and plate fixation has an increased incidence of failure in compromised bone [22]. It has been more difficult to stratify this in real-world studies. The likely reasoning behind this is due to the significant amount of variables. These variables include poor testing or definition of osteoporosis, surgical technique (i.e., type of hardware), postoperative management, age, and additional comorbidities [22]. Thus, currently, there is no excellent literature that shows osteoporosis leads to complications, but one should be highly suspicious that it may be one of many factors that cause them.

Chronic Conditions

Many patients undergoing surgery may be treated for multiple chronic conditions such as cardiovascular disease, hypertension, congestive heart failure, and chronic obstructive pulmonary disease. Most will have multiple comorbid conditions including diabetes and obesity. Patients with these conditions will oftentimes need preoperative workup such as basic lab work, CBC with differential, BMP, and INR. Additional studies such as chest X-ray, EKG, and stress test may need to be ordered, and the patient may need a referral to a specialist for surgical clearance. Most hospitals and surgery centers have set guidelines for preadmission testing that guide the evaluation of the patient and aid in determination of the appropriate tests and referrals.

Little research has been published looking at chronic conditions and their association with complications in regard to foot and ankle surgery. One study, looking at general orthopedics and the rate of mortality in inpatients, showed a 0.92% mortality [23]. Seventy-seven percent of all deaths occurred in patients more than 70 years old, and 50% of all deaths occurred in patients undergoing surgical management of hip fractures [23]. Medical risk factors associated with death included chronic renal failure, congestive heart failure, metastasis of the bone, atrial fibrillation, chronic obstructive pulmonary disease, and osteomyelitis [23]. Risk factors of diabetes, coronary artery disease, peripheral vascular disease, septic arthritis, and rheumatoid arthritis did not achieve significance [23]. In our opinion, even though there is little research in regard to chronic conditions and foot and ankle surgery, it is still important to be aware of your patient's medical conditions and risk of problems. When appropriate, consult with other medical professionals so that these patients receive optimal medical management and the risk of surgical complications can be minimized.

Autoimmune Diseases

Rheumatoid Arthritis

Patients with autoimmune diseases, particularly rheumatoid arthritis (RA), have been reported to have an increased incidence of postoperative complications, though the existing literature is inconsistent. These complications include surgical site infections (SSI), wound healing, delayed or nonunion of arthrodesis procedures, deep venous thrombosis (DVT), and RA disease flare. The potential for an increased risk of postoperative complications is multifactorial, due in part to the disease process and potentially accentuated by the medical treatment of the disease. The disease process in patients with rheumatoid and other forms of reactive arthritis results in changes in steroidogenesis, leading to low levels of cortisol and other adrenal hormones. The effect of this hormonal alteration is perpetuation of inflammation and other immunomodulating effects [24]. Alternative research suggests the possibility of inherited collagen variants that could predispose to osteoporosis and impaired wound healing [25]. Agents used in the treatment and modulation of the RA such as steroids, methotrexate, and tumor necrosis factor-alpha (TNF-alpha) inhibitory agents have immunosuppressive effects and have been thought to increase the risk of infections and healing complications in those patients under active treatment [26–28]. Additionally, patients with RA often present with polyarticular foot and ankle deformities that require multiple procedures in order to achieve an improved function and to allow the patient to maintain ambulation without significant pain. Approximately 90% of adults with chronic RA will have forefoot degeneration and/or deformity, 58–72% will have hindfoot involvement, and many will have ankle involvement [29].

It has been noted by many that patients with RA have a higher baseline risk for surgical complications [28, 30]. In a population-based, age- and sex-matched retrospective review of 609 RA and 609 non-RA subjects over a 39-year time frame from 1955 to 1994, Doran et al. [28] found that surgical patients with RA are at twice the risk of developing an infection, an infection compared to non-RA surgical patients. They found the sites of infection with the highest risk ratio were bone, joints, skin, and soft tissues. However, there are many case series showing minimal or modest surgical risks associated with RA and the drugs used to treat the disease.

Grennan et al. [25] performed a prospective randomized study of patients with RA undergoing elective orthopedic surgery to determine the incidence of postoperative infection and surgical complications within 1 year of surgery. Three hundred eighty-eight patients were divided into three cohorts: the first is consisting of 88 patients who were receiving methotrexate and continued this in the perioperative period, the second group of 72 patients had been receiving methotrexate but discontinued this 2 weeks prior to surgery until 2 weeks postoperative, and these were compared to the third group of 288 patients with RA who were not receiving methotrexate. The results showed that patients receiving methotrexate did not have an increased risk of infection or complications after elective orthopedic surgery. Other researchers have found similar results with no significant increase in complications with perioperative continuation of methotrexate in orthopedic surgery [30–33].

Another group of RA medications that are becoming more commonly seen are the biologic antitumor necrosis factor class of disease-modifying drugs. Several researchers have evaluated the incidence of postoperative complications in orthopedic surgery when anti-TNF-alpha agents were continued perioperatively. One foot and ankle-specific study [34] found that if looking at infection and healing complications independently, the TNF-alpha inhibition group did not have a significant increase compared to the group that was not receiving treatment. However, the TNF-alpha inhibition group did show a statistically higher overall complication rate ($p = 0.33$). Others [35–37] have found that continuation of anti-TNF-alpha agents did not result in a significant increase in postoperative infection rates overall. However, there is also work to support that hypothesis that continuation of anti-TNF-alpha agents does increase the incidence of postoperative infections in orthopedic surgery [38].

A systematic review and meta-analysis [39] of the literature on the perioperative management of RA treatment with respect to medication continuation or discontinuation that included 27 studies, with 5268 patients and 7933 surgeries, found that the most studied drug was methotrexate. Their recommendation was that methotrexate should be continued in the perioperative period in the absence of other risk factors that would increase the likelihood of complications (level of evidence 1c, grade D recommendation) and that biological DMARDs such as anti-TNF-alpha agents should be temporarily suspended or the surgery should be scheduled as far as possible from the last dose (level of evidence 2c, grade D recommendation).

Research has shown an increased incidence of DVT postoperatively in orthopedic surgical patients continuing anti-TNF-alpha agents perioperatively [40]. There also appears to be a link between patient age and disease duration [37, 40] and history of previous skin or wound infection [27, 36].

While there is some conflicting data, most of the research specific to the foot and ankle shows that the common antirheumatic medication methotrexate does not need to be discontinued in the perioperative period because there is not a significant increase in the infection or complication. Consideration may be given to discontinuing TNF-alpha inhibitory agents in the perioperative period, though the evidence for foot and ankle surgery is unclear with respect to this. There is also research to support that there may actually be potential detriment in discontinuation of these medications in the form of increased RA flares in the immediate postoperative period [25].

Surgeons must consider many aspects of the rheumatic patient's history with making perioperative decisions, including age, disease duration, vascular status, additional comorbidities such as diabetes and hypertension, prednisone dose, and previous SSI, all of which may play a greater role in the risk of surgical infections and complications. Surgeons must also take into account the potential risk of RA disease flare and increased pain associated with the discontinuation of RA medications including methotrexate and anti TNF-alpha agents.

Preoperative planning is very important, and medical clearance in RA patients is imperative, especially for those undergoing general anesthesia and a major reconstructive procedure. Part of this preoperative assessment is obtaining cervical spine lateral flexion-extension radiographs. C-spine disease and atlantoaxial subluxation associated with the RA must be recognized if present and the appropriate neurological evaluation performed prior to the administration of general anesthesia.

Glucocorticoids, such as prednisolone, are the main immunosuppressants used in the treatment of RA and other autoimmune conditions such as SLE. Extended use of glucocorticoids results in suppression of adrenal function, which can be potentially detrimental to the surgical patient who is exposed to surgical stress, particularly in the first 48 h postoperatively. The evidence is unclear on the need for stress dosing with hydrocortisone during the perioperative period for patients undergoing foot and ankle surgery [41, 42]. Consideration for stress dosing needs to be done on a case-by-case basis taking each individual patient's situation into account, including dose and length of steroid use and the stress that will be encountered during the surgical procedure.

Systemic Lupus Erythematosus

Systemic lupus erythematosus (SLE) is a multisystem immune complex-mediated autoimmune condition. This disease most commonly affects women ages 15–45. Patients with SLE are at increased risk of fragility fracture; avascular necrosis; infection, including osteomyelitis and septic arthritis; tenosynovitis; and tendon ruptures. The risk of AVN is the highest in SLE compared to all rheumatic diseases.

Preoperative assessment should include a cardiovascular workup due to the increased incidence of cardiovascular disease in this population as well as a chest radiograph. Laboratory workup should include liver and kidney function as this may affect the anesthetic plan. Additionally, patients with SLE are at increased risk of thrombosis and thus deep venous thrombosis (DVT) and pulmonary embolism (PE). Conversely, in certain instances, SLE patients may present with severe thrombocytopenia that can lead to excessive bleeding in invasive procedure. The foot and ankle surgeon must be aware of these two possible states and work with the patient's internist and/or rheumatologist to determine if either state exists in order to address appropriately in the perioperative period. The postoperative care of SLE patients must include constant and thorough monitoring for DVT. Consideration must be given to mechanical and medical DVT prophylaxis [42]. As noted previously, surgeons must also consider stress dosing of hydrocortisone if the patient has been on extended glucocorticoid treatment.

Human Immunodeficiency Virus (HIV) and Acquired Immunodeficiency Syndrome

Surgeons have two categories of concern with respect to complications when performing surgery on the HIV-positive patient. These include risk to the patient and risk to the healthcare team involved in the procedure. Surgical complications can be broken down into early postoperative infections and wound healing and late infections of hematogenous origin [43]. Due to the immunosuppression with HIV and AIDS, these patients are potentially more susceptible to both routine orthopedic pathogens and opportunistic organisms, such as *Mycobacterium*.

There are several clinical studies looking at the incidence of early postoperative infections in asymptomatic HIV-positive patients compared to the HIV-negative patients; however, these are largely retrospective and use historical controls rather than matched cohorts [44, 45]. These studies tended to show that that is not a significant difference in the postoperative infection rate between these two groups. Similarly there are studies looking at the incidence of infection and complications in HIV-positive patients compared to patients with AIDS [46–48]; complication rates and infection tended to be higher in those patients with AIDS.

Several authors [49, 50] have found that the most significant risk factor for postoperative infection in orthopedic surgery is a CD4 count $\leq 200/\text{mm}^3$. Hemophilia associated with HIV may also lead to an increase in postoperative infection, particularly late joint infection [43].

Late joint infection appears to be the most significant concern in the HIV/AIDS patient. In order to decrease the incidence of this disastrous complication, close follow-up, prophylactic preoperative antibiotics, and early evaluation and intervention are essential. Surgeons must be aware of the patient's medical status, including CD4 levels, serum albumin, nutritional state, and general overall health, in order to minimize serious complications [43]. While being HIV positive is not a risk factor alone, the level of immunosuppression and presence of confounding factors such as steroid use, age, and malnutrition are host risk factors that need to be closely monitored [51].

Smoking

Cigarette smoking has well been shown to have an adverse effect on tissue oxygenation and vasoconstriction from the nicotine. At the cellular level, the resultant hypoxic environment and the inhibition of oxidative metabolism of hydrogen cyanide (HCN) have been shown to affect the healing process [52, 53]. This can result in increased risk of early postoperative infection, delayed wound healing, and increased incidence of delayed and nonunion. Thevendran [52] reviewed several level 3 and 4 clinical case studies, which showed support for the role of smoking as a risk factor for nonunion in orthopedic surgery. Additionally, there is reasonable animal model research supporting the role of smoking in bone healing as well [54, 55].

The evidence also supports that smoking is a significant risk factor for wound complications and increased early postoperative, especially in high-risk incisions such as calcaneal fractures [56–60]. There is also decreased healing of skin flaps in the presence of smoking [53].

There is enough evidence on the deleterious effects of smoking on the outcomes of foot and ankle surgery that cessation should be encourage preoperatively, especially if the patient is undergoing a procedure that is already considered high risk and/or if the patient has other medical comorbidities increasing their postoperative risk of healing complications.

Alcohol Abuse

Research has shown the connection between chronic alcohol consumption and osteopenia as well as an increase rate of fracture with chronic alcohol consumption [61]. The mechanism of alcohol-induced osteopenia occurs through the suppression of new bone formation and antiosteoblastic function [61]. There has been little evidence or clinical studies showing an increase in healing complications directly related to alcohol consumption [52]. There are confounding variables associated with alcoholism that may increase the incidence of healing complications, however, including impaired nutritional status and organ damage.

References

1. Ostrander RV, Botte MJ, Brage ME. Efficacy of surgical preparation solutions in foot and ankle surgery. J Bone Jt Surg, Am Vol. 2005;87(5):980–5.
2. Golden SH, Peart-Vigilance C, Kao WH, Brancati FL. Perioperative glycemic control and the risk of infectious complications in a cohort of adults with diabetes. Diabetes Care. 1999;22(9):1408–14.
3. Rassias AJ, Marrin CA, Arruda J, Whalen PK, Beach M, Yeager MP. Insulin infusion improves neutrophil function in diabetic cardiac surgery patients. Anesth Analg. 1999;88(5):1011–6.
4. Wukich DK, Lowery NJ, McMillen RL, Frykberg RG. Postoperative infection rates in foot and ankle surgery: a comparison of patients with and without diabetes mellitus. J Bone Jt Surg, Am Vol. 2010;92(2):287–95.
5. Armstrong DG, Lavery LA, Stern S, Harkless LB. Is prophylactic diabetic foot surgery dangerous? J Foot Ankle Surg. 1996;35(6):585–9.
6. Olgaard K, Salusky IB, Silver J. The spectrum of mineral and bone disorders in chronic kidney disease, 2nd ed. Oxford; NY: Oxford University Press; 2010. xxvi, P. 590
7. Goldsmith D, Ritz E, Covic A. Vascular calcification: a stiff challenge for the nephrologist: does preventing bone disease cause arterial disease? Kidney Int. 2004;66(4):1315–33.
8. Ackland GL, Moran N, Cone S, Grocott MP, Mythen MG. Chronic kidney disease and postoperative morbidity after elective orthopedic surgery. Anesth Analg. 2011;112(6):1375–81.
9. Karaeminogullari O, Demirors H, Sahin O, Ozalay M, Ozdemir N, Tandogan RN. Analysis of outcomes for surgically treated hip fractures in patients undergoing chronic hemodialysis. J Bone Jt Surg, Am Vol. 2007;89(2):324–31.

10. Ramarapu S. Chronic kidney disease and postoperative morbidity associated with renal dysfunction after elective orthopedic surgery. Anesth Analg 2012;114(3):700; author reply
11. Sunday JM, Guille JT, Torg JS. Complications of joint arthroplasty in patients with end-stage renal disease on hemodialysis. Clin Orthop Relat Res. 2002;397:350–5.
12. Mokdad AH, Ford ES, Bowman BA, Dietz WH, Vinicor F, Bales VS, et al. Prevalence of obesity, diabetes, and obesity-related health risk factors, 2001. Jama. 2003;289(1):76–9.
13. Sabharwal S, Root MZ. Impact of obesity on orthopaedics. J Bone Jt Surg, Am Vol. 2012;94(11):1045–52.
14. King CM, Hamilton GA, Cobb M, Carpenter D, Ford LA. Association between ankle fractures and obesity. J Foot Ankle Surg. 2012;51(5):543–7.
15. Strauss EJ, Frank JB, Walsh M, Koval KJ, Egol KA. Does obesity influence the outcome after the operative treatment of ankle fractures? J Bone Jt Surg, Am Vol. 2007;89(6):794–8.
16. Stephens BF, Murphy A, Mihalko WM. The effects of nutritional deficiencies, smoking, and systemic disease on orthopaedic outcomes. J Bone Jt Surg, Am Vol. 2013;95(23):2152–7.
17. Huang R, Greenky M, Kerr GJ, Austin MS, Parvizi J. The effect of malnutrition on patients undergoing elective joint arthroplasty. J. Arthroplasty. 2013;28(8 Suppl):21–4.
18. Ritchie RF, Palomaki GE, Neveux LM, Navolotskaia O, Ledue TB, Craig WY. Reference distributions for the negative acute-phase serum proteins, albumin, transferrin and transthyretin: a practical, simple and clinically relevant approach in a large cohort. J Clin Lab Anal. 1999;13(6):273–9.
19. Moucha CS, Clyburn T, Evans RP, Prokuski L. Modifiable risk factors for surgical site infection. J Bone Jt Surg, Am Vol. 2011;93(4):398–404.
20. Warnold I, Lundholm K. Clinical significance of preoperative nutritional status in 215 noncancer patients. Ann Surg. 1984;199(3):299–305.
21. Fairfield KM, Fletcher RH. Vitamins for chronic disease prevention in adults: scientific review. Jama. 2002;287(23):3116–26.
22. Goldhahn J, Suhm N, Goldhahn S, Blauth M, Hanson B. Influence of osteoporosis on fracture fixation--a systematic literature review. Osteoporos Int. 2008;19(6):761–72.
23. Bhattacharyya T, Iorio R, Healy WL. Rate of and risk factors for acute inpatient mortality after orthopaedic surgery. J Bone Jt Surg, Am Vol. 2002;84-A(4):562–72.
24. Harle P, Cutolo M, Scholmerich J, Straub RH. Rheumatoid arthritis—pathogenetic role of neuroendocrine axes and the peripheral nervous system. Med Klin. 2002;97(12):720–9.
25. Grennan DM, Gray J, Loudon J, Fear S. Methotrexate and early postoperative complications in patients with rheumatoid arthritis undergoing elective orthopaedic surgery. Ann Rheum Dis. 2001;60(3):214–7.
26. Straub RH, Paimela L, Peltomaa R, Scholmerich J, Leirisalo-Repo M. Inadequately low serum levels of steroid hormones in relation to interleukin-6 and tumor necrosis factor in untreated patients with early rheumatoid arthritis and reactive arthritis. Arthritis Rheum. 2002;46(3):654–62.
27. Bibbo C. Wound healing complications and infection following surgery for rheumatoid arthritis. Foot Ankle Clin 2007;12(3): 509–24. vii.
28. Doran MF, Crowson CS, Pond GR, O'Fallon WM, Gabriel SE. Frequency of infection in patients with rheumatoid arthritis compared with controls: a population-based study. Arthritis Rheum. 2002;46(9):2287–93.
29. Nassar J, Cracchiolo 3rd. A. Complications in surgery of the foot and ankle in patients with rheumatoid arthritis. Clin Orthop Relat Res. 2001;(391):140–52.
30. Bibbo C, Anderson RB, Davis WH, Norton J. The influence of rheumatoid chemotherapy, age, and presence of rheumatoid nodules on postoperative complications in rheumatoid foot and ankle surgery: analysis of 725 procedures in 104 patients [corrected]. Foot Ankle Int. 2003;24(1):40–4.
31. Escalante A, Beardmore TD. Risk factors for early wound complications after orthopedic surgery for rheumatoid arthritis. J Rheumatol. 1995;22(10):1844–51.
32. Murata K, Yasuda T, Ito H, Yoshida M, Shimizu M, Nakamura T. Lack of increase in postoperative complications with low-dose methotrexate therapy in patients with rheumatoid arthritis undergoing elective orthopedic surgery. Mod Rheumatol/Japan Rheum Assoc. 2006;16(1):14–9.
33. Barnard AR, Regan M, Burke FD, Chung KC, Wilgis EF. Wound healing with medications for rheumatoid arthritis in hand surgery. ISRN Rheumatol. 2012;2012:251962.
34. Bibbo C, Goldberg JW. Infectious and healing complications after elective orthopaedic foot and ankle surgery during tumor necrosis factor-alpha inhibition therapy. Foot Ankle Int. 2004;25(5):331–5.
35. Hayata K, Kanbe K, Chiba J, Nakamura A, Inoue Y, Hobo K. Clinical factors related to the efficacy and complications of orthopedic surgery for rheumatoid arthritis with infliximab. Int J Rheum Dis. 2011;14(1):31–6.
36. den Broeder AA, Creemers MC, Fransen J, de Jong E, de Rooij DJ, Wymenga A, et al. Risk factors for surgical site infections and other complications in elective surgery in patients with rheumatoid arthritis with special attention for anti-tumor necrosis factor: a large retrospective study. J Rheumatol. 2007;34(4):689–95.
37. Berthold E, Geborek P, Gulfe A. Continuation of TNF blockade in patients with inflammatory rheumatic disease. An observational study on surgical site infections in 1,596 elective orthopedic and hand surgery procedures. Acta Orthop. 2013;84(5):495–501.
38. Giles JT, Bartlett SJ, Gelber AC, Nanda S, Fontaine K, Ruffing V, et al. Tumor necrosis factor inhibitor therapy and risk of serious postoperative orthopedic infection in rheumatoid arthritis. Arthritis Rheum. 2006;55(2):333–7.
39. Del Olmo L, Hernandez B, Galindo-Izquierdo M, Tebar D, Balsa A, Carmona L. Peri-operative management of disease modifying antirheumatic drugs: recommendations based on a meta-analysis. Revista espanola de cirugia ortopedica y traumatologia. 2012; 56(5):393–412.
40. Kawakami K, Ikari K, Kawamura K, Tsukahara S, Iwamoto T, Yano K, et al. Complications and features after joint surgery in rheumatoid arthritis patients treated with tumour necrosis factor-alpha blockers: perioperative interruption of tumour necrosis factor-alpha blockers decreases complications? Rheumatology. 2010;49(2):341–7.
41. Hicks CW, Wick EC, Salvatori R, Ha CY. Perioperative corticosteroid management for patients with inflammatory bowel disease. Inflammatory Bowel Dis. 2015;21(1):221–8.
42. Mak A. Orthopedic surgery and its complication in systemic lupus erythematosus. World J Orthop. 2014;5(1):38–44.
43. Luck Jr JV, Logan LR, Benson DR, Glasser DB. Human immunodeficiency virus infection: complications and outcome of orthopaedic surgery. J Am Acad Orthop Surg. 1996;4(6):297–304.
44. Hoekman P, van de Perre P, Nelissen J, Kwisanga B, Bogaerts J, Kanyangabo F. Increased frequency of infection after open reduction of fractures in patients who are seropositive for human immunodeficiency virus. J Bone Jt Surg. 1991;73(5):675–9.
45. Paiement GD, Hymes RA, LaDouceur MS, Gosselin RA, Green HD. Postoperative infections in asymptomatic HIV-seropositive orthopedic trauma patients. J Trauma 1994;37(4):545–50. discussion 50-1.
46. Semprini AE, Castagna C, Ravizza M, Fiore S, Savasi V, Muggiasca ML, et al. The incidence of complications after caesarean section in 156 HIV-positive women. Aids. 1995;9(8):913–7.
47. Dodson TB. Predictors of postextraction complications in HIV-positive patients. Oral Surg Oral Med Oral Pathol Oral Radiol Endod. 1997;84(5):474–9.

48. Dodson TB, Perrott DH, Gongloff RK, Kaban LB. Human immunodeficiency virus serostatus and the risk of postextraction complications. Int J Oral Maxillofac Surg. 1994;23(2):100–3.
49. Ragni MV, Crossett LS, Herndon JH. Postoperative infection following orthopaedic surgery in human immunodeficiency virus-infected hemophiliacs with CD4 counts < or =200/mm3. J Arthroplasty. 1995;10(6):716–21.
50. Guild GN, Moore TJ, Barnes W, Hermann C. CD4 count is associated with postoperative infection in patients with orthopaedic trauma who are HIV positive. Clin Orthop Relat Res. 2012;470(5):1507–12.
51. Gurkan I, Wenz JF. Perioperative infection control: an update for patient safety in orthopedic surgery. Orthopedics 2006;29(4):329–39. quiz 40-1.
52. Thevendran G, Younger A, Pinney S. Current concepts review: risk factors for nonunions in foot and ankle arthrodeses. Foot Ankle Int. 2012;33(11):1031–40.
53. Kwiatkowski TC, Hanley Jr EN, Ramp WK. Cigarette smoking and its orthopedic consequences. Am J Orthop. 1996;25(9):590–7.
54. Craig S, Rees TD. The effects of smoking on experimental skin flaps in hamsters. Plast Reconstr Surg. 1985;75(6):842–6.
55. Wing KJ, Fisher CG, O'Connell JX, Wing PC. Stopping nicotine exposure before surgery. The effect on spinal fusion in a rabbit model. Spine. 2000;25(1):30–4.
56. Ding L, He Z, Xiao H, Chai L, Xue F. Risk factors for postoperative wound complications of calcaneal fractures following plate fixation. Foot Ankle Int. 2013;34(9):1238–44.
57. Soni A, Vollans S, Malhotra K, Mann C. Association between smoking and wound infection rates following calcaneal fracture fixation. Foot Ankle Spec. 2014;7(4):266–70.
58. Folk JW, Starr AJ, Early JS. Early wound complications of operative treatment of calcaneus fractures: analysis of 190 fractures. J Orthop Trauma. 1999;13(5):369–72.
59. Abidi NA, Dhawan S, Gruen GS, Vogt MT, Conti SF. Wound-healing risk factors after open reduction and internal fixation of calcaneal fractures. Foot Ankle Int. 1998;19(12):856–61.
60. Benirschke SK, Kramer PA. Wound healing complications in closed and open calcaneal fractures. J Orthop Trauma. 2004;18(1):1–6.
61. Friday KE, Howard GA. Ethanol inhibits human bone cell proliferation and function in vitro. Metab Clin Exp. 1991;40(6):562–5.

Part II

Forefoot

Digital Surgery

7

Brian T. Dix and Kyle S. Peterson

Introduction

Lesser toe deformities can occur independently or be linked with deformities of the hindfoot, midfoot, or forefoot. In addition, they can be dynamic or static in nature. The most common cause of lesser toe deformities is credited to ill-fitting footwear, but neuromuscular and congenital origins have also been documented and should be considered [1–5].

Classically, lesser toe deformities can be characterized as a mallet toe, hammertoe, claw toe, curly toe, or crossover toe. A mallet toe deformity involves a neutral metatarsophalangeal joint (MPJ) and proximal interphalangeal joint (PIPJ) with a plantarflexed distal interphalangeal joint (DIPJ). Whereas, a hammertoe demonstrates a dorsiflexed or neutral position at the MPJ with a plantarflexed PIPJ and a dorsiflexed, neutral, or plantarflexed DIPJ. A claw toe is defined as dorsiflexion at the MPJ and plantarflexion at the PIPJ and DIPJ. A curly toe is described as neutral or plantarflexed at the MPJ with plantarflexion at the PIPJ and DIPJ. Lastly, a crossover toe consists of medial or lateral deviation at the MPJ and is neutral or plantarflexed at the PIPJ with plantarflexion, dorsiflexion, or neutral at the DIPJ [6] (Fig. 7.1).

When nonsurgical management fails, then surgery may be indicated. There is a wide array of surgical interventions described for lesser toe deformities which include soft tissue releases, tendon transfers, arthroplasty, arthrodesis, metatarsal osteotomies, or a combination of these procedures [7]. Furthermore, a lesser toe deformity may be rigid, semiflexible, or flexible at the PIPJ and/or DIPJ. If the toe can be passively corrected to a neutral position at the interphalangeal joints, then the deformity is classified as flexible. However, if the toe cannot be passively corrected to a neutral position at the DIPJ or PIPJ, then the deformity is considered rigid. The concomitant MPJ must also be assessed [1, 2, 4, 8–10]. The Kelikian push-up test loads the metatarsal head to ascertain if there is a deformity at the MPJ. In the operating room, the toe should return to a rectus position if the deformities are corrected [11].

Soft Tissue Procedures

Flexor Tenotomy

A flexor tenotomy is a soft tissue release that is indicated only in flexible toe deformities [12]. It is rarely performed as an isolated procedure in the adult except in patients with diabetes and peripheral neuropathy that have flexible toe deformities with or without ulceration. However, it has been supported after a PIPJ arthrodesis has been performed and a subsequent flexible DIPJ contracture occurs [13]. Nevertheless, it has been advocated in children or the elderly where larger surgical procedures cannot be performed [11, 14–16]. In a case study by Ross et al., he performed a flexor tenotomy on 188 curly or hammertoes in 62 pediatric patients with a 95% success rate. He concluded that in pediatric patients with solely a flexion contracture as the cause of the hammertoe, a flexor tenotomy is an effective procedure [14].

Moreover, a systematic review from Scott et al. in the *Journal of Foot and Ankle Research* in 2016 examined the effectiveness of percutaneous flexor tenotomies for the management and prevention of recurrence in diabetic toe ulcers. The only documented literature was case series designs with a total of 250 flexor tenotomies performed in 163 patients. They found good healing rates at 92–100% with recurrence rates ranging from 0 to 18% at 2 months follow-up. The authors concluded that better level of evidence is needed to confirm if a flexor tenotomy is a reliable procedure to prevent and/or heal distal toe ulcerations with flexible soft tissue contractures. The current evidence does show low recurrence

B.T. Dix
Sanford Health, Thief River Falls, MN, USA

K.S. Peterson (✉)
Suburban Orthopaedics, 1110 W Schick Rd, Bartlett, IL 60103, USA
e-mail: kpeterson@suburbanortho.com

M.S. Lee, J.P. Grossman (eds.), *Complications in Foot and Ankle Surgery*, DOI 10.1007/978-3-319-53686-6_7

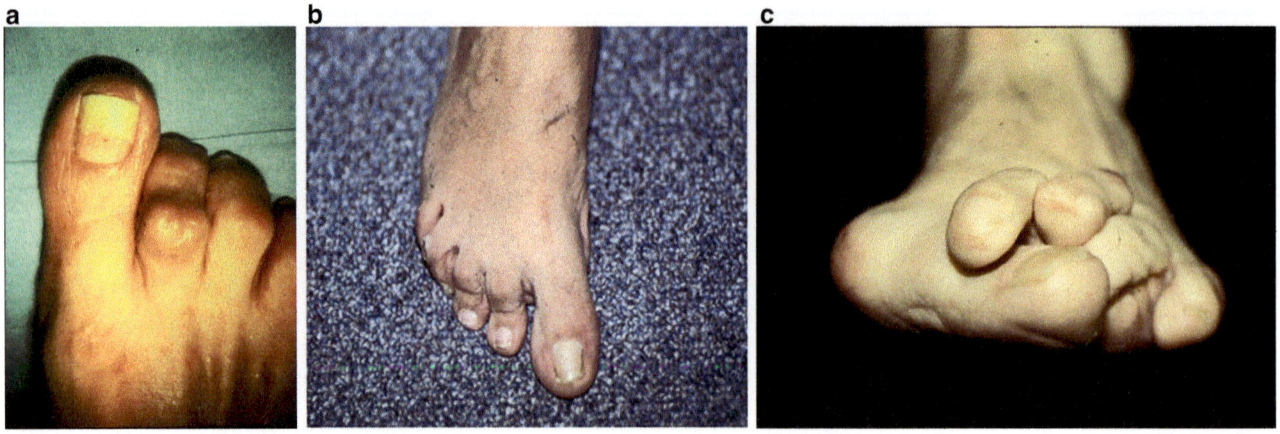

Fig. 7.1 Showing the different lesser toe deformities

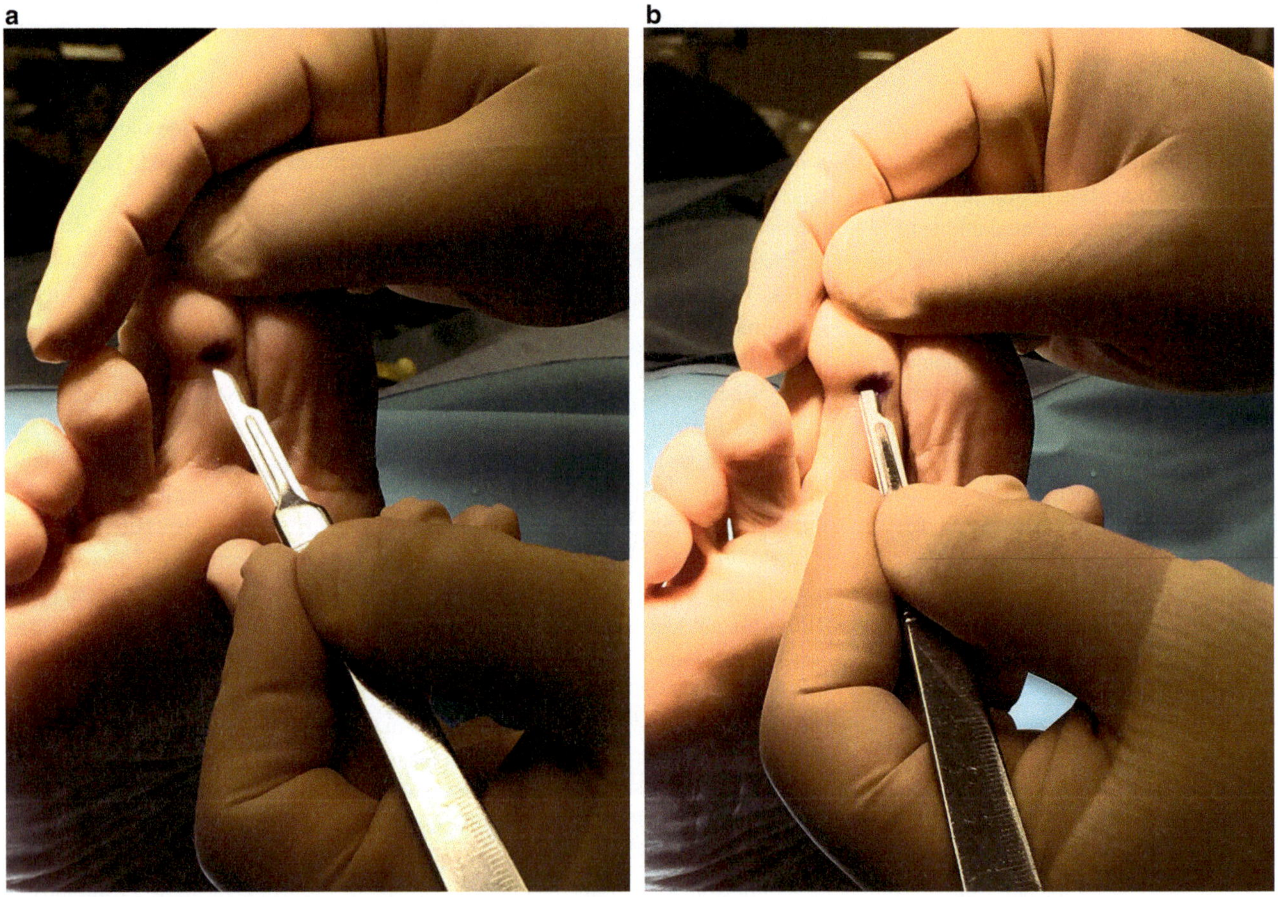

Fig. 7.2 Showing the flexor tenotomy of the 2nd toe

rates and postoperative complications with reasonably high healing rates [16].

A flexor tenotomy is performed through a small medial, lateral, or plantar percutaneous or open digital incision; the flexor digitorum longus (FDL) tendon is released at the DIPJ or the PIPJ depending on the location of the contracture [17]. Some surgeons advocate transecting the flexor digitorum brevis (FDB) tendon as well [18]. The release of the flexor tendon contracture allows the toe to assume a more neutral position decreasing pressure at the distal aspect of the toe [16] (Fig. 7.2).

As with other foot and ankle surgeries, absolute contraindications include acute or chronic infection and vascular compromise. Relative contraindications for a flexor tenotomy include the nondiabetic adult patient and rigid deformities without ancillary procedures being performed [11].

Also, there is a loading phenomenon created when a tenotomy is performed which causes the load to transfer to a neighboring tendon which can cause increased pressure to adjacent digits. This is because the four long flexors and extensors to the lesser digits start from a shared muscle belly. Thus, when one tendon is transected, each of the residual tendons will have one-third greater power. To decrease the loading phenomenon, perform a tendon lengthening or tenotomy on the remaining digits to prevent transfer lesions [11].

Flexor to Extensor Tendon Transfer

A flexor to extensor tendon transfer is rarely performed as an isolated procedure but rather an adjunct to a broader flexible hammertoe correction. This includes sequential releases beginning with the dorsal skin incision, then an extensor tenotomy or lengthening, dorsal capsulotomy, and collateral ligament release. If additional stabilization and correction are required, then a flexor to extensor transfer could be added to achieve further plantarflexory influence at the MPJ. Conversely, a flexor to extensor tendon transfer could be added to a rigid deformity after a PIPJ arthroplasty/arthrodesis with or without a shortening metatarsal osteotomy to help stabilize the MPJ [19]. The transfer of the FDL to the extensor tendons theoretically changes the FDL into an intrinsic muscle which causes dorsiflexion of the DIPJ/PIPJ with plantarflexion at the MPJ [6]. Transfer of the FDL and FDB tendons into the dorsal expansion of the extensor tendons was first described by Girdlestone in 1947 [20]. Taylor, in 1951, also performed the same surgery in 68 patients. He reported 86% of the patients had good results [21]. There are many different techniques reported for the flexor to extensor tendon transfer, but the author prefers a technique recently described by Easley. They perform the operation with two separate plantar transverse incisions and one dorsal longitudinal incision. The more proximal plantar incision is placed along the proximal skin crease and the more distal plantar incision at the DIPJ. The FDL tendon is identified in between the slips of the FDB tendon and held under traction with a hemostat. Through the second more distal incision, the FDL tendon is released from its insertion into the distal phalanx. Next, the FDL tendon is dissected out of the more proximal incision and split longitudinally into two slips. A central longitudinal dorsal incision over the PIPJ is created. The incision is normally already extended over the MPJ as a release of the MPJ is usually previously been performed. A hemostat is passed from dorsal to plantar through the slips of the FDB tendon, and the corresponding slips of the FDL tendon are transferred dorsally to the proximal phalanx. The slips are then sutured over the proximal phalanx within the extensor tendons [19] (Fig. 7.3).

The most recent meta-analysis in 2012 examined 17 articles which included 515 FDL tendon transfers with a mean ± SD follow-up of 54.21 ± 20.64 months. The total overall patient satisfaction after FDL tendon transfer was 86.7% (95% confidence interval, 81.7%–90.5%) [22].

As with any foot and ankle surgeries, absolute contraindications include acute or chronic infection and vascular compromise. Relative contraindications for a flexor to extensor tendon transfer consist of an FDL tendon transfer as the principal procedure of a rigid lesser toe deformity [6, 11].

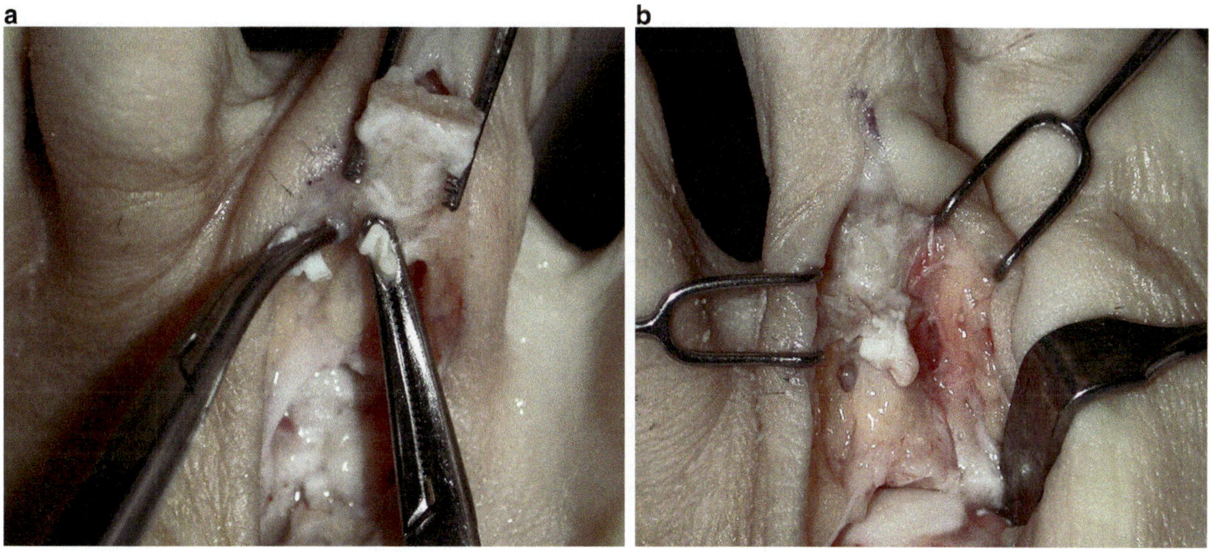

Fig. 7.3 Showing a flexor to extensor tendon transfer for hammertoe correction

Flexor to Extensor Transfer Complications

PIPJ stiffness has reported to be the highest complication when performing a flexor to extensor tendon transfer with one study reporting up to 60% of the cases had residual stiffness [23]. Furthermore, stiffness in patients with flexible hammertoe deformities is one of the chief causes for complaints postoperatively [24]. It is imperative to discuss with patients preoperatively that the operated lesser toe will not curl postoperatively and will feel stiff, but the deformity should be resolved. Recurrence of the lesser toe deformity has been described as high as 20% [19]. Swelling and numbness can also occur but usually resolve over time [2].

Recurrence of the deformity is relatively low after flexor to extensor tendon transfer but can be due to many different factors including but not limited to failure of the transfer, preoperative stiffness not sufficiently assessed, neurologic conditions, undue dorsal soft tissue scarring, or insufficient tautness of the transfer [19]. To help prevent recurrence and/or a floating toe when performing the FDL transfer, the toe should be held down at 20° of plantarflexion at the MPJ and the ankle at 90°. Moreover, if the FDL transfer is being utilized for stabilization of the MPJ, then perform the transfer toward the base of the proximal phalanx to achieve additional plantarflexory control over the MPJ. Conversely, if the FDL transfer is being performed to better stabilize the PIPJ, then the FDL tendons should be sutured toward the head of the proximal phalanx to attain added plantarflexion of the PIPJ.

Loss of blood supply to the toe can occur due to traction of the neurovascular bundle or compression due to the transfer. Deflation of the tourniquet before closure can help assess blood flow to the toe and allow much easier dissection to confirm the neurovascular bundle is not compressed if this is required. Other measures to help increase blood flow to a toe that may be compromised include applying warm gauze; removing, bending, or adjusting the K-wire; lowering the patient's leg; dorsiflexing the toe at the MPJ; injecting lidocaine around the neurovascular bundle; applying of nitropaste and heat lamps; or simply waiting [7, 19].

Osseous Procedures

Common surgical lesser toe deformity procedures include an interphalangeal joint arthroplasty or arthrodesis. Often, these are also combined with concomitant procedures, such as MPJ releases, tendon transfers, and metatarsal osteotomies. Fixation for a digital arthrodesis or arthroplasty can range from Kirschner wires, cerclage wire, intramedullary screws, resorbable pins, and many newer hammertoe-specific implant devices [25].

Complications of Osseous Procedures

Flail or Floppy Toe

One common complication following a digital arthroplasty or arthrodesis is a flail or floppy toe. This occurs with a nonunion of the interphalangeal joint following an arthrodesis or with instability of the joint and shortening of the toe following an arthroplasty, which ranges from 0 to 35% in the literature [26]. Patients with a floppy toe often complain of the lack of fine motor control in the toe and stability to maintain toe purchase to the ground, creating what Solan and Davies describe as the "toe cripple" [13] (Fig. 7.4). Surgical correction for flail or floppy toes is difficult and oftentimes can still lead patients with a sense of dissatisfaction. Preoperative discussion about the complications of lesser toe deformity surgery is imperative for good outcomes. Patient expectations should be clearly outlined to minimize complications. Often, there are patients who will never be happy with the outcome of surgery, and being able to identify these patients and avoid surgery is a crucial skill a surgeon should obtain.

If the cause of the flail toe is from a shortened PIPJ arthroplasty, then surgical PIPJ arthrodesis may be an option to stabilize the digit. However, proper patient expectations must be explained that the toe will always be shorter than the neighboring toes. If revision of a PIPJ arthrodesis is to be performed, the

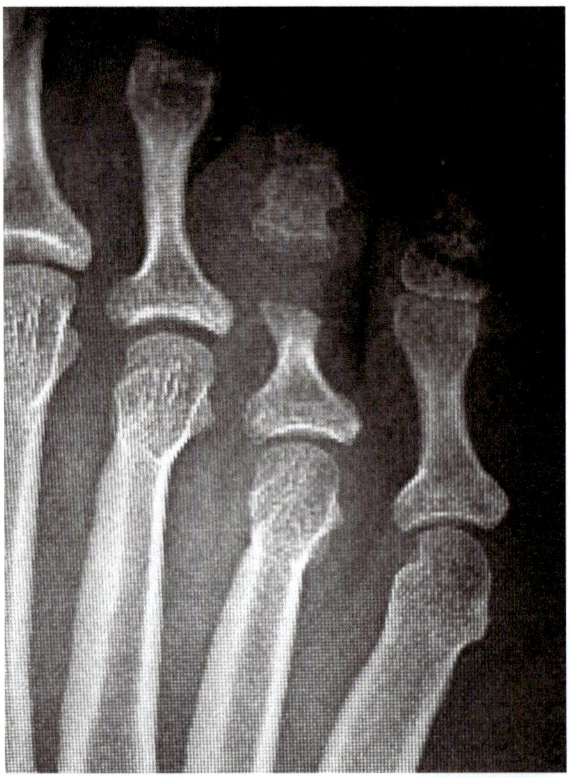

Fig. 7.4 Showing a flail/floppy 4th toe after over-aggressive digital arthroplasty

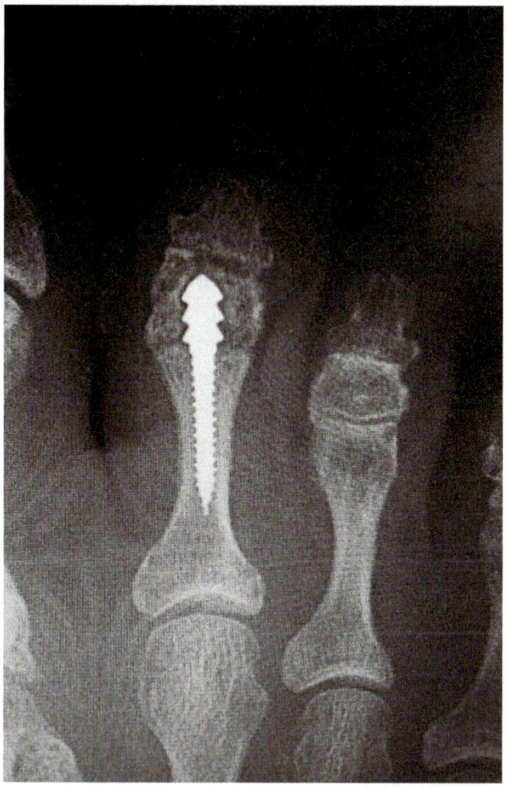

Fig. 7.5 A one-piece intramedullary fixation device for interphalangeal joint arthrodesis

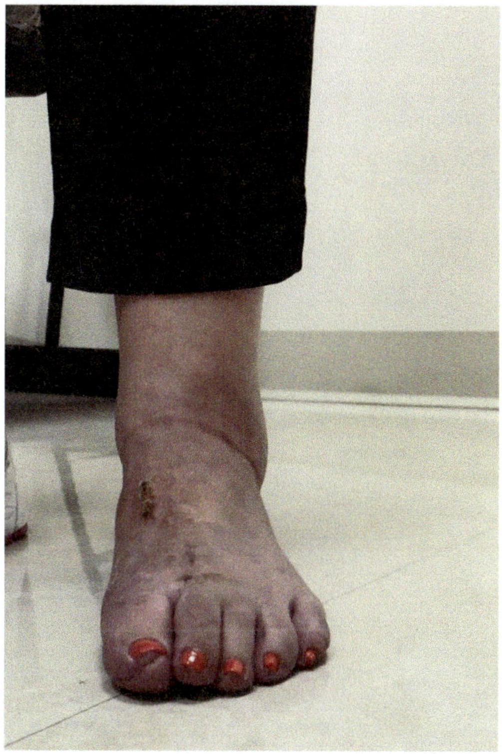

Fig. 7.6 Floating second toe that occurred postoperatively following a second metatarsal Weil osteotomy

authors advocate for the use of a permanent implantable device to maintain the stability and fusion of the interphalangeal joint (Fig. 7.5). These permanent interphalangeal devices are reported to have a high rate of bony fusion [27]. Infrequently, a second surgical option for a shortened and flail toe is to regain length with the use of a bone block graft and transfixation wire [28]. Before considering this option, the surgeon may also be able to improve the appearance of the foot by shortening the other toes through a middle phalangeal diaphyseal shortening osteotomy or through a DIPJ excision arthroplasty [13]. In some cases with significant bony loss, syndactylization to an adjacent toe is warranted. As a last resort, surgical amputation of the flail toe may also be a viable option.

The best way to elude a flail toe in the first place is to avoid excessive bone resection during the arthroplasty or arthrodesis procedure. In particular, excess shortening can often result from too much resection of the head of the proximal phalanx, compared to resection of the base of the middle phalanx. Additionally, the use of fixation for at least 4–6 weeks can also reduce the risk of flail toes in order to stabilize the interphalangeal joint with increased bony or fibrous consolidation. The authors commonly utilize Kirschner wires for fixation; however, when patients are hesitant to have fixation with these protruding wires, internal medullary devices may also be utilized.

Floating Toe

One of the most common complications following a PIPJ fusion with central metatarsal osteotomy (Weil) is a floating toe deformity [29]. The floating toe is a deformity in the sagittal plane in which the toe fails to purchase the ground in static stance (Fig. 7.6). Floating toes are often caused by lesser metatarsal osteotomies, but can also be present concomitantly in a lesser toe deformity with MPJ subluxation or dislocation. Biomechanically, floating toes have a tear or strain of the MPJ plantar plate. If the plantar plate tear and floating toe are present prior to the initial surgical procedure, it is important that this deforming force is properly repaired. Furthermore, following a Weil osteotomy, the MPJ axis is shortened and directed more plantar, which can overload the plantar plate and also cause the intrinsic muscles to act as dorsiflexors of the toe.

The incidence of a floating toe following a Weil osteotomy is reported anywhere from 15% to 33% [30–33]. Pinning the toe in plantarflexion with a Kirschner wire through the MPJ will allow temporary stabilization and scar tissue to form to maintain the position of the toe. Additionally, a flexor tendon transfer has also become a common procedure to plantarflex the toe and prevent a floating toe. An interphalangeal joint fusion must also be performed in conjunction with a flexor tendon transfer to avoid a hyperextension deformity in the toe.

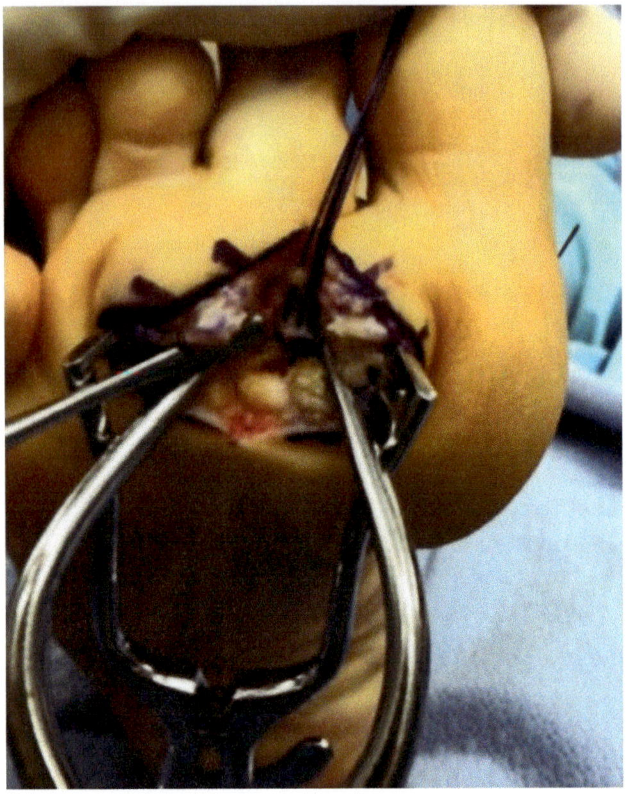

Fig. 7.7 Direct plantar approach for a plantar plate repair of the second MPJ

If a postoperative floating toe occurs, common conservative treatment measures should first be employed before revision surgery. Crossover taping of the toe or a prefabricated toe splint can stabilize the toe and provide purchase to the ground. Oral anti-inflammatory medications, topical pain and scar creams, and a custom orthotic with a metatarsal pad can also be used with success.

Surgical intervention for a postoperative floating toe should be reserved as a last resort measure as patient satisfaction is often difficult. Again, a flexor tendon transfer may be performed to stabilize the MPJ in a plantarflexion direction. A direct or indirect plantar plate repair may also be used as new techniques and instrumentation are now being performed (Fig. 7.7)

Malaligned Toe

Malaligned toes can also occur in the frontal plane. Kilmartin et al. in 2007 described a closing base wedge osteotomy of the proximal phalanx for a valgus deformity of the hammertoe. He noted 73% of the patients were completely satisfied with the end result, 27% were satisfied with reservations, and 0% were dissatisfied. Furthermore, 96% regarded their toe to be better than before the surgery [34]. However, correct bone resection from a previous failed arthroplasty with appropriate soft tissue releases is sometimes all that is required to correct the malaligned toe [13]. Additionally, Hadad et al. reported on extensor brevis tendon transfers and flexor to extensor tendon transfers in patients with a varus toe deformity. The overall recurrence rate for both procedures was 15%. He concluded that extensor brevis tendon transfers can be adequately be performed in flexible varus toe deformities, and flexor to extensor tendon transfers should be reserved for rigid varus toe deformities. As discussed earlier, stiffness was a common complaint in the flexor to extensor tendon transfers that were performed [35].

Other salvage options for a malaligned lesser toe deformity include a syndactylization or a toe amputation [36–38]. The authors advocate an elective toe amputation in the elderly where a singular hammertoe is problematic but do caution that drifting of the other toes will most likely occur.

Conclusion

Lesser toe surgery is complicated with increasing difficulty in revisional hammertoe surgery. It is imperative to properly diagnose hammertoes preoperatively and to execute correct surgical technique to avoid postoperative complications. Furthermore, it is essential that the patient understands the anticipated surgical results preoperatively to avoid postoperative dissatisfaction. Lastly, new high-quality evidence-based medicine studies need to be performed to help advance our knowledge in complications of lesser toe surgery.

References

1. Coughlin MJ. Common causes of pain in the forefoot in adults. J Bone Jt Surg Br. 2000;82(6):781–90.
2. Coughlin MJ. Lesser toe abnormalities. J Bone Jt Surg Am. 2002;84:1446–69.
3. Coughlin MJ. Operative repair of the mallet toe deformity. Foot Ankle Int. 1995;16(3):109–16.
4. Coughlin MJ, Dorris J, Polk E. Operative repair of the fixed hammer toe deformity. Foot Ankle Int. 2000;21(2):94–104.
5. Coughlin MJ, Kennedy MP. Operative repair fourth and fifth toe corns. Foot Ankle Int. 2003;24(2):147–57.
6. Coughlin MJ: Lesser toe deformities. In: Coughlin MJ, Mann RA, Saltzman CL, editors. Surgery of the foot and ankle, vol. 1, 8th ed. Philadelphia, PA: Mosby Elsevier; 2007, p. 363–464.
7. Shirzad K, Kiesau CD, DeOrio JK, Parekh SD. Lesser toe deformities. J Am Acad Orthop Surg. 2011;19:505–14.
8. Mann RA, Coughlin MJ. Lesser toe deformities. In: Jahss M, editor. Disorders of the foot and ankle. Philadelphia: WB Saunders, 1991. p. 1207–1209.
9. Mann RA, Coughlin MJ. Lesser toe deformities. Instr Course Lect. 1987;36:137–59.
10. Mann RA, Coughlin MJ. Lesser toe deformities. In: Mann RA, Coughlin MJ, editors. The video textbook of foot and ankle surgery. St Louis: Medical Video Productions, 1991. p. 47–49.
11. Banks AS, Downey MS, Martin DE, Miller SJ. McGlamary's comprehensive textbook of foot and ankle surgery, vol. 1, 3rd ed. Philadelphia, PA: Lippincott Williams and Wilkins; 2001p. 253–353.

12. Landsman A, Cook E, Cook J. Tenotomy and tendon transfer about the forefoot, midfoot and hindfoot. Clin Podiatr Med Surg. 2008;25:547–69.
13. Solan MC, Davies MS. Revision surgery of the less toes. Foot Ankle Clin N Am. 2011;16:621–45.
14. Ross ER, Menelaus MB. Open flexor tenotomy for hammer toes and curly toes in childhood. J Bone Jt Surg Br. 1984;66(5):770–1.
15. Pollard JP, Morrison PJ. Flexor tenotomy in the treatment of curly toes. Proc R Soc Med. 1975;68(8):480–1.
16. Scott JE, Hendry GJ, Locke J. Effectiveness of percutaneous flexor tenotomies for the management and prevention of recurrence of diabetic toe ulcers: a systematic review. J Foot Ankle Res. 2016;9:25.
17. Schepers T, Berendsen HA, Hok Oei I, Koning J. Functional outcome and patient satisfaction after flexor tenotomy for plantar ulcers of the toes. J Foot Ankle Surg. 2010;49:119–22.
18. Rasmussen A, Bjerre-Christensen U, Almdal TP, Holstein P. Percutaneous flexor tenotomy for preventing and treating toe ulcers in people with diabetes mellitus. Tissue Viability. 2013; 22:68–73.
19. Easley M. Operative techniques in foot and ankle surgery, 1st ed. Philadelphia, PA: Lippincott Williams and Wilkins, 2011. p. 208-215.
20. Girdlestone GR. Physiology of the foot and hand. J Bone Jt Surg. 1947;29:167–8.
21. Taylor RG. The treatment of claw toes by multiple transfers of the flexor into extensor tendons. J Bone Jt Surg. 1951;33:539–42.
22. Losa Iglesias ME, Becerro de Bengoa Vallejo R, Jules KT, Trepal MJ. Meta-analysis of flexor tendon transfer for the correction of lesser toe deformities. J Am Podiatr Med Assoc. 2012; 102(5):359–68.
23. Kirchner J, Wagner E. Girdlestone-Taylor flexor to extensor tendon transfer. Tech Foot Ankle Surg. 2004;3:91–9.
24. Cyphers SM, Feiwell E. Review of the Gridlestone-Taylor procedure for clawtoe in myelodysplasia. Foot Ankle. 1988;9:229–33.
25. Zelen CM, Young NJ. Clin Podiatr Med Surg. 2013;30:271–82.
26. Edwards WH, Beischer AD. Interphalangeal joint arthrodesis of the lesser toes. Foot Ankle Clin. 2002;7:43–8.
27. Witt BL, Hyer CF. Treatment of hammertoe deformity using a one-piece intramedullary device. J Foot Ankle Surg. 2012;51:450–6.
28. Myerson MS, Filippi J. Bone block lengthening of the proximal interphalangeal joint for managing the floppy toe deformity. Foot Ankle Clin. 2010;15:663–8.
29. Derner R, Meyr AJ. Complications and salvage of elective central metatarsal osteotomies. Clin Podiatr Med Surg. 2009;26:23–35.
30. Vandeputte G, Dereymaeker G, Steenwerckx A, et al. The Weil osteotomy of the lesser metatarsals: a clinical and pedobarographic study. Foot Ankle Int. 2000;21(5):370–4.
31. O'Kane C, Kilmartin TE. The surgical management of central metatarsalgia. Foot Ankle Int. 2002;23(5):415–9.
32. Migues A, Slullitel G, Bilbao F, et al. Floating-toe deformity a complication of the Weil osteotomy. Foot Ankle Int. 2004;25(9):609–13.
33. Beech I, Rees S, Tagoe M. A retrospective review of the Weil metatarsal osteotomy for lesser metatarsal deformities: an intermediate follow-up analysis. J Foot Ankle Surg. 2005;44(5):358–64.
34. Kilmartin TE, O'Kane C. Correction of valgus second toe by closing wedge osteotomy of the proximal phalanx. Foot Ankle Int. 2007;28:1260–4.
35. Haddad SL, Sabbagh RC, Resch S, et al. Results of flexor-to-extensor and extensor brevis tendon transfer for correction of the crossover second toe deformity. Foot Ankle Int. 1999;20:781–8.
36. Coughlin MJ. Lesser toe abnormalities. Instr Course Lect. 2003;52:421–44.
37. Gallentine JW, DeOrio JK. Removal of the second toe for severe hammertoe deformity in elderly patients. Foot Ankle Int. 2005;26:353–8.
38. Feeney S, Rees S, Tagoe M. Hemiphalangectomy and syndactylization for treatment of osteoarthritis and dislocation of the second metatarsal phalangeal joint: an outcome study. J Foot Ankle Surg. 2006;45:82–90.

Lesser Metatarsal Osteotomy Complications

8

Lowell S. Weil and Erin E. Klein

Introduction

Metatarsalgia is defined as pain in the metatarsal region. Surgical correction of metatarsalgia can be very difficult. Historically, a high rate of complications has been associated with procedures performed for the treatment of metatarsalgia. A plethora of different types of procedures have been described for the surgical management of metatarsalgia.

Surgical procedures may be classified by the region of the metatarsal bone where they are performed. Procedures can be done at the head [1–6], the neck [7–10], the shaft, or the base of the lesser metatarsal. Resectional procedures [3] of the metatarsal head or ray and implant procedures [11] have also been described. When you review what these procedures ultimately accomplish, one will find that the bone can be either shortened or elevated. Very few procedures described can both of these functions.

Early papers on surgical procedures for forefoot problems report success [1, 7, 12]. However, many subsequent papers discuss complications such as floating toes [13] and transfer metatarsalgia [14, 15]. This further illustrates the point that historically these procedures have been wrought with complications [13].

Technique Pearls and Pitfalls: To Avoid Complications (Central Rays)

The lesser MTP joint is composed of the lesser metatarsal head, the base of the proximal phalanx, the intracapsular supporting structures (collateral ligaments), the capsular supporting structures (including the plantar plate), the intrinsic musculature of the foot, and the extrinsic musculature of the foot (Fig. 8.1) [16–18].

The metatarsal head has a medial and lateral tubercle upon which the collateral ligaments originate. These structures are important not only in the stability of the joint but also in marking an anatomic location for the main blood vessels that provide arterial flow to the metatarsal head [19] (Fig. 8.2). Dissection of the metatarsal head should aim to avoid detaching the collateral ligaments from the metatarsal head for two distinct reasons. First, the collateral ligaments are important sagittal plane-stabilizing structures for the lesser MTP joint [2, 18, 20]. Second, severance of the collateral ligaments may also cause damage to the blood vessels and could, potentially, increase the risk of avascular necrosis and delayed healing to the metatarsal osteotomy site [19].

The Weil metatarsal osteotomy was originally described as an intra-articular osteotomy that is created as close to parallel to the weight-bearing surface of the foot as possible. Surgically, this means that the osteotomy is started *within* the cartilage of the metatarsal head [21]. Proper angulation of the osteotomy (typically 15°) will lead to direct proximal translation with minimal plantar translation of the capital fragment [22]. Improper angulation of the osteotomy will lead to plantarization of the capital fragment and could potentially result in continued forefoot pain postoperatively (Fig. 8.3). It is also important to avoid over-penetration of the plantar cortex of the metatarsal with the saw blade. There is a nutrient artery that enters the metatarsal plantarly that may be at risk if this occurs [19].

The Weil metatarsal osteotomy was described to shorten the metatarsal 1–3 mm in length in order to avoid plantarization of the capital fragment [1]. When the osteotomy is performed at the prescribed 15° angle, there will not be plantar translation if the bone is shortened less than 3 mm [22]. If the metatarsal is to be shortened more than 3 mm in length, a second parallel osteotomy must be created in order to avoid plantarization of the capital fragment. When a review of the literature regarding this osteotomy is undertaken, it should be noted that many studies report a shortening of 4–10 mm with

L.S. Weil (✉) • E.E. Klein
Department of Surgery, Weil Foot and Ankle Institute,
1455 Golf Road, Des Plaines, IL 60016, USA
e-mail: LWJ@weil4feet.com; EEK@weil4feet.com

M.S. Lee, J.P. Grossman (eds.), *Complications in Foot and Ankle Surgery*, DOI 10.1007/978-3-319-53686-6_8

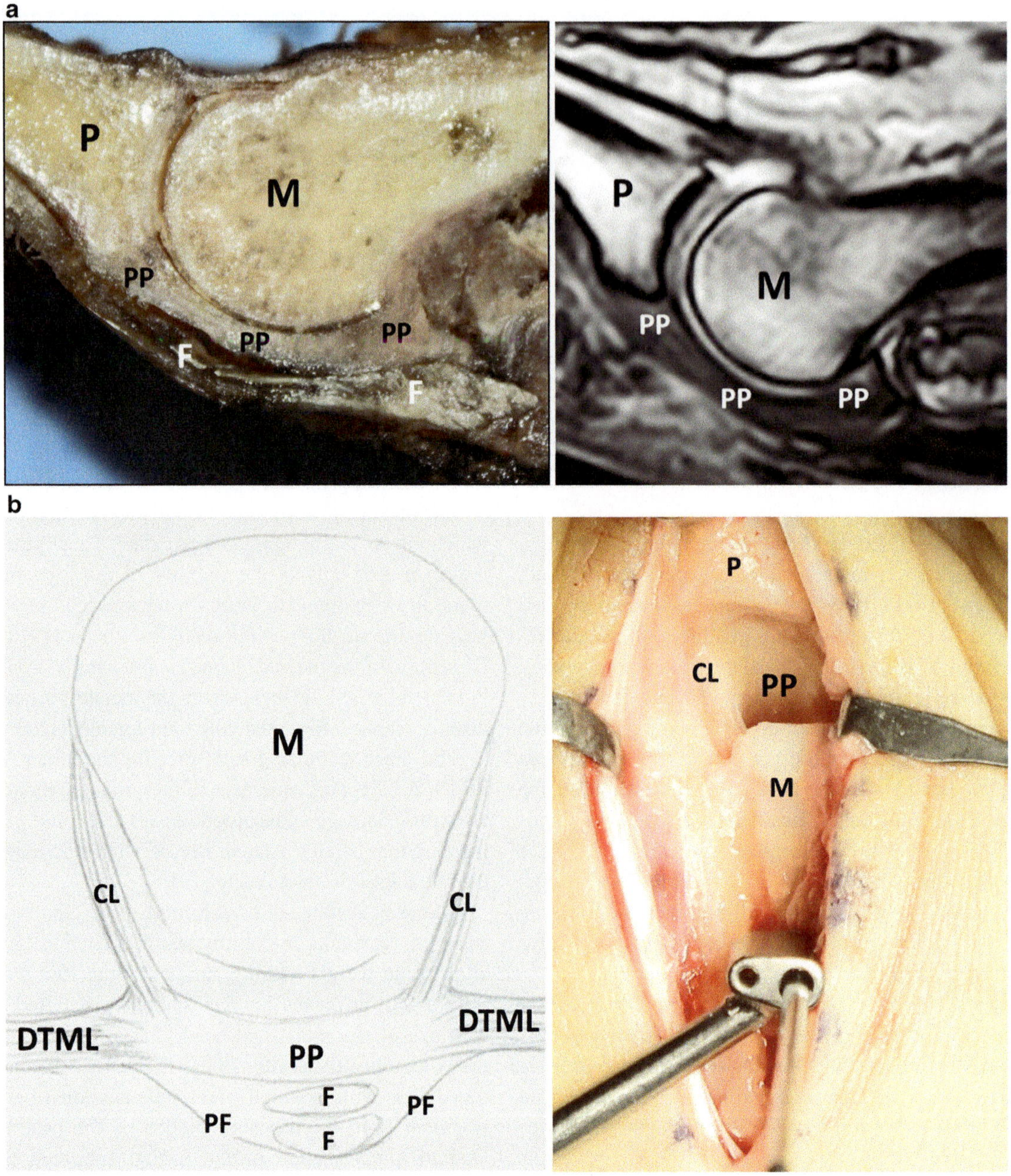

Fig. 8.1 (**a**) A cadaveric (*left*) and MRI (*right*) view of a midsection through the second metatarsal at the level of the metatarsal head. *P* base of the proximal phalanx, *M* metatarsal head, *PP* plantar plate, *F* flexor tendon. (**b**) A frontal image at the level of the metatarsal head. *M* metatarsal head, *PP* plantar plate, *F* flexor tendons, *DTML* deep transverse metatarsal ligament, *CL* collateral ligaments, *PF* deep slips of the plantar fascia

this osteotomy and a rate of postoperative floating toes as high as 36% [13, 15, 22, 23]. It should be noted that this osteotomy was not originally designed to shorten the metatarsal in that capacity and that the rate of postoperative floating toes may be related to the amount of shortening performed.

Aggressive shortening can lead to transfer metatarsalgia as the corrected metatarsal could take on a length that overloads the adjacent metatarsal(s). If there is a concern about the postoperative length of the second or the adjacent metatarsals, correcting this at the initial procedure, rather than waiting until problems develop later, may be beneficial [22].

Fixation for the Weil osteotomy should follow basic AO principles. This will assure primary bone healing and decrease the rate of nonunions that occur. As noted above, maintenance of the blood supply to the metatarsal will also decrease the incidence of this complication.

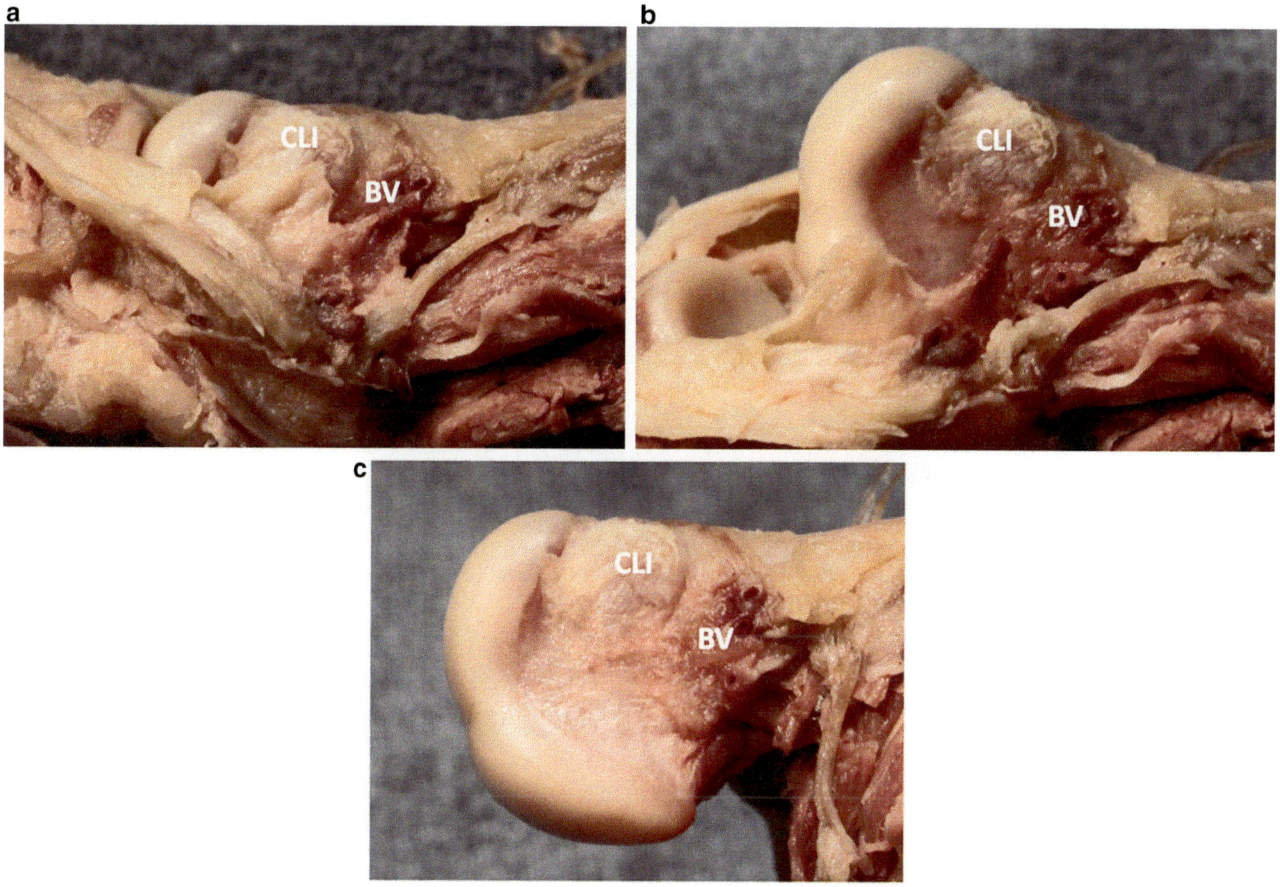

Fig. 8.2 (**a**) A cadaveric specimen of the lesser MTP joint. The proximity of the blood vessels (BV) to the collateral ligament insertion (CLI) can be seen. (**b**) The same specimen with the collateral ligaments reflected. (**c**) The same specimen with the proximal phalanx removed

As with any procedure, postoperative care is important and can vary from surgeon to surgeon. The postoperative regimen utilized in our institution [21] includes the patient being in a bandage and a surgical shoe for 7–10 days. At that time, the patients are instructed to return to athletic shoes with guarded weight bearing and aggressive physical therapy commences. Physical therapy focuses on strengthening of the intrinsic muscles of the foot and restoring the muscle balance to the MTP joint. There is a significant emphasis placed on the strength of the plantarflexory muscles and mobility in that direction. Additionally, the patient is instructed to utilizing nighttime bracing with the toe strapped in a plantarflexed position. This will decrease the amount of dorsal scar tissue that forms, theoretically decreasing the rate of floating toes that occur.

Recently, there has been a considerable emphasis on the correct diagnosis of the causative factor of metatarsalgia. Traditionally, it has been thought that the long metatarsal or "unharmonious parabola" [24] is the sole problem. However, more recent literature [18, 25–28] focuses on the plantar plate as a cause of deformity and pain in the forefoot with particular emphasis on differentiating plantar plate pain from neuroma pain [25, 28].

The plantar plate is the main stabilizer of the lesser MTP joint, particularly in the direction of plantarflexion [2, 18, 28]. This structure is approximately 2 cm in length and 1 cm in width and can vary in thickness from 2 to 5 mm [16, 17, 29]. The plantar plate is composed of a combination of type 1 (75%) and type 2 (21%) collagen that is woven together to create a fibrocartilaginous structure. The dorsal fibers of the plantar plate are longitudinally orientated, while the plantar aspect of the plantar plate has horizontally orientated fibers that are continuous with the deep transverse intermetatarsal ligament [18]. The lateral edges of the plantar plate serve as the attachment of the accessory collateral ligament and the deep slips of the plantar fascia. The plantar fascia has the additional role of providing the pulley-like structure that allows the flexor tendons to provide plantarflexion to the MTP joint (Fig. 8.4) [17].

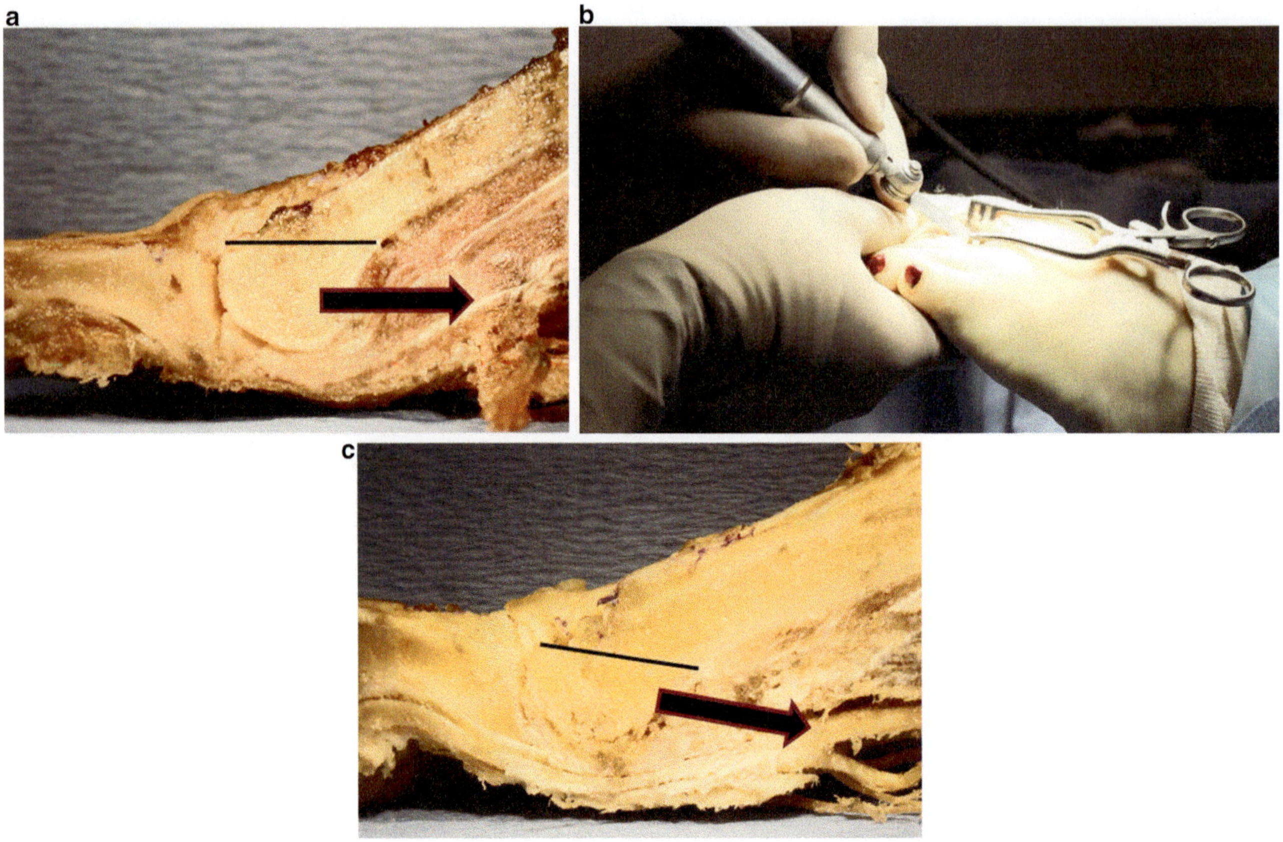

Fig. 8.3 (**a**) A cross section of a cadaver with a Weil metatarsal osteotomy performed that is angulated correctly. As the osteotomy is translated proximally, it will follow the course of the *thick black arrow*, and plantarization will not occur if the metatarsal is shortened less than 3 mm. (**b**) The intraoperative angle needed to achieve an osteotomy that is parallel to the weight-bearing surface of the foot. (**c**) A cross section of a cadaver with a Weil metatarsal osteotomy performed that is angulated incorrectly. As the osteotomy is translated proximally, it will follow the course of the *thick black arrow* and plantarization will occur

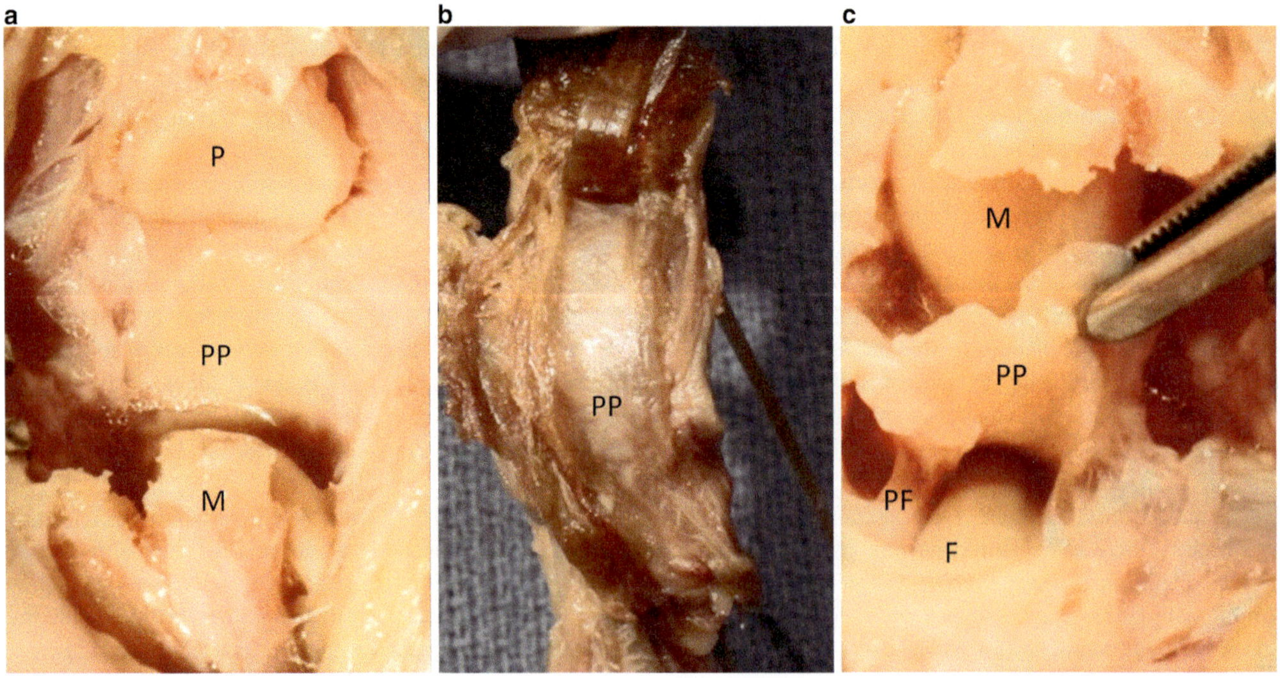

Fig. 8.4 (**a**) The plantar plate as it appears approaching it from the dorsum with longitudinal fibers in place. In this particular cadaveric specimen, the plantar plate attaches in two bundles. (**b**) The plantar aspect of the plantar plate with the transversely orientated fibers. (**c**) The slips of the plantar fascia are still attached to the plantar plate in this cadaveric specimen. This is a great illustration of the pulley system that allows plantar flexion at the MTP joint

With understanding of the anatomy of the lesser MTP joint, it is clear that the plantar plate may have a role in lesser MTP joint pain. Mann et al. [30] described a monoarticular synovitis of the lesser MTP joint capsule in 1985 and thought that this may be a new diagnosis. Now, however, it is recognized that the inflamed capsule and synovitis of the joint may actually be a prodrome to a plantar plate tear [30, 31]. If this problem is underdiagnosed or missed, an underlying osseous deformity [32] may lead to pathology in the plantar plate, collateral ligaments, or both. Ninety-five percent of patients with plantar plate pathology can be diagnosed clinically [25–27] with the symptoms of pain, edema, and a positive drawer sign. When you have a patient with a positive drawer sign and an increased lateral deviation of the third MTP joint on AP radiographs, this should alert the astute clinician to the potential presence of plantar plate pathology [26].

Management of Specific Complications

Transverse Plane Deformities

Transverse plane deformities need to be properly diagnosed as a transverse plane deviation at the MTP joint and may represent a partial lateral tear of the plantar plate, a tear of the collateral ligament, or a large interdigital neuroma (Fig. 8.5). The combination of a positive drawer test on clinical exam coupled with transverse plane deviation of the MTP joint >15° has been shown to be associated with plantar plate injuries [26]. Advanced imaging can also be useful. Both ultrasound [33, 34] and MRI [35, 36] have been shown to be useful to the diagnosis of plantar plate pathology with MRI being more useful in imaging of the collateral ligament structures [36].

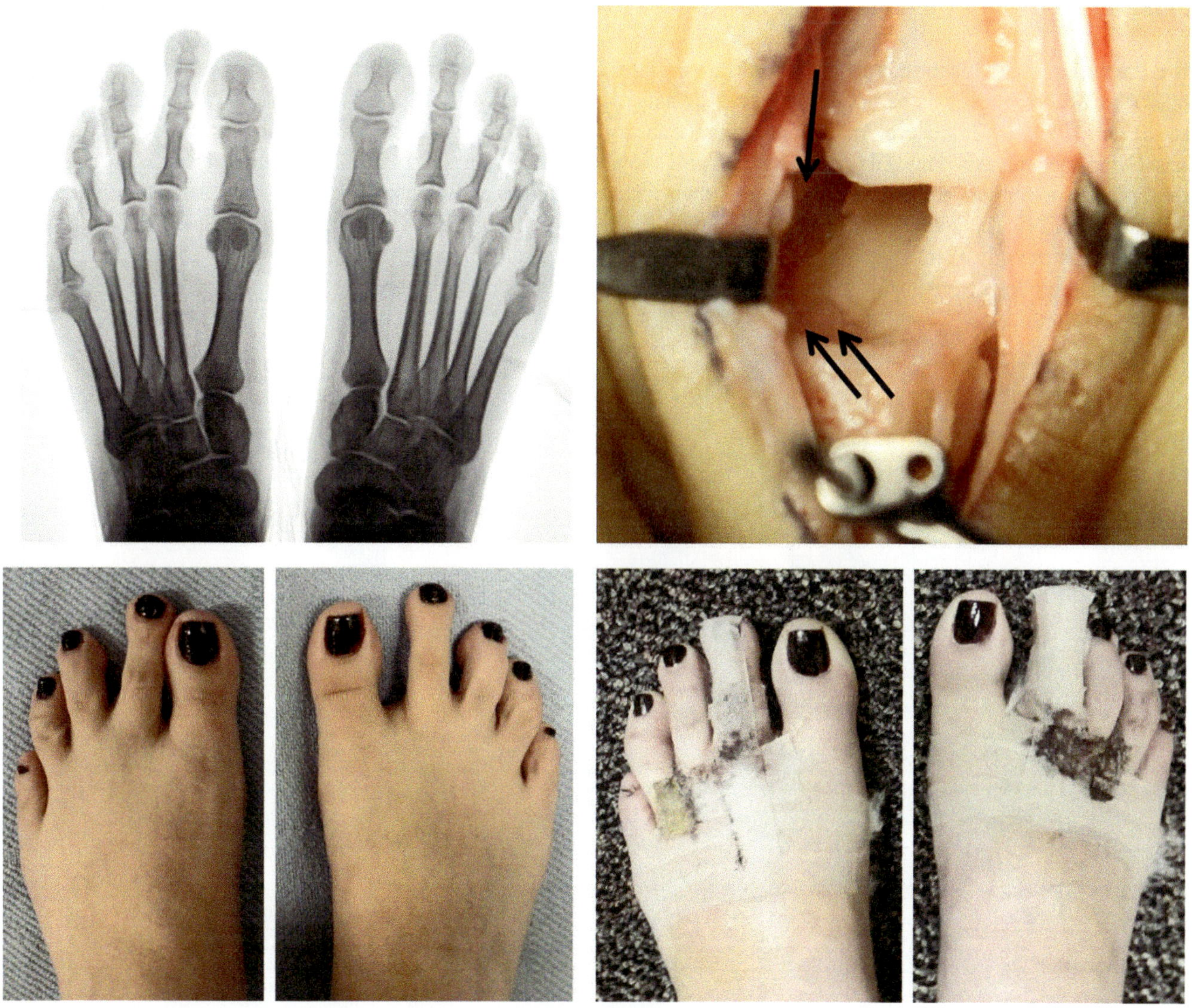

Fig. 8.5 Weight-bearing radiographs, clinical weight-bearing pre- and postoperative photographs, and intraoperative view of a patient that demonstrates transverse plane deviation of the digit. This patient was found to have both plantar plate and collateral ligament pathology

The management of the transverse plane deformity at the MTP joint is dependent on what is causing this deviation to occur. If the plantar plate is torn, surgical correction can be undertaken from the dorsal approach to repair this problem [21, 37]. Similarly, the collateral ligaments can be surgically repaired through the same approach. A repair of the plantar plate can be augmented with capsule/tendon balancing procedure or tendon transfer.

The authors of this chapter and others have been using a combined dorsal approach Weil osteotomy and plantar plate repair since 2007 with consistent results [21]. Specifically designed instrumentation has aided in the success of this approach to repair which avoids the problematic plantar incision, allows direct visualization of the plantar plate pathology, and provides precise correction of the metatarsal position with excellent tensioning of the plantar plate.

Floating Toes

It is important to remember that central metatarsal osteotomies (the Weil osteotomy, in particular) will alter the axis of the lesser MTP joint [23]. In proximally translating the metatarsal head, the joint axis is moved proximally. This will allow the intrinsic muscles to act more as dorsiflexors than plantarflexors [22, 24]. This may explain a part of the floating toe problem. Interestingly, there is also a report in the literature that a PIPJ arthrodesis combined with an osteotomy may have a higher incidence of floating toes than when these two procedures are not combined [22].

There are three distinct causes of floating toes. The first cause of the floating toe is excessive shortening of the metatarsal and/or incorrect angulation of the osteotomy. As the capital fragment of the metatarsal is proximally translated, the axis of the joint is altered allowing the extensors to have a mechanical advantage over the weak, indirect attachment of the flexor tendons. If the soft tissues around the joint (specifically the extensor tendons and the plantar plate) are not addressed properly, floating toes can occur.

The second cause of the floating toe is the presence of plantar plate pathology that is not addressed at the same time as the Weil osteotomy. As the plantar plate is the primary stabilizing structure of the lesser MTP joint, if this structure is damaged, there will be instability of the MTP joint and decreased plantarflexory strength of the MTP joint. This, again, will allow the extensors a mechanical advantage as stated above. The easiest way to correct this problem is to correct the pathology at the plantar plate.

Third, floating toes can be caused by dorsal scar tissue and adhesions that occur postoperatively. This scar tissue may be able to be prevented by aggressive postoperative brace and physical therapy. If this does occur, however, an aggressive tenotomy and capsulotomy of the scar tissue at the dorsal aspect of the MTP joint with aggressive manipulation of the toe in the direction of plantarflexion performed 6–12 months postoperatively can be helpful to treat this problem [22] (Fig. 8.6).

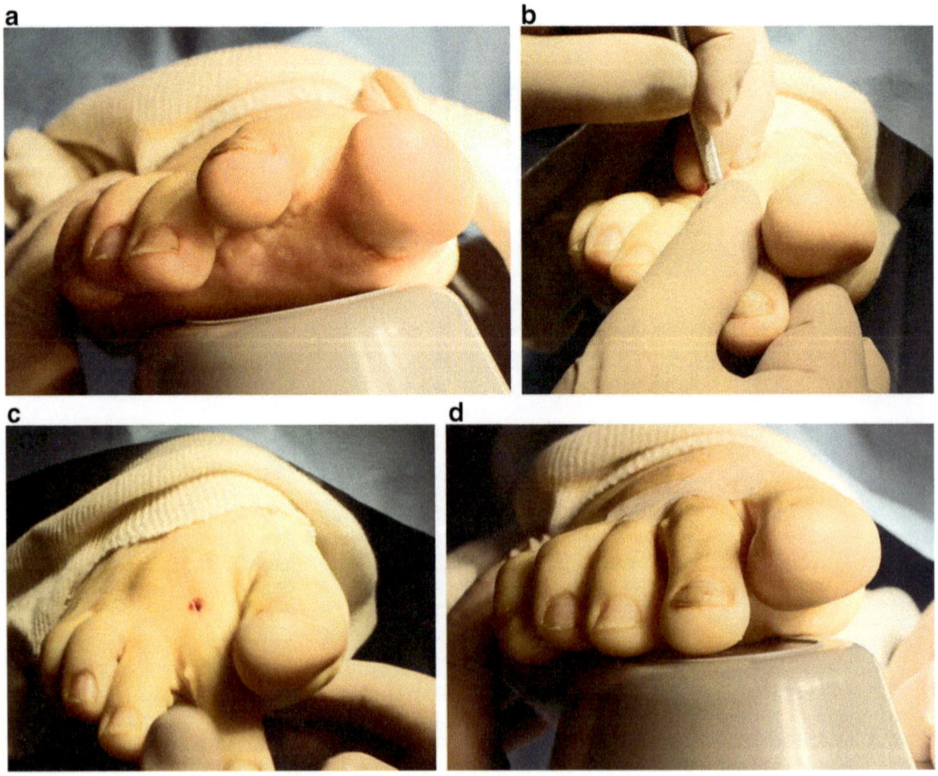

Fig. 8.6 (**a**) This patient is 12 weeks s/p plantar plate repair, and the toe is slightly elevated when the foot is loaded. (**b**) A percutaneous tenotomy and capsulotomy of the MTP joint. (**c**) Plantarflexory manipulation of the joint. (**d**) Toe purchase is obtained

Transfer Metatarsalgia

Transfer metatarsalgia typically occurs from overshortening or overelevation of the metatarsal at the time of surgery and has been cited by almost all procedural-type articles on this subject. If concerns about shortening exist during the index procedure, it may be advisable to shorten the adjacent metatarsals at that time [22].

Nonsurgical treatment of this problem can include offloading the affected metatarsal head that is prominent. However, if this fails to alleviate pain and symptoms, one may be faced with the challenge of restoring the "harmonious parabola" [24]. To do this, a critical evaluation of AP and axial radiographs as well as a computerized footprint pressure analysis (if available) must be undertaken. Once the apex of the deformity (i.e., the unharmonious metatarsal) is identified, that metatarsal must be surgically altered in a way that will restore the metatarsal parabola [51]. This may require one or more osteotomies of the adjacent metatarsals. All previous discussion of the orientation and limitations of the metatarsal osteotomy apply.

Nonunion/Malunion

This is a rare complication if this procedure is performed properly. Preservation of the blood supply to the metatarsal head (particularly maintaining the collateral ligament attachment to the metatarsal head) has been discussed. It is also important to avoid over-penetration of the plantar cortex of the bone with the sagittal saw. There is a blood vessel that enters the bone plantarly. Although this artery is not the major source of blood flow to the distal aspect of the bone, it is important to avoid damaging it.

Fixation of the osteotomy should follow AO principles. This should prevent nonunion of the osteotomy. Observing the osteotomy closing intraoperatively is important. In order to achieve this, plantarflexion of the toe with dorsal pressure of the phalanx on the plantar aspect of the metatarsal head creates compression while fixation is performed. Alternatively, one can use their thumb on the plantar surface of the foot and provide dorsal compression of the osteotomy site while the screw is being inserted. Additionally, the surgeon at the foot of the table can utilize a sesamoid or phalangeal clamp to gently grasp the capital fragment and provide dorsal force, while the surgeon at the side of the table inserts the screw. If one point of fixation is not adequate, a second point of fixation can be utilized. If a nonunion does occur, one can consider many of the modalities discussed in the nonunion chapter of this text.

In cases of malunion, one may consider a revisional osteotomy with fixation that adheres to the AO guidelines. This has not been specifically described for an elective osteotomy of the lesser metatarsals. However, it has been described with promising results for lesser metatarsal fractures that were not fixated initially [38]. Occasionally, patients may present with a hypertrophic process that produces prominence and pain on the dorsum of the foot. This can be treated with resection of the hypertrophic tissue.

Bunionette/Tailor's Bunions

There are a plethora of surgical procedures aimed at correcting deformities of the fifth ray. Head [39], neck [40, 41], shaft [42–46], base, and resectional procedures have all been described. Percutaneous [47, 48] and MIS procedures [49] have been described as well [50]. There is a classification system [43] that the Tailor's bunion deformity can be (a) an enlarged lateral prominence, (b) a metaphyseal-diaphyseal flare/deviation, or (c) a widened 4–5 IM angle. The literature related to the description of surgical procedures for this deformity are limited in nature, and many of these articles do not describe true complications of this procedure. Therefore, principles from other portions of the foot must be applied to this area.

Under-Correction

One of the limitations of the ability of a procedure to correct a larger 4–5 intermetatarsal angle or a larger lateral deviation angle is the width of the fifth metatarsal. This can lead to under-correcting the deformity with the index procedure. Larger deformities may require either a more proximal procedure or a procedure with a longer lever arm and more post-osteotomy osseous contact. If under-correction occurs and nonsurgical treatment does not alleviate the patient's post-procedural symptoms, a reevaluation of the root of the problem needs to occur.

If the recurrent problem is prominence of the metatarsal head, a lateral or plantar condylectomy (depending on the location of the problem) would likely be sufficient. However, if one has under-corrected IM and/or lateral deviation angle, a secondary osteotomy may be necessary. It may also be necessary to perform a more proximal osteotomy that has more ability to correct the remaining IM and/or lateral deviation angles. Proximal osteotomies, however, may require a prolonged healing time as the blood flow at the base of the fifth metatarsal is notoriously poor.

Shortened Ray

Creating osteotomies of the fifth metatarsal will lead to shortening of the bone in some capacity. Osteotomies that require removal of a segment of the bone shorten the fifth ray more than ones that do not. Therefore, if it is suspected that that fifth ray is shortened initially, avoiding these procedures helps limit this complication.

If the fifth ray remains shortened and this is causing significant pain to the patient, there are surgical options. First, one may consider treating this problem as one would treat a brachymetatarsia – with either a single-stage bone block lengthening procedure or with a corticotomy and callus distraction procedure. Second, one can consider shortening the fourth metatarsal in order to harmonize the parabola.

Nonunion and Malunion

Non- and malunions are not reported in the current medical literature in association with surgical procedures to correct bunionettes. However, these complications can occur with any surgical procedure that requires an osteotomy. If a nonunion does occur, one can consider many of the modalities discussed in the nonunion chapter of this text.

Malunion of the bone can also occur. If this does occur, an evaluation of the apex of the resultant deformity needs to be undertaken. If the problem is prominence of the metatarsal head, a lateral or plantar condylectomy (depending on the location of the problem) would likely be sufficient. If there is hypertrophy of any part of the bone resulting in a subcutaneous prominence, this can be removed with care being taken to remove a bit more the bone than might look immediately necessary. This will allow for osseous regrowth but hopefully prevent the subcutaneous prominence that was there previously.

Conclusion

The lesser metatarsals present surgical challenges to the astute physician. There are many complications that can occur with these procedures, particularly on metatarsals 2–4. Many of these complications can be avoided by tedious operative technique, correct procedure selection, and knowledge of the local anatomy.

References

1. Barouk L. Weil metatarsal osteotomy in the treatment of metatarsalgia. Orthopade. 1996;25(4):338–44.
2. Coughlin M. Subulxation and dislocation of the second metatarsophalangeal joint. Orthop Clin N Am. 1989;20:535–51.
3. Garg R, Thordarson D, Schrumpf M, Castaneda D. Sliding oblique versus segmental resection osteotomies for lesser metatarsophalangeal joint pathology. Foot Ankle Int. 2008;29(10):1009–14.
4. Morandi A, Dupplicato P, Sansone V. Results of a distal metatarsal osteotomy using absorbable pin fixation. Foot Ankle Int. 2009; 30(1):34–8.
5. Hamilton WG, Thompson FM. Problems of the second metatarsophalangeal joint. Orthopedics. 1987;10:83–9.
6. Helal B. Metatarsal osteotomy for metatarsalgia. J Bone Jt Surg Br. 1975;57:187–92.
7. Lui T. Percutaneous dorsal closing wedge osteotomy of the metatarsal neck in management of metatarsalgia. Foot (Edinb). 2014;24(4):180–5.
8. Bennett A, McLeod I. An adaptation of Weil's osteotomy of the lesser metatarsal neck. J Foot Ankle Surg. 2009;48(4):516–7.
9. Kennedy J, Deland J. Resolution of metatarsalgia following oblique osteotomy. Clin Orthop Relat Res. 2006;453:309–13.
10. Helal B, Greiss M. Telescoping osetotomy for pressure metatarsalgia. J Bone Jt Surg Br. 1984;66B:213–7.
11. Cracchiolo A, Kitaoka H, Leventen E. Silacone implant arthroplsty for second metatrsophalangeal joint disorders with and without hallux valgus deformities. Foot Ankle. 1988;9:10–8.
12. Muhlbauer M, Trnka H, Zembsch A, Ritchl P. Short-term outcome of Weil osteotomy in treatment of metatarsalgia. Z Orthop Ihren Grenzgeb. 2003;141:590–4.
13. Highlander P, VonHerbulis E, Gonzalez A, Brit J, Buchman J. Complications of the Weil osteotomy. Foot Ankle Spec. 2011;4(3): 165–70.
14. Winkler I, Kelaridis T. Helal's metatarsal osteotomy: indication and technic with reference to shape and function of the foot. Z Orthop Ihren Grenzgeb. 1989;127:556–60.
15. Trnka H, Kabon B, Zettl R, Kaider A, Salzer M, Ritschl P. Helal metatarsal osteotomy for the treatment of metatarsalgiaL a critical analysis of results. Orthopedics. 1996;19:457–61.
16. Johnston R, Smith J, Daniels T. The plantar plate of the lesser toes: an anatomical study in human cadavers. Foot Ankle Int. 1994; 15(5):276–82.
17. Sarafian S, Topouzian L. Anatomy and physiology of the extensor apparatus of the toes. J Bone Jt Surg Am. 1969;51(4):669–79.
18. Stainsby G. Pathological anatomy and dynamic effect of the displaced plantar plate and the importance of the integrity of the plantar plate-deep transverse metatarsal ligament tie-bar. Ann R Coll Surg Engl. 1997;79(1):58–68.
19. Petersen W, Lankes J, Paulsen F, Hassenpflug J. The arterial supply of the lesser metatarsal heads: a vascular injection study in human cadavers. Foot Ankle Int. 2000;23(6):491–5.
20. Bhatia D, Myerson MS, Curtis MJ, Cunningham BW, Jinnah RH. Anatomic restraints to dislocation of the second metatarsophalangeal joint and assessment of repair technique. J Bone Jt Surg Am. 1994;76A(9):1371–5.
21. Weil Jr L, Sung W, Weil Sr LS, Malinoski K. Anatomic plantar plate repair using the Weil metatarsal osteotomy approach. Foot Ankle Spec. 2011;4(3):145–50.
22. Migues A, Slullitel G, Bilbao F, Carrasco M, Solari G. Floating toe deformity as a complication of the Weil osteotomy. Foot Ankle Int. 2004;25(9):609–13.
23. Trnka H, Nyska M, Parks B, Myerson M. Dorsiflexion contracture after the Weil osteotomy: results of a cadaver study and three dimensional analysis. Foot Ankle Int. 2001;22:47–50.
24. Maestro M, Besse JL, Ragusa M, Berthonnaud E. Forefoot morphotype study and planning for forefoot osteotomy. Foot Ankle Clin. 2003;8(4):695–710.
25. Klein EE, Weil Jr L, Weil Sr LS, Coughlin MJ, Knight J. Clinical examination of plantar plate abnormality: a diagnostic perspective. Foot Ankle Int. 2013;34(6):800–4.
26. Klein EE, Weil Jr L, Weil Sr LS, Bowen M, Fleischer AE. Positive drawer test combined with radiographic transverse plane deformity of the 3rd metatarsophalangeal joint suggests high grade tears of the 2nd metatarsophalangeal joint plantar plate. Foot Ankle Spec. 7(6):466–70.
27. Kaz AJ, Coughlin MJ. Crossover second toe: demographics, etioogy and radiographic assessment. Foot Ankle Int. 2007;28:1223–37.

28. Doty J, Coughlin M, Jr LW, Nery C. Etiology and management of the lesser toe metatarsophalangeal joint instability. Foot Ankle Clin. 2014;19(3):385–405.
29. Deland J, Lee K, Sobel M, DiCarlo E. Anatomy of the plantar plate and its attachments in the lesser metatarsal phalangeal joint. Foot Ankle Int. 1995;16(8):480–9.
30. Mann RA, Mizel MS. Monoarticular nontraumatic synovitis of the metatarsophalangeal joint: a new diagnosis? Foot and Ankle. 1985;6:18–21.
31. G. Yu and D. DiNapoli, "Surgical management of hallux abductovalgus with concomitant metatarsus adductus," In: McGlamry ED, editor. Reconstructive Surgery of the foot and ankle: update '89. Tucker, GA: Podiatry Institute, p. 262–268; 1989.
32. Klein EE, Weil Jr L, Weil Sr LS, Knight J. The underlying osseous deformity in plantar plate tears: a radiographic analysis. Foot Ankle Spec. 2013;6(2):108–18.
33. Feuerstein CA, Weil Jr L, Weil Sr LS, Klein EE, Fleischer A, Argerakis NG. Static versus dynamic ultrasound for detection of pathology of the plantar plate. Foot Ankle Spec. 2014;15(7):259–65.
34. Klein EE, Weil Jr L, Weil Sr LS, Knight J. Musculoskeletal ultrasound for preoperative imaging of the plantar plate: a prospective analysis. Foot Ankle Spec. 2013;6(3):196–200.
35. Sung W, Weil L, Weil LS, Rolfes RJ. Magnetic resonance imaging of the plantar plate with reference to intra-operative findings. J Foot Ankle Surg. 2012;51(5):570–4.
36. Klein EE, Weil Jr L, Weil Sr LS, Knight J. Magnetic resonance imaging versus musculoskeletal ultrasound for identification and localization of plantar plate tears. Foot Ankle Spec. 2012;5(6):359–65.
37. J. Jastifer and M. Coughlin, Exposure via sequential release of the metatarsophalangeal joint for plantar plate repair through a dorsal approach without an intraarticular osteotomy. Foot Ankle Int. 2015 Mar; 36(3):335–8.
38. Murphy R, Fallat L. Surgical correciton of metatarsal malunion. J Foot Ankle Surg. 2012;51(6):801–5.
39. Cooper M, Coughlin M. Subcapital oblique osetotomy for correction of bunionette deformity: medium-term results. Foot Ankle Int. 2013;34(10):1376–80.
40. Weil LJ, Weil LS. Osteotomies for bunionette deformity. Foot Ankle Clin. 2011;16(4):689–712.
41. Legenstein R, Bonomo J, Huber W, Boesch P. Correction of tailor's bunion with the Boesch technique: a retrospective analysis. Foot Ankle Int. 2007;28(7):799–803.
42. Masquijo J, Willis B, Kontio K, Dobbs M. Symptomatic bunionette deformity in adolscents: surgical treatment with metatarsal sliding osteotomy. J Pediatr Orthop. 2010;30(8):904–9.
43. Coughlin M. Treatment of bunionette deformity with a longitudinal diaphyseal osteotomy with distal soft tissue repair. Foot Ankle. 1991;11:195–203.
44. Maher A, Kilmartin T. Scarf osteotomy for correction of tailor's bunion: mid to long term follow up. Foot Ankle Int. 2010;31(8): 676–82.
45. Glover J, Weil LJ, Weil LS. Scarfette osteotomy for surgical treatment of bunionette deformity. Foot Ankle Spec. 2009;2(2):73–8.
46. Guha A, Mukhopadhyay S, Thomas R. "Reverse" scarf osteotomy for bunionette correction: initial results of a new surgical technique. Foot Ankle Surg. 2012;18(1):50–4.
47. Michels F, Bauwhede JVD, Guillo S, Oosterlinch D, de Lavigne C. Percutaneous bunionette correction. Foot Ankle Surg. 2013;19(1): 9–14.
48. Magnan B, Samaila E, Merlini M, Bondi M, Mezzari S, Bartolozzi P. Percutaneous distal osteotomy of the fifth metatsral for correction of bunionette deformity. J Bone Jt Surg Am. 2011;93(22): 2116–22.
49. Giannini S, Faldini C, Vannini F, Digennaro V, Bevoni R, Luciani D. The minimally invasive osteotomy "S.E.R.I" (simple, effective, rapid, inexpensive) for correction of bunionette deformity. Foot Ankle Int. 2008;29(3):282–6.
50. Lui T. Percutaneous osteotomy of the fifth metatarsal for bunionette deformity. J Foot Ankle Surg. 2014;53(6):747–52.
51. Hofstaetter S, Hofstaetter J, Petroutsas J, Gruber F, Ritschl P, Trnka H. The Weil osteotomy: a seven year follow up. J Bone Jt Surg Br. 2005;87(11):1507–11.

Neuromas

9

Thomas J. Chang

Introduction

Cortisone is still the first line of treatment for nerve entrapment pain. This is commonly seen in primary neuromas, recurrent neuromas, as well as post-traumatic neuromas [1–3]. The benefits and side effects of cortisone are well understood, and repetitive injections with cortisone to the same area should be avoided. There has been a significant interest in sclerosing agents such as 4% medical ethyl alcohol to kill the nerve and take away the consistent burning pain from these injured nerves. Dockery has published 89% success for intermetatarsal neuromas and this has revolutionized the treatment for these chronic problems [2]. Others have stated mixed results. We have utilized the same approach for superficial cutaneous nerves of the foot and ankle which have post-traumatic or chronic pain syndromes, and the success is also worth noting. The recommendation is to do a minimum of three weekly injections up to a maximum of seven. After seven injections, symptoms are usually dramatically improved. Regardless of the percentage of relief noted, studies have shown that there is no statistical benefit to doing more than seven injections. When injected around the nerve, the alcohol has an affinity to nerve tissue and does not appear to cause any damage to other soft tissues in the area. From anecdotal observation, we have seen that when nerves which have been injected with the alcohol treatment are later surgically removed, the nerve appeared to be thinner as the alcohol must have some denaturing effect on them.

Thicker incisions can be painful with gentle palpation or stimulation due to sensory or deeper nerve adhesions. Silicone gel sheeting has been used for many of these thicker incisions with much success. Although the mechanism of action is not clear, there is consistent softening of the incision and ultimately, the deeper soft tissues soften and this serves to release scar tissue along these cutaneous nerve branches. The gel sheets are used for up to 3 months for maximum success.

T.J. Chang (✉)
Redwood Orthopedic Surgery Associates, Inc.,
208 Concourse Blvd #1, Santa Rosa, CA 95403, USA
e-mail: thomaschang14@comcast.net

Resection of Recurrent Neuromas

The most common location of recurrent neuromas is in the metatarsal interspaces after primary resection. There are several reasons for recurrence in these situations. Some surgeons will make a small incision at the level of the sulcus and try and find the nerve in the distal interspace. In this scenario, the initial resection may be inadequate, and the remaining end of the intermetatarsal nerve gets scarred down and often adheres within the capsular tissues of the metatarsal-phalangeal joint, causing recurrent pain. Also, there are often small branches of this main nerve that will give off branches which travel to the metatarsal head and the joint capsule. When surgeons pull distally on the nerve and attempt to resect the nerve as proximal as possible, the hope is the nerve will then retract a moderate amount proximally and lie within the intrinsic muscles (Fig. 9.1). What often happens is the nerve will actually be tethered by these small nerve fibers. These adjacent branches will often prevent it from retracting proximally (Fig. 9.2). This remaining distal position of the nerve will again be scarred down along the capsule of the adjacent tissue as well. During the evaluation process, a diagnostic injection of the amputation neuroma in the proximal interspace is important to confirm that relief is predictable after a possible revisional nerve resection.

We have also seen a dramatic increase of amputation neuromas within the second interspace as well. Many patients who present with second metatarsal stress syndrome, predislocation syndrome, or central metatarsal overload are diagnosed with second interspace neuroma. There may be some neuroma symptoms as swelling from the joint capsule may often irritate or put pressure on the nerves. Some of these patients are diagnosed with both second and third

M.S. Lee, J.P. Grossman (eds.), *Complications in Foot and Ankle Surgery*, DOI 10.1007/978-3-319-53686-6_9

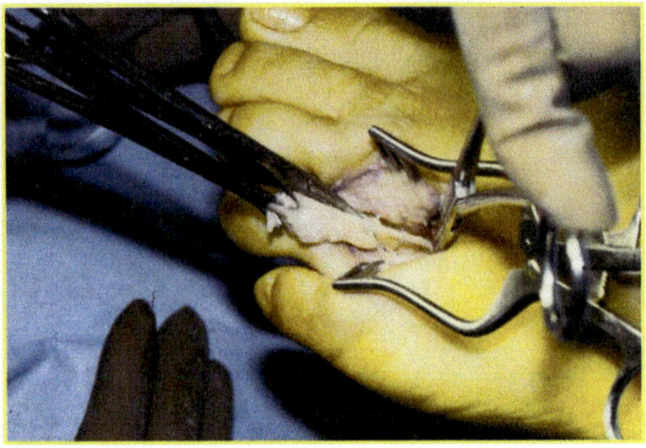

Fig. 9.1 Third interspace nerve being pulled distally in efforts to allow retraction of the cut end into the proximal muscle layer

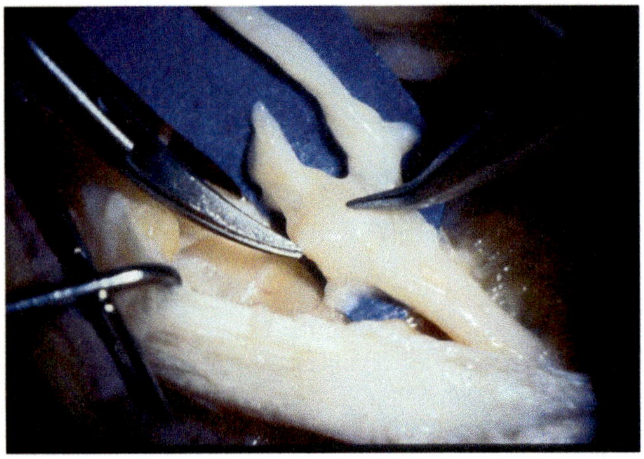

Fig. 9.2 Small nerve branches may tether the distal nerve to adjacent soft tissue and prevent retraction of the nerve more proximal upon resection. This may be the case with small distal incisions where the small side branches are not visualized

interspace neuromas and treated by removal using two dorsal incisions. Since the second metatarsal base is locked securely within the proximal articulations at Lisfranc joint, it is difficult to separate the second interspace for an adequate proximal resection. Due to this anatomy, these will often result in secondary amputation neuromas arising after nerve resection at the distal metatarsal level.

The best approach in resolving the chronic recurrent nerve syndrome is to resect the nerve more proximally and most likely implant it into a muscle or bone. Nerves exhibit a property called "neurotropism." When a nerve is cut, there are chemotactic factors which are transmitted from the cut end in an attempt for the nerve fibers to find its other end and repair itself. As the nerve does so, it forms a mass of randomly directed nerve tissue, and hence an "amputation neuroma" is born. The importance of nerve implantation is the ability for the nerve to calm down and not attempt to reconnect to its other end. If the nerve can be placed within richly innervated tissues, like a skeletal muscle or bone, then this will serve to turn off these chemotactic factors, suppress the regeneration potential of the transected nerve, and increase the chances of a successful outcome [4–7]. It is best to approach this revision with surgery through a plantar incision. The incision can either be longitudinal or in a curvilinear fashion. A curvilinear incision may be better to minimize scarring within the plantar aspect of the foot since this incision is oblique to the relaxed skin tension lines versus the longitudinal incision being perpendicular to these lines. In clinical practice, there is no clear difference in how these two different incisions heal, as long as they are protected non-weightbearing for 3–4 weeks. If dealing with multiple interspaces with amputation neuromas, then a curvilinear approach will offer better medial to lateral visualization for adjacent interspaces. After the skin incision is made, it is important to dissect down to and find the deep fascia, which is the plantar fascia in this area of the foot. It is important to keep the retracted skin full thickness, keeping the subcutaneous tissues attached to the skin. There will be natural septations within the distal plantar fascia which will divide out and insert at each metatarsal-phalangeal joint. There is a separation between the bands of the plantar fascia that can easily be found, and this separation can be extended more proximally, and the nerve is often visualized immediately underneath the plantar fascia. If there is any difficulty finding the nerve in question, look more superficially than deeply. The nerve may even be found adhered to the underside of the plantar fascia. In the third interspace, it is important to look for nerve branches from both the medial and lateral plantar nerves as they will both contribute into this interspace (Figs. 9.3, 9.4, 9.5, 9.6, 9.7, 9.8, 9.9, 9.10, 9.11, and 9.12).

The goal of revision is to transect this nerve as proximally as possible so it will lie within the intrinsic soft tissues of the plantar muscles of the foot. If there is adequate surrounding muscle, then this nerve can just be transected and allowed to sit within an area of the intrinsic muscle [1, 3–5, 7–10]. Other techniques involve performing an epineuroplasty and then transposing and anchoring the nerve into either skeletal bone or an adjacent muscle to make sure the regeneration potential of the nerve is suppressed. With the epineural approach, it is possible to use 6-0 Prolene to tag the cuff of thin wispy tissue and use this to mobilize the nerve and also to anchor the nerve into the muscle effectively. The skeletal bone is also richly innervated and can serve to suppress the regeneration tendency of the nerve [5, 6].

When the nerve is implanted into the muscle, several principles exist. First, sutures which are used to help mobilize the nerve should not pierce the nerve itself. The sutures should only purchase the epineural tissue to assist in nerve mobilization. Secondly, the nerves should be anchored under minimal to no tension. This will prevent further irritation to the nerve

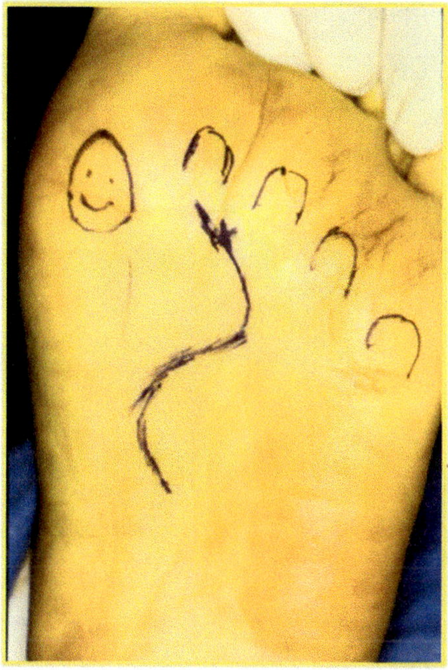

Fig. 9.3 Curvilinear incision oblique to RSTL to allow a wider field of vision and exposure. This approach is preferred for access to multiple nerves and/or interspaces

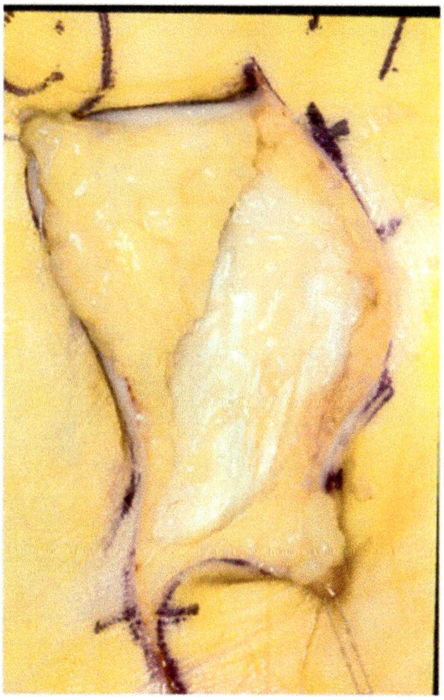

Fig. 9.4 Full-thickness skin flaps with dissection to help maintain vascularity to the skin edges

branch with movement of the foot and ankle and during ambulation. Resect the nerve as distally as possible and then loop the nerve proximally to minimize tension during implantation. And third, authors have also stated that it is ideal

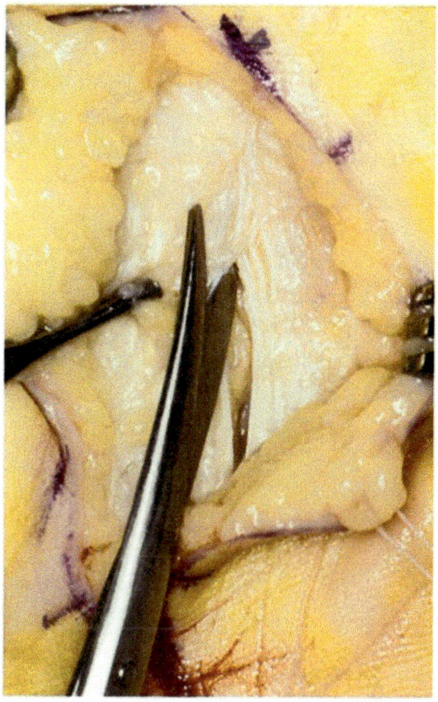

Fig. 9.5 Once the deep fascia is exposed, there are natural septations which divide to the separate MPJ's. This is helpful to help guide the surgeon for dissection directly into the interspace of choice

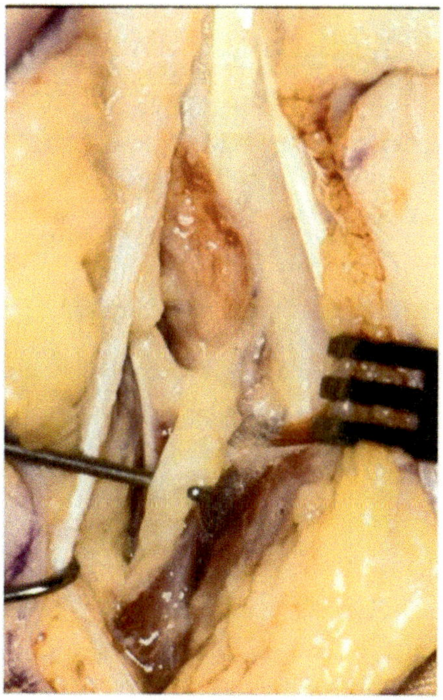

Fig. 9.6 A typical entrapped nerve found directly upon dissection along the natural separation of the deep fascia septations

to place the nerve into a muscle that has the least amount of excursion [11]. On the plantar aspect of the foot, this is the transverse head of the adductor hallucis. For plantar approaches

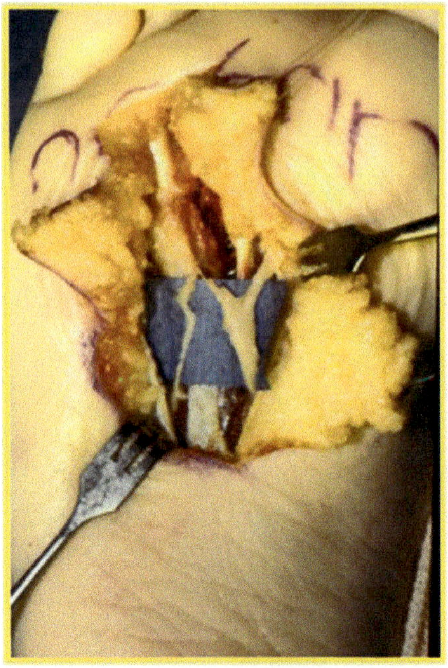

Fig. 9.7 Example of the nerve contributions from both the medial and lateral plantar nerves into the third interspace

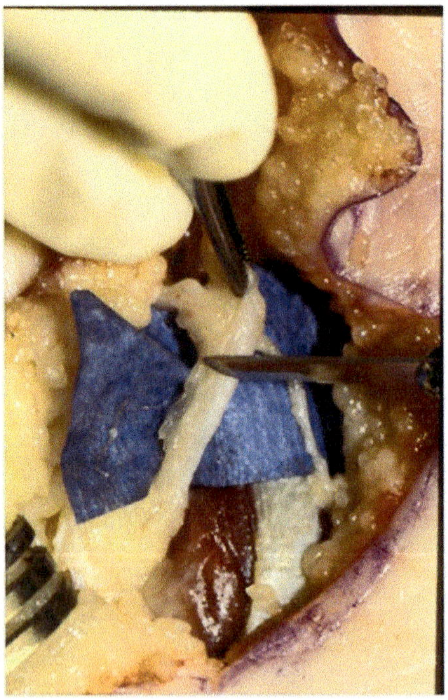

Fig. 9.8 Gentle scraping of the epineural sheath with a #15 blade to form a cuff of epineural tissue for anchoring the suture for muscle implantation

into the bottom of the foot, the intrinsic muscles are readily available, and there is no clear benefit to finding the adductor when the other muscles are all present. In the posterior ankle/leg area, this is the soleus muscle.

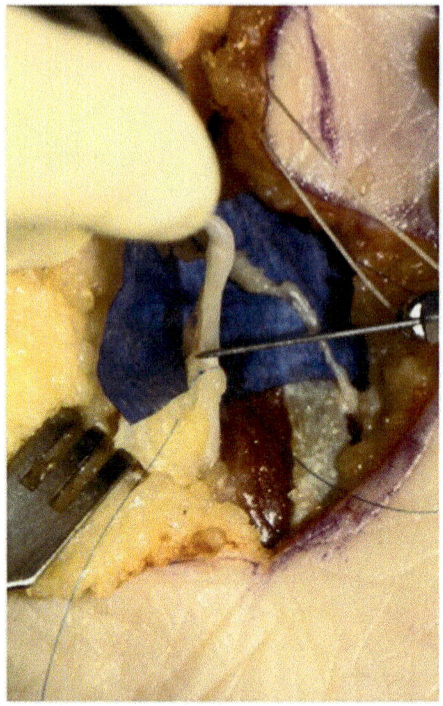

Fig. 9.9 Example of the epineural cuff tagged with two knots of 6-0 Prolene. This cuff of tissue is thin and wispy in appearance, but strong enough to hold the suture well

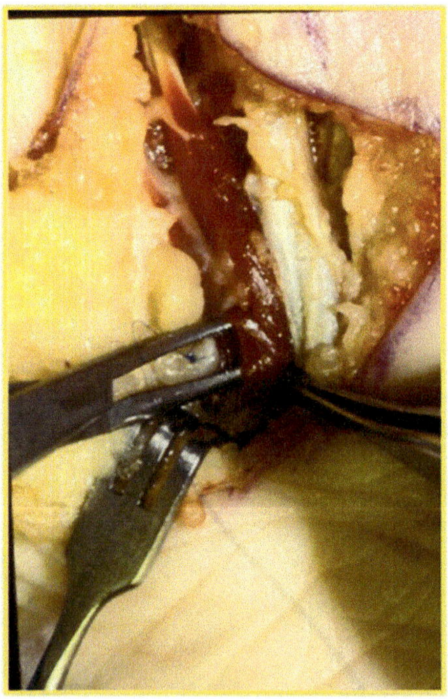

Fig. 9.10 Preparation of a tunnel within a nearby muscle for anchoring of the resected nerve. Implantation of the nerve into this richly innervated tissue will help to turn off the regeneration potential of the nerve

This approach for intermetatarsal nerve entrapment can also be used for the lateral dorsal cutaneous nerve (sural) and IDCN and MDCN entrapments after traumatic crush injuries or iatrogenic nerve damage to the dorsum of the foot. This is

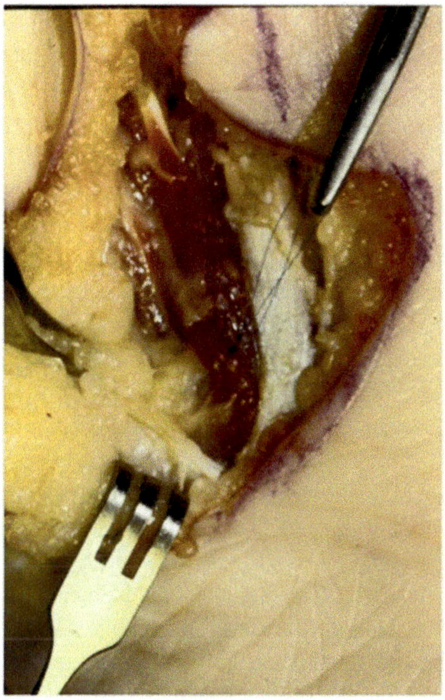

Fig. 9.11 The nerve anchored successfully into adjacent muscle tissue. The nerve is dragged with the sutures into the tunnel created within the muscle and the sutures are tied on the opposite side

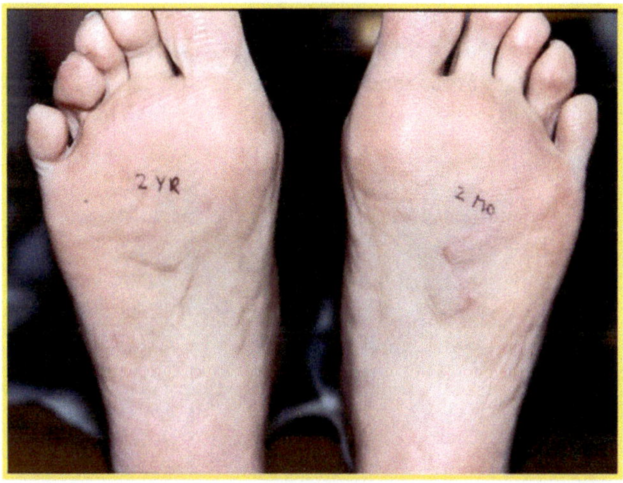

Fig. 9.12 Post-op incisions which heal very well on the plantar aspect of the foot. Three week non-weightbearing is essential to allow the soft tissues to heal fully before pressure is applied to the foot

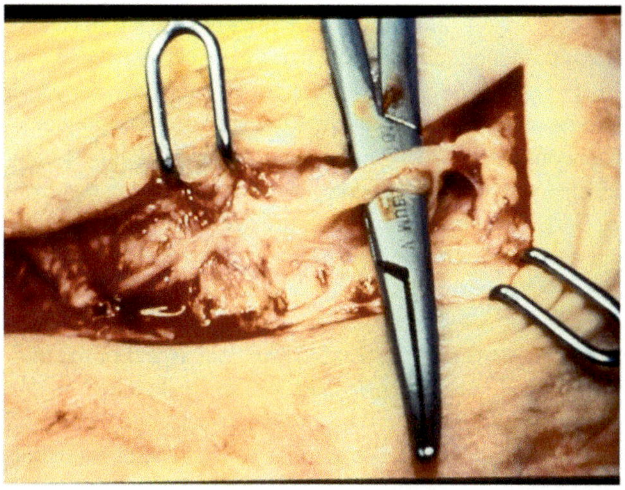

Fig. 9.13 Example of a sural nerve neuroma status post prior triple arthrodesis with scarring along the lateral subtalar joint incision

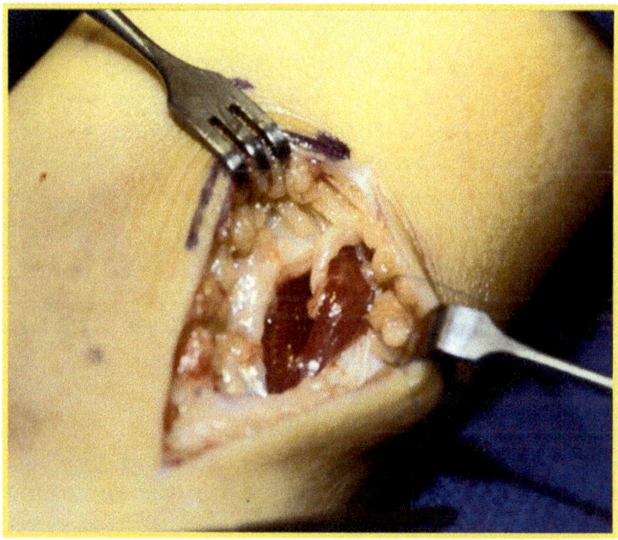

Fig. 9.14 Resection of the sural nerve with epineuroplasty and muscle implantation into the soleus muscle belly

also seen with sural nerve entrapments, as these are fairly common after lateral ankle or lower limb surgery. Often there are situations of nerve entrapment after flatfoot surgery or calcaneal fracture repair, where incisions are made on the lateral hindfoot (Fig. 9.13). In chronic cases of suspected sural nerve entrapment pain, a diagnostic injection can be very helpful to confirm and isolate the nerve pain and then discuss removing the painful sensation of nerve entrapment. If the initial injection works well, then usually we can often duplicate this relief to try and guarantee an improved situation for the patient. A diagnostic injection can easily be done with 3 mL of local anesthesia on the posterior distal one third of the leg and then resection and implantation is done with a slightly more proximal oblique incision. Once the nerve if safely found, scar tissue can be removed and then the nerve mobilized and placed into the soleus muscle (Fig. 9.14). The soleus muscle is known to have the least excursion of the extrinsic muscles in the lower leg and is an ideal choice for sural nerve implantation. The lateral fibula can also be used for nerve implantation if desired, and this can be done through a simple drill hole in the posterior lateral portion of the fibula. A comparison study between muscle placement and fibular burial shows better relief of pain after bone burial of the sural nerve [5].

There are also situations in the anterior aspect of the ankle where the superficial and deep nerves can be involved chronically. Crush injuries to the top of the foot can result in chronic nerve injuries to the medial and intermediate dorsal cutaneous nerves. The nerves can again be diagnostically injected and isolated and then placed in a muscle in the distal leg through an incision through the deep fascia covering the anterior muscle group. There is not a preferred muscle choice with this approach, but the nerve will often calm down when resected and allowed to lie within the anterior musculature. One example is pain seen at the proximal aspect of the bunion incision. Chronic proximal incision pain after bunion surgery at the level of the first metatarsal cuneiform joint may be secondary to damage to the medial dorsal cutaneous nerve (MDCN). If this pain is relieved with a superficial wheal of local anesthesia placed at this site, then the diagnosis of MDCN damage is made. The nerve can be resected with burial of the end into the medial cuneiform or resected locally at this level [6]. Since there is not abundant skeletal muscle at the dorsal aspect of the foot, bone implantation in this area is a good alternative. Although more aggressive, the MDCN can be resected at the distal aspect of the lower leg and buried into the anterior leg musculature. This is also a good approach to chronic injuries to the IDCN. Deep peroneal nerve entrapment is also seen at times on the anterior dorsal aspect of the foot. The best way to isolate the deep peroneal nerve diagnostically is to place 1–2 cc of local anesthesia between the EHL and EDL at the distal tibia. Inject through the skin, contact the distal tibia, withdraw the needle a few millimeters, and then aspirate before injecting.

If you are in the right location, this should provide anesthesia from this level out to the first interspace dorsally. If the entrapment is at the level of the dorsal foot, then surgically this can be released by resecting the EHB at the level of Lisfranc joint (Fig. 9.15). The release of pressure can free up adhesions on the nerve similar to a carpal tunnel release or EDIN procedure. Another approach would be to resect the nerve at the anterior compartment of the leg and leave the nerve end to lie deep within this compartment. The nerve resected from this area of the distal leg will not result in any motor weakness of the ankle as the motor nerve branches come off more proximal. I have found it is not necessary to perform muscle implantation at this level as the nerve will naturally be surrounded by the skeletal muscles of the anterior muscle group.

A difficult problem in nerve complications is a recurrent nerve entrapment to the tarsal tunnel area. There is varied success in performing a revisional tarsal tunnel release, yet it may often depend on the technique used for the primary release. Dellon et al. have described the importance of an aggressive distal release of the calcaneal tunnels of the terminal branches of the tibial nerve under the abductor hallucis muscle belly [12, 13]. If the initial release was essentially a limited release of only the retro-malleolar area and not extending distally under the muscle, then a revisional release with attention to the calcaneal tunnels will often result in improvement for the patient. These tunnels include the medial and lateral plantar nerve tunnels as well as the infracalcaneal nerve (aka Baxter's nerve). This nerve is the first muscular branch off the lateral plantar nerve and will often dive deep to the abductor hallucis muscle proximally to the lateral plantar nerve (Fig. 9.16). Proper release of the separate tunnels starts off with a longitudinal release of the superficial fascia of the abductor hallucis muscle. The muscle is now reflected off the deep fascial covering, and the muscle can be mobilized both dorsally and plantarly to visualize the deep fascia or the fascia covering the backside of this muscle. This deeper fascial layer is much thicker than the superficial fascial layer of this muscle and is a

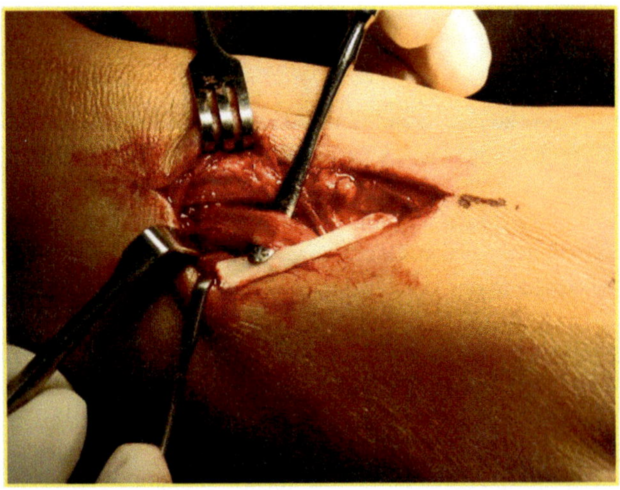

Fig. 9.15 Surgical release of the deep peroneal nerve over the medial metatarsal cuneiform joints with resection of the EHB muscle/tendon traveling over this area

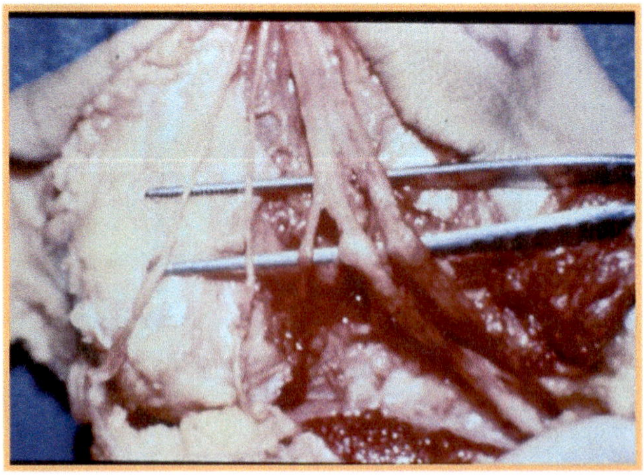

Fig. 9.16 Nerve branches to be familiar with in surgical dissection of the tarsal tunnel area. The medial and lateral plantar nerves are depicted. The first muscular branch of the lateral plantar nerve is the infracalcaneal nerve (aka Baxter's nerve). The two smaller branches on the left are the superficial sensory calcaneal nerves

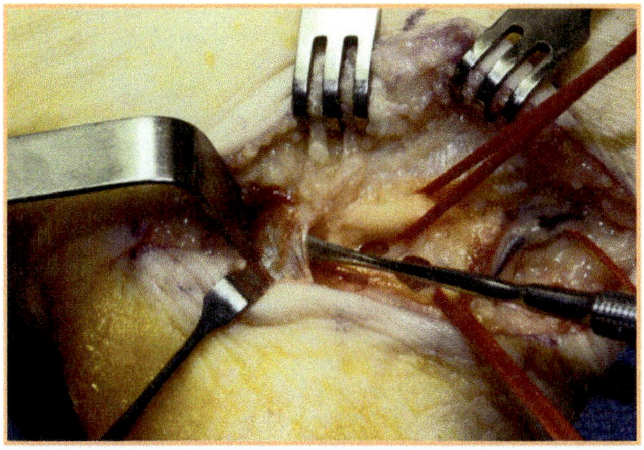

Fig. 9.17 The dense tissue shown is the deep fascial covering of the abductor hallucis muscle. This tissue is the roof of all the calcaneal tunnels. Aggressive release of this dense layer is vital to a successful tarsal tunnel release

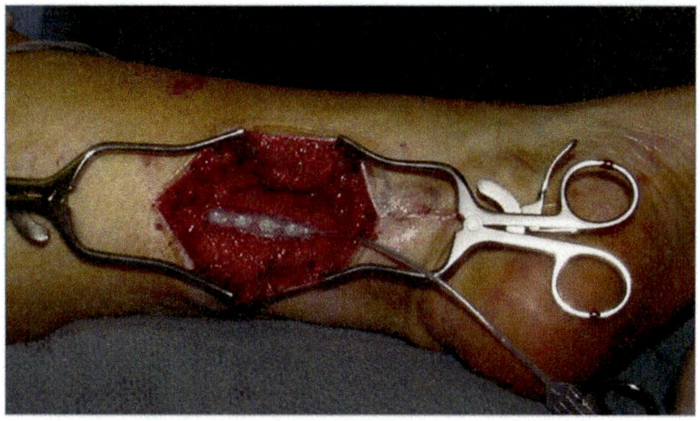

Fig. 9.18 Surgical placement of the neuro-stimulator along the posterior tibial nerve

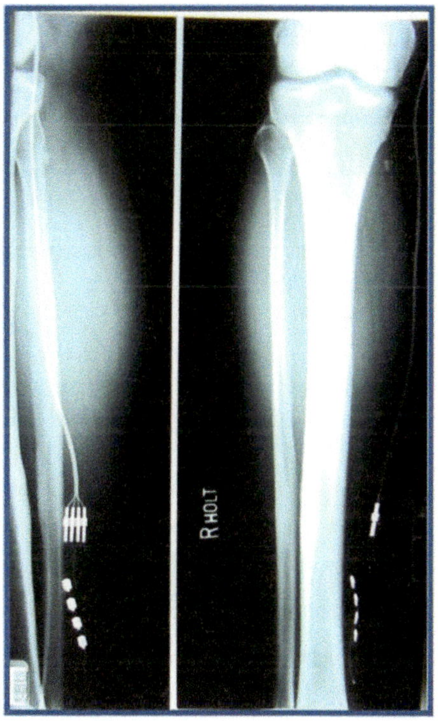

Fig. 9.19 X-ray image of the neuro-stimulator in place at the posterior medial ankle area

dense tissue which has been shown to put pressure onto the distal tarsal tunnel. This layer is the roof of the separate nerve tunnels, with the medial wall of the calcaneus being the floor of the tunnel compartment (Fig. 9.17). The nerves should be followed from proximal and seen to dive deep to this thick layer of tissue. Careful release of this deep layer is now performed along the whole course of the nerve as it enters the plantar medial vault of the foot [13]. The muscle should be retracted as plantarly as possible and this deep fascial layer is released as distal as possible. For a more complete release, the muscle can then be retracted upward, and the remainder of this layer can now be released from the bottom upward. If there is scar tissue surrounding the main portion of the tibial nerve, there are anatomic nerve barriers which may be helpful such as nerve wraps. Amniotic tissue has also been used recently to help minimize adhesions along the nerves during the healing period [14].

It is not recommended to resect the tibial nerve at the ankle level in cases of chronic tibial nerve entrapment. This will destroy the motor function to the plantar foot and serve to denervate all of the intrinsic musculature. Implantable nerve stimulators have been used for purposes of blunting the nerve pains from these chronic situations. More commonly, the stimulators are implanted at the level of the spinal cord and can be adjusted when needed for maximal effect. There are also smaller stimulators which may be implanted along the tibial nerve for the same purposes (Figs. 9.18 and 9.19). Ideally due to their size, they are usually placed along the distal thigh, yet placing them along the tibial nerve just proximally to the ankle has also been described [11, 15]. Schon et al. has presented acceptable outcomes with this approach in the end stage chronic nerve entrapment patients [11, 15].

At times, patients may also exhibit pain along the tarsal tunnel incision, especially when the incision is placed slightly more proximal or anterior in the retro-malleolar region. There is a recurrent articular branch of the saphenous nerve which has been shown to become entrapped in incisions around the medial malleolus [16]. If this can be confirmed by a diagnostic injection along the posterior aspect of the saphenous nerve, this nerve can be resected, transposed, and implanted into the soleus muscle to alleviate the pain from this entrapment. The soleus muscle is usually the muscle of choice for implantation in the lower leg.

Over the years, there have been several natural barriers explored in an attempt to assist in blocking nerve regeneration. Cryoprecipitate and calcium chloride and thrombin have been mixed together to form a drop of glue which will harden once placed in contact with each other within the epineural sleeve. The sleeve is then sutured closed in an effort to entrap the nerve and prevent regeneration. Studies have shown that although some of the biological barriers have some success, the best outcomes consistently occur when the chemotactic factors of the nerve are turned off by placing the nerve into the skeletal muscle or bone tissue [4, 7].

References

1. Barrett JP, Downey MS, Hillstrom HJ. Retrospective analysis of neurapraxia and axonotmesis injuries of select peripheral nerves of the foot and ankle and their conservative and surgical treatment (external neurolysis and neurectomy). J Foot Ankle Surg. 1999;38(3):185–93.
2. Dockery GL. The treatment of intermetatarsal neuromas with 4% alcohol sclerosing injections. J Foot Ankle Surg. 1999;38(6):403–8.
3. Mann RA, Reynolds JC. Interdigital neuroma—a critical clinical analysis. Foot Ankle. 1983;3(4):238–43.
4. Banks AS, Vito GR, Giorgini TL. Recurrent intermetatarsal neuroma. A follow-up study. J Am Podiatr Med Assoc. 1996;86(7):299–306.
5. Chiodo CP, Miller SD. Surgical treatment of superficial peroneal neuroma. Foot Ankle Int. 2004;25(10):689–94.
6. Miller SD. Dorsomedial cutaneous nerve syndrome: treatment with nerve transection and burial into bone. Foot Ankle Int. 2001;22(3):198–202.
7. Wolfort SF, Dellon AL. Treatment of recurrent neuroma of the interdigital nerve by implantation of the proximal nerve into muscle in the arch of the foot. J Foot Ankle Surg. 2001;40(6):404–10.
8. Adams Jr SB, Peters PG, Schon LC. Persistent or recurrent interdigital neuromas. Foot Ankle Clin. 2011;16(2):317–25.
9. Colgrove RC, Huang EY, Barth AH, Greene MA. Interdigital neuroma: intermuscular neuroma transposition compared with resection. Foot Ankle Int. 2000;21(3):206–11.
10. Ferkel E, Davis WH, Ellington JK. Entrapment neuropathies of the foot and ankle. Clin Sports Med. 2015;34(4):791–801.
11. Schon LC, Anderson CD, Easley ME, Lam PW, Trnka HJ, Lumsden DB, Levin G, Shanker J. Surgical treatment of chronic lower extremity neuropathic pain. Clin Orthop Relat Res. 2001;389:156–64.
12. Gould JS. Recurrent tarsal tunnel syndrome. Foot Ankle Clin. 2014;19(3):451–67.
13. Mullick T, Dellon AL. Results of decompression of four medial ankle tunnels in the treatment of tarsal tunnels syndrome. J Reconstr Microsurg. 2008;24(2):119–26.
14. Fairbairn NG, Randolph MA, Redmond RW. The clinical applications of human amnion in plastic surgery. J Plast Reconstr Aesthet Surg. 2014;67(5):662–75.
15. Schon LC, Lam PW, Easley ME, Anderson CD, Lumsden DB, Shanker J, Levin GB. Complex salvage procedures for severe lower extremity nerve pain. Clin Orthop Relat Res. 2001;391:171–80.
16. Kim J, Dellon AL. Pain at the site of tarsal tunnel incision due to neuroma of the posterior branch of the saphenous nerve. J Am Podiatr Med Assoc. 2001;91(3):109–13.

10 Complications of Metatarsal Fractures

J. Randolph Clements

The First Metatarsal and First Metatarsophalangeal Joint

The first metatarsal is considerably wider and stronger than the lesser metatarsals. It is thought that one third of the body weight is transferred through the first metatarsophalangeal joint during gait [1]. The first metatarsal has cartilage surfaces both proximally and distally. The proximal aspect is reniform, or kidney-shaped, and articulates with the first cuneiform. The distal aspect articulates with the base of the proximal phalanx and the sesamoid complex. The distal aspect is round to allow for sagittal plane motion of the first metatarsophalangeal joint. The first metatarsophalangeal joint has a vertical and transverse axis. The vertical axis allows for abduction and adduction while the transverse axis allows for dorsiflexion and plantar flexion. During propulsion, approximately 65° of dorsiflexion is needed at the first metatarsophalangeal joint [1, 2]. The sesamoid complex is held in position by the medial and lateral flexor hallucis brevis muscles. The two heads of the abductor hallucis are attached on the lateral side of the fibular sesamoid. A portion of the adductor hallucis inserts on the medial side of the tibial sesamoid. The deep transverse intermetatarsal ligament also contributes to sesamoid stabilization and helps to maintain the sesamoids relationship to the lesser metatarsals. This unique anatomic relationship makes minimal displacement of the sesamoid complex intolerable. The topic of turf toe injuries will not be discussed in this chapter. However, the authors believe a brief review of first metatarsophalangeal joint biomechanics is important in order understand reconstruction of complications of metatarsal fractures.

Injuries to the first metatarsophalangeal joint are typically caused by direct trauma. The majority of trauma involving the first metatarsophalangeal joint occurs from hyperdorsiflexion mechanisms [2, 3]. These mechanisms can create dislocations with or without an osseous component.

Osteochondral fractures can occur at the base of the head of the first metatarsal secondary to trauma. However, few descriptions of osteochondral fracture of the first metatarsophalangeal joint have been reported. All of the previously described lesions have been localized to the first metatarsal head, rather than the phalangeal base. A review of the literature failed to reveal any fractures occurring at the base of the proximal phalanx of the hallux [2].

Malunion of a first metatarsal fracture can result in angular, rotational, or shortening of the metatarsal. Dorsiflexory malunions can be caused by poor intraoperative fixation, loss of fixation postoperatively due to premature weight bearing, or catastrophic failure. There is a paucity of literature on the rate and incidence of malunions following first metatarsal fractures treated either operatively or nonoperatively. The treatment course for a malunion depends upon patient's symptoms, which may include pain, difficulty with ambulation, and transfer metatarsalgia [4].

Central Metatarsal Fractures

The central metatarsals consist of the second, third, and fourth metatarsals. Each metatarsal consists of a head, neck, shaft, and base. The head of each metatarsal articulates with the base of the corresponding proximal phalanx. The neck serves as the junction of the epiphysis and the diaphysis. The diaphysis is the largest segment of the metatarsal. The bases of the second and third metatarsals articulate with the middle and lateral cuneiform respectively. The fourth metatarsal articulates with the medial articular surface of the cuboid.

There are differing opinions on the importance of open reduction and internal fixation for lesser metatarsal fractures. There is little emphasis placed on performing open reduction and internal fixation of displaced central metatarsal fractures. There are a variety of fracture patterns which affect the

J. Randolph Clements (✉)
Carilion Clinic Orthopaedics, Virginia Tech Carilion School of Medicine, 3 Riverside Circle, Roanoke, VA 24014, USA
e-mail: jrclements@carilionclinic.org

M.S. Lee, J.P. Grossman (eds.), *Complications in Foot and Ankle Surgery*, DOI 10.1007/978-3-319-53686-6_10

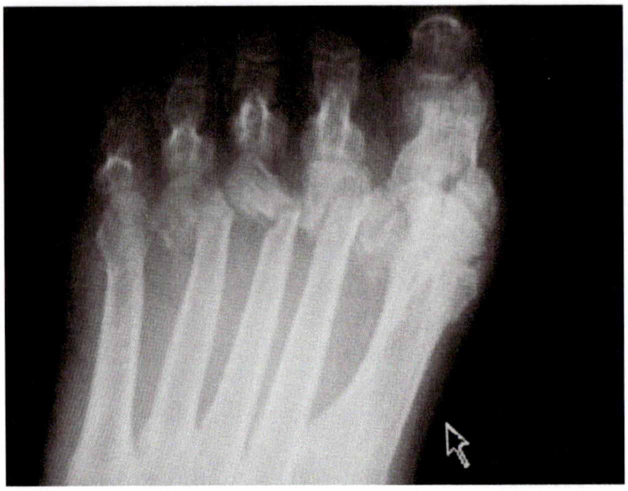

Fig. 10.1 AP radiograph demonstrates central metatarsal fractures that exceed the acceptable criteria for non surgical treatment

central metatarsals, but the majority of fractures involving the metatarsal head or neck are treated nonoperatively. The plane of deformity is paramount in making this decision. Patients with significant transverse plane deformity can have satisfactory results with nonsurgical care. However, sagittal plane displacement is less acceptable. Rockwood and Green's reported greater than 3–4 mm of displacement or 10° of sagittal plane deformity should be treated aggressively to avoid a painful plantar keratosis and metatarsalgia [5, 6] (Fig. 10.1).

Complication of these injuries can result in osteochondral defects, avascular necrosis, or more commonly sagittal plane malunion. Osteochondral injuries are often caused by axial load, and the cartilage surface sustains a shear-type injury. The majority of the literature pertains to reconstruction of avascular necrosis. However, several authors have described a variety of applicable treatments for osteochondral defects of the metatarsal head [2, 7–10]. These treatments include debridement, excision, synovectomy, and dorsal closing-wedge osteotomy. The treatment depends on the size of the fragment. If the fragment is small, simple excision is sufficient treatment. If the articular insult is large, excision is not recommended and more advance reconstructive techniques should be considered. Rotational dorsal wedge osteotomies have shown to be an excellent option. These osteotomies use the viable and uninjured plantar cartilage to interface with the base of the proximal phalanx. A dorsal wedge is removed from the metatarsal head, and the viable plantar cartilage is rotated dorsally (Fig. 10.2).

Fixation of osteochondral fractures and these reparative osteotomies present another challenge to the surgeon. If the fixation is inadequate, the potential for avascular necrosis and subchondral fatigue fracture increases [7, 11]. Absorbable pin fixation has improved the surgeon's ability to achieve mechanical stabilization of these injuries. Two crossed absorbable pins provide excellent stability for these revision osteotomies

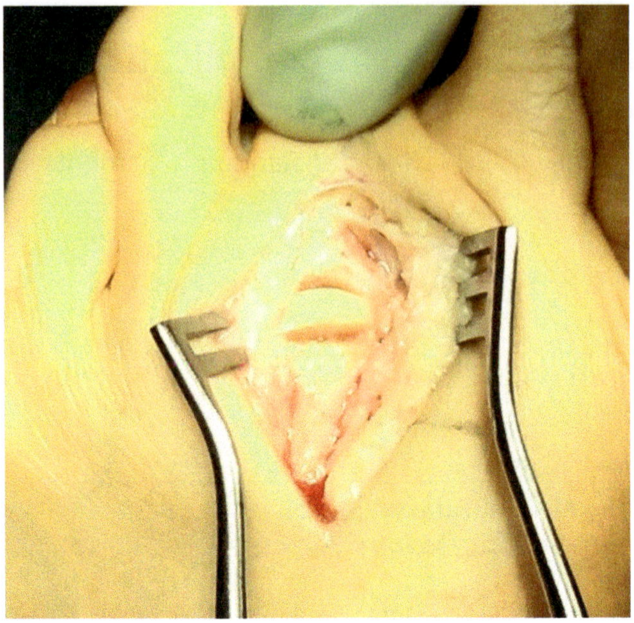

Fig. 10.2 This image is an intraopertaive depiction of a dorsally based wedge. This wedge is removed in to allow the metatarsal head to rotate cephalad to improved the articulation with the proximal phalgeal base

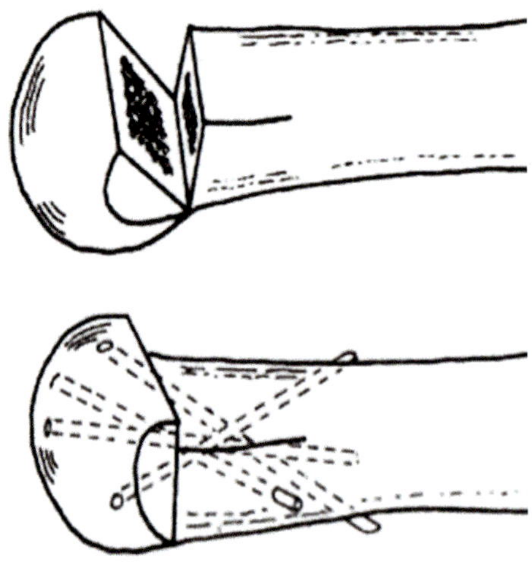

Fig. 10.3 These illustrations show the dorsally based wedge osteotomy in the metatarsal head. This osteotomy allows for dorsal rotation of the articular surface. The second illustration depicts the use of absorbable fixation to stabilize the osteotomy. This illustration shows the dorsally based wedge osteotomy in the metatarsal. This osteotomy allows for dorsal rotation of the articular surface

[7, 9]. Zhongguo et al. reported complete union in all subjects who underwent revision dorsal wedge osteotomy with absorbable fixation [9] (Figs. 10.3, 10.4, and 10.5).

Central metatarsal head malunions and intra-articular metatarsal head fractures are rare. Retroversion of the fracture segment is more uncommon but has been described by Atik [10].

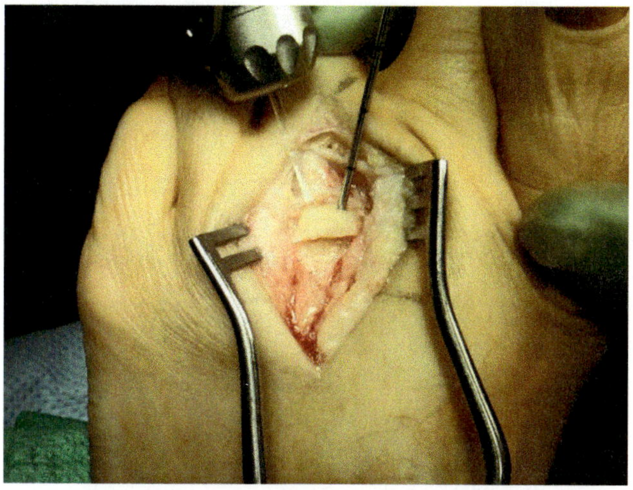

Fig. 10.4 Intraoperative image of fixation technique. The absorbable pins should be placed in a converging orientation. The use of predrill is recommended to simplify the insertion of the absorbable pin. Both steps are shown in this image

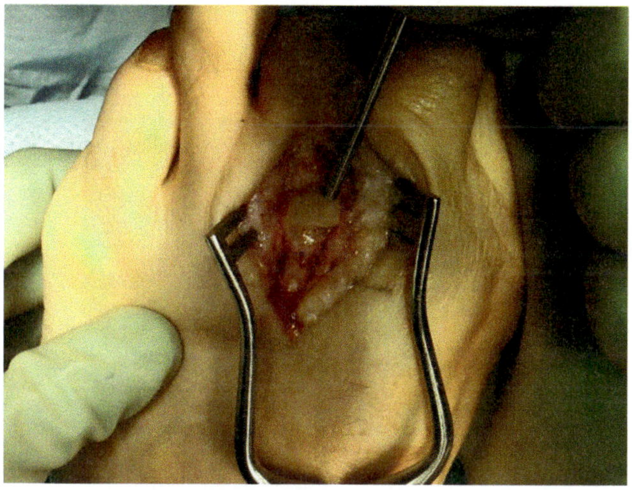

Fig. 10.5 A small tamp is used to recess the pin below the cartilage

Corrective osteotomies for metatarsal fractures have been described in Avian literature [12]; however, this author does not see the clinical relevance in including their findings in this text.

Complications of central metatarsal fractures are usually a result of failure to realign the metatarsal heads and the metatarsal parabola [6]. Corrective realignment osteotomies are used in cases of symptomatic metatarsalgia from malunion. The surgeon should focus on restoration of anatomic alignment for resolution of pain and disability [13]. The surgeon must realize that despite the diligence of restoring the metatarsal parabola, this does not always result in asymptomatic gait.

Fractures of the central metatarsal diaphysis are often treated nonsurgically as well. Certain fracture patterns of the metatarsal shafts are more appropriately treated with surgical stabilization. When the fracture is displaced and surgical treatment is being considered, the pattern of the fracture helps determine the most appropriate fixation. A vertical oriented fracture can be treated in with a 0.062 in. or 0.045 in. retrograde Kirschner wire. Spiral fractures should be stabilized with interfragmentary fixation. The perpendicular placement of this screw is challenging due to inference of the adjacent metatarsals. Because of this, additional dorsal plating is recommended for neutralization. Deviation from this technique can lead to healing complications including nonunion and malunion. Bridge plating works well for comminuted metatarsal shaft fractures. Bridge plating allows the surgeon to "bridge or span" the comminuted segment while concurrently receiving osseous stability from the bone proximal and distal to the area of comminution. This provides stabilization of the fracture without disrupting the biology around the fracture. Another option for stabilizing these fractures is external fixation. This technique is most useful in highly comminuted or open fractures. The surgeon should pay close attention to the metatarsal declination angle when using external fixation. The external fixation bars should be oriented parallel to the long axis of the metatarsal. This will prevent sagittal plane malposition of the metatarsal. Much like metatarsal head malunions, a sagittal plane malunion of the shaft is corrected with realignment osteotomies. When there is a dorsiflexory sagittal plane malunion, the patient will present with symptomatic metatarsalgia juxtaposition to the malunited metatarsal. The treating physician may be tempted to address the symptomatic metatarsal; however, correcting the malunited metatarsal is more prudent. Highly comminuted or segmental fractures of the metatarsal diaphysis can result in painful nonunion. Several techniques have been described to revise these nonunions. The preferred method of revision treatment is intercalary autogenous bone grafting and dorsal plating.

Stress Fractures of the Central Metatarsals

Stress fractures rarely occur due to acute trauma. In most cases the patient has an underlying foot deformity that is aggravated by recurrent and repetitive activity. Other underlying biological issues should be considered as prodromal. These include osteoporosis, vitamin D deficiency, menopause, and obesity. Patients with forefoot pain and stress fracture should also be evaluated for equinus. A tight heel cord can increase the forefoot pressures resulting in stress fracture. This concept is often overlooked as a cause of metatarsal stress fractures. Most stress fractures can be treated nonoperatively. Typically 4–6 weeks in an orthopedic walking boot is sufficient. In some cases, these develop into nonunion and are treated with bone grafting and dorsal plating.

Fifth Metatarsal Fractures

Fractures of the fifth metatarsal are common injuries. Studies have shown that greater than 50% of all metatarsal fractures occur in the fifth metatarsal [14–16]. The majority of these fractures involve the base of the fifth metatarsal, but distal fifth metatarsal fractures involving the head, neck, and diaphysis occur regularly. The decision to operate or treat nonsurgically depends upon the fracture location, angular deformity, and displacement. A moderate amount of transverse plane angulation of the distal fragment is acceptable, but again sagittal plane position of the distal fragment should be carefully scrutinized on the lateral radiograph.

Isolated fractures of the metatarsal head usually occur secondary to a direct trauma. These injuries are typically treated conservatively unless significant sagittal displacement of the head is present. The patient is immobilized in a below-knee cast or fracture boot for 4–6 weeks. If the fracture fails to unite or subsequently displaces enough to become symptomatic, a resection of the fifth metatarsal head can be considered. However, this is not suggested as a primary treatment.

Diaphyseal fractures of the fifth metatarsal are usually a short oblique and oriented proximal- dorsal to distal-plantar [5, 14, 17]. This fracture is commonly referred to as a dancer's fracture. The fracture occurs as a result of ground reactive forces acting distally against a stable proximal metatarsal base. This is often associated with a moderate degree of displacement and shortening due to the obliquity of the fracture. This fracture pattern is more unstable than transverse fractures in the same location. Conservative treatment with short leg casting may be considered if the fracture is well aligned. Open reduction with internal fixation may also be accomplished with the use of small cortical screws or small plating systems (Figs. 10.6 and 10.7).

Comminuted fractures of the fifth metatarsal may also respond well to nonsurgical treatment. In the presence of heavy comminution, achieving mechanical stability of the fracture is often difficult. Bridge plating is very useful in situations of comminution. There are several plating systems available that offer versatile screw orientation.

Fractures of the proximal diaphyseal portion of the fifth metatarsal are often referred to as a "Jones fracture." These are typically caused by an inversion force, creating an avulsion at the base of the fifth metatarsal. A true "Jones fracture" is an acute fracture at the proximal portion of the shaft near the metadiaphyseal junction. If the fracture is treated nonoperatively, reports show up to 66–93% chance of healing [14, 15]. It is important to note that these fractures should be non-

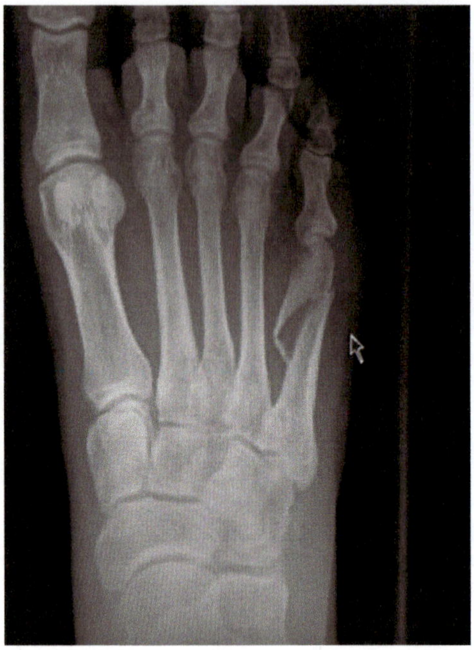

Fig. 10.6 5th metatarsal diaphyseal fracture showing significant displacement

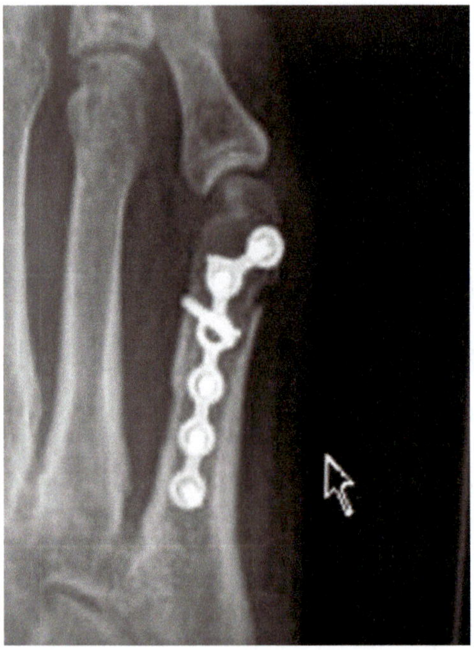

Fig. 10.7 This picture shows the use of a small cortical interfragmetary screw with a neutralization plate

displaced. Non-displaced or unicortical fractures should be treated for 6 weeks in a non-weight bearing short leg cast with gradual transition to weight bearing in an orthopedic walking boot.

Traditionally, surgical treatment has been reserved for high performance athletes. However, fractures of the base of the fifth metatarsal should be given careful consideration to all patients due to its limited vascular supply. Because of this, operative management in these fractures may be performed despite significant deformity or displacement. Intramedullary solid screw fixation is recommended. Cannulated screws can be used but do not offer equivocal strength to solid screws. Cannulated screws are less technically demanding. This author recommends using cannulated instrumentation but inserting a solid screw. This is generally achieved by using a standard cannulated guide wire followed by the appropriate cannulated drill bit. After countersinking and measuring, the cannulated guide wire is removed and the appropriate size solid screw is inserted. Since there are minimal discrepancies in drill bit size and outer diameter of the screw, this technique allows the surgeon to use cannulated instrumentation for a solid screw. No statistically significant differences have been reported between titanium and stainless steel.

Smaller avulsion fractures can be treated with tension band wiring. When fracture fragments are too small to accommodate a standard screw, the tension band technique is the best option. The tension band technique is achieved by placing two parallel K wires through the avulsion fracture. Next a pilot hole is drilled in the diaphysis of the fifth metatarsal. An 18- or 20-gauge surgical wire is then used to provide compression and neutralization to the fracture. The use of three small wires to fixate a fifth metatarsal fracture has also been described [17]. This technique allows for a more minimally invasive approach while still providing adequate stabilization. If this technique is used, the surgeon should be conscientious of the orientation of the wires. The wires should be in multiple planes to optimize neutralization.

Fractures of the proximal fifth metatarsal metaphysis (i.e., the Jones fracture) can be problematic because of a high incidence of nonunion and recurrence with nonoperative treatment. In some cases, mainly athletes, reinjury or nonunion can occur despite operative stabilization. This is often attributable to hardware of insufficient strength, aggressive postoperative rehabilitation, or biologic insufficiency at the fracture site (Figs. 10.8 and 10.9).

Hunt et al. recommend revision fixation with a large, solid screw (5.5 mm or larger) with autogenous bone grafting [16]. Additional investigation remains necessary to determine

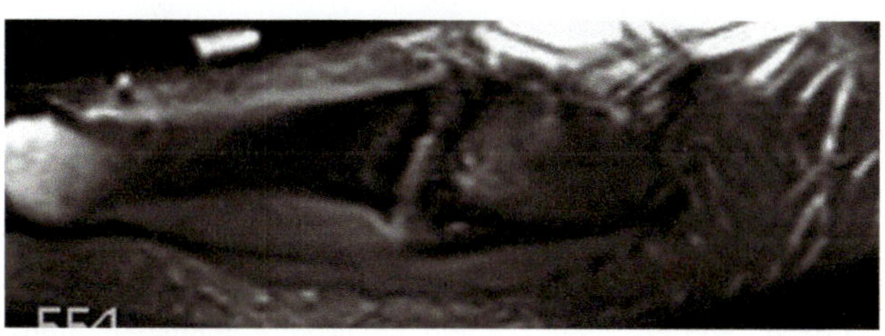

Fig. 10.8 T1 weighted MRI (sagittial and transverse) shows nonunited Jones fracture

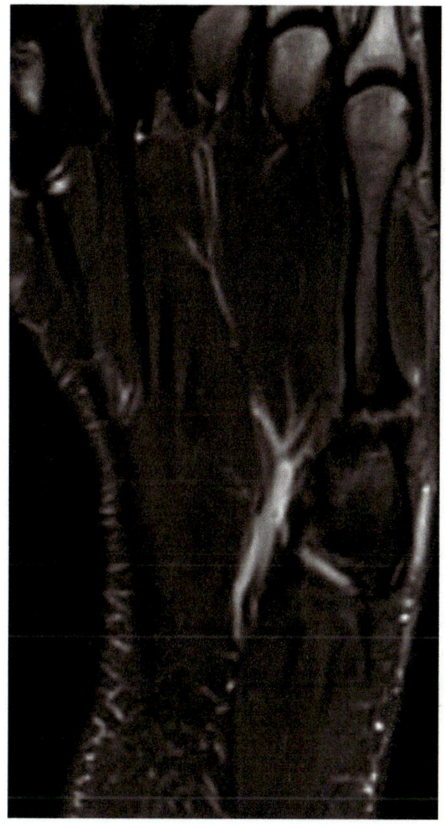

Fig. 10.9 T1 weighted MRI (Tranverse Plane) showing same non-united Jones Fracture

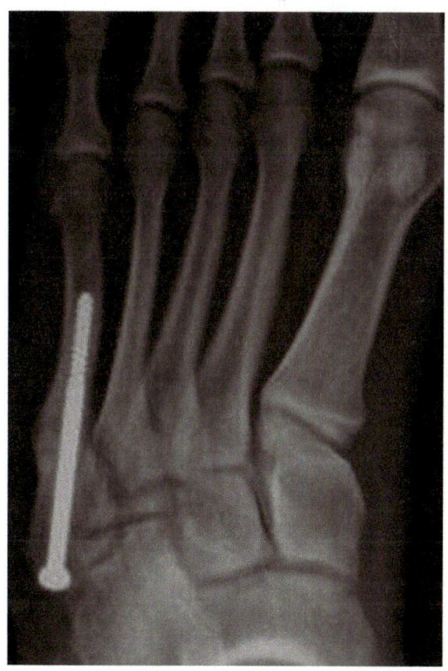

Fig. 10.10 1 year post operative AP foot xrays healed left 5th metatarsal shown previously as non united

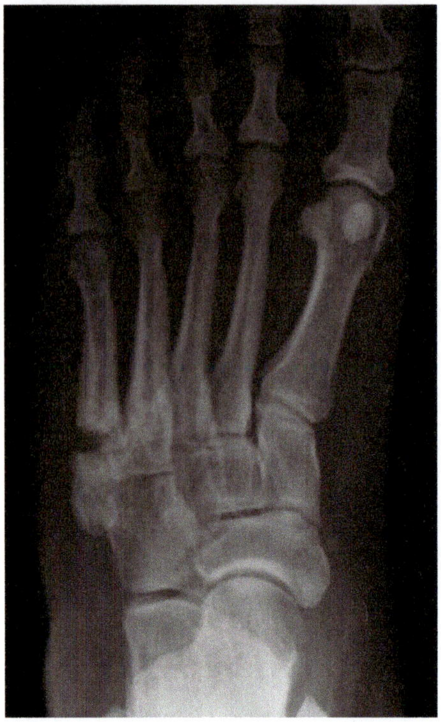

Fig. 10.11 AP radiographof the left foot shows nonunited 5th metatarsal with increased fracture gap

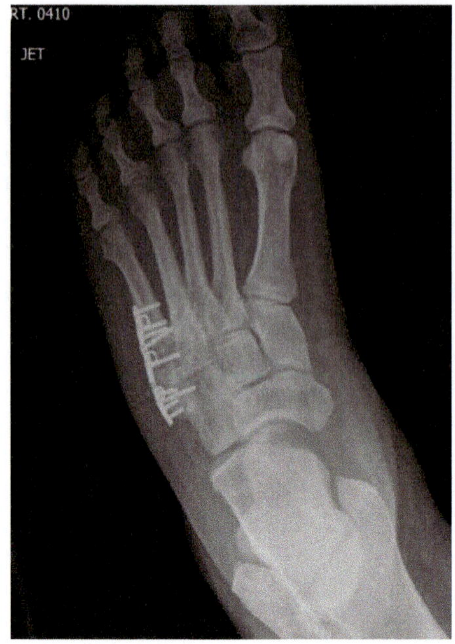

Fig. 10.12 Post operative radiographs show internal fixation with autogenous bone graft

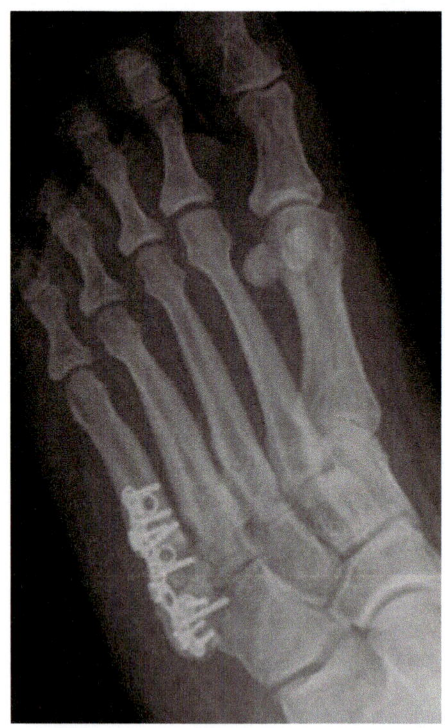

Fig. 10.13 1 year follow up showing complete osseous consolidation of autogenous bone graft

whether bone marrow aspirate with demineralized bone matrix is an effective substitute for cancellous autograft [16] (Fig. 10.10).

If nonsurgical treatment results in nonunion and further displacement of the fragment, the treating surgeon may consider autogenous bone grafting. This technique resembles the one previously described in the central metatarsal fracture section. The appropriate size intercalary graft may be harvested from the calcaneus or other locations depending on the defect. The proximal and distal aspects of the bone are debrided to viable margins, and the defect is filled with the autogenous graft. A bridge plate construct is suitable to provide necessary mechanical stabilization [18] (Figs. 10.11, 10.12, and 10.13).

Finally, the exigencies of the athletic and leg-based working population require prompt return to play or work. This need can be met by providing intramedullary fixation as primary treatment. This practice of avoiding the complication of nonunion in this cohort may remain the most prudent treatment of fifth metatarsal metadiaphyseal fractures as it provides better, quicker, and more reliable recovery for the patient [14–16, 18]

Technique Pearls and Pitfalls

Although cannulated instrumentation makes operative treatment of a fifth metatarsal fracture easier for the surgeon, the cannulated design of the screw is weaker than a solid screw. This author supports cannulated screws if the screw is larger than 5.5 mm in diameter. If the screw is less than 5 mm in diameter, a solid screw should be used. Cannulated guide wires, drill bits, and depth gauges can be used if smaller screws are required. However, if the cannulated instrumentation is used, a solid screw should be placed.

Conclusion

In general, complications of metatarsal fractures are unusual. However, given the dynamic mechanical requirement of the first metatarsophalangeal joint, functional need for well-maintained metatarsal parabola, and biologic factors, metatarsal fractures can create challenging clinical scenarios. Since the peer-reviewed literature does not offer a great deal of direction for metatarsal fracture complications, the surgeon should rely on sound surgical principles and an understanding of pedal biomechanics for guidance.

References

1. Root ML. An approach to foot orthopedics. J Am Podiatr Assoc. 1964;54:115–8.
2. Wertheimer SJ, Balazsy JE. A unique osteochondral fracture of the first metatarsophalangeal joint. J Foot Surg. 1992;31(3):268–71.
3. Coker TP, Arnold JA, Weber DL. Traumatic lesions of the metatarsophalangeal joint of the great toe in athletes. Am J Sports Med. 1978;6(6):326–34.
4. Becker A. First Metatarsal Malunion. Foot Ankle Clinic. 2009;14(1):77–90.
5. Tornetta P, Brown C, Heckman JD, McKee M, McQueen MM, Ricci W. Fractures and dislocations of the midfoot and forefoot, rockwood and green. 8th ed. Philadelphia, PA: Lippincott, Williams and Wilkins; 2015. p. 2689–97.
6. Alepuz E, Carsi V, Alcantara P. Fractures of the central metatarsal. Foot Ankle Int. 1999;17(4):200–3.
7. Lee HJ, Kim JW, Min WK. Operative treatment of Freiberg disease using extra-articular dorsal closing-wedge osteotomy: technical tip and clinical outcomes in 13 patients. Foot Ankle Int. 2013;34(1):111–6.
8. Mereddy PK, Molloy A, Hennessy MS. Osteochondral fracture of the fourth metatarsal head treated by open reduction and internal fixation. J Foot Ankle Surg. 2007;46(4):320–2.
9. Zhongguo X, Fu C. Effect evaluation of treating Freiberg's disease with dorsal wedge osteotomy and absorbable pin fixation. Jian Wai Ke Za Zhi. 2009;23(6):651–3.
10. Atik A, Ozyurek S, Cicek EI, Kose O. Isolated slipped-retroverted osteochondral fracture of second metatarsal head. Foot. 2013;23(4):176–9.
11. Capar B, Kutluay E, Mujde S. Dorsal closing-wedge osteotomy in the treatment of Freiberg's disease. Acta Orthop Traumatol Turc. 2007;41(2):136–9.
12. Rahal SC, Teixeira CR, Pereira-Júnior OC, Vulcano LC, Aguiar AJ, Rassy FB. Two surgical approaches to fracture malunion repair. J Avian Med Surg. 2008;22(4):323–30.
13. Murphy R, Fallat LM. Surgical correction of metatarsal malunion. J Foot Ankle Surg. 2012;51(6):801–5.
14. Clapper MF, O'Brien TJ, Lyons PM. Fractures of the fifth metatarsal. Analysis of a fracture registry. Clin Orthop Relat Res. 1995;315:238–41.
15. Zogby RG, Baker BE. A review of nonoperative treatment of Jones' fracture. Am J Sports Med. 1987;15(4):304–7.
16. Hunt KJ, Anderson RB. Treatment of Jones fracture nonunions and refractures in the elite athlete: outcomes of intramedullary screw fixation with bone grafting. Am J Sports Med. 2011;39(9): 1948–54.
17. Banks AS, Downey MS, Martin DE, Miller SJ. Metatarsal fractures, McGlamery comprehensive textbook of foot and ankle surgery. Philadelphia, PA: Lippincott, Williams and Wilkins; 2001. p. 1775–90.
18. McBryde Jr AM. The complicated jones fracture, including revision and malalignment. Foot Ankle Clinic. 2009;14(2):151–68.

Part III

The First Ray

Complications of Hallux Valgus Surgery

11

Christopher L. Reeves and Amber M. Shane

Hallux valgus deformity is one of the most common pathologies seen by a foot and ankle surgeon, with an estimated incidence of 23% in adults aged 18–65 years and 35.7% in patients over 65 years [1]. With such a high prevalence of hallux valgus deformity, surgical correction is commonplace for foot and ankle surgeons. With a large volume of procedures being performed, minor and major complications can arise. The complication rate throughout the literature has a wide range extending from 1% to 55% following hallux valgus surgery in general [2–4]. There are a multitude of factors that contribute including physician experience, procedural selection, and patient selection. Meticulous attention to detail in the preoperative, intraoperative, and postoperative setting can reduce the incidence of complications. Prevention of complications begins with a thorough history and physical examination and detailed radiographic evaluation. It is imperative that the surgeon assesses concomitant deformities such as pes planovalgus deformity, hypermobility of the first ray, metatarsus adductus, equinus, second metatarsal pathology with instability, and evidence of other biomechanical factors such as plantar callosities, as the presence of any of these plays a role in procedure selection and is directly attributed to postoperative success. Intraoperative assessment of positioning, careful attention to fixation techniques, and emphasizing postoperative compliance is essential. Defining a complication or operative failure is also important, because what appears corrected to the surgeon clinically and radiographically can still be deemed a failure if the patient is not satisfied. A discussion of the postoperative plan, expectations, and possible long-term complications is paramount in the preoperative setting. Knowing the patient's, the procedure, and the surgeon's limitations is vital in limiting complications.

With over 150 different techniques documented since the first surgical correction of a hallux valgus deformity by Gernet in 1826, we will generalize them into three different categories for the scope of this chapter: metatarsal head, metatarsal shaft, and metatarsal base procedures (first tarsometatarsal joint arthrodesis will be discussed in a later chapter) [1].

Certain osteotomies are inherently more stable than others. Stable osteotomies allow for direct transfer of weight from the capital fragment to the stable fragment simply by the nature of the osteotomy. Unstable osteotomies, on the other hand, have limited resistance implemented by the boney construct and rely on internal fixation for stability. The Chevron osteotomy is more stable than other distal metatarsal procedures and as it was first described does not require fixation due to the stable construct. Although it does not require fixation, this is not common practice today due to the increased incidence of malunion and dorsal displacement of the capital fragment without fixation. When compared with other metatarsal head procedures, the Mitchell osteotomy was found to have the highest incidence of dorsal instability, shortening, as well as increased rates of malunion and nonunion (Fig. 11.1a, b) [2, 5–7].

On the other hand, base procedures are inherently less stable than head procedures secondary to biomechanical factors. The metatarsals are the only long bones in the body that support a significant amount of the body weight perpendicular to the longitudinal axis of the bone; therefore, base osteotomies are subjected to greater forces and have increased rate of malunion, persistent pain at the osteotomy site, and nonunion. The Mau osteotomy is documented to be the most intrinsically stable of the proximal osteotomies [8]. Lagaay et al. looked at 270 Chevron osteotomies compared to 34 closing base wedge osteotomies and documented reoperation rate for Chevron osteotomies to be 5.56% compared to closing base wedge osteotomy 8.82% [9].

Regardless of the location, shape, or construct of the osteotomy complications such as avascular necrosis, shortened first ray and first ray insufficiency can be encountered. Each of these may present with similar biomechanical findings derived from varying etiologies. Transfer lesions and metatarsalgia are common complications after first ray sur-

C.L. Reeves (✉) • A.M. Shane
Orlando Foot and Ankle Clinic, Teaching Faculty, Florida Hospital East Orlando Residency Program, Orlando, FL 32804, USA
e-mail: docreeves1@yahoo.com; ambershanereeves@yahoo.com

M.S. Lee, J.P. Grossman (eds.), *Complications in Foot and Ankle Surgery*, DOI 10.1007/978-3-319-53686-6_11

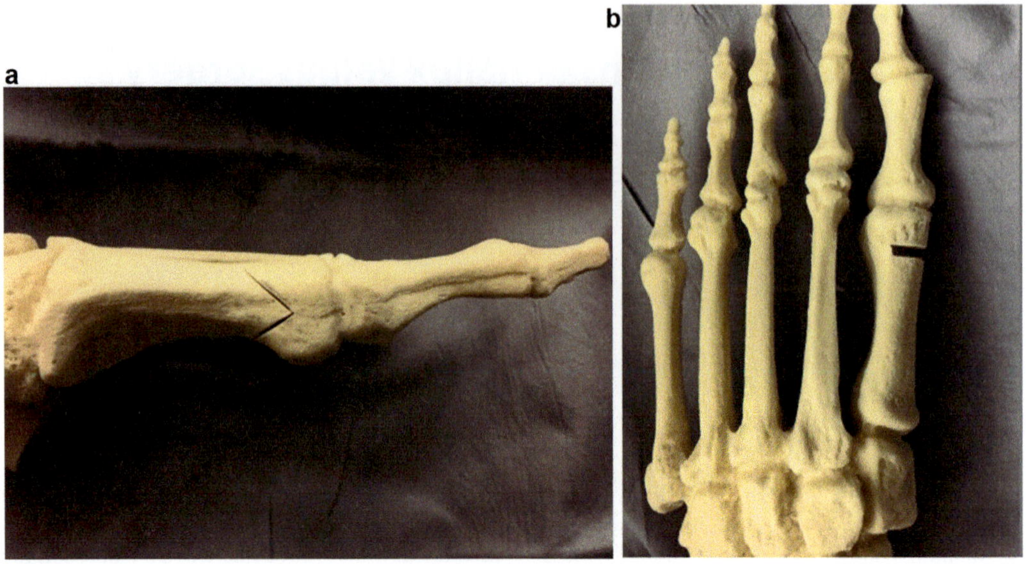

Fig. 11.1 (**a**, **b**) Comparison of inherent shortening of the Chevrons vs. Mitchell verse osteotomy

gery. Studies have documented that approximately 6% of patients have transfer lesion and 7% have metatarsalgia following distal first metatarsal osteotomies. The metatarsal parabola and the length of the first ray need to be assessed in the preoperative setting. With 64% of the total ground reactive forces being transferred through the first and second metatarsophalangeal joint during push off, minor alteration to the weight-bearing surface can be the difference between a successful outcome and an unsatisfied patient. The second metatarsal head is approximately half the size of the first metatarsal, leading to increased load and increasing callus formation or stress fracture secondary to the transfer of weight [5, 10]. The presence of sub-lesser metatarsal head hyperkeratosis with pain on palpation may be indicative of insufficiency and must be evaluated preoperatively. If a lesion is present, and radiographic signs of a short first metatarsal or long second metatarsal are noted, one may opt for lesser metatarsal osteotomy to balance the forefoot.

First Ray Shortening

Inevitably with any osteotomy, the surgeon will experience some aspect of shortening typically one to two millimeters of shortening with each pass of the saw blade. As a result, meticulous surgical technique is imperative to minimize iatrogenic shortening. Additionally, different osteotomies inherently result in various amounts of shortening. The literature reports shortening as little as 2.0–2.5 mm following a Chevron bunionectomy and up to 3–7 mm of shortening in the Mitchell bunionectomy [3, 4]. Banks et al. documented 1.1–2.5 mm of shortening following closing base wedge bunionectomy [11]. Patients with a wider metatarsal will expect to get increase shortening with a closing base wedge bunionectomy. When comparing the angulation of the cut with respect to the long axis, the obliquity does not influence the amount of shortening [11]. Opening base wedge bunionectomy, on the other hand, theoretically may maintain metatarsal length. Budny et al. reported an increase in length following an opening base wedge bunionectomy of 0.47–1.35 mm depending on the size of the graft inserted from 2 to 6 mm [12].

Patients with an iatrogenic shortened first metatarsal can be asymptomatic; however, common symptoms often include transfer metatarsalgia especially with barefoot walking, elevated hallux with pain on range of motion of the first metatarsophalangeal joint, and the discomfort can be to a point which inhibits the patient from enjoying the same lifestyle and performing daily activities prior to surgery (Fig. 11.2a–c). In these cases, standard dorsoplantar and lateral radiographs should be obtained to compare to preoperative radiographs. In the instance that the surgeon does not have access to preoperative radiograph, utilization of contralateral films is used for comparison. Once the surgeon has identified the patient's specific symptoms, they may address the causative agent both conservatively and surgically. Oral anti-inflammatory medications along with shoe modification and orthotic management may be implemented. A rigid sole shoe with a rocker bottom will offload the forefoot during push off. Orthotic management with medial posting or the addition of a Morton's extension may be utilized. If conservative treatment is unsuccessful or not compatible with the patient's lifestyle, surgical management may be required. Prior to initiating surgery, a patient must be well informed that they may not return to all previous activities.

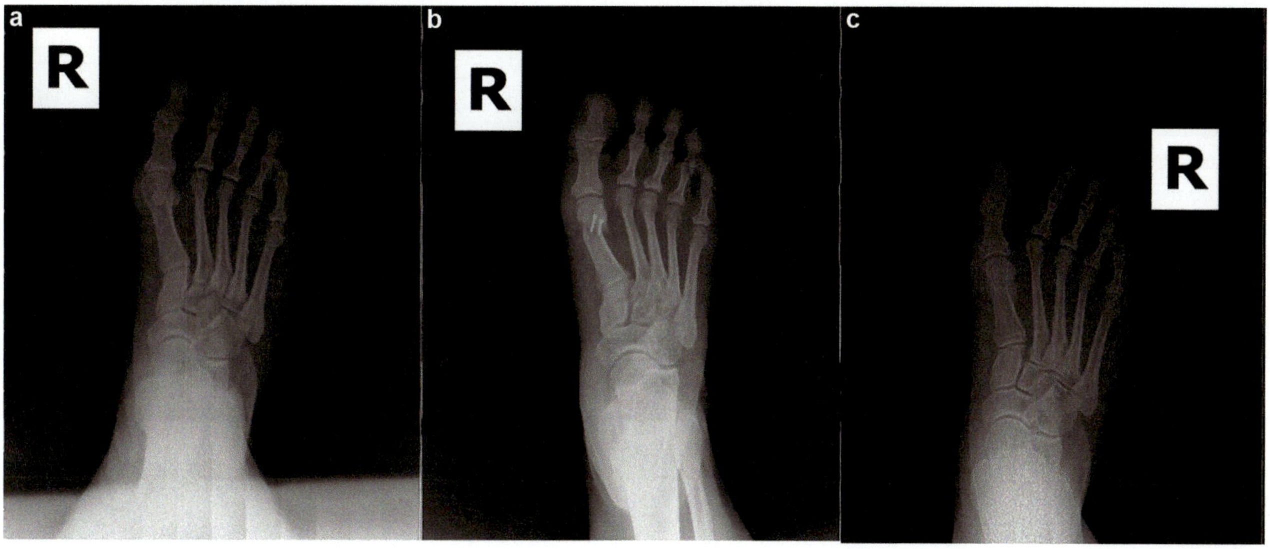

Fig. 11.2 (**a–c**) Iatrogenic shortening of the first ray following early weight bearing and malunion of a distal metatarsal osteotomy

Surgical correction of a shortened first metatarsal can be performed utilizing a lengthening osteotomy, callus distraction, or functional lengthening with a first metatarsophalangeal joint arthrodesis. Single-stage lengthening with a bone graft or callus distraction can be implemented but correlates with higher rates of stiffness of the first metatarsophalangeal joint depending on the amount of lengthening required. It is recommended that single-stage procedures be performed when less than 15 mm of length is required [4, 5, 13, 14]. If subsecond metatarsal pain is the primary complaint, restoration of the metatarsal parabola with a second metatarsal shortening osteotomy can address the deformity.

Goldberg et al. described a step cut first metatarsal osteotomy, where a Scarf-type osteotomy is performed and translated distally and fixated. When performing this procedure, the Scarf type of osteotomy must be made with the long arm of the metatarsal parallel with the long axis of the bone and not parallel with the weight-bearing surface, to avoid elevation of the metatarsal head. Gudipati et al. documented early-onset arthritis of the first metatarsal phalangeal joint following Scarf lengthening osteotomy, which required arthrodesis within 2 years following the procedure [5, 15]. With lengthening procedures, one must not neglect the soft tissues; tissue advancements and extensor hallucis longus tendon lengthening may be necessary. Even after corrective procedures to address the short first metatarsal, patients still may require shoe modifications and other conservative managements. Singh and Dudkiewicz found following Scarf lengthening procedure that only 6 out of 16 patients had good pain relief following the procedure and 4 no longer required orthotic management. Following the study they concluded that patients with less than 10 mm of length had poor outcomes. Less than 50% success rate was noted with lengthening less than 8 mm [16].

Callus distraction is a viable option if a large amount of lengthening is required or there are significant soft tissue contractures or compromise. A single plane monorail external fixator can be placed along the medial border of the first metatarsal. Then a small longitudinal incision is made on the dorsal aspect of the first metatarsal, and a corticotomy is performed. A 7- to 14-day latency period is observed, and then distraction at a rate of 1 mm/day is performed until the desired length is achieved; the monorail is left in place an additional 2–4 weeks to allow consolidation. Although callus distraction can be utilized, commonly we encounter increased first metatarsophalangeal joint stiffness and symptoms following these lengthening techniques; therefore, it is the author's preference to address shortening with functional lengthening via an end-to-end arthrodesis or interpositional bone block arthrodesis. We have found that, in most cases, enough length is available to achieve the desired correction with an arthrodesis. Once the fusion has consolidated, the functional length of the first metatarsal extends to the interphalangeal joint of the hallux.

When the deformity has been present for a prolonged amount of time, contractures, joint stiffness, or degenerative changes can be seen to the first metatarsophalangeal joint. At this point, an arthrodesis is the preferred method of treatment. Typically, we find that a primary end-to-end first metatarsophalangeal joint arthrodesis can be performed, thus increasing the functional lever arm of the first metatarsal to the interphalangeal joint. In instances with excessive shortening, interpositional bone block arthrodesis should be performed, which will be discussed later in this chapter. Primary first metatarsophalangeal joint arthrodesis is performed through a standard dorsal medial incision; limited medial and lateral dissection is required at this point. Once the extensor hallucis longus has been identified, sharp dissection is utilized to create a single soft tissue layer dissected off of the osseous structure. Any previously applied hardware should be removed, and periosteal elevator can by utilized to free plantar adhesions, to allow the surgeon to better access the joint. Preparation of the arthrodesis site can be performed with the use of curettage, reaming, or saw resection. It is the authors' preference to utilize curettage or reaming to decrease shortening and increase ability to position the arthrodesis site in the appropriate position. Following resection, the articular cartilage of the head of the first metatarsal and base of the proximal phalanx the joint is irrigated to remove any cartilaginous or soft tissue debride within the joint. Subchondral drilling is performed with a 1.5 mm drill bit, and the autogenous cancellous graft from the drill bit is left within the arthrodesis site (Fig. 11.3). The ideal positional of the arthrodesis is variable throughout the literature and is patient dependent, with the most widely accepted angles being 10–15° of dorsiflexion, 10–15° of abduction, and neutral in the frontal plane. In the intraoperative setting, simulated weight bearing is performed by evenly loading the forefoot on a lid from a hardware tray and positioning the hallux parallel to a rectus second digit and slightly elevated on off of the platform (Fig. 11.4). A periosteal elevator can be utilized to elevate the hallux just off the weight-bearing surface to allow an appropriate amount of plantar clearance upon ambulation. Temporary fixation is applied from the proximal phalanx into the metatarsal and positioned out of the way of planned definitive fixation. Fluoroscopy is utilized intraoperatively to confirm satisfactory alignment of the hallux and arthrodesis site, and an interfragmentary 3.5 solid sore or cannulated screw is applied from the medial aspect of the metatarsal to the lateral aspect of the proximal phalanx utilizing lag technique. The ideal starting point for the screw is just proximal to the previously resected medial eminence (Fig. 11.5). After good interfragmentary compression is achieved, a low-profile dorsal plate is applied.

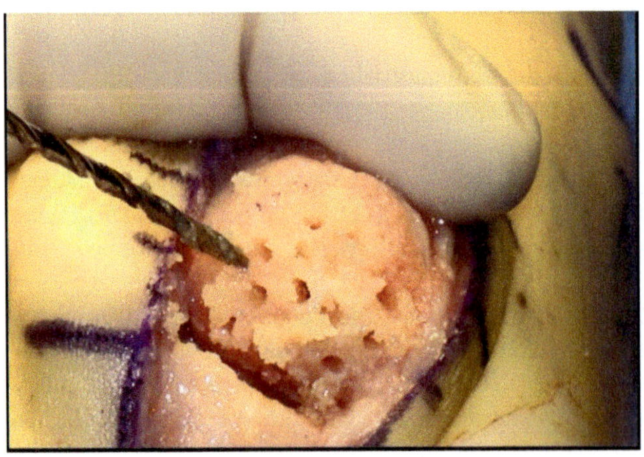

Fig. 11.3 Preparation for fusion at the first metatarsal head via subchondral drilling

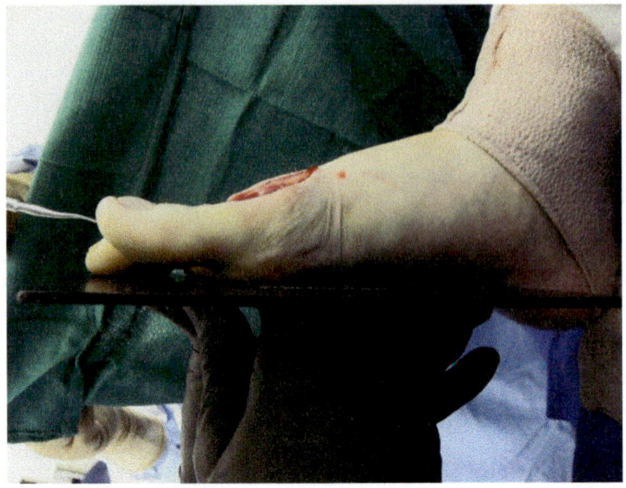

Fig. 11.4 Intraoperative positioning of first MTPJ arthrodesis using the hardware tray lid to simulate weight bearing

Multiple hardware configurations from Kirschner wires, Steinmann pins, screw fixation, screw and plate fixation, plate fixation alone, multiple stacked plates, staples, external fixation, and combinations of the above have been described in the literature with similar fusion rates ranging from 87% to 100%, with most consensus of 95% fusion rate [10]. When evaluating the various configurations for fixation of the first metatarsophalangeal joint, an interfragmentary screw with dorsal plate was found to be the strongest construct by Politi et al. when they compared to crossed Kirschner wires, interfragmentary screws, and dorsal compression plate without interfragmentary screws. An interfragmentary screw with dorsal compression plate is our preferred construct especially in revisional surgery [17].

Avascular Necrosis

Avascular necrosis (AVN) is bone death secondary to impaired circulation and can be seen in any bone in the body. It can be the result of iatrogenic causes, traumatic injury, or systemic issues, such as metabolic disorders, hemoglobinopathies, tobacco abuse, alcohol abuse, and systemic or injectable corticosteroid use. AVN can be seen associated with or independent of a nonunion. The incidence in the literature varies from 0% to 76% depending on surgical technique and amount of periosteal stripping [3, 4]. The vascular supply to the first metatarsal is an intricate network of vessels that anastomose with one another along the entire course of the first metatarsal. Along with the nutrient artery, a periosteal capillary network and metaphyseal capital vessels contribute to the blood supply. These vessels all stem from the first dorsal metatarsal artery, first plantar metatarsal artery, and superficial branches of the medial plantar artery

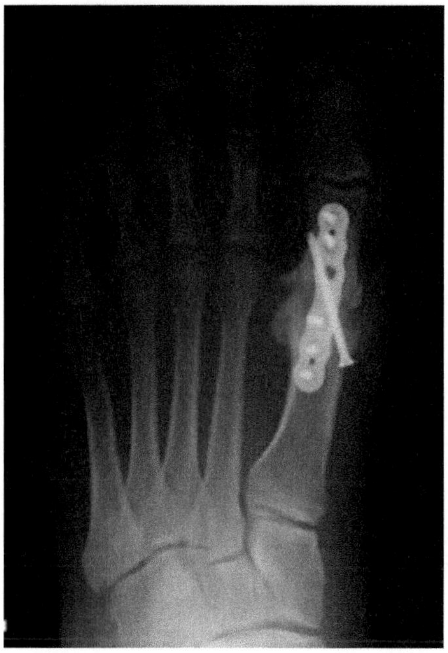

Fig. 11.5 Ideal positioning of the interfragmentary screw from the medial head of the first metatarsal to proximal phalanx of the hallux

[6, 8, 18]. Every osteotomy can potentially cause AVN, as it is disrupting the blood supply, but distal metatarsal head osteotomies have a higher prevalence due to the location of the nutrient artery of the first metatarsal, which enters through the dorsolateral aspect of the distal two thirds of the first metatarsal. The nutrient artery of the first metatarsal branches into a proximal and distal segment. It then anastomoses with the metaphyseal capital vessels at the junction of the head and neck of the first metatarsal. The capital fragment also has periosteal vessels attaching around the attachment of the capsule, and capsular vessels penetrate the head segmentally [4, 7, 8, 18, 19].

During early investigation, authors recommended limiting the lateral release during a distal first metatarsal osteotomy, as it was thought to be the only remaining blood supply to the capital fragment. Recent anatomic studies contradict the previous allegations and states that lateral release can be performed without causing significant vascular insult. Kuhn and Lippert performed a study where intraoperative intraosseous blood flow was measured after medial capsulotomy, adductor tenotomy, lateral release, and Chevron osteotomy. There was significant difference in blood flow at each portion of the procedure; the most notable insult was after medial capsulotomy with average decrease of 45% of baseline, lateral release another 13% decrease (58% total), and osteotomy another 13%. Even with this documented amount of vascular insult, all 20 patients healed without complication postoperatively [18]. There is no doubt that the blood supply to the first metatarsal is disrupted; the real questions are as follows: Is the vascular insult permanent or can it be reversed? And if this is the case, what are the different factors that make a patient more susceptible to this complication?

Since the intraosseous blood supply is compromised during a metatarsal osteotomy, special care should be taken in all aspects of the surgical procedure in order to limit the potential of AVN. The metatarsal has a significant capacity to withstand and compensate for the vascular insult, but limited capsular and periosteal stripping to preserve extraosseous and capsular vascular supply should be implemented. Care should be made to not allow the saw blade to plunge through the lateral cortex into the intermetatarsal space when performing the osteotomy. When dissecting the medial capsule, limiting trauma and cauterization of the plantar vasculature is important. It has been previously reported that when performing the osteotomy thermal necrosis to the bone can be seen if temperatures of 50°C maintained for 1 min or longer. The addition of saline irrigation to the saw bone interface has been suggested to limit temperatures. Hall et al. reviewed 112 first metatarsal osteotomies in cadaver bones and found that the addition of saline irrigation while the osteotomy was being performed resulted in a mean decrease in cutting temperature of 2.96 ± 7.32°C. However, temperatures with or without saline did not approach a level that would be consistent with thermal damage. The greatest change from base temperatures in the study was 43.7°C. The average peak temperature demonstrated in the study was 30.47° [19, 20]. As a result, we feel that it is really surgeon's preference as to whether one should use saline while performing the osteotomy.

Avascular necrosis to the capital fragment of the first metatarsal can be minor without collapse or major with collapse following a bunionectomy. The patient's clinical presentation may vary. Diagnosis in the early postoperative period is difficult, as the symptoms resemble those similar to postoperative healing process, with edema, erythema, irritability, and increased tenderness surrounding the joint. This reaction is a result of the body attempting to repair the devascularized bone. As with clinical diagnosis, radiographic evaluation in the immediate postoperative period is also difficult. In the early stages of AVN, the metatarsal may demonstrate subchondral radiolucency and focal cystic changes and may appear mottled; these radiographic changes can be seen on average within the first 2 months of surgery (Fig. 11.6). As the pathology progresses, degeneration of the capital fragment, subchondral collapse, and joint space narrowing is noted (Fig. 11.7). Magnetic resonance imaging (MRI) is the most sensitive modality with a 90–100% sensitivity for diagnosing AVN. Due to this sensitivity, the MRI can have high false-positive findings in the early postoperative period. Common appearance on MRI consists of decreased signal intensity on T1-weighted images, secondary to decreased cancellous bone content and increased T2 signal intensity due to hyperemia and edema. The double-line sign on a

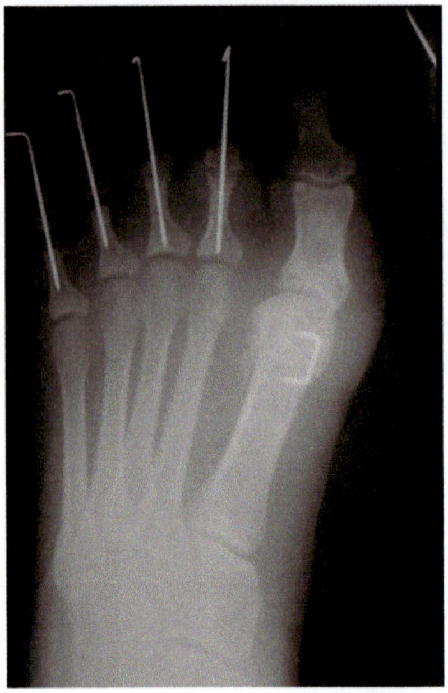

Fig. 11.6 Early radiographic signs of AVN with cystic changes to the first metatarsal head

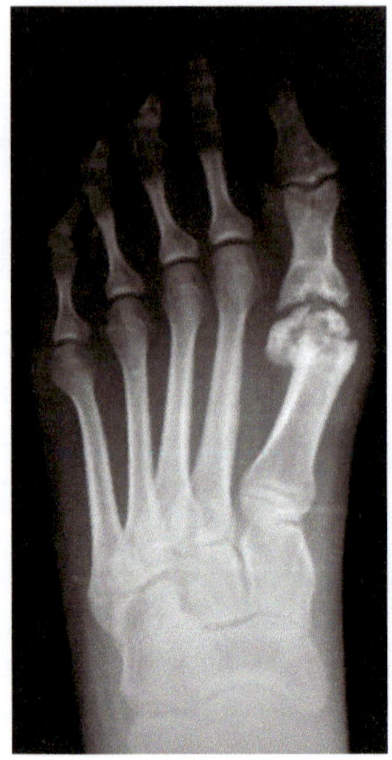

Fig. 11.7 Late-stage AVN with complete collapse of the first metatarsal head

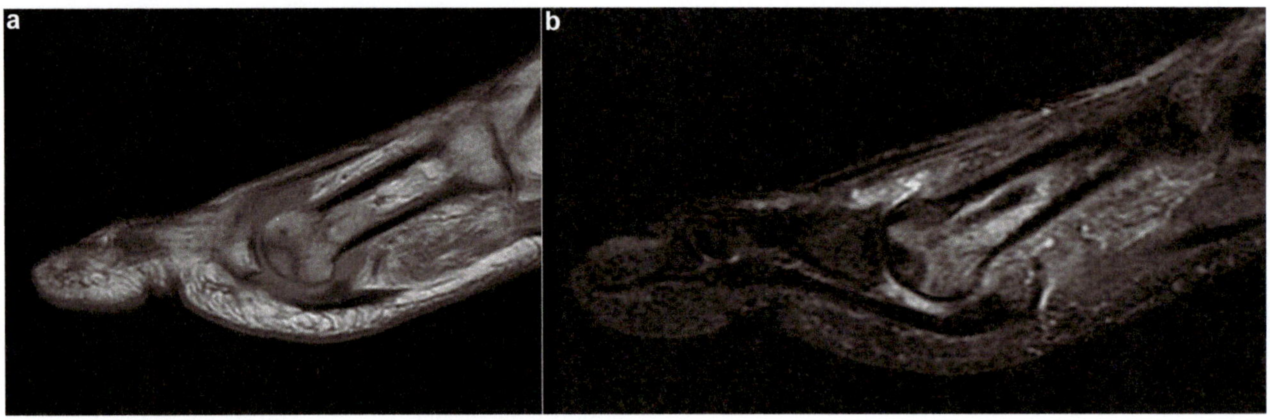

Fig. 11.8 (**a**, **b**) MRI of AVN of the first metatarsal showing a decrease signal intensity on T1 image and a corresponding increased signal intensity on double on T2-weighted image with a double-line sign

T2-weighted image is diagnostic and is seen on the periphery of the boney infarct. This consists of a line of increased signal intensity surrounded by an outer line of decreased signal intensity (Fig. 11.8a, b). Osteochondral fragmentation and degenerative changes are also noted in the later stages. Technetium-99m bone scintigraphy can be used in the postoperative period but is only 85% sensitive and is nonspecific. Scintigraphy will demonstrate changes in response to the initial osteotomy, so it is recommended that the surgeon wait a minimum of 4 weeks prior to imaging in order to be able to better differentiate between the initial vascular insult and AVN [6, 8, 19]. Wallace et al. performed a review of 13,952 patients who underwent first metatarsal head osteotomies, and 15 (0.11%) developed avascular necrosis. Thirteen out of fifteen (87%) had Chevron bunionectomy; two (13%) had Scarf procedure. On average, AVN was documented 4 months postoperatively. There was no increased incidence noted with respect to fixation type. All 15 patients responded to conservative treatment consisting of non-weight bearing in a cast and nonsteroidal anti-inflammatory medication [8].

Conservative treatment should start with off-loading and limiting the stresses on the first metatarsal phalangeal joint with orthotic management or shoe modifications. Partial or complete non-weight bearing may be beneficial in the initial stages. The majority of patients respond to conservative treatment, but those that do not may require surgical intervention. If the osseous integrity is still preserved and collapse of the capital fragment has not resulted secondary to the AVN, the patient's symptoms may resolve with synovectomy and subchondral drilling. Moderate to severe cases will require first metatarsophalangeal joint arthrodesis with or without interpositional grafting [19]. When determining if the use of interpositional graft is necessary, the overall bone stock, viability, and length of the first metatarsal need to be taken into account. If after resection greater than 1 cm of bone loss is noted or cosmetic appearance of the shortened first ray is not favorable, an interpositional graft should be utilized. With an end-to-end first metatarsophalangeal joint arthrodesis, the overall functional length of the metatarsal is extended to the level of the interphalangeal joint.

There are multiple locations for harvest of an autogenous corticocancellous graft including the lateral wall of the calcaneus, middle third of the fibular shaft, or the iliac crest. Multiple allografts are available on the market today. The most commonly utilized allografts consist of the iliac crest, patellar wedge, or femoral head. In revisional cases, autogenous graft is preferable as it not only supplies the osteoconduction or scaffolding properties that allografts provide but also has the benefit of osteogenesis and osteoinduction by transporting living cells to the area and transporting bone morphogenic protein (BMP) and other growth factors to the arthrodesis site [13, 17, 21–26]. Mankovecky et al. performed a systematic review of the incidence of nonunion of the first metatarsophalangeal joint arthrodesis with the autogenous iliac crest after failed Keller-Brandes arthroplasty and found a 4.8% nonunion rate. On the other hand, Myerson et al. performed a similar study and demonstrated a high 21.9% nonunion rate when performing an interpositional arthrodesis for salvage of failed Keller arthroplasty, failed replacement arthroplasty, and previous osteotomy [13, 25]. The previously documented high donor site morbidity following iliac crest graft harvest is not supported by recent literature; similar postoperative morbidity is noted at other autogenous graft sites, the calcaneus, tibia, and iliac crest.

Primary arthrodesis in patients with minimal comorbidities has shown similar fusion rates with the use of allogenic bone graft verse autogenous graft. Anderson et al. compared primary first metatarsophalangeal joint end-to-end arthrodesis rates with local autogenous graft versus mesenchymal stem cell (MSC) impregnated allograft and found no significant difference in fusion rate and patient satisfaction. They concluded that autograft and allogenic bone graft with MSC are both viable options for the foot and ankle surgeon to use when a bone void deficit is noted [21]. In the setting of AVN or other revisional cases, autogenous graft is utilized due to its additional properties to promote healing. Autogenous grafts have been shown to consolidate at a more rapid pace and elicit higher union rates due to the lack of immunogenicity. Allografts, however, have the benefit of decrease operative time and donor site morbidity. When using allogenic bone graft to augment arthrodesis, it is important to maintain as large of a host to graft interface. If thick allografts are utilized, the possibility of a large avascular aspect of the graft is increased as consolidation takes place primarily at the host-graft interface. Bone grafts can be utilized to maintain and restore length, provide angular correction, and augment and promote osseous consolidation [13, 17, 21–26].

Autogenous corticocancellous grafts can be taken from the dorsal lateral wall of the calcaneus, middle third of the fibular shaft, or iliac crest. The location preferred by the authors is the dorsal lateral wall of the calcaneus in which a bicortical structural bone graft can be easily harvested from the superior lateral aspect of the calcaneus. In addition, after removal of the corticocancellous graft, further cancellous

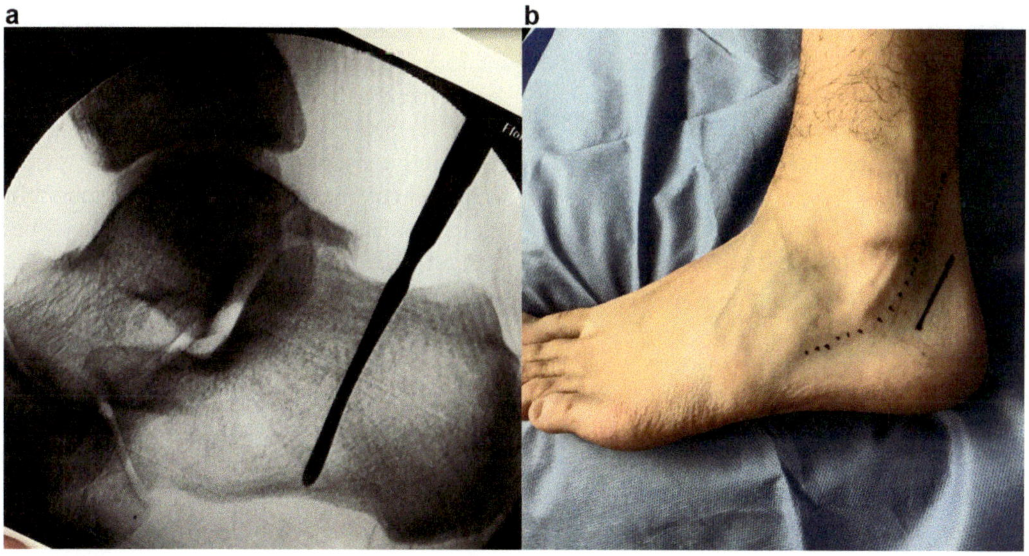

Fig. 11.9 (**a**, **b**) Fluoroscopic guidance and incision placement for calcaneal bone graft harvest

a b c

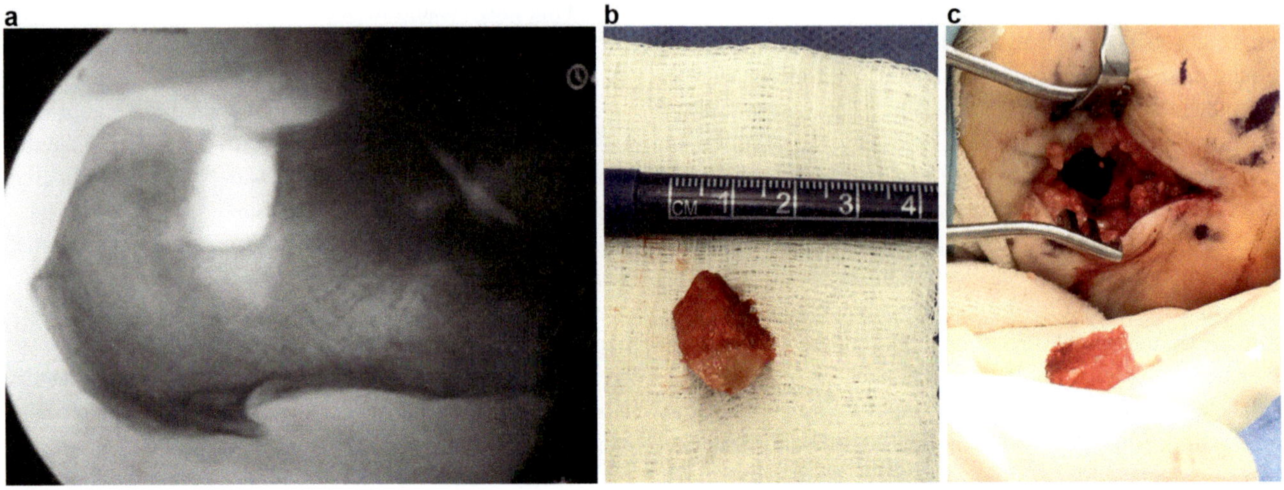

Fig. 11.10 (**a–c**) Harvest of bicortical calcaneal bone graft from the dorsolateral wall

graft can be harvested from the calcaneal body. Surgical technique includes a 3–4 cm oblique incision extending from just proximal to the superior aspect of the calcaneus, centered between the posterior facet and the posterior tuberosity of the calcaneus (Fig. 11.9a, b). The use of fluoroscopy can be utilized to confirm location intraoperatively. Blunt dissection through the subcutaneous tissue to the lateral wall of the calcaneus is utilized to limit trauma to the sural nerve. The periosteum is elevated from the superior lateral aspect of the calcaneus, and two Kirschner wires can be utilized to mark the inferior border of the donor site. These wires are placed 1.5 cm inferior to the superior border and 1 cm from posterior to anterior. The depth of the graft is approximately 1 cm from lateral to medial. Next, with the use of a sagittal saw and osteotomes, the lateral half of the calcaneus is osteotomized. A curved osteotome can be utilized from the superior aspect of the calcaneus to remove the bone from the superior lateral aspect of the calcaneus (Fig. 11.10a–c). Upon removal of the graft, further cancellous bone can be harvest from the body of the calcaneus. It is the author's preference to backfill the donor site with allogenic or synthetic bone graft substitute; however, this is not required (Fig. 11.11a–e).

Interpositional First Metatarsophalangeal Joint Arthrodesis Technique

A standard dorsal longitudinal incision is made over the first metatarsal phalangeal joint. When planning the incision, the previous surgical incision site may be utilized, but due to the increased need for hardware, it is beneficial to extend the previous incision at least a centimeter in both the proximal and distal aspect of the incision. Myerson et al. did not utilize a tourniquet as to be able to appreciate the aspect of bleeding healthy bone margin intraoperatively, and if in a case with overdistraction, blanching of the skin was noted and could be addressed [13]. It is the surgeon's preference to utilize a tourniquet to assist in visualization and limit operating time. After dissection is performed and previous hardware is removed, the tourniquet is deflated to assess resected margins. As with any revisional surgical procedure, a large amount of scar tissue will be noted. Limiting superficial dissection is imperative to limit devascularization of the cutaneous tissue to help decrease postoperative wound complications. Once the extensor hallucis longus is identified, a single soft tissue layer should be reflected off of the first metatarsophalangeal joint. On inspection of the first metatarsal head, any nonviable soft tissue and bone must be resected to the level of healthy bleeding tissue, along with a synovectomy. Resection is most commonly performed with the use of a saw or osteotomes in a "flat cut fashion" to ease graft application. Whalen proposed the use of conical reamers to prepare the arthrodesis and graft interface. If this technique is to be implemented, special care should be taken as the reamer can be aggressive, and if poor bone stock is evident, overaggressive resection can be a possibility. After resection to a level of healthy osseous tissue, subchondral drilling should be performed with a 1.5 mm drill bit. It is the author's preference to subchondral drill utilizing a drill rather than a Kirschner wire to assist in decreasing thermal injury and to also assist in bringing autogenous bone graft to the arthrodesis site. A smooth laminar spreader can be inserted into the arthrodesis site to distract the first ray out to the desired length, and then measurement of the required graft size is performed. In the author's experience, 10–15 mm is the average size graft utilized. Myerson et al. had an average graft size of 22 mm ranging from 11 to 35 mm; however, secondary to resected margins, the radiographic evaluation of increased length was not proportionate with the mean average of additional length postoperative, which was 13 mm

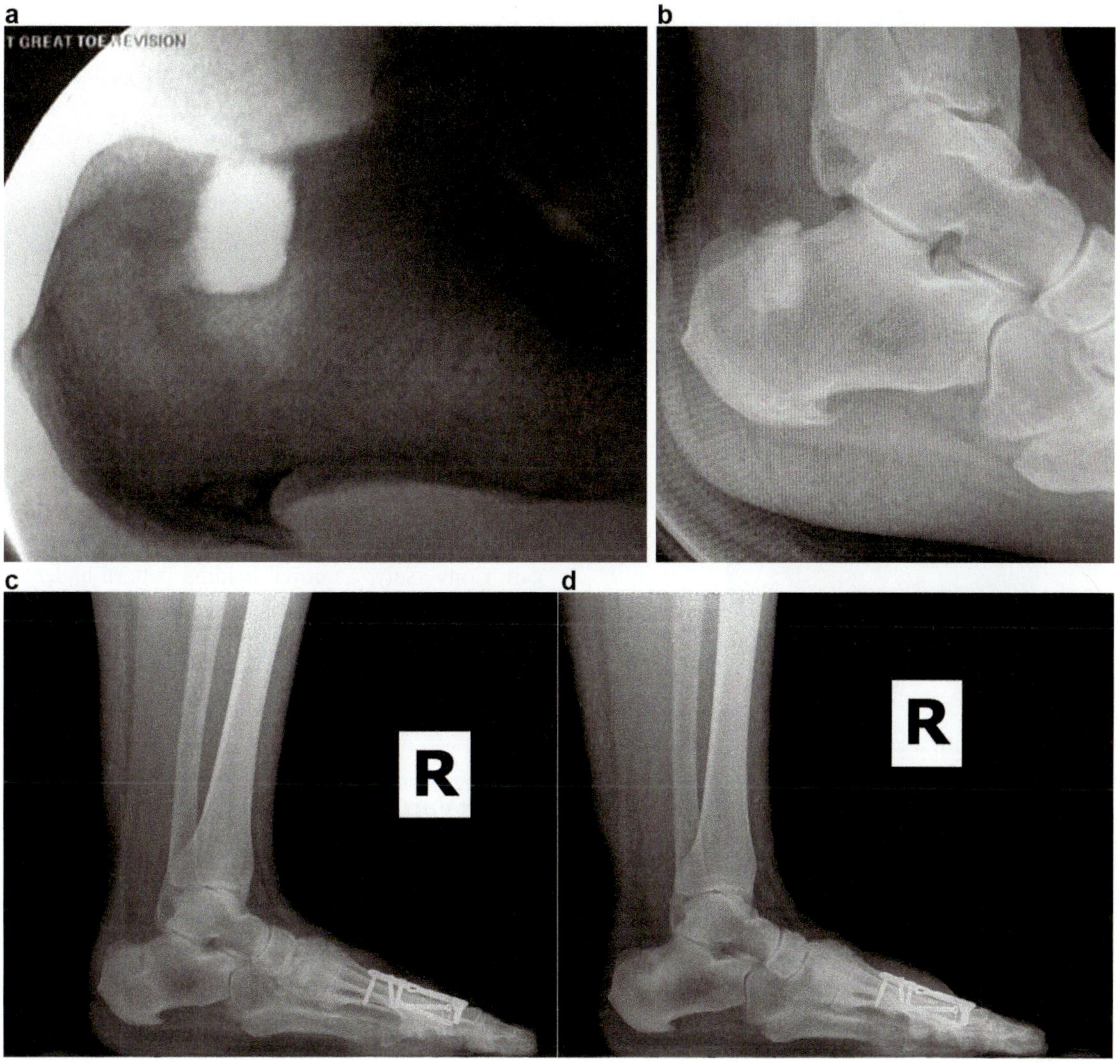

Fig. 11.11 (**a**, **b**) Backfilling the calcaneal graft harvest site with synthetic bone graft. (**c**, **d**) Synthetic graft incorporation at the harvest site at 2, 3, and 7 months

ranging from 0 to 29 mm [13]. The surgeon can now cut the graft to size and place it within the arthrodesis site. The graft is temporary fixated with the use of a Kirschner wire to ensure good restoration of length and proper alignment (Fig. 11.12). The recommendation of 10–15° of dorsiflexion, 10–15° of valgus, and neutral frontal plane alignment has been discussed previously in the literature. The appropriate amount of dorsiflexion at the first metatarsophalangeal arthrodesis sight has been debated in the literature with authors recommending a range of dorsiflexion from 10° to 40°. It is standard protocol for the author to load the forefoot with the lid from a hardware tray and position the hallux parallel to second digit and slightly elevated (Figs. 11.4 and 11.13). Too little valgus may predispose the interphalangeal joint to early degenerative change and dorsal hallux irritation secondary to shoe gear. Fixation of this arthrodesis may be performed with a variety of constructs from threaded Steinmann pins, screws, staples, dorsal plate, and any combination thereof, but it is recommended that a dorsal plate be used to augment any fixation. Depending on bone quality, it is the authors' preference to use one or two inter-

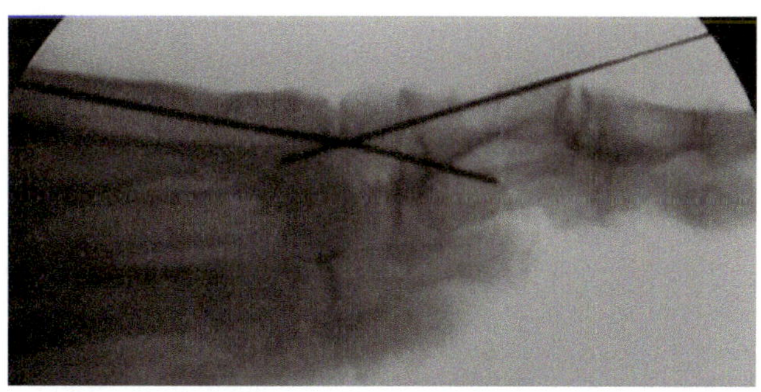

Fig. 11.12 Intraoperative placement and temporary fixation of the interpositional bone graft

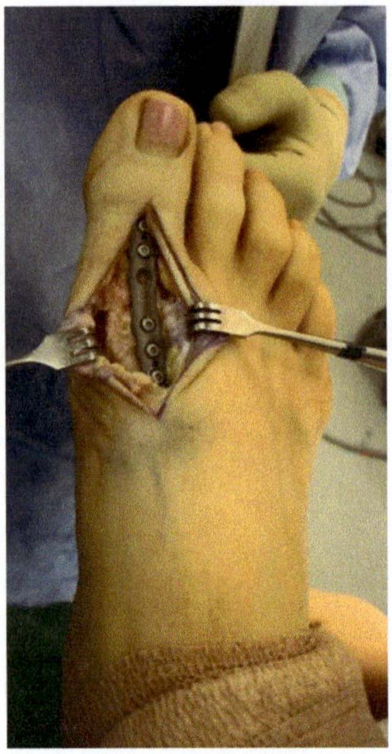

Fig. 11.13 Postoperative alignment of the hallux parallel to the second digit

fragmentary screws with a low-profile dorsal locking plate. However, static manual compression with plate to graft fixation is adequate in select cases. The construct of a dorsal plate and interfragmentary screw has been documented in the literature to be the most stable construct for in situ arthrodesis. When determining the appropriate plate for fixation, the remaining length of the proximal phalanx after resection must be taken into account to not cause jamming of the interphalangeal joint with dorsiflexion. With distraction and previously incised hypertrophic scar tissue, wound complications can be of concern postoperatively, so overall bulk of the dorsal plate has to be accounted for to ensure there will be adequate soft tissue coverage. Even with distraction arthrodesis, the lesser metatarsals may need to be addressed with shortening osteotomies depending on the overall metatarsal parabola and biomechanical accommodation and adaptation (Figs. 11.14 and 11.15).

Bhosale et al. demonstrated 8/10 patients were satisfied with their outcome following first metatarsophalangeal joint interpositional arthrodesis. The two dissatisfied patients had prominent hardware or hardware failure. Four patients required removal of implants. Due to extent of distraction and soft tissue contractures, Z lengthening of the extensor hallucis longus (EHL) tendon or sectioning of the extensor hallucis brevis may be necessary. Myerson et al. documented that 18/24 of his patients required EHL tendon lengthening. Postoperatively patients remained strictly non-weight bearing in a short-leg cast for 4 weeks. Dorsoplantar and lateral radiographs were obtained at 4-week intervals. Progressive weight bearing was allowed in a cast or walking boot when clinical and early radiographic union was evident. Brodsky et al. documented an 11-/12-fusion rate at an average of 12 weeks, with the AOFAS score 3 excellent, 4 good, 4 fair, and 1 poor post-op outcome. None of the patients were completely pain-free postoperatively, but all but one had mild occasional discomfort. Patients were not limited in activity of daily living, and the majority of patients were able to return to recreational activity. Three postoperative complications were noted with two wound complications and one nonunion. The literature reports successful primary arthrodesis rates range from 77% to 100% with various techniques. The average length of time to radiographic union reported is 2–4 months, with an average of 2.5 months.

Some surgeons prefer a resection arthroplasty with synovectomy. Though this procedure can help to alleviate pain, however it does not yield a stable, load-bearing, functional great toe. Patients have decreased overall walking velocity, longer stance phase, and shorter single-limb stance phase of gait. Conversely, a normal loading pattern under the lesser metatarsal heads and toes is seen with arthrodesis of the first metatarsophalangeal joint. Arthrodesis has favorable outcomes and allows for resection of the nonviable bone and also creates a stable platform [13, 27, 28].

Hallux Varus

Iatrogenic hallux varus is a surgical complication often resulting from overcorrection of a bunion deformity. McBride first described hallux varus following his initial procedure with resection of the medial eminence, medial capsulorrhaphy, and fibular sesamoidectomy; he documented an incidence of 5%. Now with the addition of first metatarsal osteotomies for correction of hallux valgus deformities and the large amount of research that has been published on hallux varus, the incidence in the literature ranges from 2% to 17% and can result from an imbalance in osseous, tendon, capsule, or ligamentous structures [29, 30]. Although there are multiple causes of hallux varus deformity, we are going to focus on the iatrogenic hallux varus and its correction. To properly correct a hallux varus deformity, one must understand the pathogenesis of the deformity. Hallux varus can result when one "pushes the limits" of a procedure when a more powerful procedure is indicated. More common etiologies include overaggressive resection of the medial eminence (staking of the first metatarsal head) and overcorrection of the intermetatarsal angle (negative IM angle). Soft tissue imbalance can also be a causative agent resulting in hallux varus including an overaggressive lateral release, medial capsulorrhaphy, postoperative bandage, resection of the medial head of the flexor hallucis brevis, resection of the conjoined adductor tendon, and fibular sesamoidectomy. Once the deviation of the hallux progresses past midline, the long extensor and flexor tendons become a progressive force

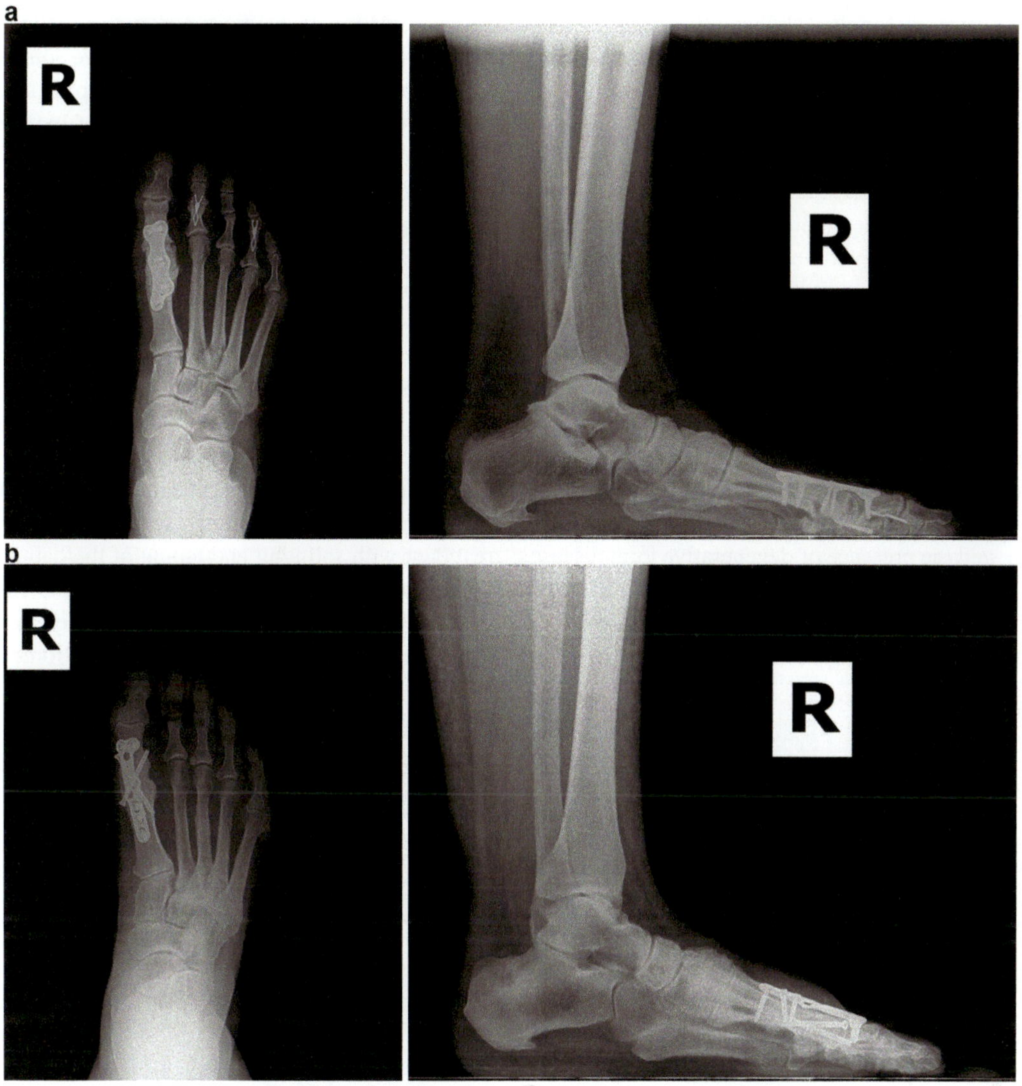

Fig. 11.14 (a, b) Various fixation options for interpositional first metatarsophalangeal joint arthrodesis

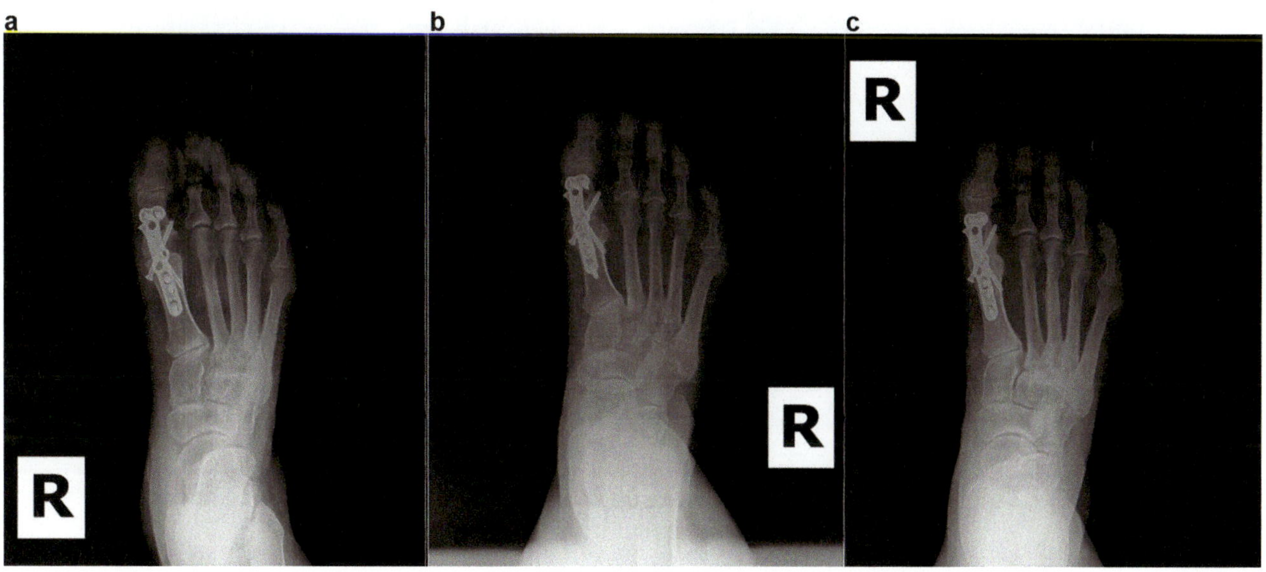

Fig. 11.15 (a–c) Interpositional graft with fixation showing immediate postoperative images, 2 months postoperative and 7 months postoperative images

to increase the varus deformity. Hallux varus deformity is usually multifactorial and a result of a combination of these etiologies. Most commonly this is a triplane deformity with medial deviation of the hallux with hammering at the interphalangeal joint and supination of the digit (Fig. 11.16).

Physical examination should consist of a weight-bearing and non-weight-bearing assessment to evaluate if the deformity is reducible or rigid and to appreciate if there is a dynamic aspect or progression with the presence of the pull of the long flexor and extensor tendon with weight bearing. The first metatarsophalangeal joint should be taken through range of motion and assess for pain or crepitus on range of motion present. Radiographic evaluation with standard dorsoplantar and lateral and medial oblique radiographs should be taken to assess the presence of staking of the head of the first metatarsal, overcorrected intermetatarsal angle, sesamoid position, and the presence of degenerative joint disease and bone quality. The authors also recommend the addition of contralateral radiographs when assessing the varus deformity. Most patients are asymptomatic if there is <10° of medial deviation of the digit; however, a maligned joint will increase the progression of degenerative joint disease and should be assessed. Patients that are symptomatic experience joint pain on palpation, pain on range of motion, pain with shoe gear, unacceptable cosmetic appearance, instability, and weakness with push off [31].

Once a hallux varus deformity is identified, prompt management of the deformity is imperative. Although many patients will tolerate a slight varus deformity, the probability of progression of the deformity if left untreated is high, due to the previous mentioned muscular imbalance. Management of hallux varus in the initial 4 weeks postoperatively can be treated nonoperatively with a moderate success rate depending on the causative agent of the varus deformity. However, a low threshold of surgical intervention is prudent as the deformity progresses and becomes more stiff and rigid. Initial treatment with splinting and taping of the hallux in a valgus position should be implemented. If edema is controlled and patient can tolerate and can be safely placed in normal shoe gear, a tennis shoe will help to apply lateral forces to the digit.

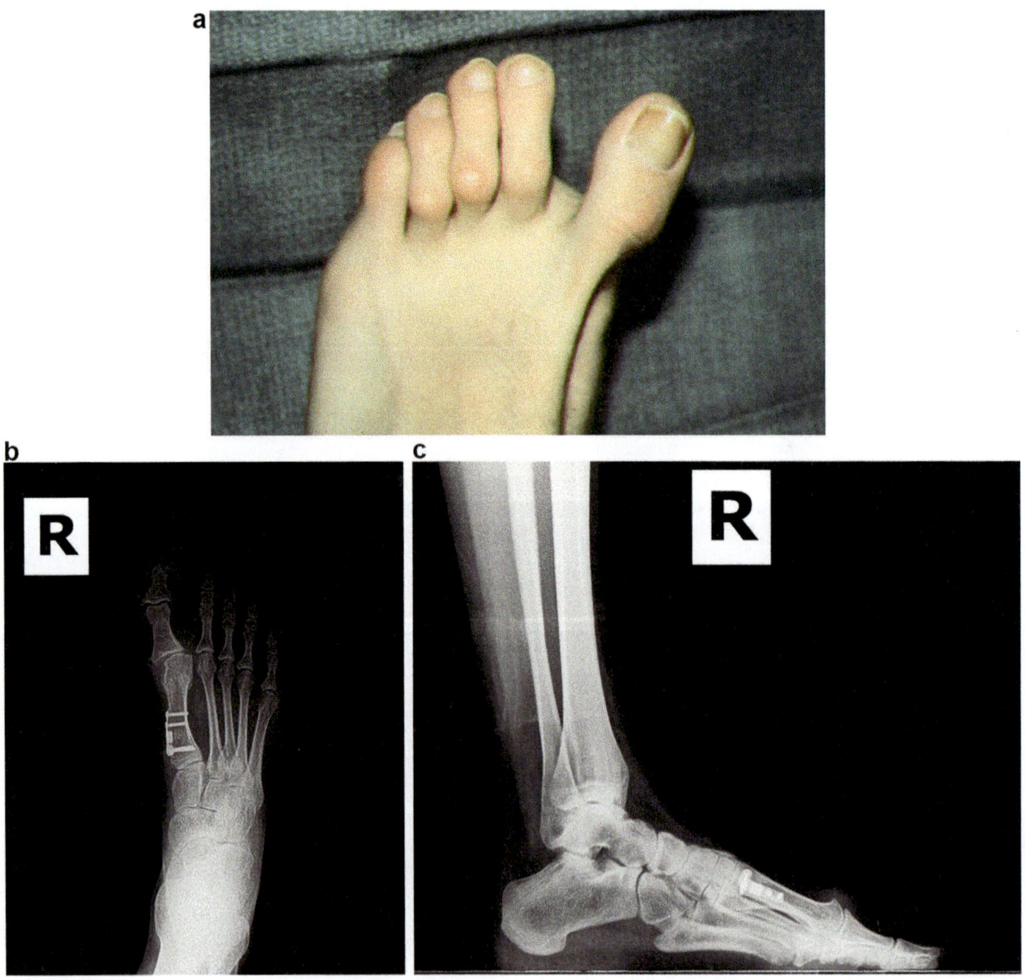

Fig. 11.16 (**a**) Triplane deformity of hallux varus following overcorrection. (**b**, **c**) Development of joint degeneration following unaddressed hallux varus

If the patient does not respond to taping and night splints after 6 weeks, a return to the operating room is warranted. Even if the patient is not currently symptomatic and if progression of the deformity is noted, surgical intervention is necessary to correct the deformity to help decrease the progression of degenerative joint disease. If a flexible deformity is still noted and soft tissue in nature, correction can be performed with minimal downtime to the patient, and this should be explained to the patient preoperatively. Once progression to a rigid deformity is noted with or without the presence of arthritis, the corrective procedures are more extensive and will require osseous correction and significant postoperative recovery in some cases [29, 32]. Determining the appropriate corrective procedure is imperative as one does not want to compound the failure with another failure. Determining the etiology of the varus deformity is paramount when making the decision between conservative, soft tissue, and osseous correction.

In the presence of a flexible deformity with a normal intermetatarsal angle without the presence of degenerative joint disease, soft tissue corrective procedures with capsular release, tendon transfer, tenodesis, direct repair with ligamentous balancing, or supplementation can be used. Many tendon transfers have been described in the literature, with transfer of the abductor hallucis tendon to the lateral side of the proximal phalanx, routing it deep to the deep transverse intermetatarsal ligament. Detachment of the first dorsal interosseous tendon from the second proximal phalanx and routing it through a drill hole in the lateral aspect of the first proximal phalanx has also been described, but the size of this tendon is a deterring factor. The extensor hallucis longus tendon transfer was first described with detachment of the entire extensor hallucis longus and transfer under the deep transverse intermetatarsal ligament to the lateral aspect of the proximal phalanx, but this resulted in an unopposed pull from the long flexor hallucis, resulting in a mallet deformity. Therefore, this procedure has been adjusted to a split extensor hallucis longus tendon transfer, where only the lateral aspect of the extensor hallucis longus is transferred in a similar fashion. The use of a right angle hemostat can be used to assist in transferring the distal lateral aspect of the tendon proximally deep to the intermetatarsal ligament. Then a 4 mm bone tunnel is made 1.5 cm proximal to the metatarsophalangeal joint and oriented oblique from dorsal medial to plantar distal lateral. The deformity is corrected and the tendon tensioned and secured by suturing it to the proximal aspect of the extensor hallucis longus. This soft tissue adjustment to the procedure is preferable compared to performing a proximal interphalangeal joint arthrodesis to address the mallet toe deformity. If these soft tissue procedures fail to correct the deformity, joint destructive procedure with first metatarsophalangeal joint arthrodesis is always a salvage procedure. With that being said, first metatarsophalangeal joint arthrodesis is better tolerated if the interphalangeal joint is still available to compensate [4, 29, 32].

The extensor hallucis brevis transfer has also been described as detaching from its insertion and reinserting through a lateral to medial bone tunnel in the proximal phalanx (Fig. 11.17). Lateral ligament augmentation and repair can be implemented with primary repair of the lateral structures and medial capsulorrhaphy. However, if after the previous surgical intervention the lateral structures are not suitable for repair, augmentation with allograft or synthetic graft can be implemented. A suture button technique was first described by Pappas and Anderson and has been described multiple times in the literature with positive outcomes. In this procedure a medial capsular release is performed, and then a bone tunnel is performed parallel with the weight-bearing surface in the proximal phalanx from distal medial to proximal lateral and a second bone tunnel is made in the metatarsal neck from proximal medial to distal lateral. A 1.6 mm Kirschner wire with intraoperative fluoroscopy can be utilized to ensure placement, followed by a 2.7 mm cannulated drill bit to create the bone tunnels. The suture button is passed through the bone tunnels, and the digit is held in a corrected position while the suture button is tightened and secured in place (Fig. 11.18) [33].

If radiographic evaluation demonstrates staking of the metatarsal head or a negative intermetatarsal angle, soft tissue correction will not be sufficient and osseous alignment must be addressed with a realignment osteotomy or first metatarsophalangeal joint arthrodesis. Rochwerger et al. proposed an osseous buttress with recreation of the medial aspect of the first metatarsal head with iliac crest bone graft `that is fixated in place, but this is not common practice for the authors. Of all of the osseous procedures that can be performed for reduction of an intermetatarsal angle, the reverse

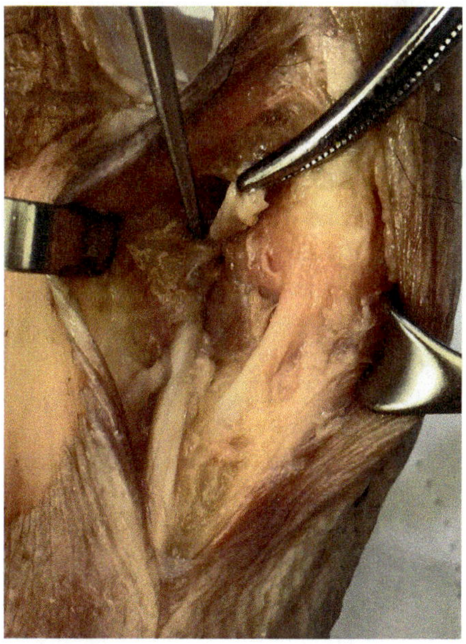

Fig. 11.17 Extensor hallucis longus tendon transfer deep to the transverse intermetatarsal ligament

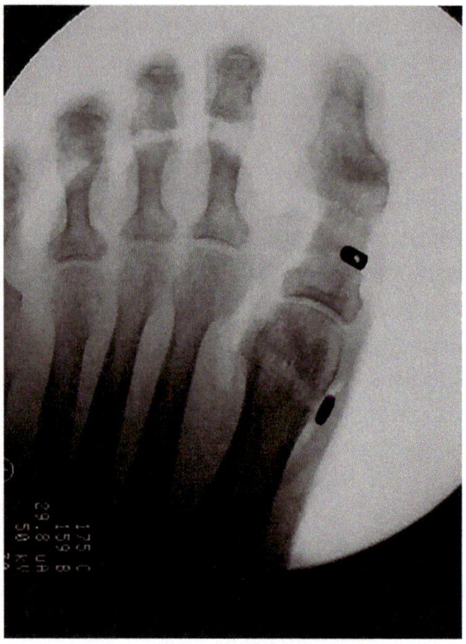

Fig. 11.18 Suture button correction for hallux varus

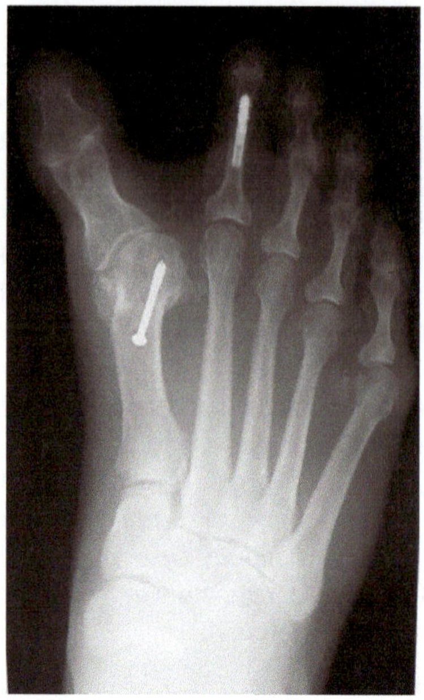

Fig. 11.19 Long-standing hallux varus with degenerative changes and rigidity at the first metatarsophalangeal joint

can be done to increase the intermetatarsal angle. Reverse Chevron osteotomy in conjunction with a medial capsular release is the most documented of these osteotomies in the literature [30]. If a negative distal articular set angle is identified, a lateral closing reverse Reverdin osteotomy may be beneficial. As described previously the first metatarsal length must be assessed preoperatively; however, decompression of the joint in some instances is beneficial, particularly if a stiff joint is noted secondary to the varus deformity. Additionally, a reverse Akin osteotomy can be employed to further align the great toe and improve overall function.

If the varus deformity has been present for a prolonged amount of time and is non-reducible with joint stiffness or degenerative changes are noted radiographically and clinically, successful outcomes even after realignment of the joint are relatively low (Fig. 11.19). In this instance, arthrodesis of the first metatarsophalangeal should be considered. Resection arthroplasty, although not preferred, can be beneficial in older very low-demand patients. After prolong varus deformity of the hallux is noted, the lesser digits start to deviate in a similar direction; therefore, assessment with shortening osteotomies or metatarsal head resections may be necessary in conjunction with correction of the first metatarsophalangeal joint.

Conclusion

Given the high incidence of hallux valgus corrections performed by foot and ankle surgeons, complications are bound to arise. Possible complications should be discussed with patients preoperatively and never hidden after the fact. Complications such as first ray insufficiency, hallux varus, and avascular necrosis are some of the most challenging complications seen. Taking proactive preventative measures in the preoperative setting is key to avoiding negative outcomes. A thorough and individualized presurgical examination is paramount to selecting the proper patient and procedure. Determining the etiology of the complication is necessary in order to make an appropriate decision between conservative care, soft tissue correction, and osseous correction. Surgical technique and proper procedure selection is imperative to ensure favorable outcomes. When the inappropriate procedure is selected and there is an attempt to force correction, complications commonly arise. When looking to address complications, the surgeon must take into account patient's activity level, chief complaint, and expectations to help produce the most favorable outcome.

Occasionally the undesirable result can be rectified conservatively, but often an additional surgical procedure is needed. A joint-sparing procedure with correctional osteotomies or tendon transfers can often be utilized, but if the deformity is rigid or degenerative changes are present, then joint destruction procedures such as first metatarsophalangeal joint arthrodesis may be necessary and result in a more predictable outcome.

References

1. Trnka H. Osteotomies for hallux valgus correction. Foot Ankle Clin North Am. 2005;10:15–33.
2. Belczyk R, Stapleton J, Grossman J, Zgonis T. Complications and revisional hallux valgus surgery. Clin Podiatr Med Surg. 2009;26:475–84.
3. Lee K, Park Y, Jegal H, Lee T. Deceptions in hallux valgus. Foot Ankle Clin North Am. 2014;19:361–70.
4. Lehman D. Salvage of complications of hallux valgus surgery. Foot Ankle Clin North Am. 2003;8:15–35.
5. Goldberg A, Singh D. Treatment of shortening following hallux valgus surgery. Foot Ankle Clin North Am. 2014;19:309–16.

6. Laughlin T. Complications of distal first metatarsal osteotomies. J Foot Ankle Surg. 1995;34:524–31.
7. Viehe R, Haupt J, Heaslet M, Walston S. Complications of screw-fixated Chevron osteotomies for the correction of hallux abductovalgus. J Am Podiatr Med Assoc. 2003;93(6):499–502.
8. Vora A, Myerson M. First metatarsal osteotomy nonunion and malunion. Foot Ankle Clin. 2005;10:35–54.
9. Lagaay P, Hamilton G, Ford L, Williams M, Rush S, Schuberth J. Rates of revision surgery using Chevron–Austin osteotomy, lapidus arthrodesis, and closing base wedge osteotomy for correction of hallux valgus deformity. J Foot Ankle Surg. 2008;47:267–72.
10. Moon J, McGlamry M. First metatarsophalangeal joint arthrodesis: current fixation options. Clin Podiatr Med Surg. 2011;28:405–19.
11. Banks A, Cargill R, Carter S, Ruch J. Shortening of the first metatarsal following closing base wedge osteotomy. J Am Podiatr Med Assoc. 1997;87:199–208.
12. Budny A, Masadeh S, Lyons M, Frania S. The opening base wedge osteotomy and subsequent lengthening of the first metatarsal: an in vitro study. J Foot Ankle Surg. 2009;48:662–7.
13. Myerson M, Schon L, McGuigan F, Oznur A. Result of arthrodesis of the hallux metatarsophalangeal joint using bone graft for restoration of length. Foot Ankle Int. 2000;21:297–306.
14. Whalen J. Interpositional bone graft for first MTPJ fusion. Foot Ankle Int. 2009;30:160–2.
15. Gudipati S, Sunderamoorthy D, Harris N. Early arthritis of the first MTPJ without AVN of the metatarsal head: a complication following lengthening SCARF osteotomy for transfer metatarsalgia. Foot Ankle Online J. 2013;6(8):2.
16. Singh D, Dudkiexicz I. Lengthening of the shortened first metatarsal after Wilson's osteotomy for hallux valgus. J Bone Joint Surg (Br). 2009;91-B(12):1583.
17. Politi J, John H, Njus G, Bennett G, Kay D. First metatarsal-phalangeal joint arthrodesis: a biomechanical assessment of stability. Foot Ankle Int. 2003;24:332–7.
18. Kuhn M, Lippert F, Phipps M, Williams C. Blood flow to the metatarsal head after Chevron bunionectomy. Foot Ankle Int. 2005;26:526–9.
19. Edwards W. Avascular necrosis of the first metatarsal head. Foot Ankle Clin North Am. 2005;10:117–27.
20. Hall P, Landsman A, Banks A, Dalmia L. Thermal properties of first metatarsal osteotomies. J Foot Ankle Surg. 2009;48:432–8.
21. Anderson J, Jeppesen N, Hansen M, Brady C, Gough A. First metatarsophalangeal joint arthrodesis: comparison of mesenchymal stem cell allograft versus autogenous bone graft fusion rates. Surg Sci. 2013;4:263–7.
22. Desai S. Bicortical structural autograft harvest during medializing calcaneal osteotomy: technique tip. Foot Ankle Int. 2011;32:644–7.
23. Ebraheim N, Elgafy H, Xu R. Bone-graft harvesting from iliac and fibular donor sites: techniques and complications. J Am Acad Orthop Surg. 2001;9:210–8.
24. Fitzgibbons T, Hawks M, McMullen S, Inda D. Bone grafting in surgery about the foot and ankle: indications and techniques. J Am Acad Orthop Surg. 2011;19:112–20.
25. Mankovecky M, Prissel M, Roukis T. Incidence of nonunion of first metatarsal-phalangeal joint arthrodesis with autogenous iliac crest graft after failed keller-brandes arthroplasty: a systemic review. J Foot Ankle Surg. 2013;52:53–5.
26. Wallace G, Bellacosa R, Mancuso J. Avascular necrosis following distal first metatarsal osteotomies: a survey. J Foot Ankle Surg. 1994;33(2):167–72.
27. Bhosale A, Munoruth A, Blundell C, Flowers M, Jones S, Davies M. Complex primary arthrodesis of the first metatarsophalangeal joint after bone loss. Foot Ankle Int. 2011;32:968–72.
28. Brodsky J, Ptaszek A, Morris S. Salvage first MTP arthrodesis utilizing ICBG: clinical evaluation and outcome. Foot Ankle Int. 2000;21:290–6.
29. Davies M, Blundell C. The treatment of iatrogenic hallux varus. Foot Ankle Clin North Am. 2014;19:275–84.
30. Lee K, Park Y, Young K, Kim J, Kim K, Kim J. Reverse distal Chevron osteotomy to treat iatrogenic hallux varus after overcorrection of the intermetatarsal 1-2 angle: technique tip. Foot Ankle Int. 2011;32:89–91.
31. Donley B. Acquired hallux varus. Foot Ankle Int. 1997;18:586–92.
32. Bevernage B, Leemrijse T. hallux varus: classification and treatment. Foot Ankle Clin North Am. 2009;14:51–65.
33. Gerbert J, Traynor C, Blue K, Kim K. Use of the mini tightrope for correction of hallux varus deformity. J Foot Ankle Surg. 2011;50:245–51.

12 Recurrent Hallux Valgus

Luke D. Cicchinelli and David Granger

Obtaining effective long-term results for the surgical correction of hallux valgus perhaps epitomizes most of any deformity within the foot and ankle, the adage that surgery is both art and science. The effective long-term correction of recurrent hallux valgus therefore adds levels of complexity and challenges both technically for the surgeon as well as expectation wise for the patient. Patients electing to undergo surgery for the correction of their painful bunion deformity have fairly basic desires. They would like the correction to look good, feel good, and be lasting with minimal disruption to their everyday life. By its very presence, the outcome of an index surgery that later necessitates a second intervention has failed all those patient desires. This heightens tremendously the importance of effective surgeon-patient communication and realistic appraisals by the surgeon as to their own personal skill set, knowledge base, and specifically those patient's expectations. A viable outcome formula characterizing the interplay between these variables may be considered as outcome = surgeon knowledge multiplied by surgical execution divided by patient expectations. Clinical experience by the author has led to the additional surgical adages of a prudent reconstructive effort that seeks "to do the least possible and yet the most necessary" and the realization that "almost everything can work—incompletely, and almost nothing works—completely."

This chapter does not seek to repeat nor simply reiterate previously published material on this topic. The reader is referred to two excellent background resources for a general and specific overview on this: Complications in Hallux Abducto Valgus Surgery by Molly Judge in the fourth edition of *McGlamry's Comprehensive Textbook of Foot and Ankle Surgery* and Recurrent Hallux Valgus: Treatment Considerations by Michael Lyons et al. in the 2009 Update of The Podiatry Institute [1, 2]. Rather this chapter seeks to clinically and radiographically illustrate the authors' and several other seasoned clinicians' experiences and results in addressing this challenging deformity while expounding on in case format style the variety of technical and patient-specific considerations that lead to the only thing a patient cares about—a satisfying and lasting result. To avoid duplication of material to be covered in other chapters of this text and complete clarity on the specific clinical contribution the authors wish to share, the authors have made several assumptions. The cases discussed deal only with under-corrected metatarsal osteotomies in which the bone healing was uneventful with no failure of internal fixation or nonunions, or avascular necrosis, or infectious processes. Recurrent hallux valgus specific to the use of the Lapidus procedure as the initial choice of the index correction is similarly excluded although the Lapidus will be discussed as a frequently viable definitive solution to the recurrent deformity of under-corrected intermetatarsal angles in general. As well, complications of hallux valgus surgery primarily causing elevation and shortening of the first ray and insufficiency issues that require plantarflexory osteotomies or callus distraction type approaches are excluded. Those deformities are necessarily included when there has been an under-corrected osteotomy or intermetatarsal angle or unrecognized hypermobility that may even require additional surgery beyond the first ray.

The cases will specifically go beyond the X-rays and consider in detail the importance of the true chief complaint of a patient now dealing with a failure of a previous surgery as the author has found this to be perhaps the single most important factor in ensuring a successful outcome and patient satisfaction. This includes as well the consideration as to whether the original surgeon is performing the revisional surgery or a new surgeon is taking on the revisional case due to patient dissatisfaction. This can factor tremendously into effective solutions for these cases and procedural selection. For example, a patient may be more amenable to the original

L.D. Cicchinelli (✉)
Centro Clinico Quirurgico,
Pintor Colmeiro 10 bajo, Vigo 36210, Spain
e-mail: luke@cicchinelli.com

D. Granger
OSS Health, 1855 Powder Mill Road, York, PA 17402, USA

M.S. Lee, J.P. Grossman (eds.), *Complications in Foot and Ankle Surgery*, DOI 10.1007/978-3-319-53686-6_12

surgeon "tweaking" or "redoing" a portion of the previous surgery such as adding in a phalangeal osteotomy as a second intervention due to under-correction, whereas an upset and dissatisfied patient seeking a new provider may be much more demanding toward a complete overhaul or redo of the original surgery. Many years of clinical practice with high volumes of hallux valgus surgery have taught that both approaches can work. This underlies the continued importance of awareness to the previously mentioned outcome formula and in particular to the denominator which is patient expectations. The higher they are, as a denominator, the more difficult is a highly positive outcome. The lower they are, a higher positive outcome is more likely.

Recurrent hallux valgus and residual hallux valgus are essentially interchangeable terms. The patient expected a definitive resolution of their bunion deformity and did not receive one. Clearly the critical step of assessment for the revisional surgery is why didn't they? Anatomically and radiographically this requires an inventory approach to what the patient started out with, what they presently have, and how will what was done allow or not allow an effective second surgery. Initially the surgeon should contemplate whether the original procedure ever had a chance of working or rather was there insufficient attention to the interplay between dynamic soft tissue forces and structural first ray issues. The lack of a structural repair such as an under-shift of an osteotomy typically will recur more quickly, while the lack of accurate soft tissue balancing may produce a more delayed recurrence. Which component, the soft tissue or the structural component, has the dominant residual effect on the recurrence? There has been substantial debate over the last several years as to whether lateral soft tissue releases are necessary in the surgical correction of hallux valgus. It bears emphasis that this debate is more pertinent to the initial surgery and that in revisional cases there is almost always a necessity for releases of deforming soft tissue forces. Inappropriate procedural selection for a deformity just too severe for what was done and poor execution of a reasonable procedure are factors to entertain as well. For example, if there was adequate procedural selection but inadequate correction obtained, is it possible that the same procedure may simply be redone? These preoperative queries require thoughtful consideration of whether it is better to avoid a redo surgery through the zone of a previous osteotomy which may also increase the likelihood of more scar tissue and joint contractures or bone healing issues or is it preferable to choose a completely new procedure for the revision. The surgeon should do a careful assessment of the presence of systemic factors un- or underappreciated at the time of the original surgery such as spasticity, undiagnosed arthritides, suprastructural biomechanical forces such as torsional issues and pes valgo planus, and unstable hindfeet or even pregnancy and ligamentous laxity. Was there unrecognized hypermobility of the first ray segment? There may be very specific unrecognized deformities or factors purely within the foot segment such as metatarsus adductus, a long hallux, flatfoot deformity, and PASA or distal articular set angle deviations that are harbingers for recurrence (Figs. 12.1, 12.2, 12.3, 12.4, 12.5, 12.6, 12.7, and 12.8).

The exam of the patient considering reoperation for recurrent hallux valgus mirrors the exam of an initial surgery patient with the addition of heightened thoroughness and inspection as to whether anything has changed or developed since the initial surgery. Within the PMH for example, has the patient become a diabetic or developed rheumatoid arthritis since the initial surgery? Of primary and utmost importance is the elicitation by the clinician of what exactly is the patient's chief complaint. This should be obtained now, at the beginning of the overall exam, and then repeated at the end for comparison and confirmation by the clinician that they are focused squarely on resolving the issue at hand and physical limitation from the patient's perspective and not myopically treating the X-rays solely or their own subjective and conditioned tendencies with hallux valgus surgery. The margin of error for a successful and pleasing result for the patient is much slimmer than an initial surgery. Is the chief complaint recurrence of the prominence of the first metatarsal head? Pressure and pain on the medial aspect of the second toe due to persistent hallux abductus? Is there metatarsal-sesamoid pain? Is hallux limitus or rigidus the primary complaint?

A full standing exam follows with careful evaluation for any torsional or suprastructural postural forces that may be impacting the foot. Does the patient have a valgus knee that may increase pronatory forces on the foot segment or have they had a proximal joint replacement from the ankle up that may affect favorably or negatively their mobility and functional demand? The standing foot-specific exam must identify the presence or absence of hindfoot and midfoot forces and dynamics that may have been undertreated or unrecognized with the initial surgery. Does the patient have a hindfoot valgus or adult-acquired flatfoot? Is there bowstringing of the extensor halluces tendon? Is there significant flexor substitution which may contribute to deforming pronatory and flexor forces? Is there metatarsus adductus present that contributes to lateralizing compensatory musculotendinous forces? The seated exam may begin distally at the foot segment and specifically the hallux. Is the hallux abnormally long relative to the second toe? This has been implicated as a causative factor in recurrent hallux valgus due to shoe pressure medially and may increase the vector forces of EHL and FHL on the first mtp joint in a lateral direction. Progressing proximally is evaluation of the first mtp joint and not only the quantity of range of motion but also the quality. Frequently the quantity is emphasized over the quality when in reality a lower yet painless total range of motion may be more tolerable by a patient versus larger yet painful excur-

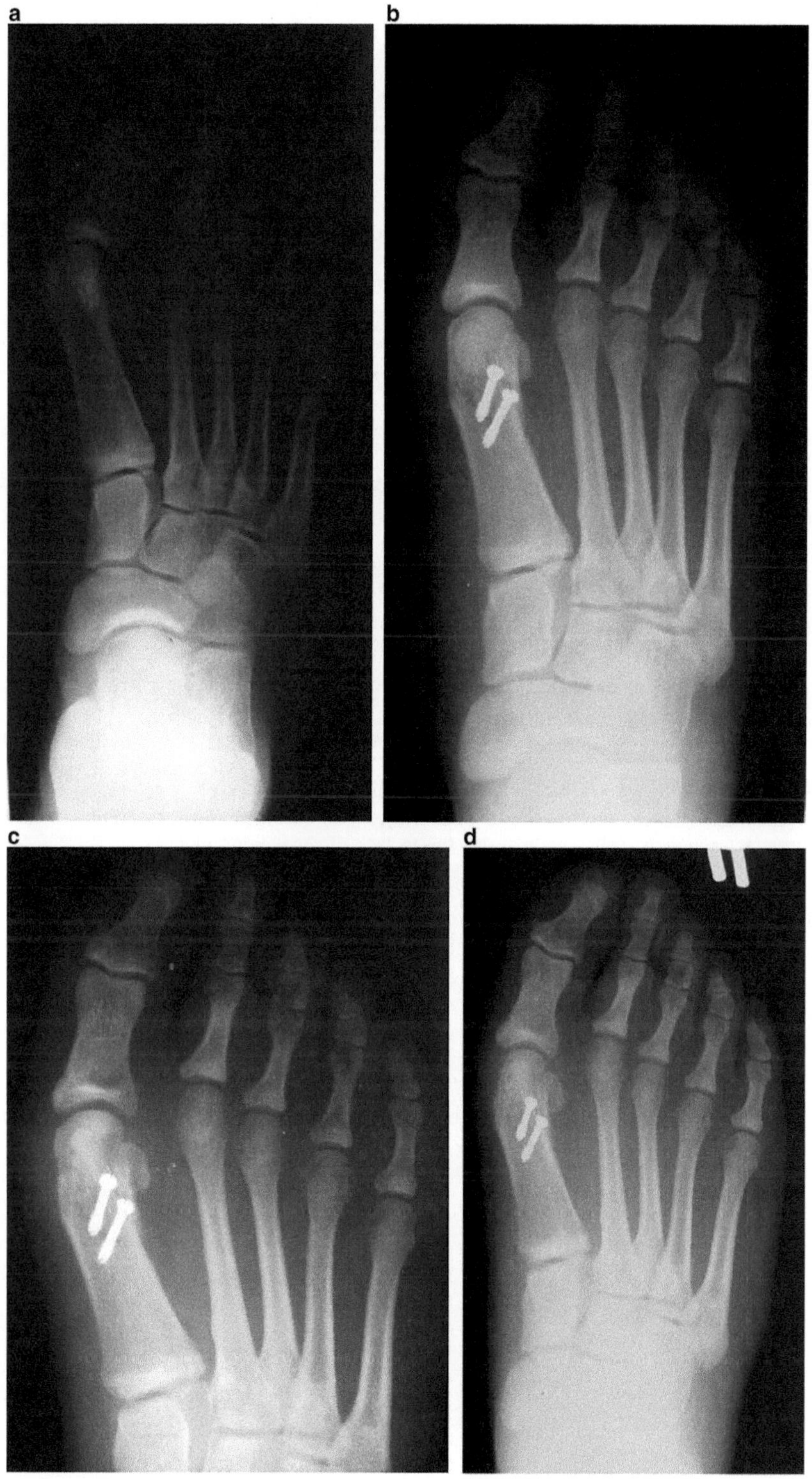

Fig. 12.1 (**a**) Case courtesy of Margo Jimenez preoperative X-ray of HAV deformity. (**b**) Five days post-op with good reduction of the intermetatarsal angle, the metatarsal head well aligned on top of the sesamoids and a congruous mtp joint. (**c**) At 6 weeks post-op, the beginning of recurrence is noted by opening of the IM angle and early lateral drift of the hallux. (**d**) At 3 months postoperatively the patient has a definitive prompt recurrence of the hallux abducto valgus deformity

sions of the joint. Is there metatarsal-sesamoid pain along the medial plantar joint line signifying osteoarthritic changes as a part of the chief complaint? An overall assessment of the mobility of the first ray and reducibility of the deformity is critical here and determines the role of the first tarsometatarsal joint in later procedural correction. Was underlying hypermobility missed during the initial surgery? The reducibility or lack thereof of the deformity assists in determining if the residual effect of soft tissue deforming forces is primary or is it more the latent structural deformity of persistent metatarsus primus varus.

The X-rays must be studied thoroughly and correlated with the physical exam with an eye now toward procedural selection. It is an error to study the X-rays too early in the exam prior to a complete overview of the patient and the determination exactly of what is their chief complaint.

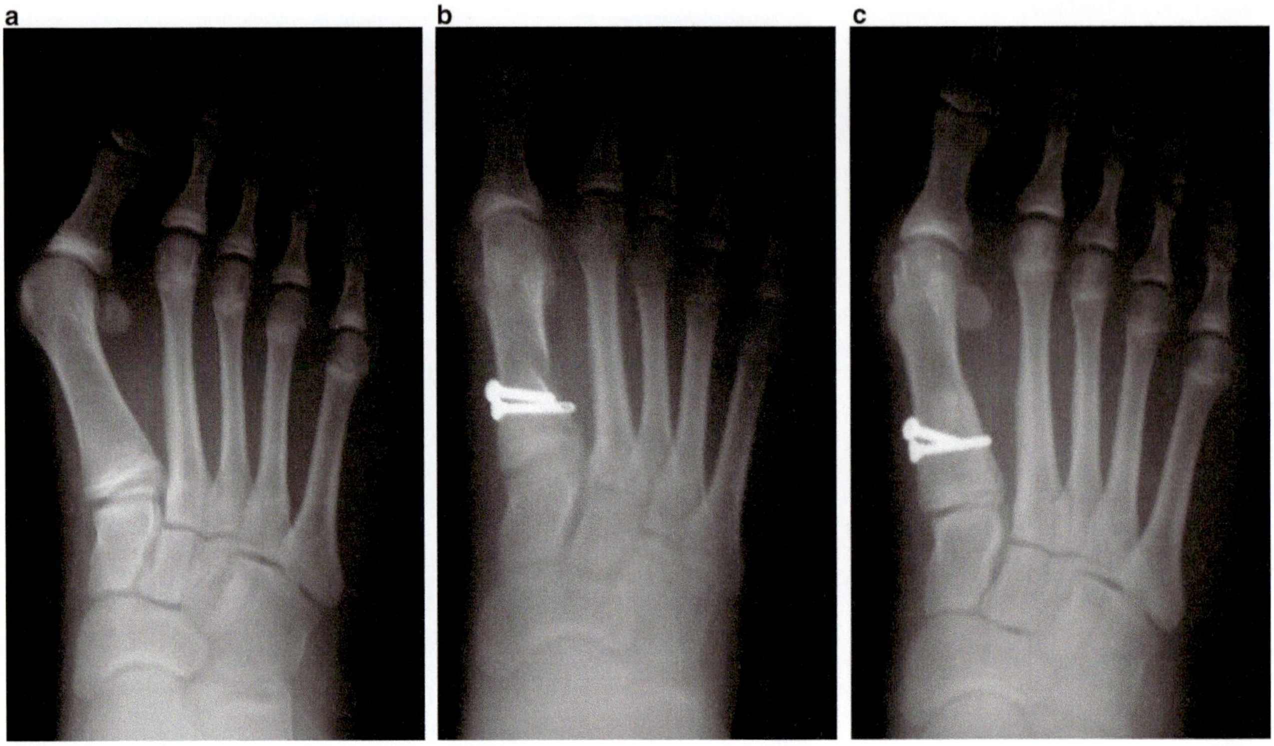

Fig. 12.2 (**a–c**) In this adolescent hallux valgus case, in spite of excellent initial alignment via a base wedge osteotomy, 1 year later there is a clear recurrence as well. This may be due to lack of recognition of deforming forces such as an overlying flatfoot and faulty hindfoot mechanics or an untreated equinus deformity

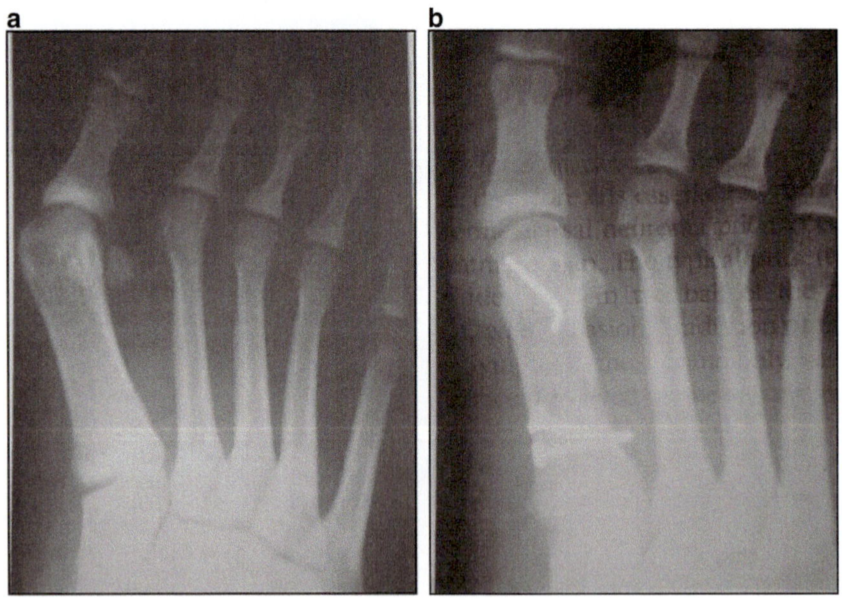

Fig. 12.3 (**a**, **b**) It is well recognized and recommendable in a modern approach to adolescent hallux valgus to include a distal articular set realignment procedure in addition to a proximal osteotomy of choice to discourage late recurrence of the deformity

A global view of the state of the first mtp joint is critical. Is the joint congruous, deviated, or subluxed? As the base of the phalanx deviates, do the sesamoids deviate as well? Are they grossly subluxed signifying resultant or recurrent soft tissue forces that must be neutralized? Again, is the proximal phalanx relatively longer than normal, and was there a previous phalangeal osteotomy performed that may have left an osseous deformity within the phalanx? Are there clear degenerative or erosive changes? Has the metatarsal head been excessively staked which may factor into the practicality of revisional osseous procedures. A rudimentary assessment of any articular set deviation of the metatarsal head cartilage is important with recognition that this must later be substantiated via intraoperative inspection. Next the metatarsal segment is studied. In the case of a previously performed metatarsal osteotomy, is there an identifiable apex of the recurrent deformity? Is there retained hardware that will need to be retrieved thereby affecting the consideration of revisional first metatarsal osteotomies? It is always wise to obtain either an MRI or a CT scan of the first mtp joint as part of the revisional surgery planning to ascertain the state of the cartilage of the metatarsal phalangeal joint as well as the metatarsal-sesamoid joint.

a b

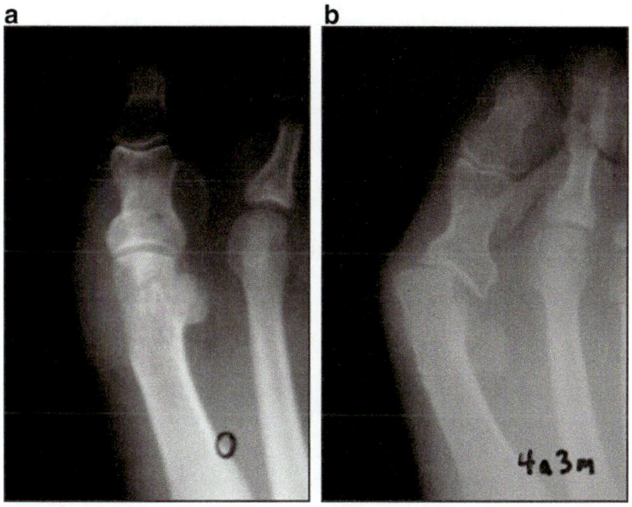

Fig. 12.4 (**a**, **b**) In this minimal incision surgical approach to hallux valgus surgery, a percutaneous Akin osteotomy was performed with a medial eminence exostectomy of the first metatarsal. Four years and 3 months later, there is tremendous recurrence and in fact worsening from the preoperative condition due to the osseous angular deformity created in the proximal phalanx which has affected the vectors of pull of the extrinsic muscles and the weakening of the medial capsule

Procedural planning and procedural selection are best approached via an inventory checklist method that culls any findings from the physical and radiographic exam into a workable and viable suggested surgical approach that will effectively resolve the patient's chief complaint. The inventory list of pertinent clinical and radiographic findings is now collated and assessed directly against a revisitation of the patient's explicit chief complaint. Only now may procedural selection begin. The goal of revisional surgery in a general sense is similar to initial hallux valgus surgery, that is, a well-aligned first ray with reduction of metatarsus primus varus, a congruous first mtp joint, the metatarsal head displaced back directly over the sesamoids, and an aesthetically pleasing and functional alignment of the great toe in relation to the lesser toes. The surgeon must also play a social worker role during procedural selection to the extent that although some patients may be eager and desirous of complying completely with postoperative requirements, they may be situationally noncompliant in the sense that their living and daily arrangements and responsibilities simply do not allow them to comply with certain postoperative instructions.

The overriding goal of the procedural selection phase of the revisional surgical treatment is to err on the side of being aggressive and definitive. A one-stage lasting correction and an end to the frequently frustrating saga are the goal for the surgeon and the patient alike. A simple starting point is the determination of whether the first mtp joint can be saved or not. In the spirit of definitive treatment, if it cannot, a fusion may be considered immediately, and it is clearly understood that the first mtp fusion reliably corrects the intermetatarsal angle as well. If the first mtp joint can be saved, a definitive structural correction of the first ray deviation, intermetatarsal angle recurrence, and unrecognized hypermobility via the

a b c

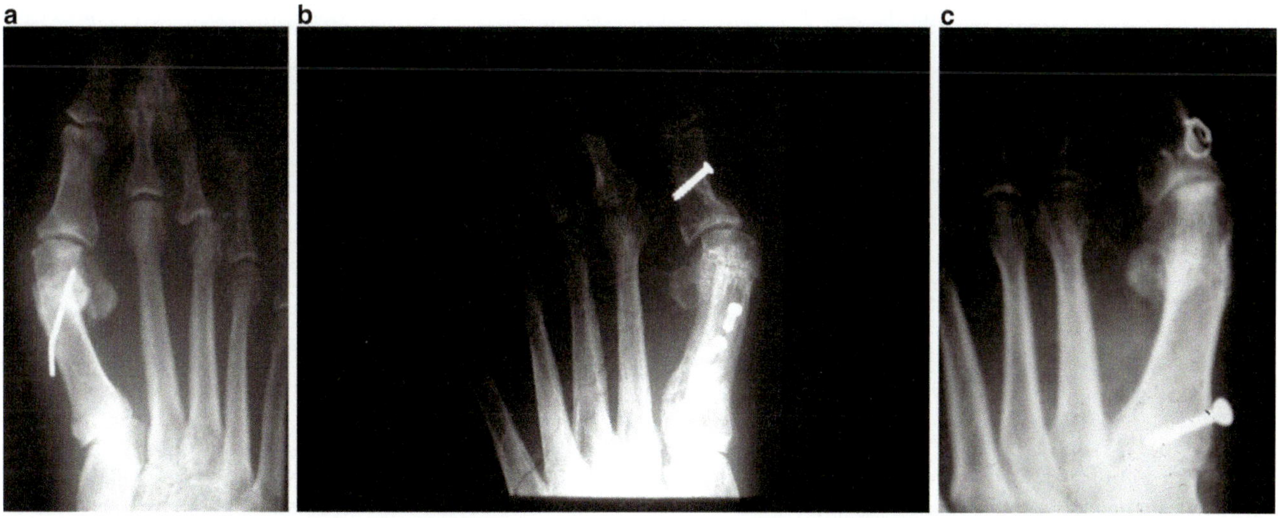

Fig. 12.5 (**a**) Recurrence of the intermetatarsal angle may come from with performance of a distal osteotomy and perhaps inadequate release of soft tissue contractures or (**b**) and (**c**) with diaphyseal osteotomies and phalangeal and proximal osteotomies that have not accounted sufficiently for stabilization of the first ray segment or considerations of hypermobility of the first ray and first TMT joint

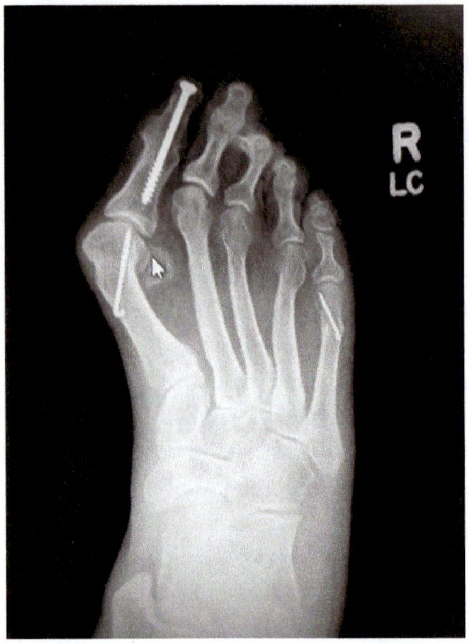

Fig. 12.6 The performance of a distal metatarsal osteotomy and the unappreciated underlying deformity of metatarsus adductus have led predictably here to a recurrent deformity

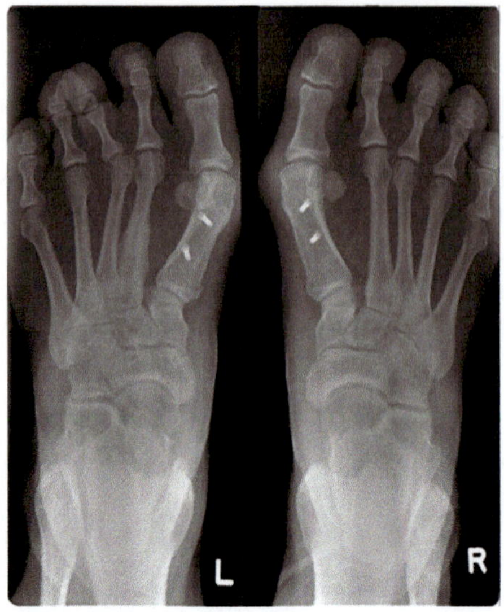

Fig. 12.7 Bilateral recurrent hallux valgus deformity secondary to poor surgical execution where scarf diaphyseal osteotomies were performed but never translated laterally and therefor never reducing the intermetatarsal angle

Fig. 12.8 Recurrent deformity due to the failure of the internal fixation choice, in this case an endobutton and suture construct, whose use has provoked a stress fracture in the neck of the second metatarsal and reopening of the intermetatarsal angle

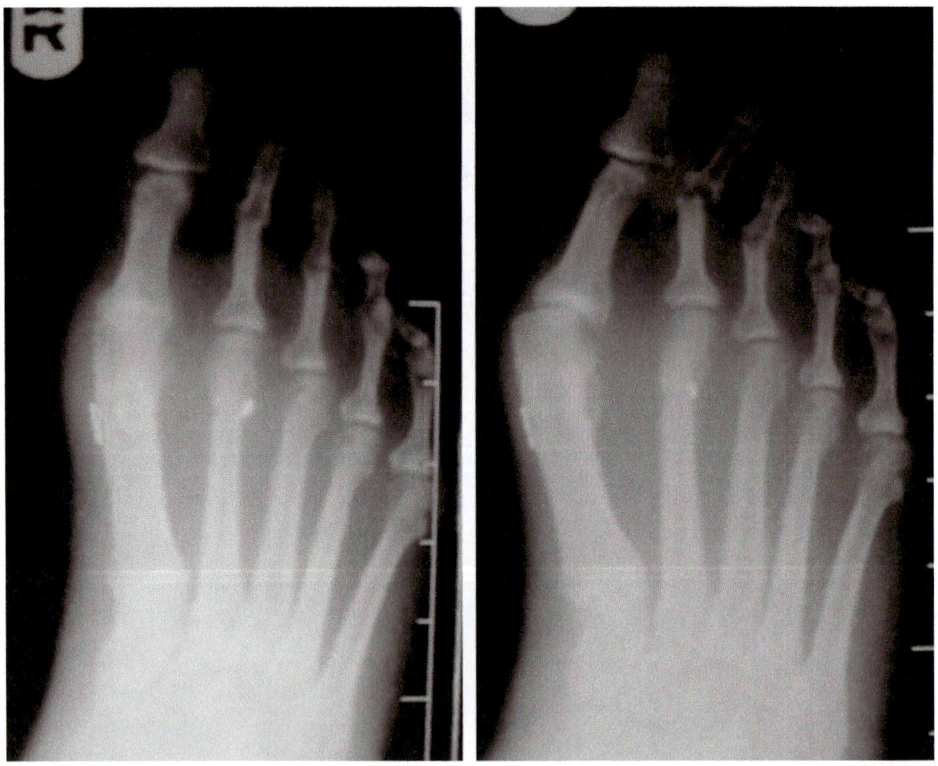

Lapidus fusion may be considered. An intermediary option between a fusion at the mtp joint or TMT joint is the performance of a first metatarsal osteotomy and especially if none was performed previously or a proximally based one if a distal one was performed previously. Lastly, deformities of the midfoot or hindfoot and even recessions of the gastrocnemius should be corrected when deemed influential in the cause of the recurrence. Although it may be attractive to go straight to the Lapidus as the treatment of choice for all recurrent cases, the author cautions that the principle of $N = 1$ dictates that

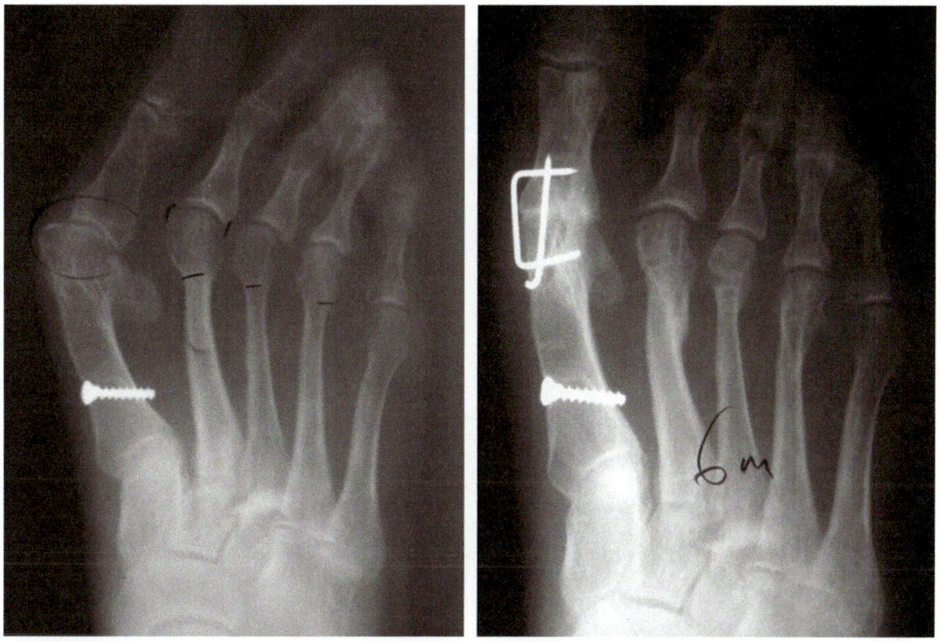

Fig. 12.9 First mtp fusion for non-salvageable first mtp joints is a definitive and reliable method to resolve permanently the deformity of recurrent hallux valgus. Note the reduction in the IM angle via the fusion and neutralization of the reverse buckling forces on the first ray. This fusion was performed with staple, K-wire, and absorbable pin fixation, and, as is frequently the case in revisional bunion surgery, other forefoot procedures were required as well. Multiple Weil osteotomies were performed on the second, third, and fourth rays to harmonize and decompress the parabola

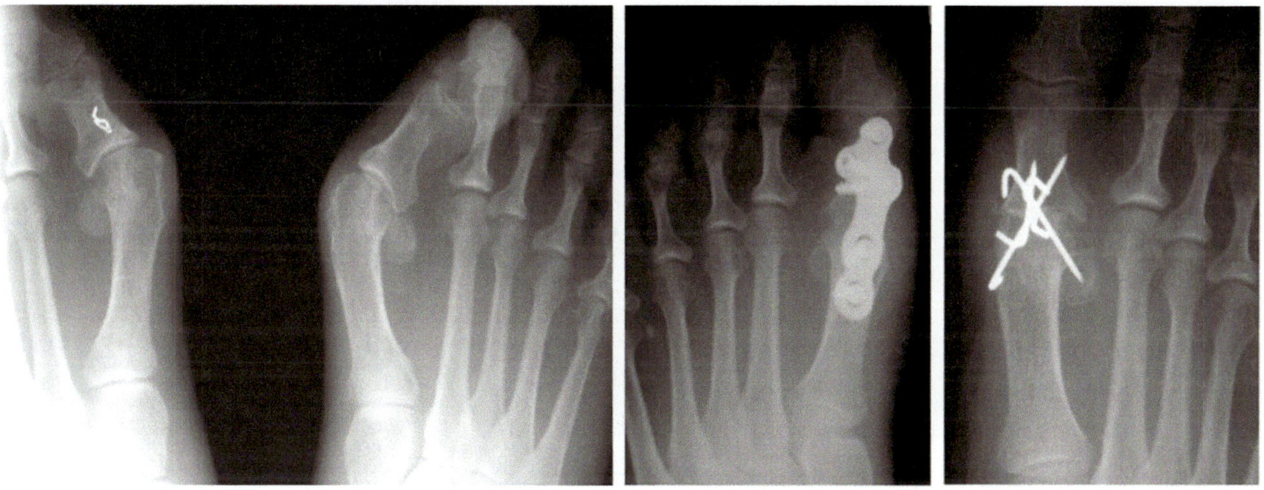

Fig. 12.10 This case of bilateral recurrent hallux valgus was resolved with first mtp fusions with plate and screws on one foot and crossed multiple K-wires on the other

factors such as surgeon skill, surgeon experience, technical execution, and patient desires and expectations allow for other creative and effective ways to resolve the recurrent hallux valgus dilemma for patients. The remainder of the chapter will illustrate all these options via case presentations and in several specific categories.

The first category is the non-salvageable first mtp joint addressed via first mtp joint fusion (Figs. 12.9, 12.10, and 12.11). The second is the salvageable first mtp joint addressed via a Lapidus fusion (Figs. 12.12, 12.13, and 12.14). The third is the use of basal osteotomies, either opening or closing wedge types for effective recurrent intermetatarsal angle correction, and occasionally a distal osteotomy (Figs. 12.15, 12.16, 12.17, 12.18, 12.19, 12.20, 12.21, and 12.22). Fourth is the manipulations of the scarf or Z-type diaphyseal osteotomy that allow more case-specific corrections of recurrent hallux valgus to be entertained (Figs. 12.23, 12.24, 12.25, 12.26, and 12.27). The fifth category is illustration of examples of cases where a pivotal portion of the revisional correction was the correction of a concomitant midfoot or hindfoot deformity or unrecognized structural issue (Figs. 12.28 and 12.29). Lastly, the sixth and final category embraces the concept of $N = 1$ and demonstrates cases in which careful analysis of all elements and variables in the outcome formula described at the outset of this chapter has allowed for very patient-specific procedural selection and combinations of traditional and less traditional

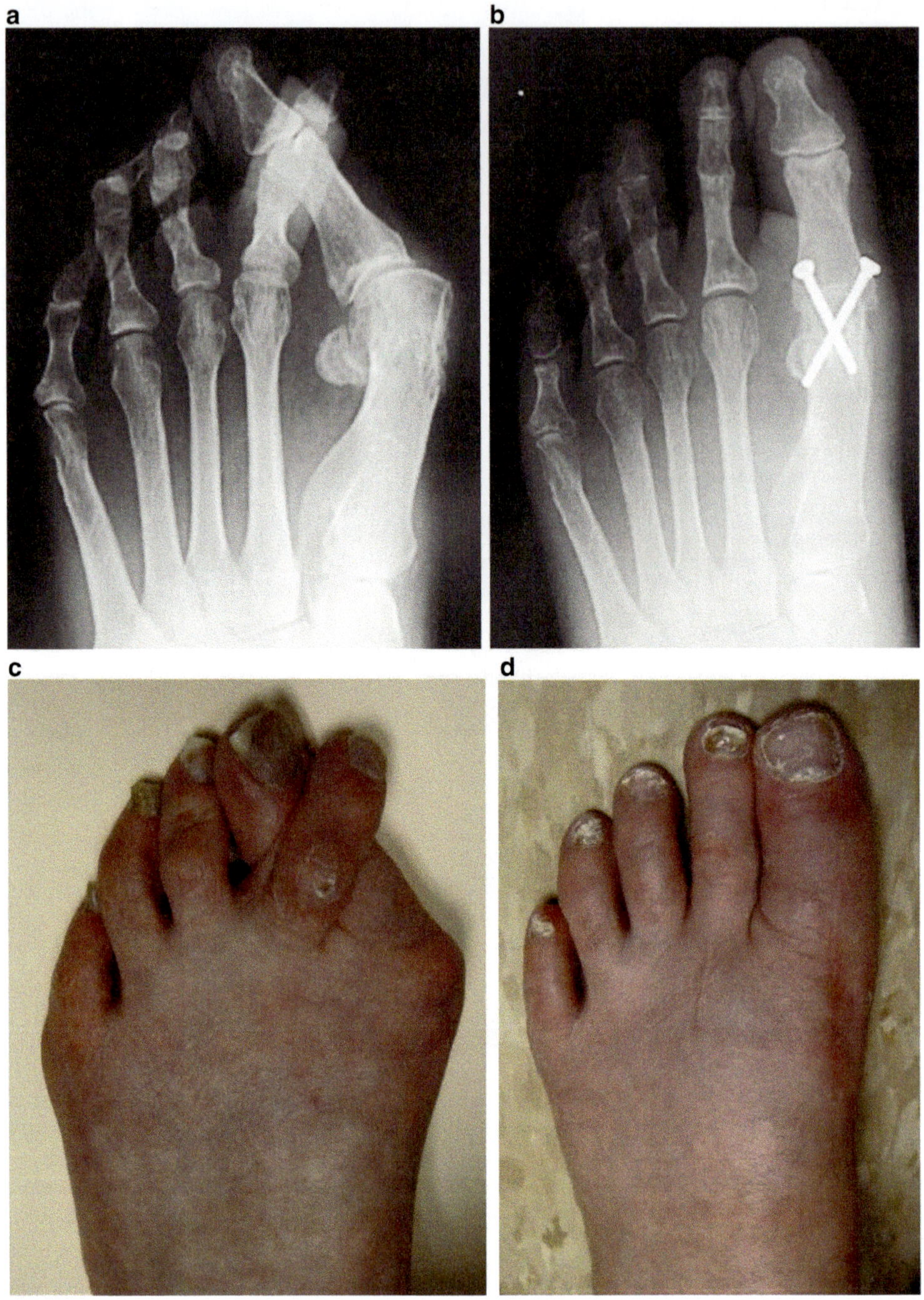

Fig. 12.11 (**a**, **b**) Case courtesy of Craig Camasta. Severe subluxation and recurrent hallux abducto valgus after a failed basilar procedure that was effectively corrected with a crossed screw fixation of the first mtp. (**c**, **d**) Preop and post-op clinical photos of the patient

approaches to still solve their chief complaint (Figs. 12.30, 12.31, 12.32, 12.33, 12.34, and 12.35).

In summary, the authors find it interesting that patients with recurrent hallux abductus with satisfactory reduction of the IM angle are still fairly satisfied. To a lesser extent, patients are seen as well with recurrent IM malalignment who have no pain. It is possible they have had some compromise of the medial dorsal cutaneous nerve or redundant scar tissue in the medial capsule, but sometimes they do not have pain. In those cases, our preference is not to intervene. In practices that see a fair amount of second opinions, we are not likely to attempt heroics with a second/third/fourth surgery if there is not significant pain just to make a radiograph look better.

Although there has been for year the thought of the Akin osteotomy as a "cheater Akin," we find it very valuable as an adjunct. It serves to realign the center of rotation of angulation (CORA) of the great toe joint and realign the pull of the EHL and FHL tendons to discourage abduction.

PASA and articular set deviations also have an understated difficulty in both rotational and translational osteotomy work. When this is not corrected, testing range of

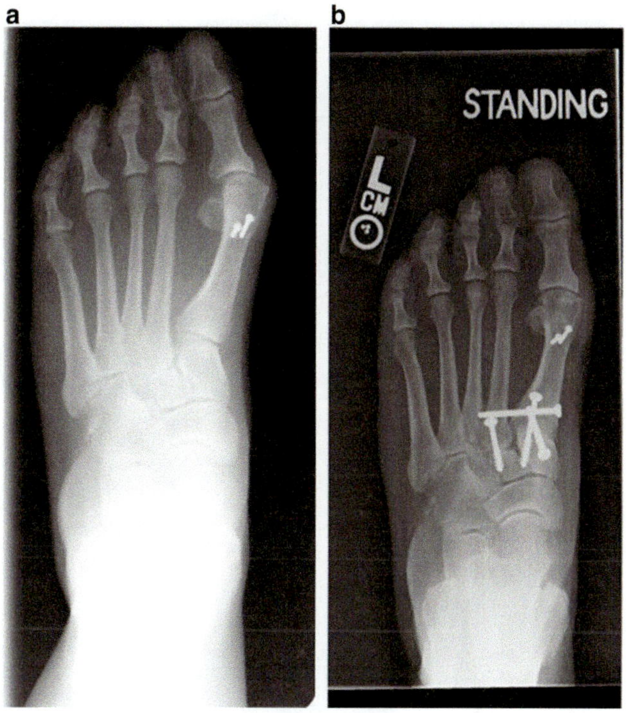

Fig. 12.12 (**a**, **b**) Case courtesy of David Granger. Recurrent hallux valgus deformity by attempted distal osteotomy. First ray hypermobility was unrecognized in the initial surgery and corrected by a Lapidus fusion incorporating intermetatarsal base fixation as well

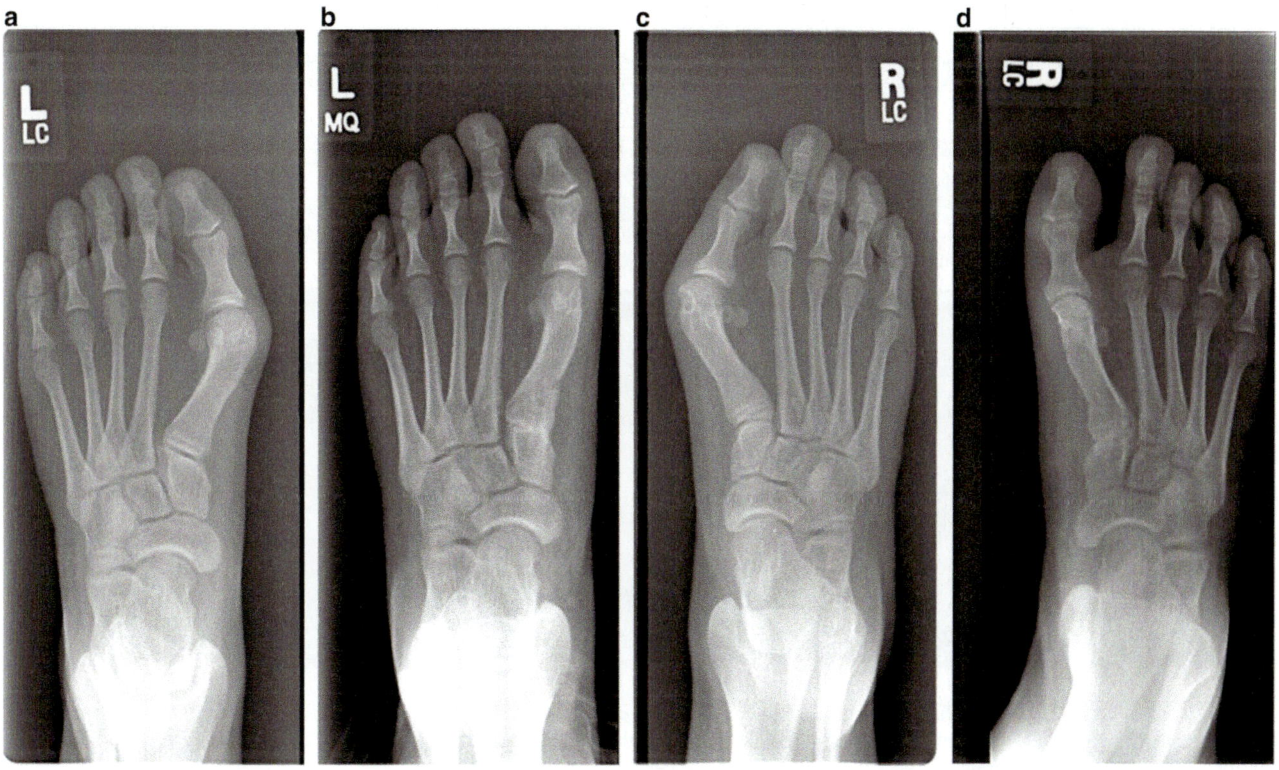

Fig. 12.13 (**a**) Juvenile hallux valgus surgery via poor surgical selection of a distal osteotomy and unrecognized first ray hypermobility of the first tmt joint. (**b**) Correction by revisional surgery and a Lapidus fusion with absorbable screw fixation. (**c**, **d**) The contralateral foot of the same patient with the same presentation and revisional correction via Lapidus fusion with absorbable fixation and distal Reverdin osteotomy

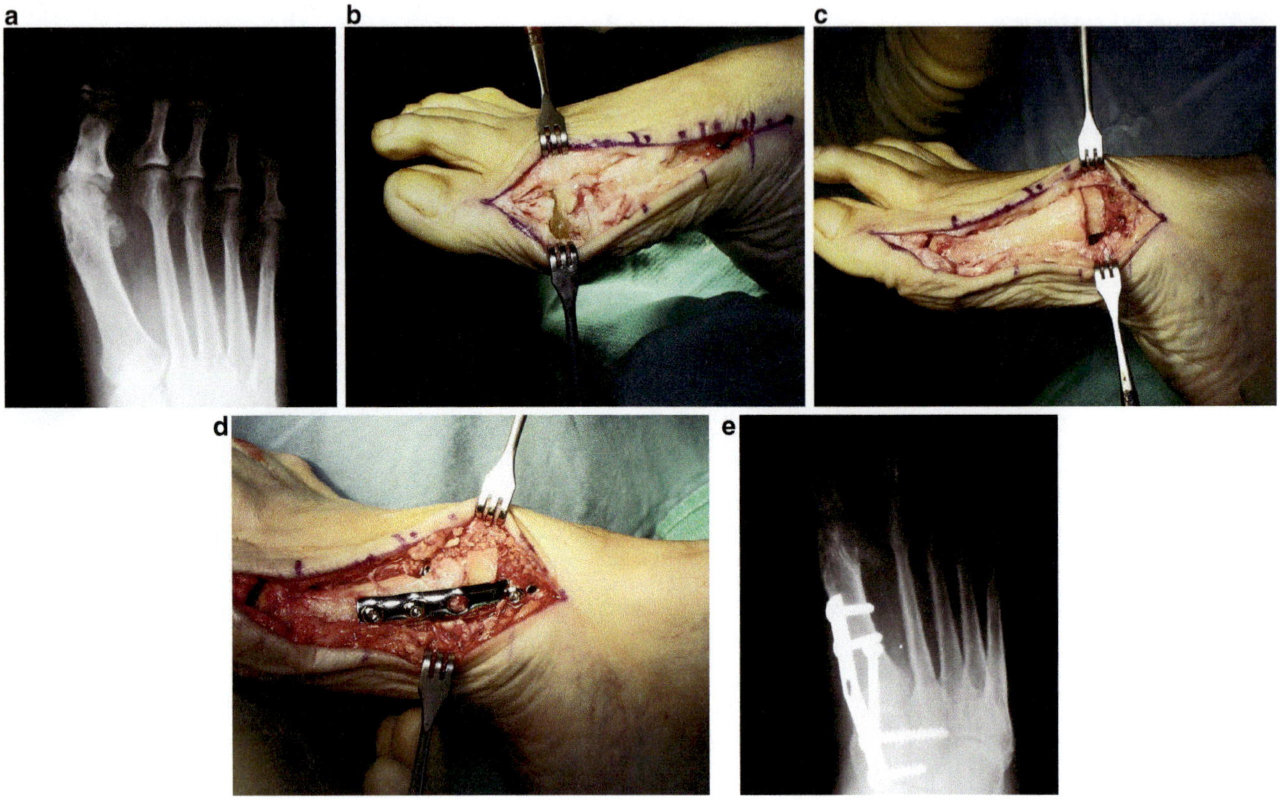

Fig. 12.14 (**a**) Case courtesy of Michael McGlamry. Recurrent hallux valgus with untreated first ray hypermobility and use of a Silastic hemi-implant that cannot provide any structural alignment to the first mtp joint. (**b**) Intraoperative view of failed Silastic hemi-implant. (**c**) Interpositional bone block Lapidus fusion to gain length to the first ray and stabilize the medial column. (**d**) Interfragmentary and plate fixation of the first tmt joint. (**e**) Radiographic view of consolidation bone block Lapidus fusion with removal of Silastic implant and conversion to a Keller resectional arthroplasty of the first mtp joint

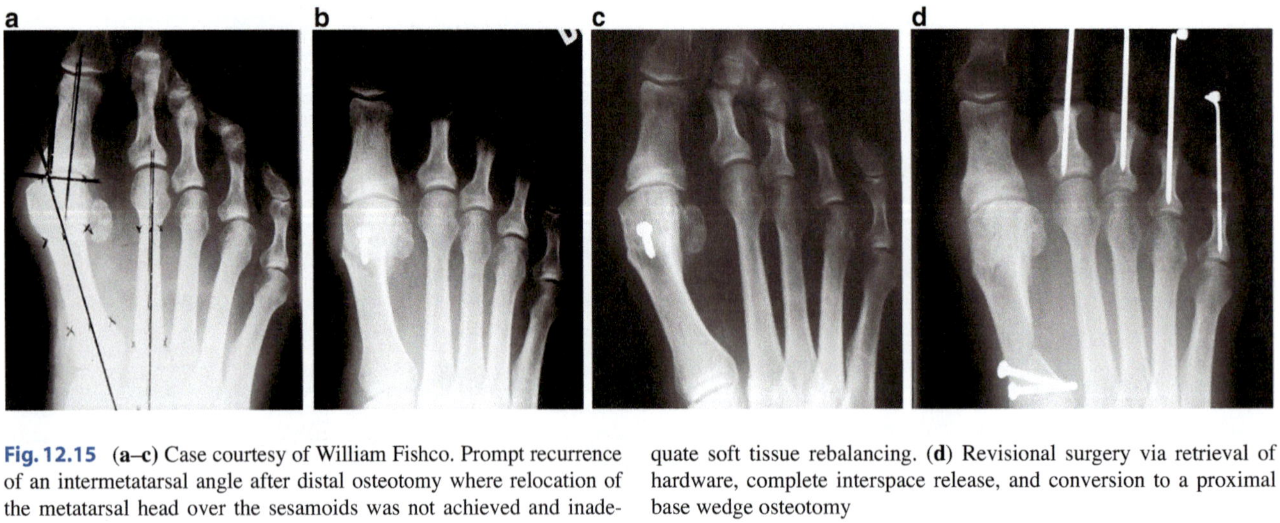

Fig. 12.15 (**a–c**) Case courtesy of William Fishco. Prompt recurrence of an intermetatarsal angle after distal osteotomy where relocation of the metatarsal head over the sesamoids was not achieved and inadequate soft tissue rebalancing. (**d**) Revisional surgery via retrieval of hardware, complete interspace release, and conversion to a proximal base wedge osteotomy

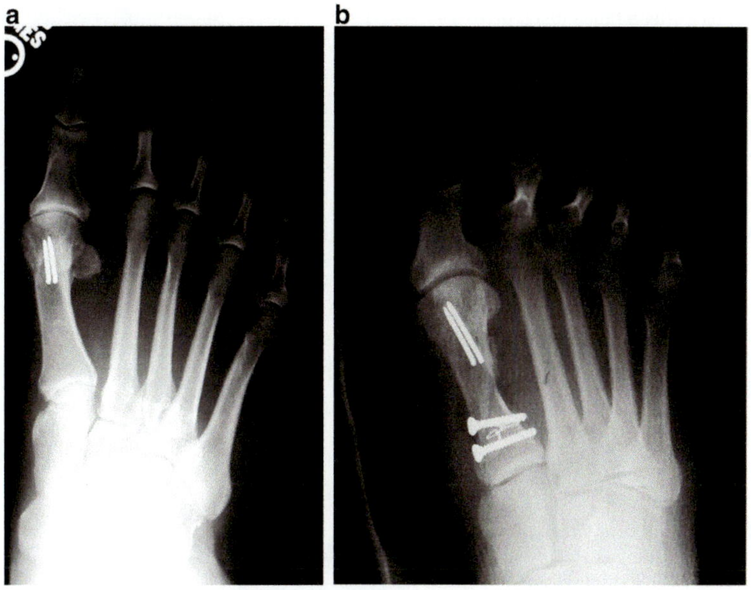

Fig. 12.16 (**a**, **b**) Case courtesy of Annette Filiatrault. Recurrent hallux valgus after distal osteotomy revised via a closing base wedge osteotomy where clinically it was not deemed that first ray insufficiency was clinically relevant

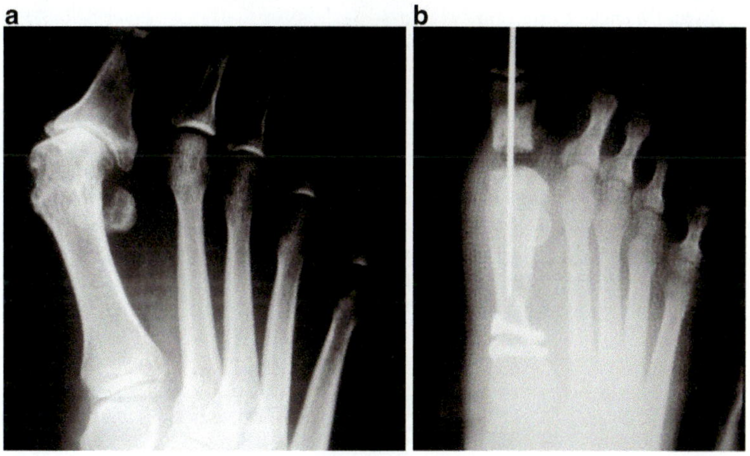

Fig. 12.17 (**a**, **b**) Recurrent hallux valgus from a previous distal metatarsal osteotomy. Although a first mtp joint fusion would have been a reasonable choice here, this case was addressed via resectional arthroplasty of the first mtp joint and closing base wedge osteotomy

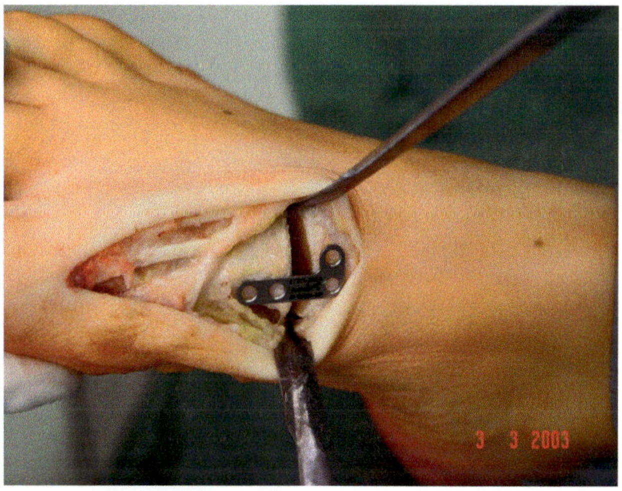

Fig. 12.18 An example of an opening wedge plate for basilar osteotomies that can be particularly helpful in revisional surgery and specifically in the case of a recurrent IM angle or previous first metatarsal osteotomy that has resulted in a short first ray

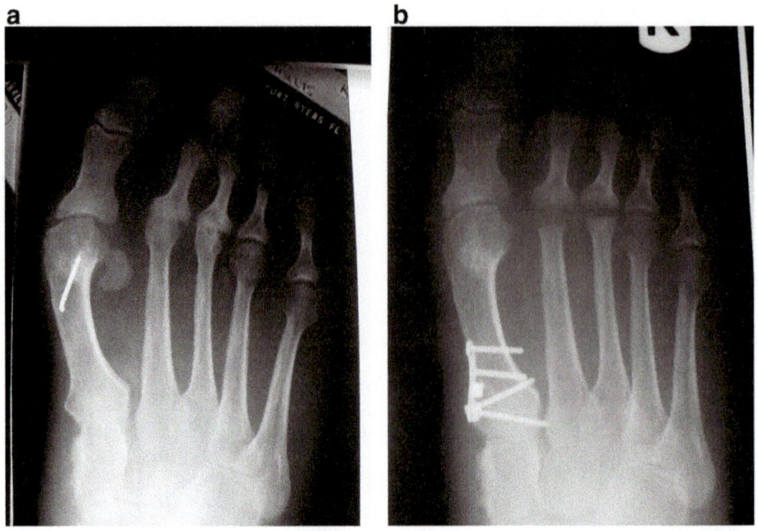

Fig. 12.19 (**a**, **b**) Case courtesy of Brad Castellano. Revisional surgery after a failed distal first metatarsal osteotomy via an opening wedge base osteotomy that allows for preservation of first metatarsal length and closure of the IM angle. Notice in this case ancillary procedures were required as well in the form of partial metatarsal head resections of rays 2 and 3

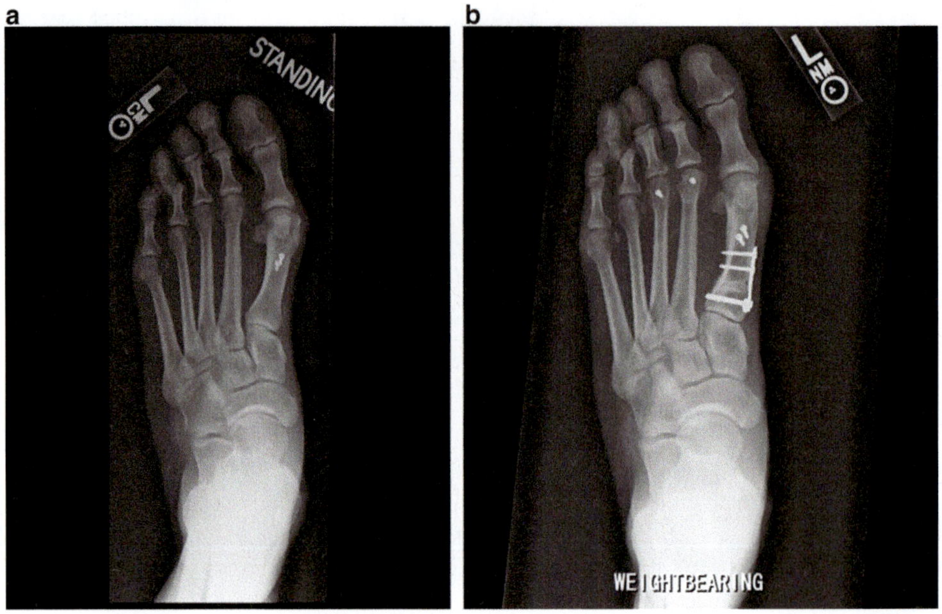

Fig. 12.20 (**a**, **b**) Case courtesy of David Granger. Recurrent hallux valgus after a distal osteotomy that left an incongruous first mtp joint and a persistent IM angle. Correction via an opening wedge proximal osteotomy that has clearly regained metatarsal length while closing the IM angle. Decompressive osteotomies of the second and third were also required. This case may have benefited from a phalangeal osteotomy as well for more rectus alignment of the hallux

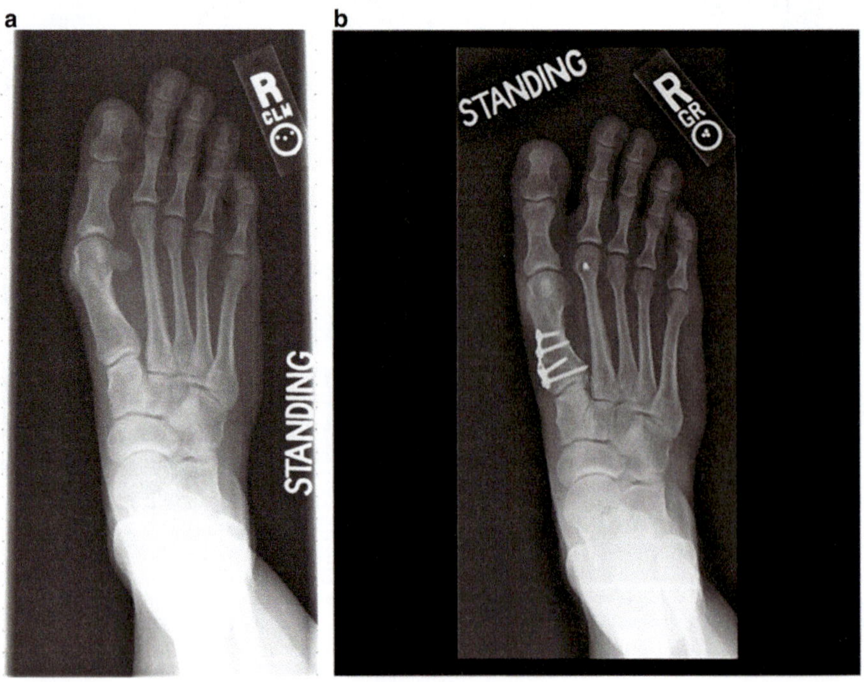

Fig. 12.21 (**a**, **b**) Case courtesy of David Granger. Recurrent deformity after a distal first metatarsal osteotomy revised via a proximal opening wedge osteotomy and shortening osteotomy of the second ray

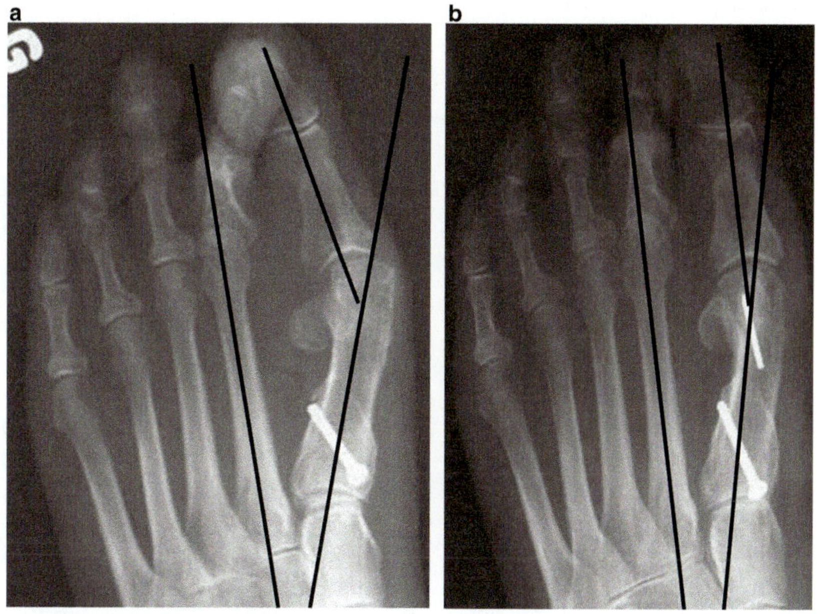

Fig. 12.22 (**a**, **b**) Case courtesy of Craig Camasta. Recurrent deformity after a proximal osteotomy. Inadequate soft tissue release was performed initially, and there was sufficient flexibility of the intermetatarsal angle to allow revision via a more complete soft tissue release and distal osteotomy. This is a much less common option but demonstrates the importance of continued intraoperative assessment and evaluation of the reducibility of the deformity after the soft tissue release

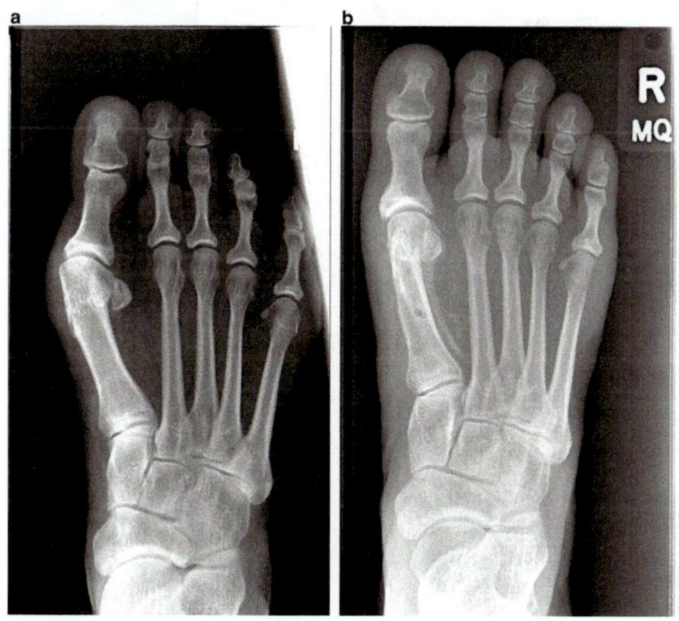

Fig. 12.23 (**a**, **b**) Recurrent hallux valgus after simple exostectomy and no attempt to reduce the IM angle. A full-length scarf osteotomy with absorbable fixation was utilized and also swiveled proximally to allow for distal articular set correction of the PASA deformity. The scarf diaphyseal cut allows for translation laterally of the first ray and realignment over the intrinsic musculature of the medial column

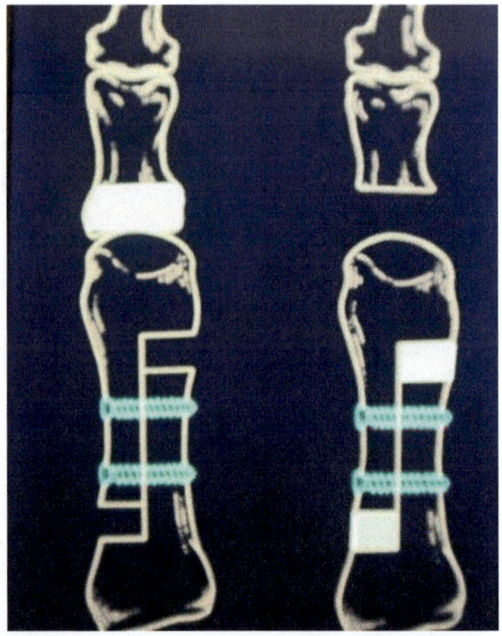

Fig. 12.24 The scarf cut may be manipulated to allow for lengthening of the first ray as well

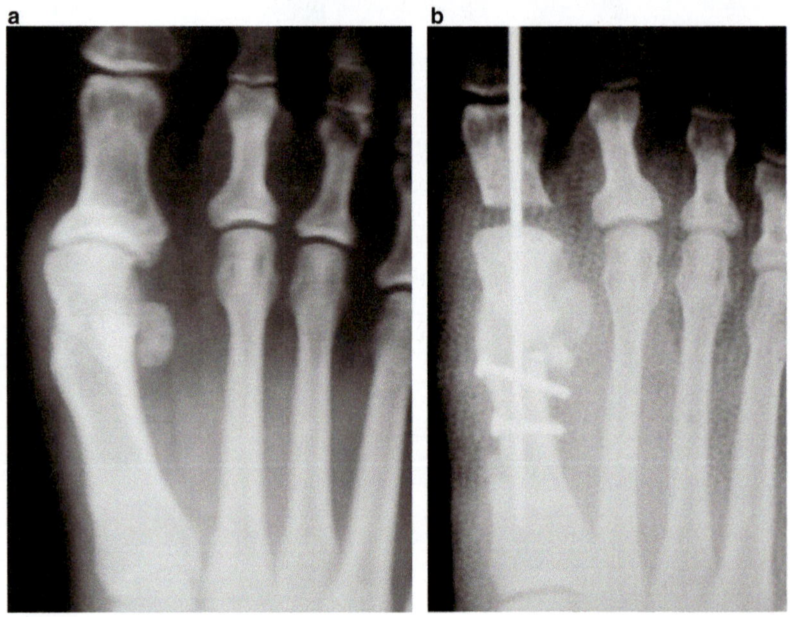

Fig. 12.25 (**a**, **b**) By removing a section of bone from the mid-diaphyseal region, recurrent IM angle may be reduced while simultaneously lengthening the first ray. Here the residual osseous deformity in the proximal phalanx from previous osteotomy and the compressive effect of lengthening of the first ray are addressed via Keller resectional arthroplasty

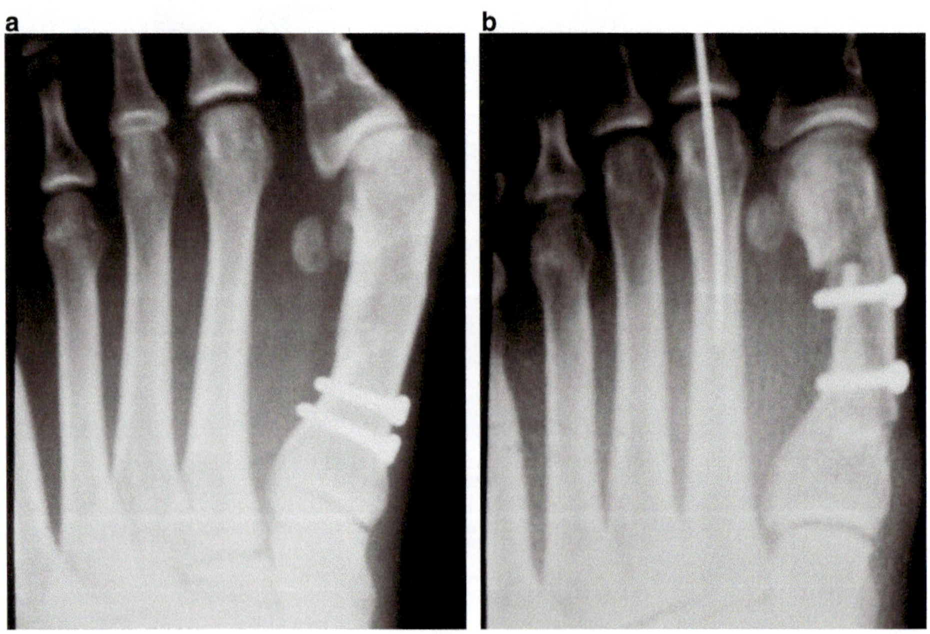

Fig. 12.26 (**a**, **b**) In a similar fashion to case 25, here a midshaft manipulation of the scarf osteotomy is used to reduce the IM angle and plantarflex the first ray. No Keller resectional arthroplasty was required

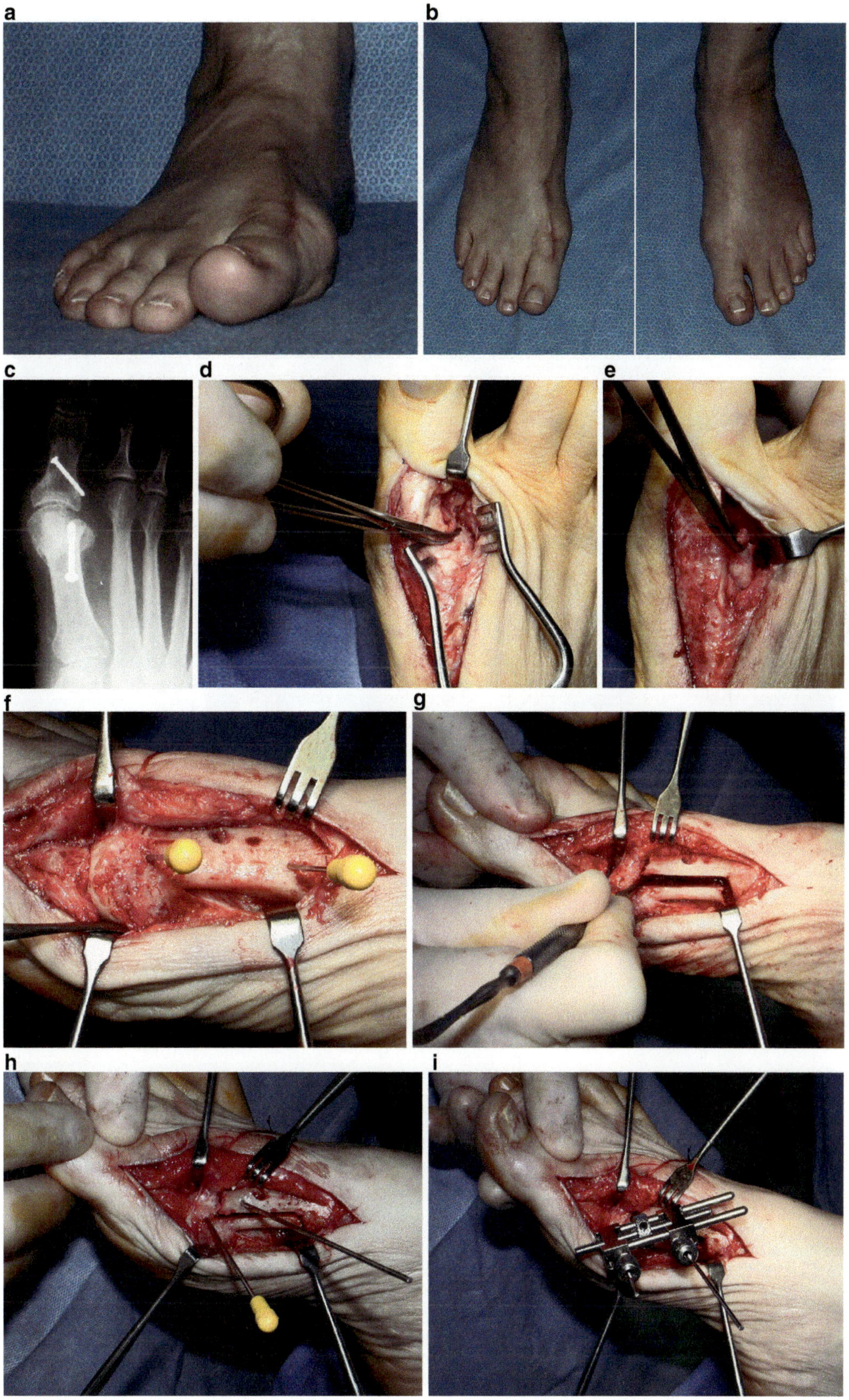

Fig. 12.27 (**a, b**) Case courtesy of John Ruch. Clinical photos of recurrent hallux valgus and residual IM angle increase in spite of previous surgery. (**c**) Residual IM increase secondary to swiveling of the capital osteotomy. (**d, e**) The first step in revising this case was a complete identification and release of the abductor tendon. (**f**) Planning with axis guides for a midshaft scarf osteotomy. (**g**) The scarf osteotomy is cut

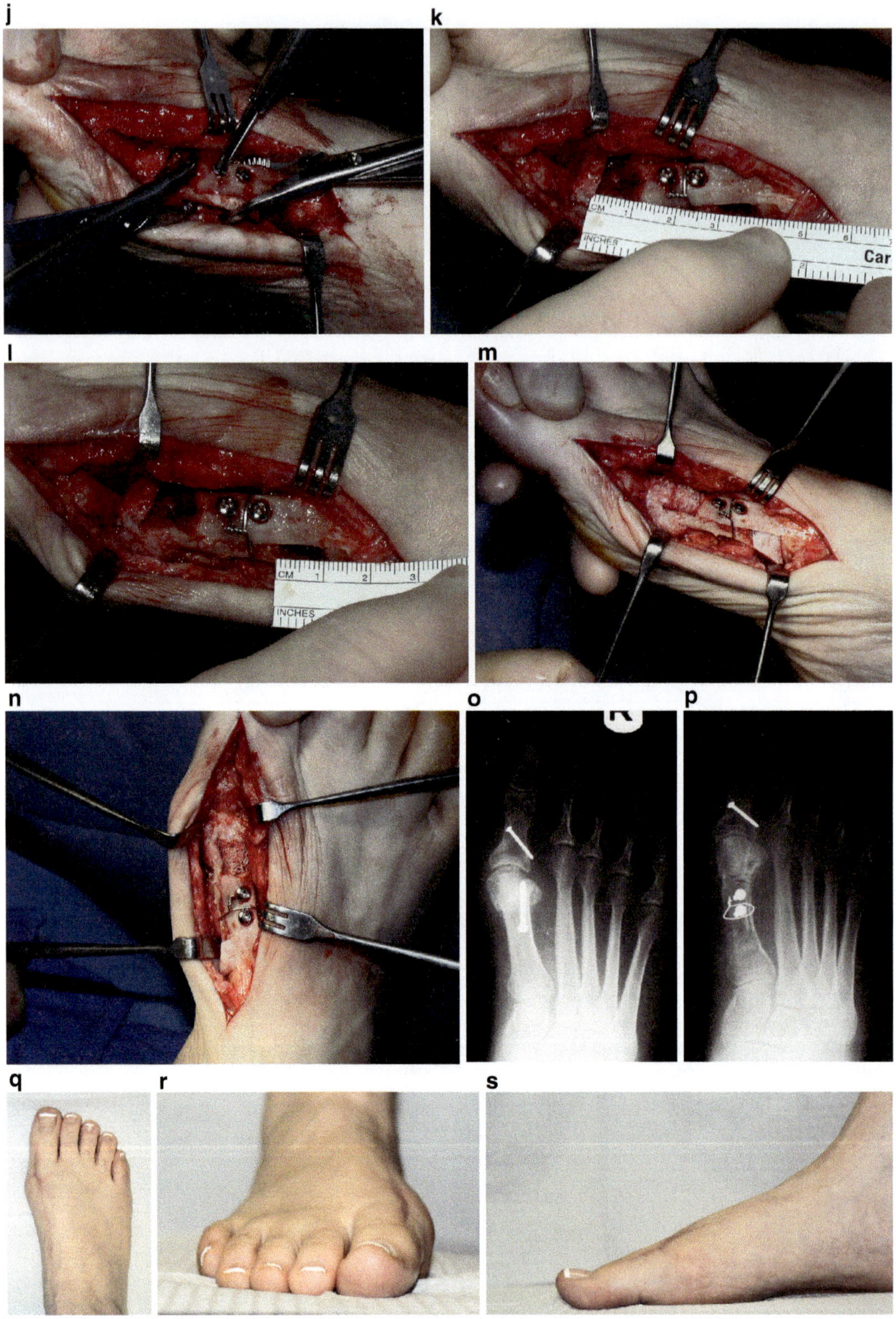

Fig. 12.27 (continued) and initial manipulation and distraction begun. (**h**, **i**) The pins are placed for a mini distractor to assist in manipulations of the scarf osteotomy to allow for reduction of the residual IM angle as well as lengthening of the first ray. (**j**) The osteotomy is clamped and fixated with standard AO technique. (**k**, **l**) Careful measurements are taken determining the amount of interpositional bone graft required to fill the gaps created by the lengthening. (**m**, **n**) Bone graft in place both proximally and distally on AP and lateral views. (**o**, **p**) Preoperative X-rays with comparison to postoperative X-rays after consolidation of the bone graft. (**q–s**) Multiple clinical pictures at the 7 month mark postoperatively

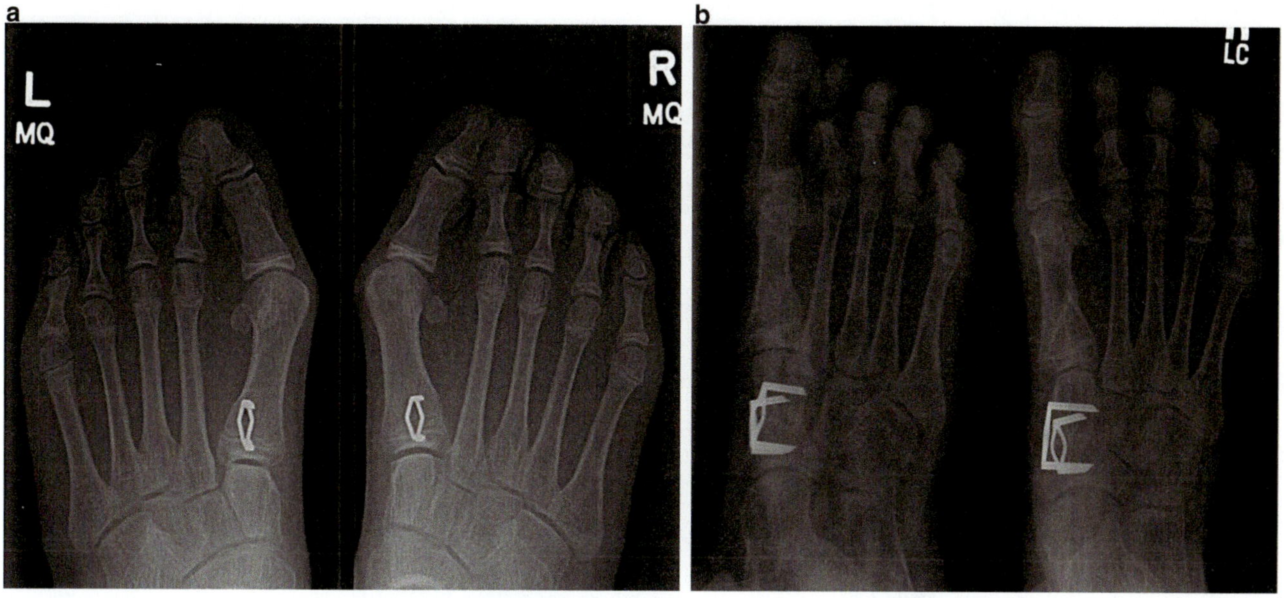

Fig. 12.28 (**a**) Failed epiphysiodesis in a juvenile patient with the resultant residual/recurrent hallux valgus deformity. (**b**) Complete revision of the failed case with attention to an unstable midfoot as a primary deforming force that was not addressed during the initial surgery. A navicular cuneiform fusion was performed with a closing base wedge osteotomy and distal Reverdin capital osteotomy

motion of the joint can feel similar to a soft tissue limitation, and yet an appropriate radiograph will reveal the deformity is osseous. This is one of the preferences for the scarf osteotomy by one author as PASA corrections and swiveling are much easier than with chevron-type cuts. The thoroughness of the lateral soft tissue release including the lateral head of flexor halluces brevis is very important, but PASA must be corrected simultaneously. Fibular sesamoidectomy is considered more readily in revisional surgery as well and allows the surgeon to more easily gauge the digital correction of the hallux abductus when performing osteotomy work. Lastly, the use of fluoroscopy is emphasized as critical during revisional surgery and can be misleading. It is not unusual for the foot to be supinated during fluoroscopy shots and be misleading as to the actual correction of the IM angle.

Recurrent hallux valgus deformities require, both in their evaluation and considerations for correction via revisional surgery, a sensible, practical, and empathic mixture of prudence, surgical skill and experience, and attention to detail.

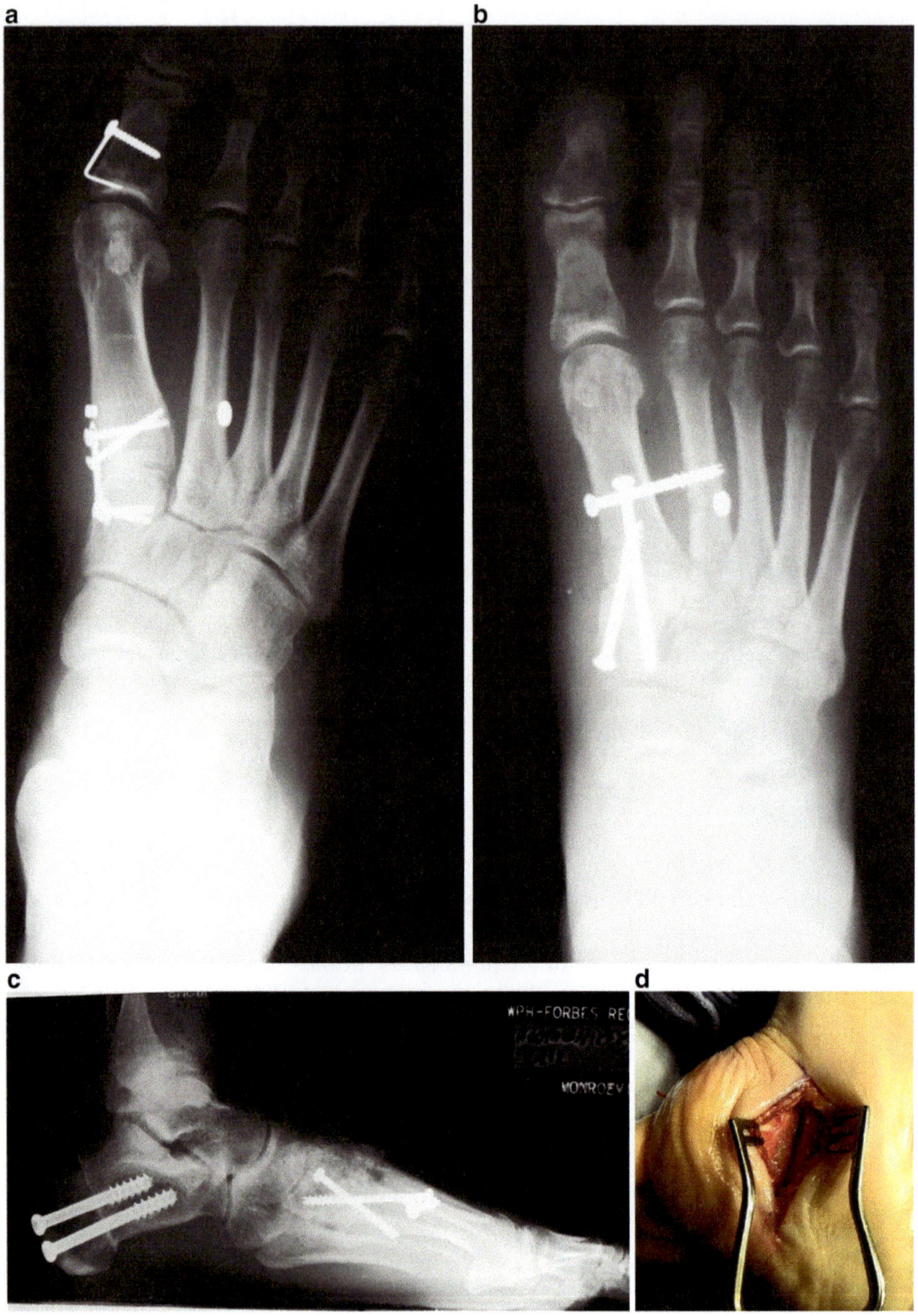

Fig. 12.29 (**a**) Case courtesy of Alan Catanzariti. Recurrent hallux valgus with attempt at Lapidus fusion and proximal endobutton technique that was insufficient to control the deforming forces of the hindfoot. (**b–d**) Revisional Lapidus fusion with fixation between the bases of the metatarsals and correction of the unstable hindfoot pronatory forces via medial displacement calcaneal osteotomy

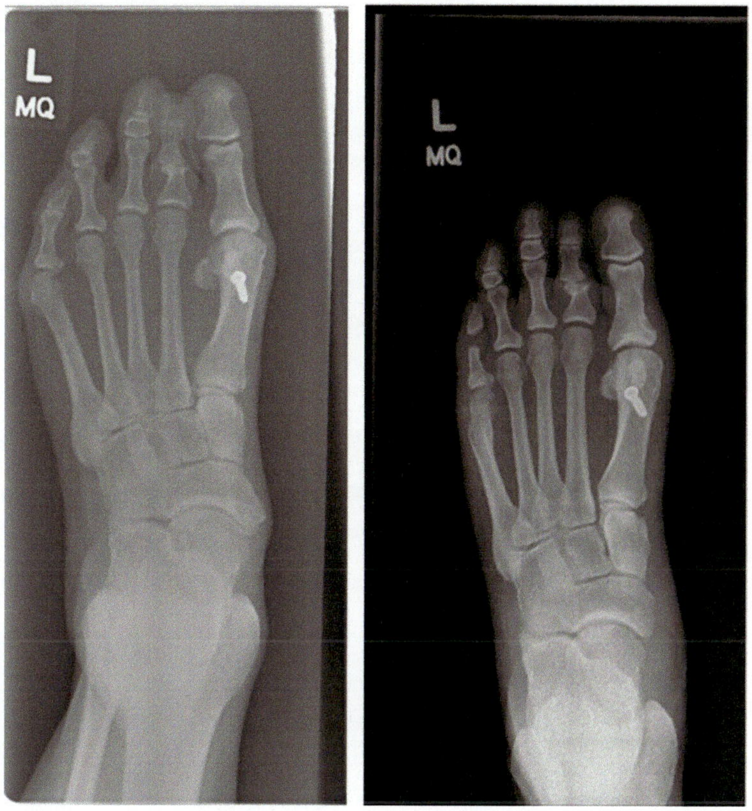

Fig. 12.30 (**a**, **b**) In the case, the patient's specific complaint was pressure between the first and second toe, and she had learned to live with the resultant recurrent prominence of the bunion. By focusing squarely on the patient's chief complaint, this case was satisfactorily resolved by a simple Akin osteotomy fixed with absorbable pins. The b photo is 3 years postoperative. In this case the forefoot was narrowed sufficiently by the performance of a fifth metatarsal osteotomy for tailor bunion correction and was accepting of her residual prominence of the first metatarsal head, and therefore it was not addressed

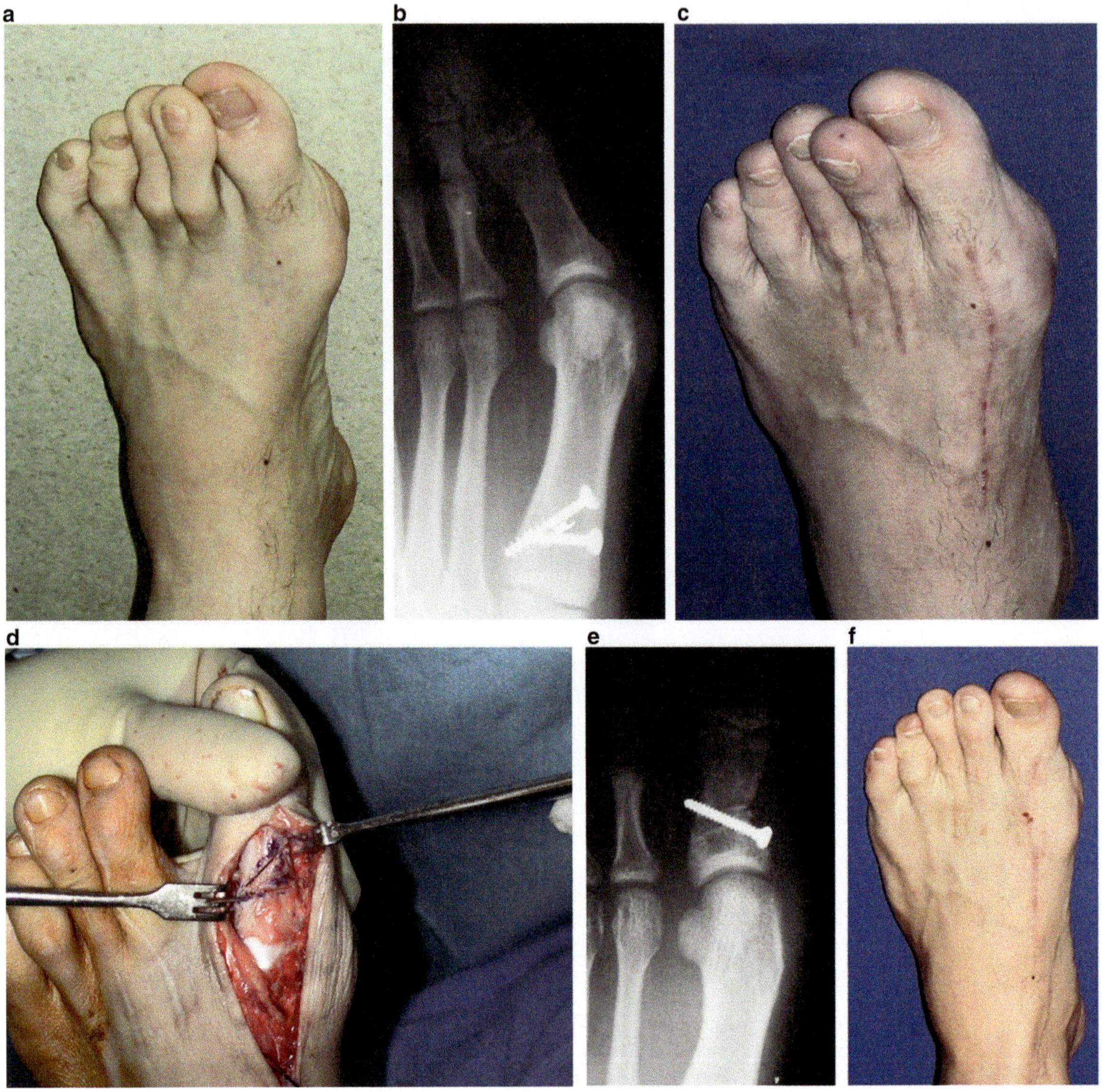

Fig. 12.31 (**a–c**) Case courtesy of Molly Judge. (**a**) Recurrent hallux valgus after base wedge osteotomy. Note the flexor power on the adjacent toes. (**b**) Radiograph of excellent IM angle correction although the patient still has **c** substantial hallux abductus. (**d–f**) The performance of an Akin osteotomy and the clinical photo 2 years later. In this case specific attention was paid to the patient's chief complaint of the deviation of the great toe due in part to its unnaturally length. This also allowed for the avoidance of a first metatarsal osteotomy on a well-aligned and reduced IM angle and a faster rehab and resolution of the real concern

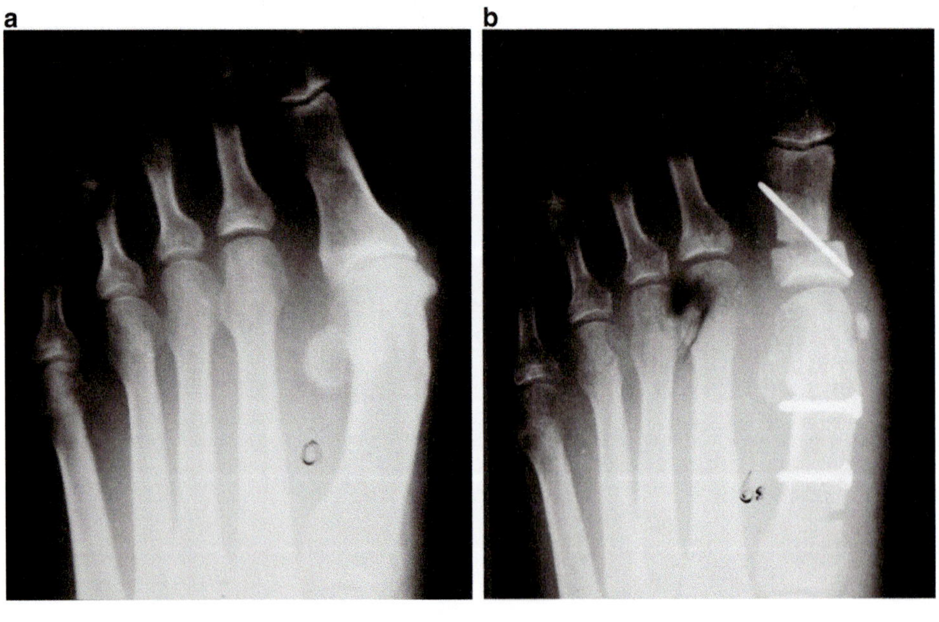

Fig. 12.32 (**a**, **b**) This recurrent deformity was corrected with a shortening scarf osteotomy and a Regnauld decompressive proximal phalangeal osteotomy. This patient was not interested in a first mtp joint fusion which also would have been a viable option

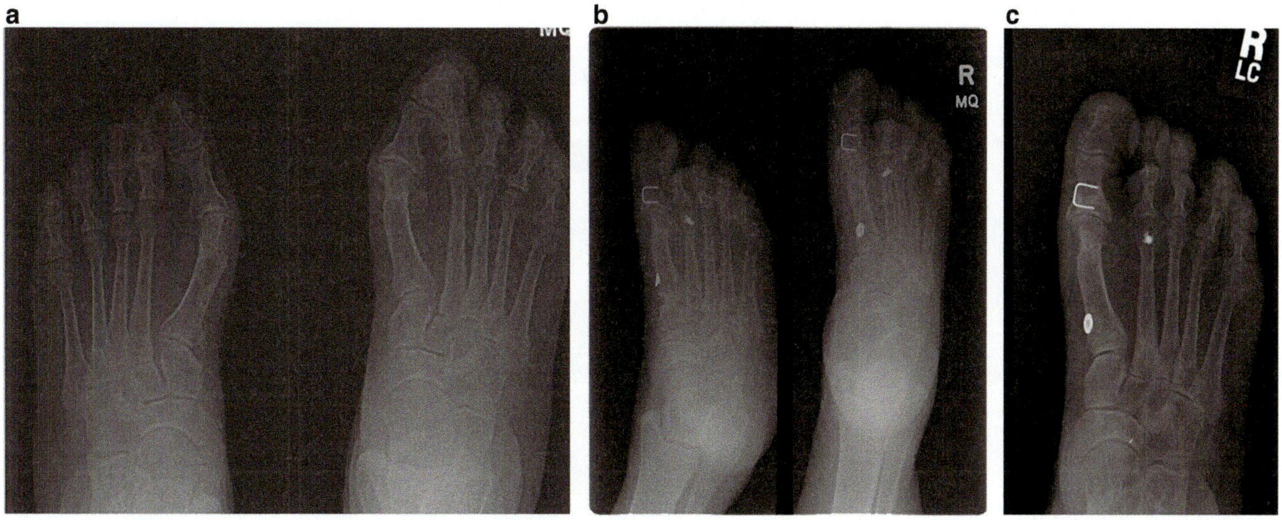

Fig. 12.33 (**a**) Recurrent hallux valgus deformity with severe staking of the metatarsal heads. There is little bone to work with essentially eliminating the possibility of a distal metatarsal osteotomy. (**b**, **c**) This patient was not a candidate for any non-weightbearing procedures nor a first mtp fusion and had low functional demand. She was a high-BMI individual. Her primary complaint was irritation between the first and second toes from the severe hallux abductus. An effective and lasting correction, c, which is 3 years post-op, was achieved via proximal endobutton repositional correction combined with an Akin and a second metatarsal decompressive osteotomy

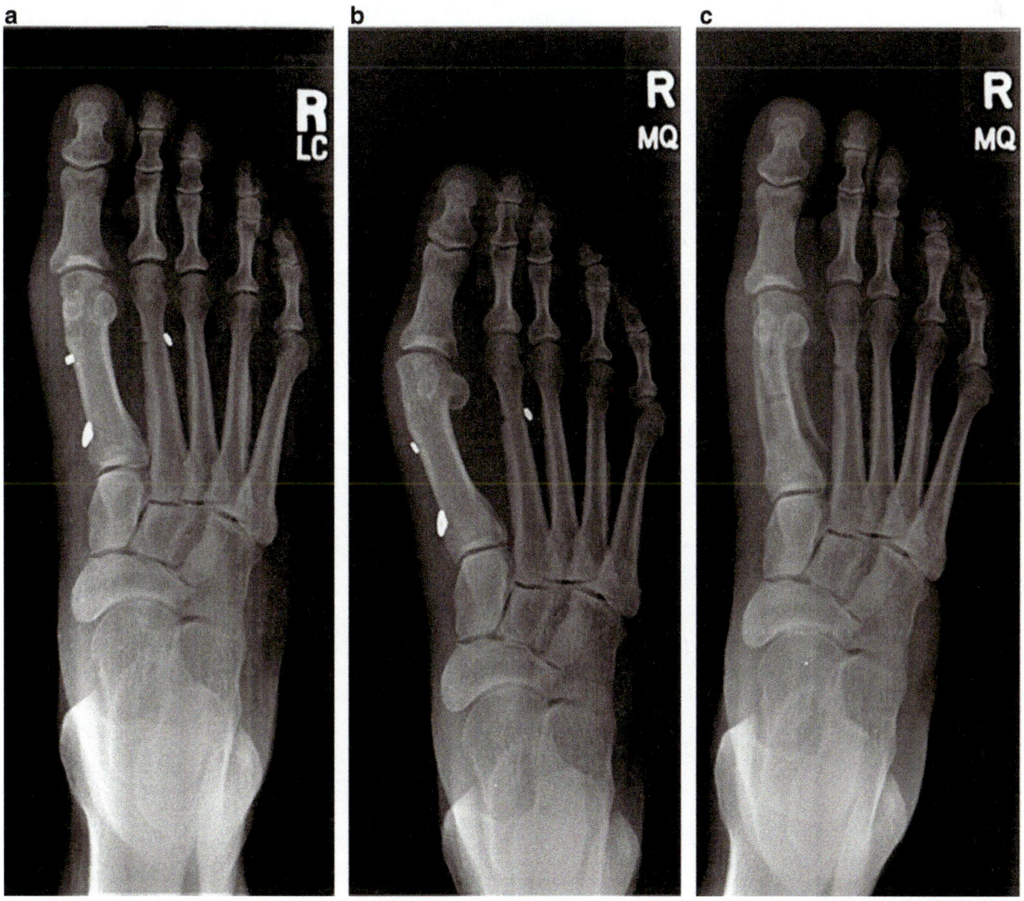

Fig. 12.34 (**a–c**) Failure and recurrence of the intermetatarsal angle after a double row suture and endobutton repair where the suture broke. The patient was highly accepting of the revisional correction via scarf osteotomy as no osteotomy had been performed on the first ray prior as well as the original surgeon did the revisional surgery as well. Strong patient-doctor communication and confidence can have a profound effect on procedural selection

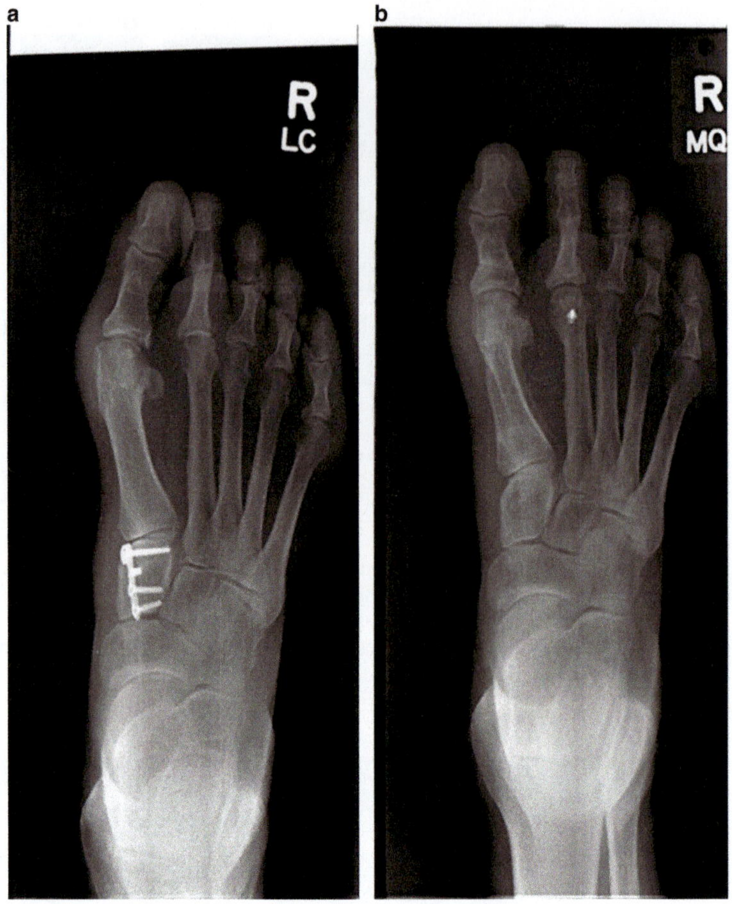

Fig. 12.35 (**a**, **b**) This patient had a recurrence of her hallux valgus deformity after an attempt at distal McBride and opening medial wedge osteotomy of the medial cuneiform. Similar to the case 34, this patient was highly amenable to reoperation which included a scarf osteotomy of the first ray, proximal phalangeal osteotomy, and decompressive Weil osteotomy of the second metatarsal. Again, additional procedures within the forefoot are frequently required in revisional hallux valgus surgery. In this case the patient was unhappy with the previous surgeon and therefore more agreeable to the additionally required procedures

References

1. Judge M. Complications in hallux abducto valgus surgery (excluding hallux varus). In: McGlamry's comprehensive textbook of foot and ankle surgery. 4th ed. Wolters Kluwer/Lippincott Williams & Wilkins; 2013.
2. Lyons MC, et al. Recurrent hallux valgus: treatment considerations. The Podiatry Institute; 2009. Chapter 26

Complications of First Metatarsophalangeal Joint Arthrodesis

13

Mark H. Hofbauer and Joshua D. Thun

First metatarsophalangeal joint (MTPJ) arthrodesis has long been established as an effective surgical procedure for treatment of many different pathologies. These commonly include severe hallux valgus, chronic joint instability, neuromuscular disease, avascular necrosis, and arthritic conditions such as hallux rigidus, post-traumatic osteoarthritis, infective arthritis, gouty arthritis, and rheumatoid arthritis [1–25]. First MTPJ arthrodesis has also been indicated for failed procedures of the first ray including previous hallux valgus osteotomies, hallux varus deformity, and salvage of replacement and resectional arthroplasties [20, 26–38]. As with any surgical procedure, complications of first MTPJ arthrodesis may arise postoperatively, which may include infection, wound dehiscence, osteomyelitis, ischemic limb, nerve entrapment hematoma, seroma, failed hardware, delayed union, nonunion, malunion, and hallux interphalangeal joint (HIPJ) arthritis [4, 5, 13, 14, 19, 39–44]. Amputation or loss of limb may be a catastrophic sequelae as a result of one of the aforementioned complications.

Complications can often be avoided with thorough history and physical exam, proper screening of surgical candidates, and thoughtful surgical planning. Although most postoperative complications of the first MTPJ are considered mild to moderate, management can often be challenging for the surgeon. The intent of this chapter is to provide helpful insight for the prevention and management of first MTPJ arthrodesis complications, namely malunion and nonunion.

Preventing first MTPJ arthrodesis complications involves taking the necessary steps to reduce potential risk in obtaining a satisfactory outcome for the patient. There are two principles in avoiding risk. The first principle is to minimize risk exposure. One must recognize the patient-dependent risk factors and select only those patients who have factors favorable for a successful outcome. The second principle is to embrace risk in accordance with one's capacity and skill level as a surgeon. He or she must adhere to procedural indications and not veer from them. Complications tend to occur when risk exposure does not match risk capacity.

Evaluating risk factors that lead to postoperative first MTPJ arthrodesis complications breaks down into two categories: patient-dependent risk factors and surgeon-dependent risk factors. As complications arise, we tend to blame the patient-dependent factors. It is, however, the surgeon's responsibility to identify the patient-dependent risk factors when electing to operate on an individual. It is also the surgeon's responsibility to critically evaluate the surgeon-dependent risk factors that may have contributed to a complication. This may illuminate a flaw of the surgeon in question.

There are different categories of patient-dependent risk factors. The systemic dependent risk factors include obesity, diabetes, rheumatoid arthritis, vascular disease, neuromuscular disease, and nutritional deficiencies. The social patient-dependent risk factors include smoking, alcohol, and illicit drug use. The educational level, hygiene, home support network, job requirements, and socioeconomic status of patients can also be factors that influence surgical success. One may also consider a patient's expectations as a patient-dependent risk factor. If the patient and surgeon's expectations do not coincide, then a complication is probable.

A major focus of this chapter will be the surgeon-dependent risk factors that lead to complications. The procedure should be based on the patient's risk capacity and the surgeon's capacity level. The procedural execution should match the surgeon's risk capacity. Critical decision making in the preoperative, intraoperative, and/or postoperative course can ultimately lead to a negative outcome. It is the author's belief that problems begin to develop more commonly with poor decisions made during the preoperative and intraoperative settings.

M.H. Hofbauer (✉) • J.D. Thun
Monongahela Valley Hospital,
1163 Country Club Road, Monongahela, PA 15063, USA
e-mail: hofdude30@gmail.com

M.S. Lee, J.P. Grossman (eds.), *Complications in Foot and Ankle Surgery*, DOI 10.1007/978-3-319-53686-6_13

Malunion

A malaligned first MTPJ arthrodesis and its sequelae can be more frustrating for the surgeon and patient than the preoperative pathology. In our experience, a malunion occurs due to one of two reasons: poor surgical execution or the patient's inability to comply with postoperative protocol. Positioning of the hallux is critical to obtain optimal shoe fit and foot function. A malunion can occur in one or more combinations of the sagittal, frontal, and transverse planes (Fig. 13.1). Sagittal plane malalignment can be either in a plantar or dorsiflexed position. Excessive dorsiflexion is poorly tolerated by the patient due to increased plantar pressure at the MTPJ, sesamoiditis, pain over the dorsal HIPJ, pain with shoegear, and HIPJ contracture with resultant arthritis (Fig. 13.2) [45–48]. Biomechanically, lack of hallux purchase requires excessive pronation at the subtalar joint which leads to internal rotation of the leg, causing patellar malalignment and medial knee pain.

A plantar flexed arthrodesis can place increased pressures on the plantar hallux during step-off in gait resulting in plantar hallux ulceration, difficulty with step-off during ambulation, and increases stress at the HIPJ possibly leading to HIPJ degenerative changes (Fig. 13.3) [45, 47, 48]. It is not uncommon for the patient to experience lesser metatarsal pain, in particular the fifth metatarsal, caused by compensatory forefoot varus. The plantar flexed fusion leads to dysfunctional gait patterns including functional equinus, lack of dorsiflexion at the ankle during push-off, and resultant genu recurvatum.

Frontal plane rotation of the hallux can leave a patient with painful medial or lateral callosities as well as painful nail deformities. Transverse abduction or "valgus" malunion of the joint can crowd the lesser digits, cause painful interdigital rubbing, and even over or underlapping of the hallux with the second toe. Failure to recognize hallux interphalangeus when positioning interoperatively may lead to a painful and cosmetically unsatisfactory result with abutment against the medial second toe (Fig. 13.4). In transverse adduction or "varus" malunion, the most common complaint

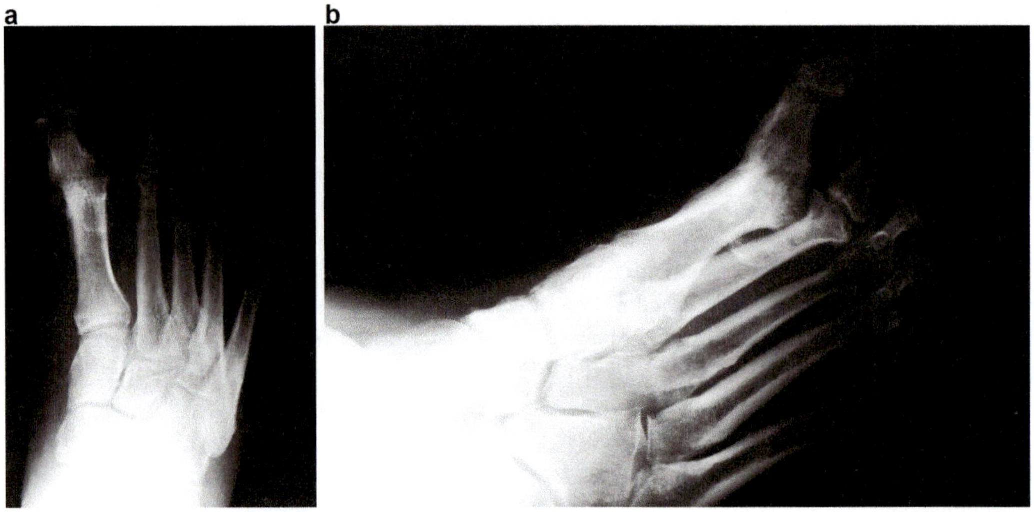

Fig. 13.1 (**a**, **b**) Radiographs of multi-planar nonunion

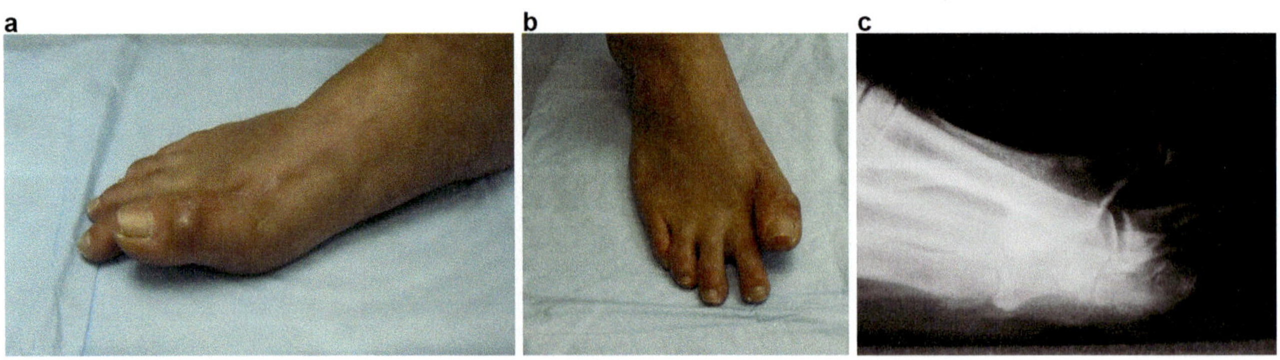

Fig. 13.2 (**a**, **b**) Clinical example of a dorsiflexed malunion. (**c**) Lateral radiograph of a dorsiflexed malunion

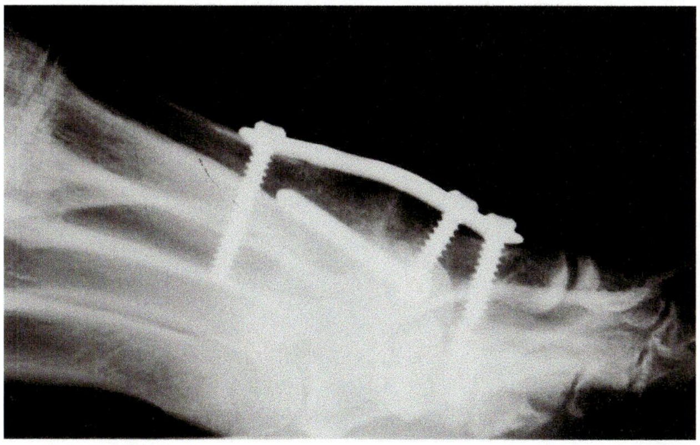

Fig. 13.3 Lateral radiograph of a symptomatic plantarflexed malunion

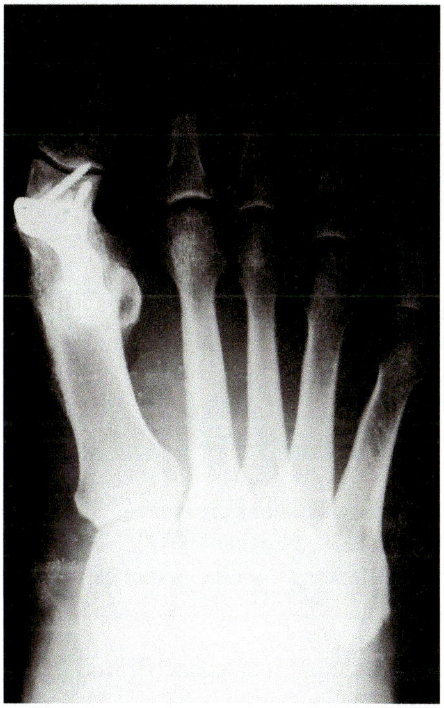

Fig. 13.4 Radiograph demonstrating symptomatic malunion with unaddressed interphalangeus

is fitting into shoegear, with irritation of the distal and medial portions of the hallux.

Significant shortening of the first ray following attempted arthrodesis is, in the mind of the authors, a malunion complication, regardless of any associated planar deformity. Excessive shortening is almost always associated with lack of hallux purchase, an abnormal push-off gait, abnormal shoe fit, and lack of patient satisfaction secondary to cosmetic appearance.

Positioning of the hallux intraoperatively is the single most important factor in avoiding malunion. Unfortunately, many of the anatomic plating systems for first MTPJ fusion are designed with what we believe is an excessive amount of

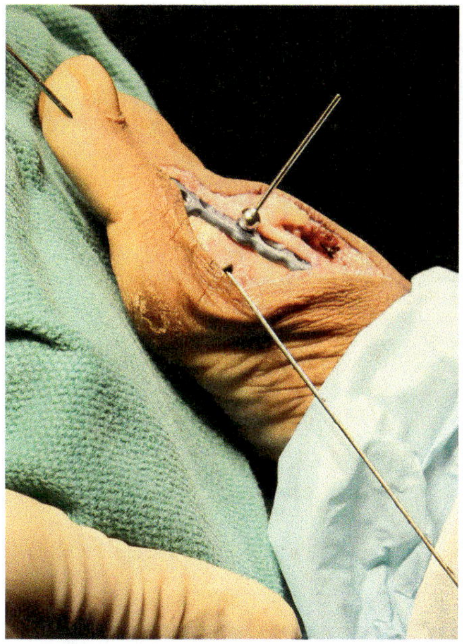

Fig. 13.5 Intraoperative maneuver simulating weight bearing, appropriate positioning of hallux

dorsiflexion. The resulting dorsiflexed malunion complication may not be detected until well into the postoperative course. There is a growing popularity among experienced surgeons today to utilize plating systems that have gone away from the 8–10 degrees of dorsiflexion to a more rectus position of 4–5 degrees. It has been suggested that the ideal position of the hallux is in 10–15 degrees of valgus and 15–30 degrees of dorsiflexion relative to the first metatarsal [1, 3, 4, 19, 28, 46, 47, 49–57]. Clinical dorsiflexion has also been recommended to be less than 15 degrees relative to the weight bearing surface (Fig. 13.5) [47, 58]. However, with these reported angles, patient function and specific foot type are not taken into account. In a study of 39 first MTPJ fusions, Aas et al. [45] measured arthrodesis positions radiographically and clinically along with the distribution of pressure under the foot using insoles with pressure sensors. While an increase in local pressure was observed under the pulp of the great toe in all patients, clinical measurements of 10 degrees of plantar flexion to 15 degrees of extension revealed a weak correlation between position and clinical outcome. In the author's opinion, the hallux should be positioned parallel to the second toe in the transverse plane without any frontal plane rotation and light hallux purchase on the ground while weight bearing. The unrecognized complication when fusing the hallux off of the weight bearing surface is that the fixed position of the sesamoids following arthrodesis elevates the entire first ray, leading to lack of hallux purchase and ultimately a painful HIPJ flexion contracture.

Treatment of HIPJ flexion contracture may require flexor hallucis longus tenotomy, HIPJ arthroplasty, or fusion. Treatment of a dorsiflexed HIPJ complication may require

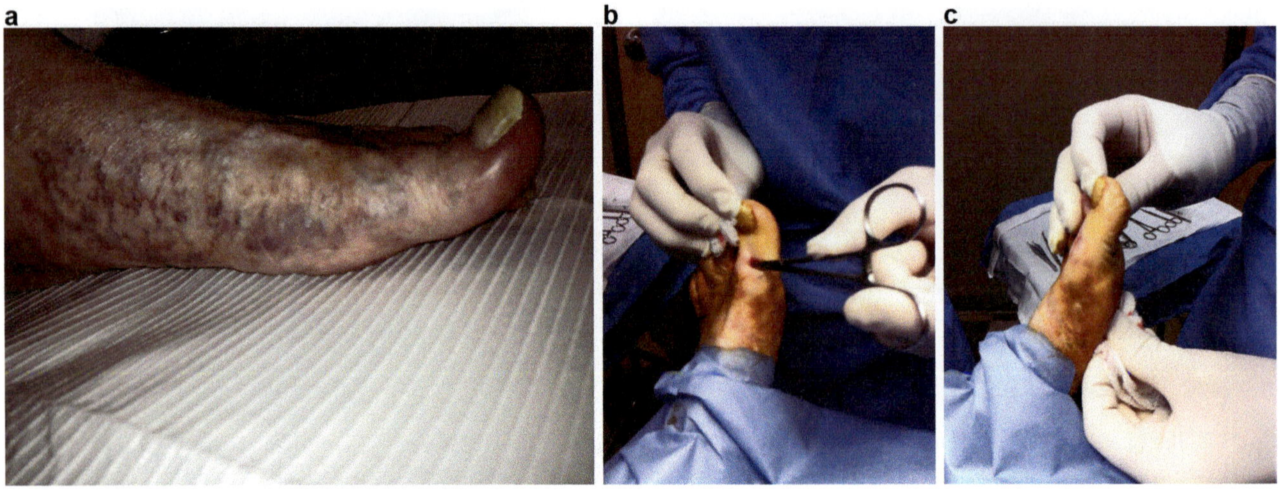

Fig. 13.6 (**a**) Clinical post first MTPJ arthrodesis with hallux extensus. (**b**, **c**) Intraoperative extensor hallucis longus tenotomy

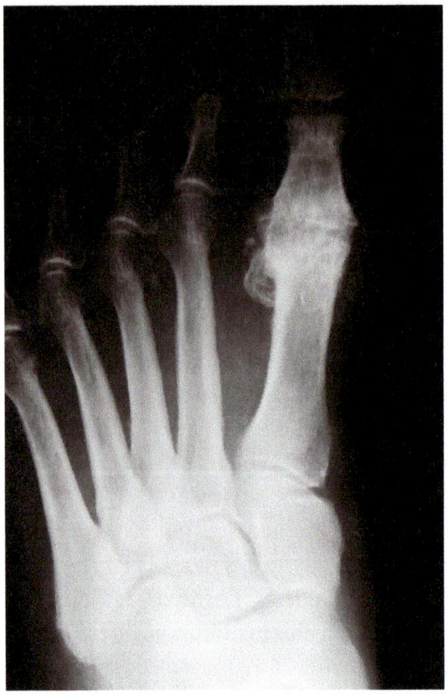

Fig. 13.7 Radiograph demonstrating HIPJ arthroplasty with first MTPJ arthrodesis

extensor hallucis longus tenotomy, HIPJ arthroplasty, or fusion (Figs. 13.6 and 13.7). Patient variants of first metatarsal declination angle should discourage the surgeon from basing their fusion off of radiographic angles, but rather clinical positioning of the hallux. When utilizing minimal fixation constructs for attempted fusion, such as crossing K-wires, staples, or cannulated screws, patient noncompliance, specifically early weight bearing, may contribute to malunion as well.

Conservative treatment for a malunion should include accommodative shoegear, orthotics, toe spacers, and routine callus care (Fig. 13.8). When conservative measures fail, surgical intervention should be considered. In a systematic review, Roukis [14] reported a 6.1% (39 of 640) malunion rate with dorsal malalignment accounting for a majority 87.1% and valgus malunion occurring in the remaining instances. No mention was made as to the number of symptomatic malunions or the need for revision.

Revisional first MTPJ arthrodesis secondary to malunion is scarcely reported and researched. Sagittal plane malunions can be revised utilizing a plantar wedge osteotomy, crescentic osteotomy [59], dorsal opening wedge osteotomy [48], or trapezoid osteotomy. All of these techniques are extremely technical and require thoughtful surgical consideration. Quite often, these malunions are multi-planar in nature.

A truly dorsiflexed malunion will require a plantarly based wedge osteotomy from a medial to lateral approach, with care to maintain a dorsal hinge. The surgeon should begin with minimal wedge resection to prevent excessive plantarflexion. Reciprocal planning will allow for final positioning of the hallux. Hesitation during execution of the osteotomy may lead to thermal necrosis of an already high-risk fusion site, leading to further complication.

Multi-planar malunions often require a through-and-through osteotomy to achieve correct anatomical positioning. Execution of this osteotomy requires thoughtful planning as to prevent excessive shortening of the toe.

However, rare, bone grafting may be necessary in a malunion complication where the initial attempt at fusion was performed via saw resection with residual shortening of the first ray where the patient is left with a multi-planar residual hallux valgus deformity. In such cases, bone grafting may be required to (1) restore length, (2) re-establish anatomical alignment, and (3) to accommodate secure plate fixation when minimal proximal phalanx is available. The advantages of utilizing a structural bone graft for restoring length of the first ray will be discussed later in this chapter. When re-establishing first ray length in a patient with a

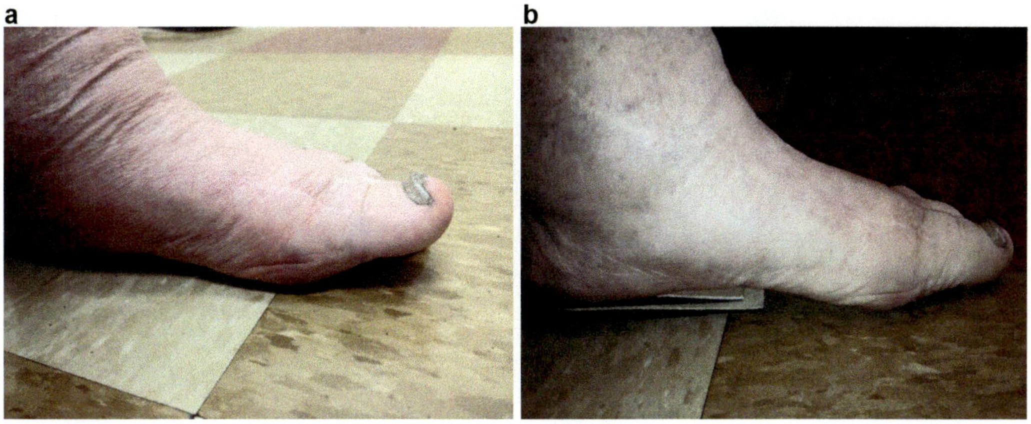

Fig. 13.8 (**a**, **b**) Conservative affect of heel lift for a dorsiflexed malunion of the first MTPJ

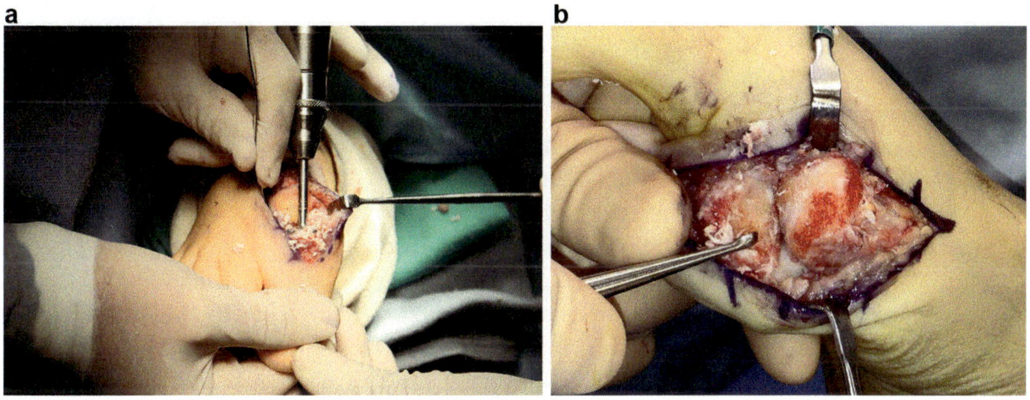

Fig. 13.9 (**a**) Joint preparation with conical reamers. (**b**) Joint preparation with curettage

long-standing malunion, adaptive soft tissue changes may lead to flexion or extensor contracture at the level of the HIPJ. Prophylactic soft tissue balancing and possibly HIPJ arthroplasty or fusion should be considered.

It goes without saying that a well-planned, secure fixation construct designed to prevent rotation and provide compression at the arthrodesis site is paramount in any revision.

Nonunion

Nonunion of a first MTPJ arthrodesis is a potential complication encountered postoperatively. While rates of nonunion have been documented between 0 and 23% [31–33, 60–62], the most commonly reported and accepted nonunion rate is approximately 10% [14, 19, 20, 29, 30, 46, 54, 58, 63–72]. With advancements in surgical technique and fixation devises, the rate of nonunion has decreased [14]. In a systematic review performed by Roukis [14], 2818 first MTPJ arthrodesis procedures were evaluated to determine if nonunion rates were different than the historical value of 10%. Inclusion criteria included studies utilizing modern osteosynthesis techniques that had a minimum of 30 ft. Exclusion criteria involved studies involving only patients with rheumatoid arthritis or use of structural bone graft [14]. He found lower incidence of nonunion at 5.4% when utilizing modern osteosynthesis techniques, concluding that the historical rate of 10% is inaccurate.

Even with advancements in surgical fixation devises, higher incidence of nonunion can occur without proper joint preparation. Numerous joint preparation techniques such as conical reamers, high-speed burrs, flat cuts, and curettage have been described (Fig. 13.9) [58, 73, 74]. It has been hypothesized that increased bone temperature caused by high levels of friction created by saws, high-speed burrs, and conical reamers may lead to aseptic thermal necrosis and decrease the odds of successful fusion (A16) [75–78]. The use of saline water irrigation, reamer-irrigator-aspirator systems, and even subaqatic reaming has all been shown to dissipate heat to prevent thermal necrosis of bone [75, 79, 80]. Iatrogenic shortening of the first ray from overzealous joint resection can also be a consequence of powered instrumentation. The author's preferred techniques include manual curettage or cortical reaming without power to a level of raw bleeding bone surface. Further preparation by fish-scaling and drilling of the bone surfaces with a 1.5 mm drill is

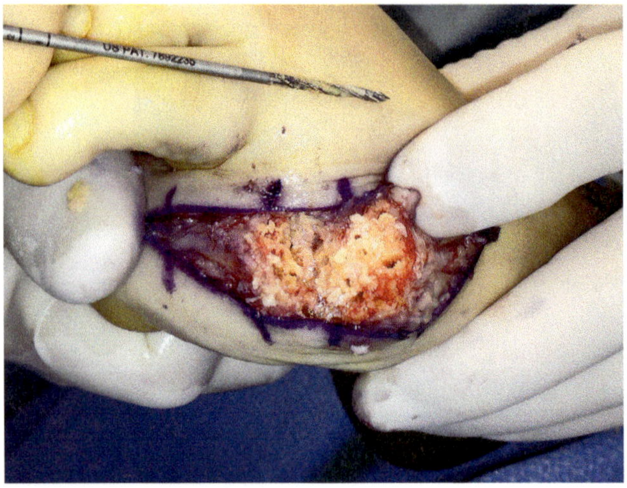

Fig. 13.10 Drill fenestration with a 1.5 mm drill bit

suggested (Fig. 13.10). While a K-wire is commonly used for fenestration of the joint surface, we believe that thermal necrosis may be induced utilizing this method [81–83]. Likewise, the act of K-wire fenestration may produce a sterile subchondral plug preventing the intent of active bleeding. By using a drill, the fluted tip allows churning of the cancellous bone below the subchondral plate allowing for release of cancellous bone and pluripotent stem cells into the fusion site, believed to aid in the arthrodesis process.

During the process of joint preparation, attention to the position and abnormal anatomy of the sesamoids should be considered. Quite often, the sesamoids are degenerative, hypertrophic, and at times adhered to the first metatarsal head. This pathological condition can prevent adequate bone apposition plantarly, leading to a nonunion of the plantar one-third of the joint or a dorsiflexed malunion of the hallux. Debridement, mobilization, planning, and even removal of the sesamoid may be needed in this situation.

Fixation failure is another important factor when understanding nonunions. Often, we may ask ourselves if the nonunion was caused by hardware failure or hardware failure from the nonunion. To this, we suggest that hardware does not fail on its own, but must have deforming forces driving the process. Motion at the arthrodesis site is the most plausible force causing hardware deformation and ultimately leading to its failure (Figs. 13.11 and 13.12). Therefore, the hardware used to strengthen and protect the surgical site must be able to withstand these forces.

Mini-external fixation has long been accepted as a possible fixation construct for first MTPJ arthrodesis. Caution should be exercised when using this approach due to the high incidence of malunion and nonunion. In the author's opinion, proper positioning of the half-pins is paramount for a successful outcome. Due to the complex nature of the joint anatomy, compression at the fusion site can lead to abnormal

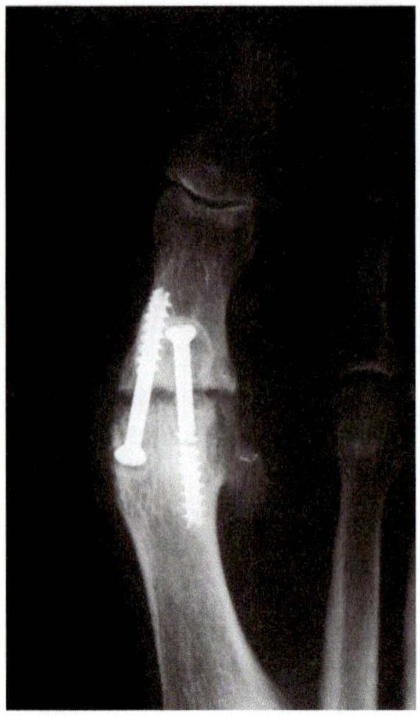

Fig. 13.11 Improper AO technique with hardware failure due to motion at the first MTPJ

anatomical alignment of the hallux if perfect positioning of the half-pins has not been achieved. The technical difficulty of placing half-pins correctly, while at the same time visualizing the three dimensional spacial orientation of the first MTPJ during compression through the fixator is what we believe leads to a high malunion and nonunion rate (Fig. 13.13).

Certain plate constructs such as a non-conformed plate are not anatomic and require bending prior to placement. When bending of the plate is needed, the required location of this bend is most commonly found at the fusion interface. This is the site where motion is most likely to occur postoperatively. Likewise, this area is undergoing bone remodeling and revascularization and is most vulnerable to deforming forces. The authors have seen this fixation type fail most commonly at the bend site and it has even been reported in the literature (Fig. 13.14) [70]. Pre-conformed anatomical plates allow for a rigid construct that can disperse these deforming forces better than other forms of fixation.

As the trend for early to immediate weight bearing continues, a solid fixation construct, such as pre-conformed anatomical plates, is an important consideration in avoiding complications [68]. The ideal plate construct should provide the following: (1) mechanically generated cross joint compression through the plate, (2) lobe contour and screw positioning that resists rotation in all four planes, (3) the ability for a locking component, and (4) length sufficient to dissipate the weight bearing load off of the fusion site to more proximal and distal uninjured bone (Fig. 13.15). Plating that incorporates these four components will provide a fixation construct stable enough to protect the fusion site during the

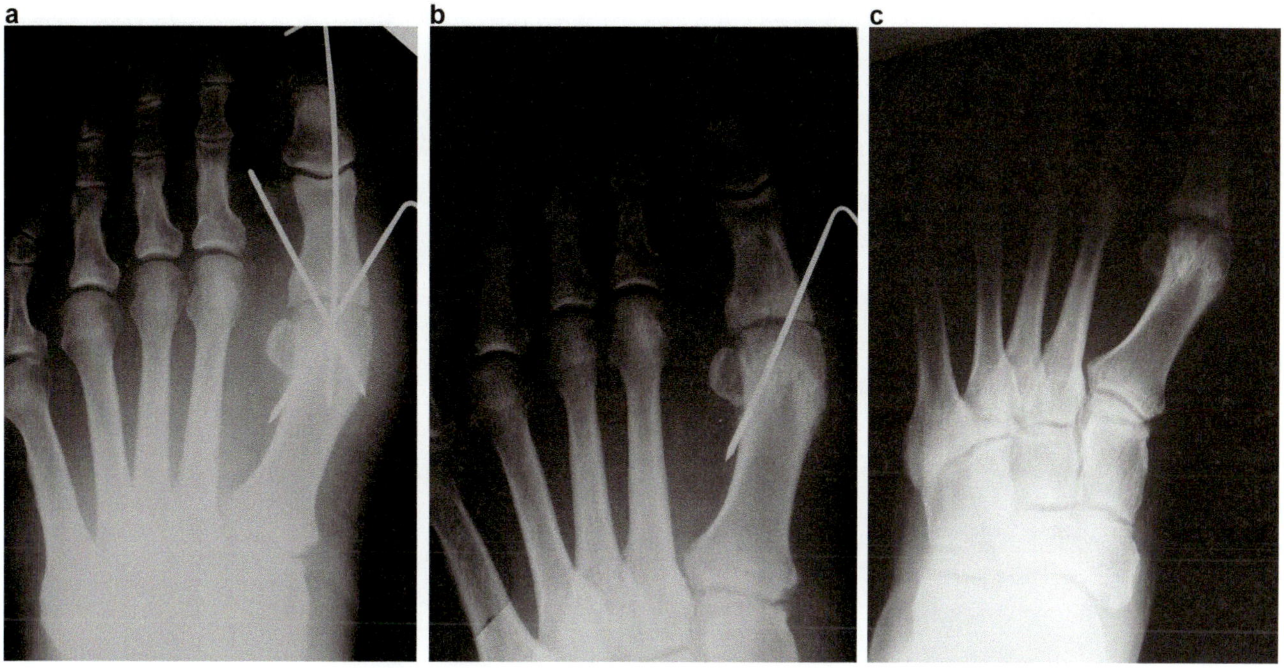

Fig. 13.12 (**a–c**) Nonunion of the first MTPJ as a result of premature K-wire removal destabilizing the fixation construct

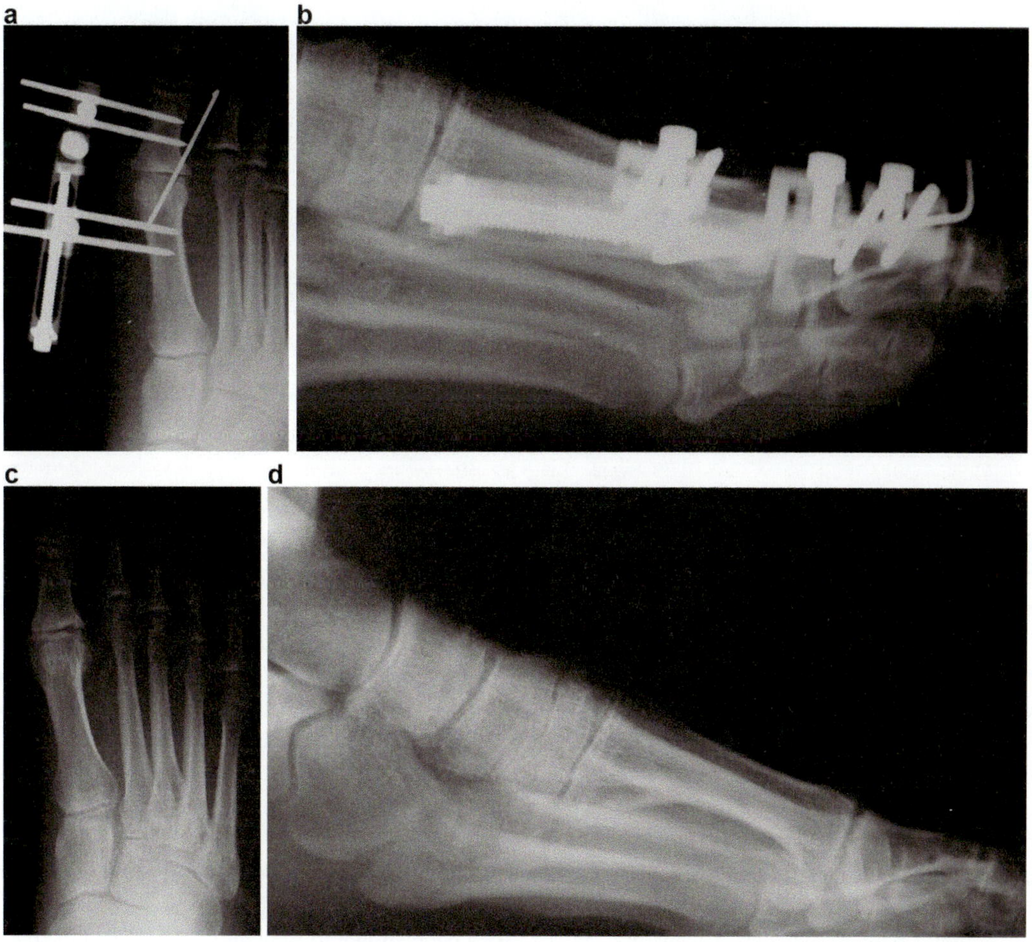

Fig. 13.13 (**a–c**) External fixator attempt at first MTPJ fusion with plantar gapping and ultimately resulting in nonunion

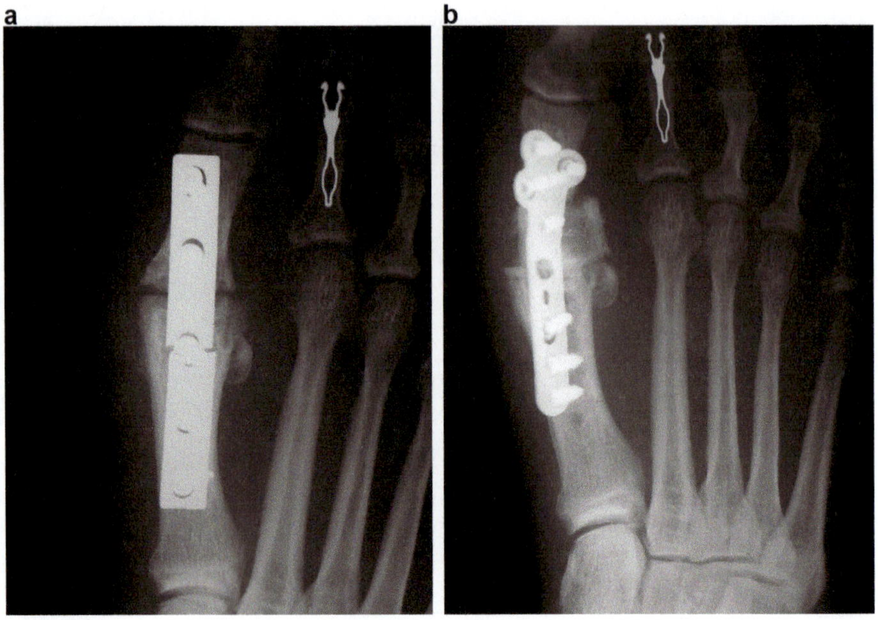

Fig. 13.14 (**a**) Painful nonunion with broken one-third tubular plate. (**b**) Revisional fusion with iliac crest interpositional bone autograft with spanning revisional anatomical locking plate

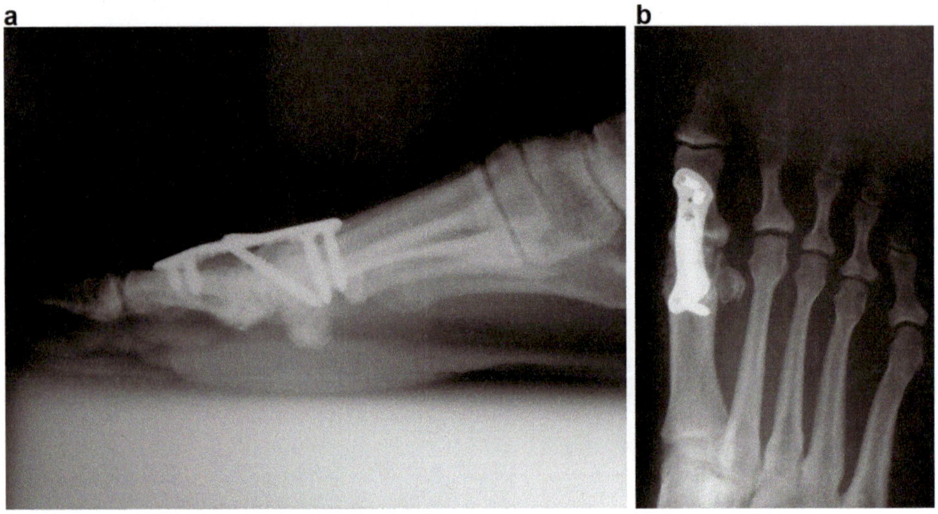

Fig. 13.15 (**a**, **b**) Plating construct demonstrating stabilizing first MTPJ fusion in all four planes

initial phases of bone healing while allowing immediate postoperative weight bearing. We believe that immediate weight bearing decreases the risk of deep venous thrombosis and increases micro-motion at the fusion site promoting the neovascularization necessary for bony union. In patients where the bone quality is poor, osteoporotic, or incapable of accepting screw and plate fixation such as in a patient with rheumatoid arthritis, a 3 crossing K-wire or Steinman pin fixation construct may be a necessary and acceptable fixation method [46, 53, 55, 84, 85].

Other co-morbidities such as diabetes, deformity type, nicotine use, endocrine disorders, vitaminosis D, and other nutritional deficiencies may lead to nonunion. In a study evaluating 76 diabetic patients who underwent first MTPJ arthrodesis by Anderson et al. [86], those with peripheral neuropathy were found to be at higher risk for complication. In total, 80% of neuropathic patients resulted in nonunion and concluded that although first MTPJ arthrodesis is an effective and beneficial procedure in patients with diabetes, caution must be exercised in this population. Shibuya and colleagues [87] evaluated factors in diabetic patients leading to nonunion, delayed union, and malunion and reported that surgical duration, peripheral neuropathy, and hemoglobin A1c levels greater than seven were all contributors. They noted that peripheral neuropathy had the strongest association with bone healing complications.

Metabolic and endocrine abnormalities should be considered when evaluating patients with a nonunion. Vitamin D has been shown to play an essential role in fracture healing, specifically mineralization, which is a key component during hard callus formation and bone remodeling. Although not specific to nonunions of first MTPJ arthrodesis, vitaminosis D has been associated with bony nonunions [88–92].

Brinker et al. [92] evaluated a series of patients who experienced an unexplained nonunion without technical error, poor reduction, or other obvious etiology. They found that of the 37 patients that met their criteria, 31 of them had one or more newly diagnosed metabolic or endocrine abnormalities. Vitaminosis D was present in 68% of these patients. Other diagnosed abnormalities included central hypogonadism, thyroid disorders, calcium imbalances, and parathyroid hormone disorders. Of these patients, eight went on to achieve bony union with medical treatment alone. We recommend routine screening and coordinated care with an endocrinologist in this patient population. We have also observed that regional factors such as areas with less daylight may be a contributing factor in vitaminosis D.

The effects of smoking on musculoskeletal healing are well documented. Postoperative complications including wound healing, increased infections, delayed unions and nonunions have been shown to be associated with smoking [93–97]. Smoking cessation of 3–4 weeks prior to surgery has been shown to effectively reduce the overall postoperative complication rate substantially [96, 97].

Effect of underlying first MTPJ pathology has also been discussed as a possible influence on union rates. Korim and Allen [67] observed an 8.2% nonunion rate in 134 patients. 100% of the nonunions reported were found in patients with hallux valgus. They suggested that fixation may have difficulty resisting the deforming forces of the adductor hallucis, flexor hallucis brevis, and extensor hallucis longus. They also noted that bone in patients with hallux rigidus is often more sclerotic and may offer a stronger fixation construct and screw purchase. Grimes and Coughlin [30] reported a 12% nonunion rate for first MTPJ arthrodesis for failed hallux valgus surgery. Of the four nonunions, only one was symptomatic and underwent successful revision.

Severity of the hallux valgus deformity provides for difficult rectus positioning with increased strain on the fixation due to soft tissue adaptation. Significant deformity often requires resection of bone versus curettage. By doing so, stable fixation becomes more difficult due to the amount of hard subchondral bone resected which is required for adequate screw purchase. This may be less of a concern when plating is utilized as opposed to crossed screw fixation.

Ruling out underlying osteomyelitis is important before considering revision (Fig. 13.16). There should always be a high suspicion of such an underlying process. Radiographic evidence of lucency and erosions at the nonunion site coupled with clinical suspicion requires appropriate lab work and ultimately a bone biopsy. Computer assisted tomography and white blood cell labeled bone scans can assist in the diagnosis. If osteomyelitis is found, antibiotic therapy, hyperbaric oxygen therapy, resection of infected bone, or amputation may be indicated.

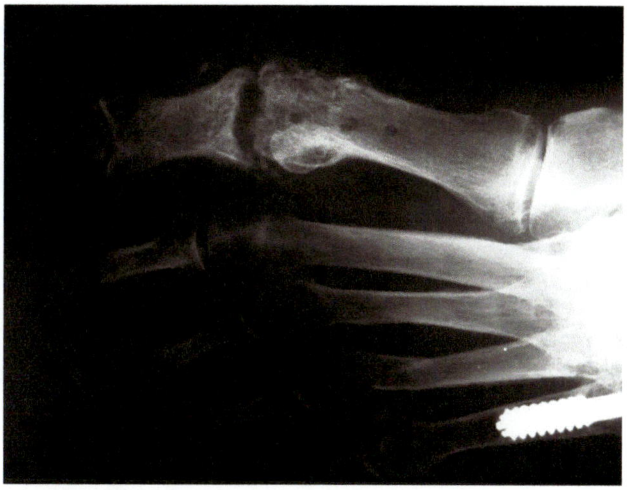

Fig. 13.16 Radiograph of a nonunion with suspicion for osteomyelitis

Nonunion of the first MTPJ can either present as being symptomatic or asymptomatic. The authors encounter asymptomatic nonunions more often than symptomatic. This clinical observation is also documented by others in the literature. In a systematic review, 50 out of 153 (32.7%) nonunions were reported as symptomatic [14]. A pseudoarthrosis formation of the first MTPJ and breakage of internal fixation is sometimes well tolerated without further intervention needed (Fig. 13.17) [46, 70]. When symptomatic, conservative measures such as prolonged immobilization and the use of a bone stimulator are limited. These patients ultimately will require revisional surgery. The patient's activity level, job demands, and expectations are all factors that need careful consideration when choosing a procedure. One of the most difficult decisions for a surgeon in managing a nonunion is determining when to surgically revise. Sometimes just a little time and patient education is all it may take for bony union to occur.

Identifying the underlying factors which led to a nonunion of the first MTPJ is imperative when determining revision surgical options for these patients. Identifiable co-morbidities such as a history of smoking, uncontrolled diabetes, peripheral neuropathy, nutritional deficiencies, and chronic steroid use have an increased likelihood to fail a revisional arthrodesis. This population may benefit more from removal of hardware and joint debridement with or without implant arthroplasty. Hope and colleagues [98] reviewed their treatment of 12 symptomatic nonunions. Eleven of twelve patients elected to undergo removal of hardware and joint debridement. Four of these patients went onto painful pseudoarthrosis and required either revision fusion or first MTPJ replacement. They concluded that removal of hardware and joint debridement alone is a reasonable option to offer as a

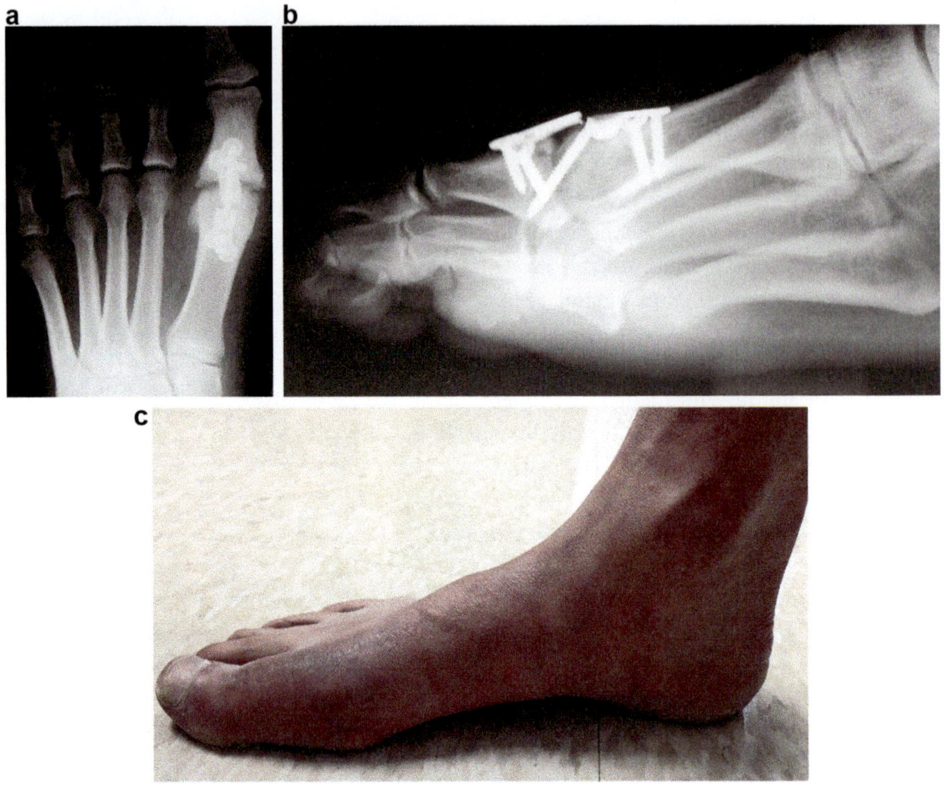

Fig. 13.17 (**a–c**) Example of an asymptomatic nonunion with hardware failure

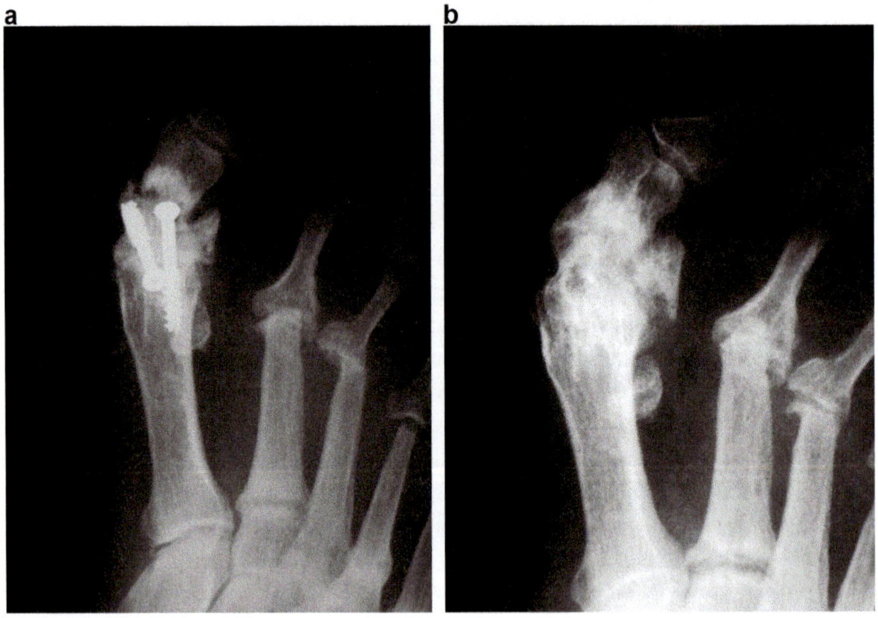

Fig. 13.18 (**a**, **b**) Example of a rheumatoid nonunion with painful hardware revised with hardware removal and debridement resolving pain

relatively minor procedure following failed arthrodesis. It is important to discuss preoperatively with the patient that this surgical procedure often leaves a short, non-functional, floppy toe, with the primary goal being relief of pain (Fig. 13.18).

In a retrospective chart review performed by Thun and colleagues [99], 77 consecutive first MTPJ arthrodesis procedures were divided into two groups consisting of 34 K-wire and 43 modern osteosynthesis fixation techniques with a minimum follow-up of 10 months. Modern osteosynthesis was defined as compression screws, dorsal plating, or dorsal plate with compression screw fixation. All other fixation methods were excluded from this study. They hypothesized that the nonunion rate would be lower in fusions utilizing modern osteosynthesis techniques. The overall nonunion rate was 6.5%. The K-wire group nonunion and delayed

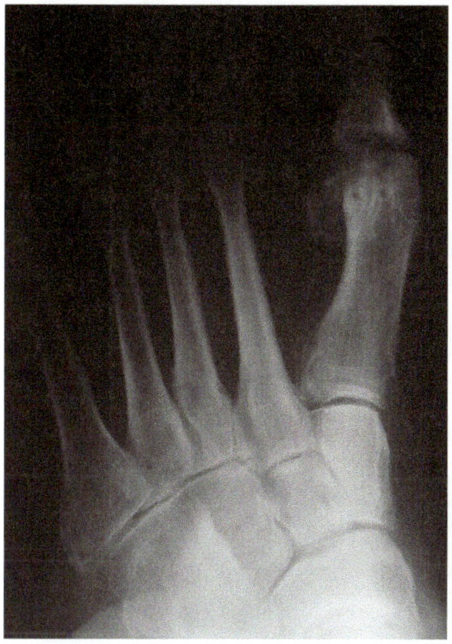

Fig. 13.19 Asymptomatic nonunion after K-wire removal for first MTPJ arthrodesis

union rate was 11.76% and 5.88%, respectively. Modern osteosynthesis nonunion and delayed union rates were both 2.33%. Co-morbidities identified prior to surgery were diabetes mellitus (14.2%), smoking (10.4%), and previous surgery (13%). Of the five nonunions, two (40%) were smokers and three (60%) were diabetic with peripheral neuropathy. One of the patients was both a smoker and diabetic. Fusion was achieved in all patients with a previous surgery. Two of the five (40%) nonunions were symptomatic requiring a second surgery (one revisional first MTPJ fusion with autogenic bone graft and one hardware removal with debridement) resulting in resolution of pain. Of interesting note, 75% of the nonunions found in the K-wire group were asymptomatic (Fig. 13.19). This may be in part due to the fact that these patients did not have any retained hardware postoperatively. As a failed arthrodesis results in pseudoarthrosis, motion at the first MTPJ occurs. These patients often experience irritation provoked by the retained hardware. Similar to Hope's [98] findings, it should come as no surprise that removal of hardware and debridement alone may be a reasonable solution for some patients where relief of pain is the primary goal. There was only one nonunion within the modern osteosynthesis group. This nonunion was painful and required removal of hardware and debridement. Resolution of pain was achieved postoperatively (Fig. 13.20).

Revisional arthrodesis is usually reserved for a symptomatic nonunion in an active, healthy individual where an iatrogenic cause or poor postoperative adherence is identified. Examples of iatrogenic causes include poor surgical technique or fixation failure. With this knowledge, the surgeon can attempt revision with more confidence. Takacs and Swierstra [100] described the use of a turnaround inlay graft for first MTPJ pseudoarthrosis with union occurring in 23 of 25 patients. This technique negates the need for joint debridement or use of autogenous grafting in the presence of shortening. Although these authors had an overall successful outcome with this revisional technique, our preferred approach includes resection of the symptomatic nonunion with interpositional structural autograft.

A standard dorsal incisional approach is performed to the nonunion site (Fig. 13.21). This allows adequate visualization of the nonunion and the most advantageous approach for hardware removal (Fig. 13.22). After removal of hardware and resection of the nonunion, a 1–3 cm deficit is usually noted (Figs. 13.23a–d). There are conflicting opinions with regards to the advantage of deflating the tourniquet at this point. The obvious advantage of deflation is to observe the nonunion site and evaluate for healthy, bleeding bone. The disadvantage is creating a bloody field, delay in procedure, and possible difficulty in soft tissue closure over plate fixation due to swelling within the tissues. Shortening of the first ray is a common issue encountered by the surgeon in the presence of a nonunion and can be restored by interposing a structural bone graft (Fig. 13.24). The authors recommend the use of autogenous graft either harvested from the iliac crest or posterior calcaneus (Figs. 13.23e, f and 13.25). Harvest from these sites has been described with success, low surgical complication, and minimal morbidity [101–112]. While not specific for revisional first MTPJ arthrodesis, many articles have reported the successful use of tricortical autogenous bone graft in restoring length of the first ray with favorable fusion rates [26, 27, 29–32].

Once the autogenous graft has been properly fashioned into the surgical site, temporary fixation is placed across the graft for stabilization (Fig. 13.23g–i). Again, positioning of the hallux is vital in avoiding a painful malunion (Fig. 13.23j). Spanning the graft with a locking anatomic reconstruction plate is the author's preferred fixation method (Figs. 13.23k–n and 13.26). A locking screw through the plate and into the graft prevents displacement and eliminates the need for transfixation techniques, which often results in splitting of the graft. Although structural allografts are commonly used in fusions and even some revisional arthrodesis procedures of the foot and ankle, we do not recommend it for use in first MTPJ revisional arthrodesis. In the author's opinion, the use of cadaveric bone in an already failed fusion of the first MTPJ is at high risk for repeated nonunion and should be avoided. Should allograft be used, we highly recommend combination with biologics that incorporate osteoinductive and conductive properties. Another acceptable option for revisional arthrodesis when a structural graft is needed is the use of a mini-external fixator. It is important to utilize a fixator that has the ability to compress and manipulate in

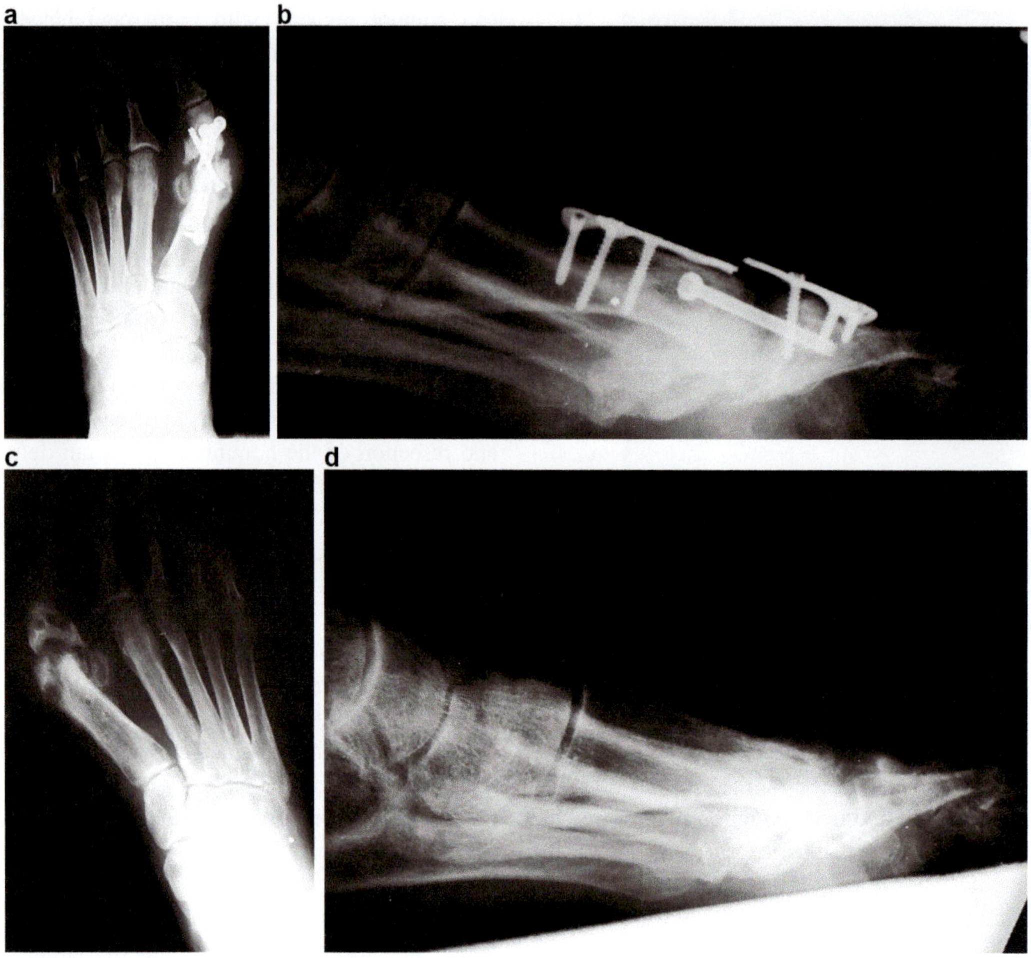

Fig. 13.20 (**a**, **b**) Painful nonunion, smoker, rheumatoid arthritis. (**c**, **d**) Resolvement of pain with hardware removal and debridement

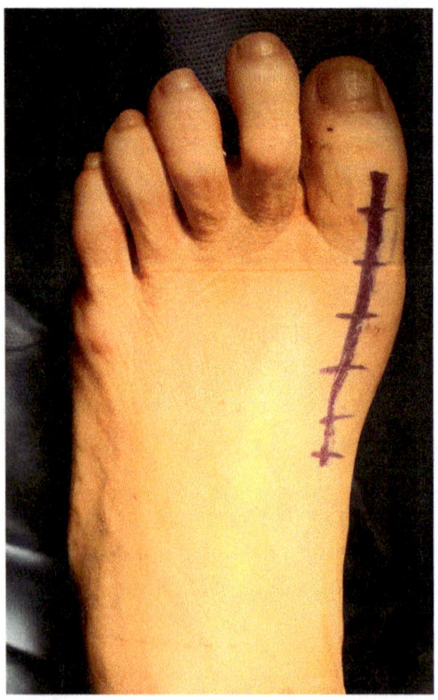

Fig. 13.21 Standard dorsal revisional approach

multiple planes in order to accomplish proper positioning of the hallux. If a fixed, uniplanar mono-rail system is used, position of the hallux is compromised when compression is achieved (Fig. 13.27).

In acute cases where hardware failure is observed with the need for intervention, shortening of the first ray may be avoided, thus negating the need for structural graft. In this situation, removal of hardware, minimal debridement of the joint, and a spanning anatomical plate fixation may be all that is needed (Fig. 13.28). Autogenous cancellous bone or bone marrow aspirate may be used in the revisional surgery and can be easily harvested from the distal tibia or calcaneus (Fig. 13.29).

In any revisional first MTPJ arthrodesis, the surgeon will likely encounter questions regarding fixation options. Commonly, removal of previous hardware will leave large bone deficits where screws were used. To avoid complications associated with this, the need for spanning plate fixation into previously untouched bone is necessary in providing a stable revisional construct by transferring the deforming

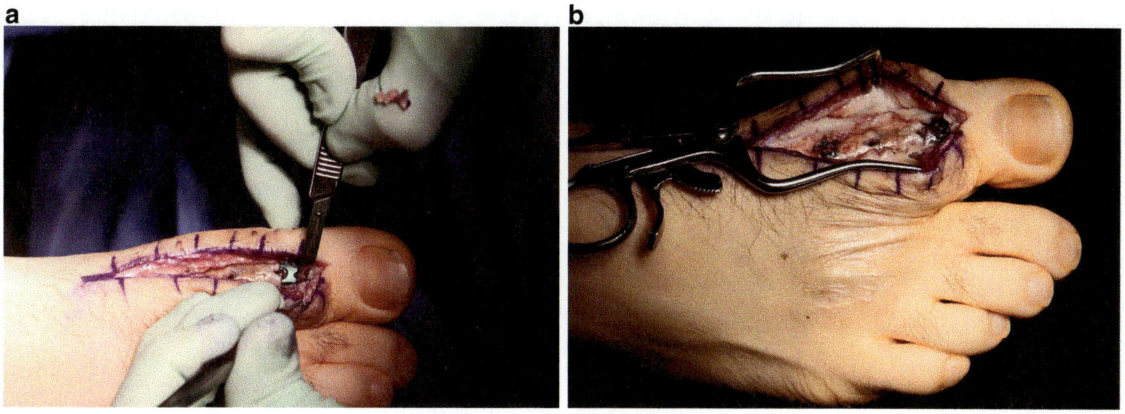

Fig. 13.22 (**a**, **b**) Approach allowing direct visualization of hardware and nonunion site

forces away from the fusion site. In a revision where bone quality is poor or compromised due to previous surgical procedures and a structural graft is not incorporated, the use of K-wire fixation may be a necessary and acceptable fixation method. Strict non-weight bearing with cast immobilization for 6–8 weeks is recommended with progression into a postoperative boot for an additional 4 weeks. Utilization of a bone stimulator should be considered as an adjunct treatment starting immediately after surgery (Fig. 13.30) [113–123].

Failure of a revisional first MTPJ arthrodesis leaves limited treatment options for the surgeon and patient. Again, identifying the factors leading to another nonunion is key in directing the surgeon towards further intervention. Revisional arthrodesis of an already failed fusion is rarely seen and has little to no mention in current literature but may be reasonable for certain patients where hardware failure or poor surgical technique has been demonstrated. Other surgical options include removal of hardware and conversion to a joint arthroplasty with implant (Fig. 13.31) [124]. Conversion to a true Keller arthroplasty with pinning is not an option because the head of the first metatarsal has previously been resected. While these options are less than ideal, at this point the goal of treatment should be focused on resolution of pain with salvage of the toe. In some patients, amputation of the hallux or first ray is a reasonable option (Fig. 13.32).

Conclusion

Complications of first MTPJ arthrodesis can be devastating to the patient and the surgeon. The high demand required of the hallux for normal foot function makes the first MTPJ a vital part of one's overall lifestyle and well-being. Proper biomechanical function of the hallux that leads to a normal pain free gait should trump cosmesis regardless of the patient's age, activity level, or desire for certain shoegear.

We cannot overstate the preoperative assessment of risk factors, both patient-dependent and surgeon-dependent. Patient education appears to be overrated in that the literature supports the fact that our patients only comprehend 25% of what we tell them [125].

Avoid the temptation to perform a high-risk procedure in a high-risk patient. Patients with multiple risk factors that require multiple procedures will have inherent biomechanical risk, which will increase the likelihood of complications exponentially. Furthermore, these types of patients and complications are a nightmare to fix when things go bad. Remember that in managing first MTPJ nonunions, you can drill them, you can graft them, you can attempt stimulation, you can plate them or triple plate them, but if the patient lacks the biological requirements to heal on a cellular level, the joint will never fuse.

Eliminate risk by evaluating your patient properly. Select your procedure with risk capacity and risk exposure in mind. Execute the procedure perfectly and follow the basic principles. Conceptualize your fixation construct and keep things simple.

Managing complications of first MTPJ arthrodesis prove difficult and challenging. However, through a thorough evaluation and systematic approach, many of these complications can be managed with acceptable outcomes. Sound surgical techniques and principles can provide the patient with their desired outcome.

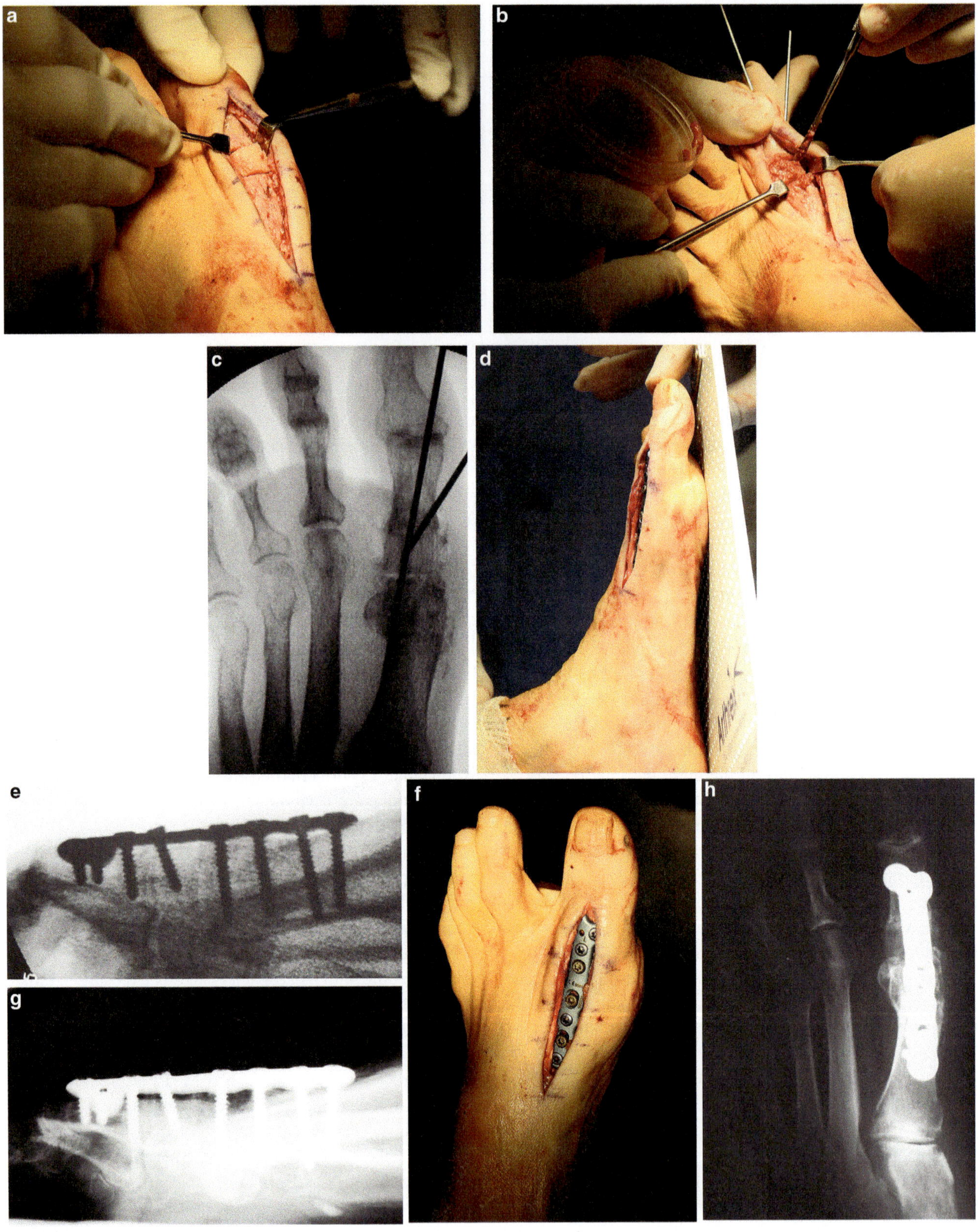

Fig. 13.23 (**a–d**) Resection of nonunion resulting in a shortened first ray. (**e, f**) Harvest of structural autograft from the posterior calcaneus. (**g–i**) Placement of the structural autograft with temporary fixation and packed with bone marrow aspirate. (**j**) Intraoperative positioning of the hallux. (**k, l**) Placement of graft spanning anatomic reconstruction locking plate. Note the placement of a screw from the plate to the graft. (**m, n**) Six month postoperative radiographs of revision

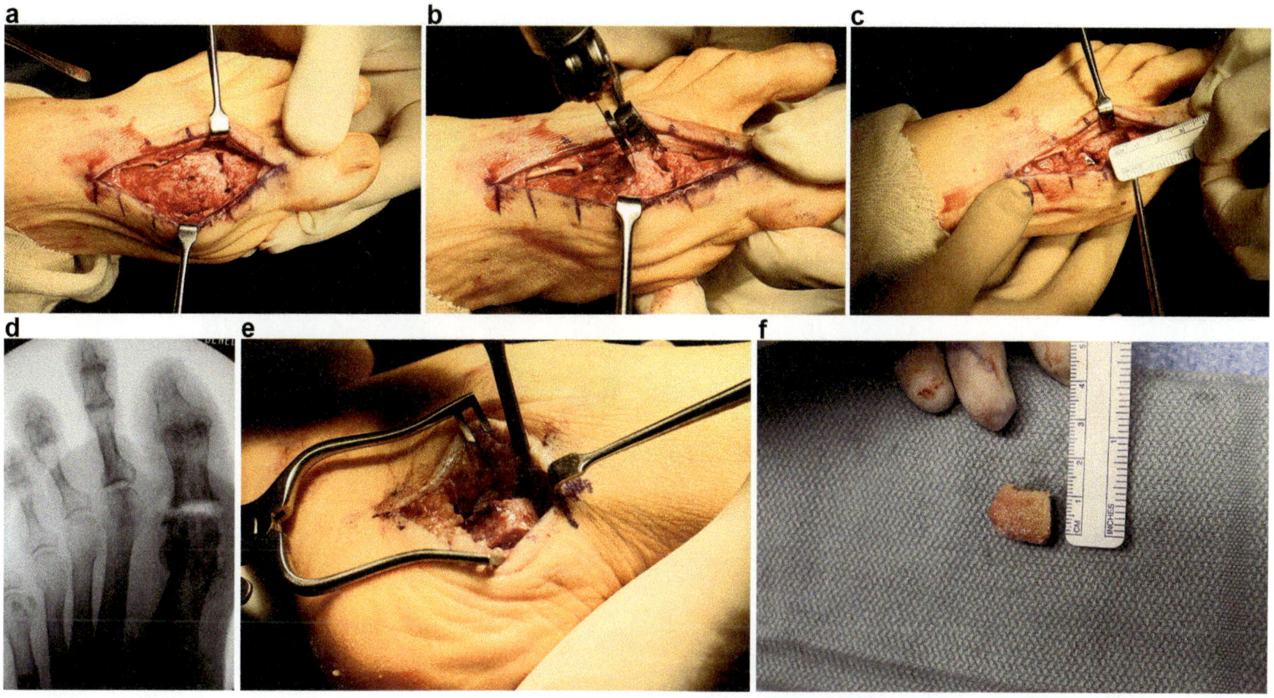

Fig. 13.24 (continued)

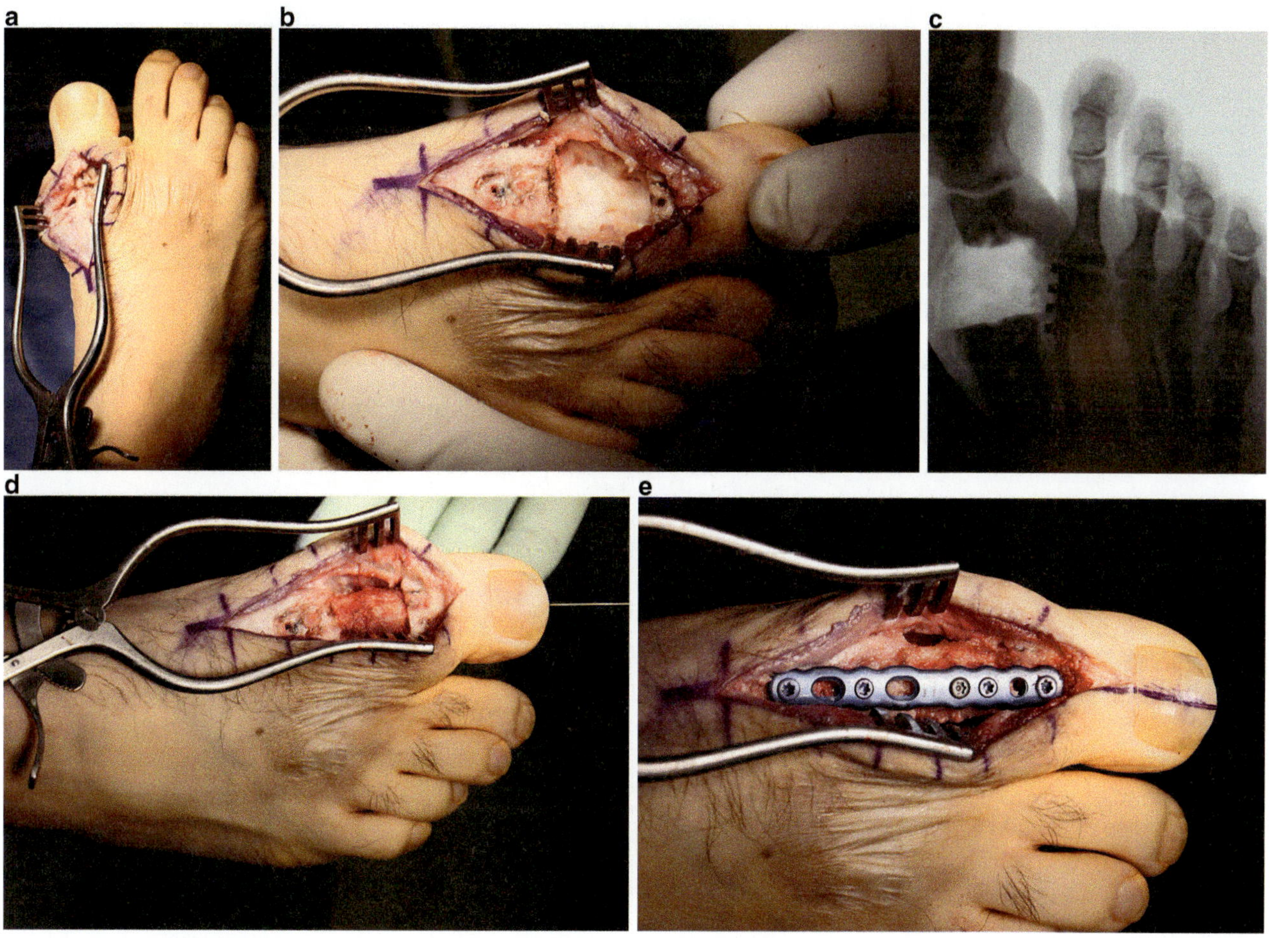

Fig. 13.24 (a–c) Intraoperative pictures demonstrating shortening of the first ray after resection of nonunion. (d, e) Placement of iliac crest interpositional autogenous bone graft with graft spanning reconstruction plate to restore length to the first ray

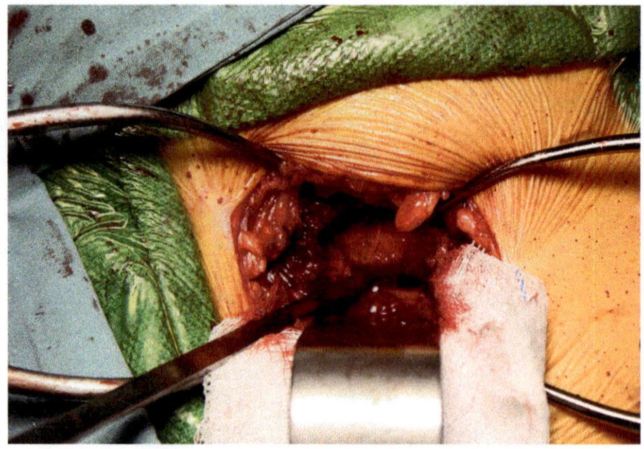

Fig. 13.25 Harvest of iliac crest for autograft

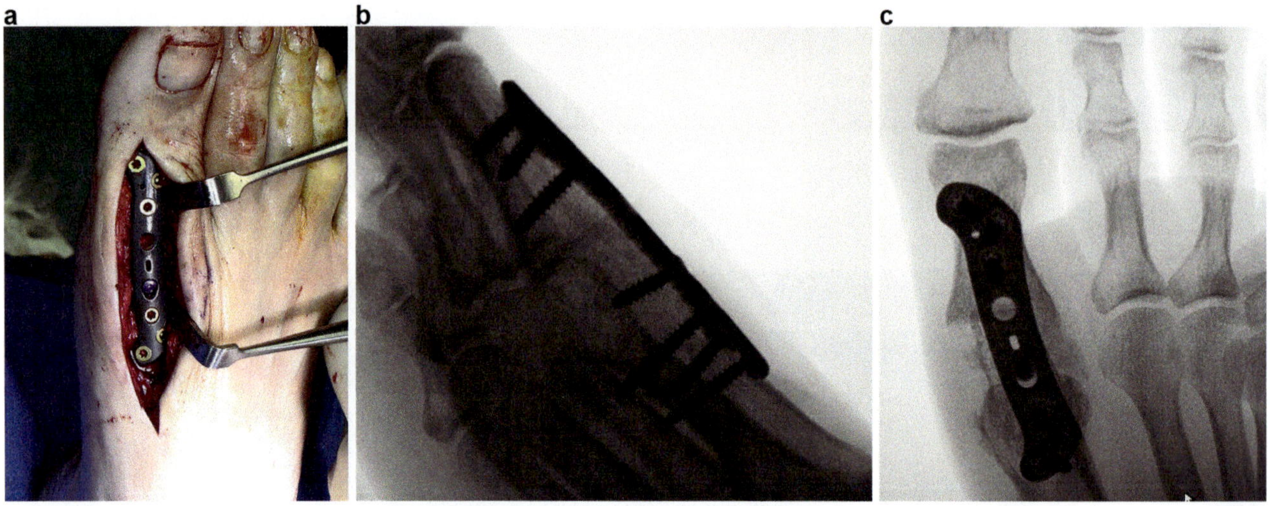

Fig. 13.26 (**a–c**) Example of a graft spanning locking anatomic reconstruction plate with locking screw through plate into graft

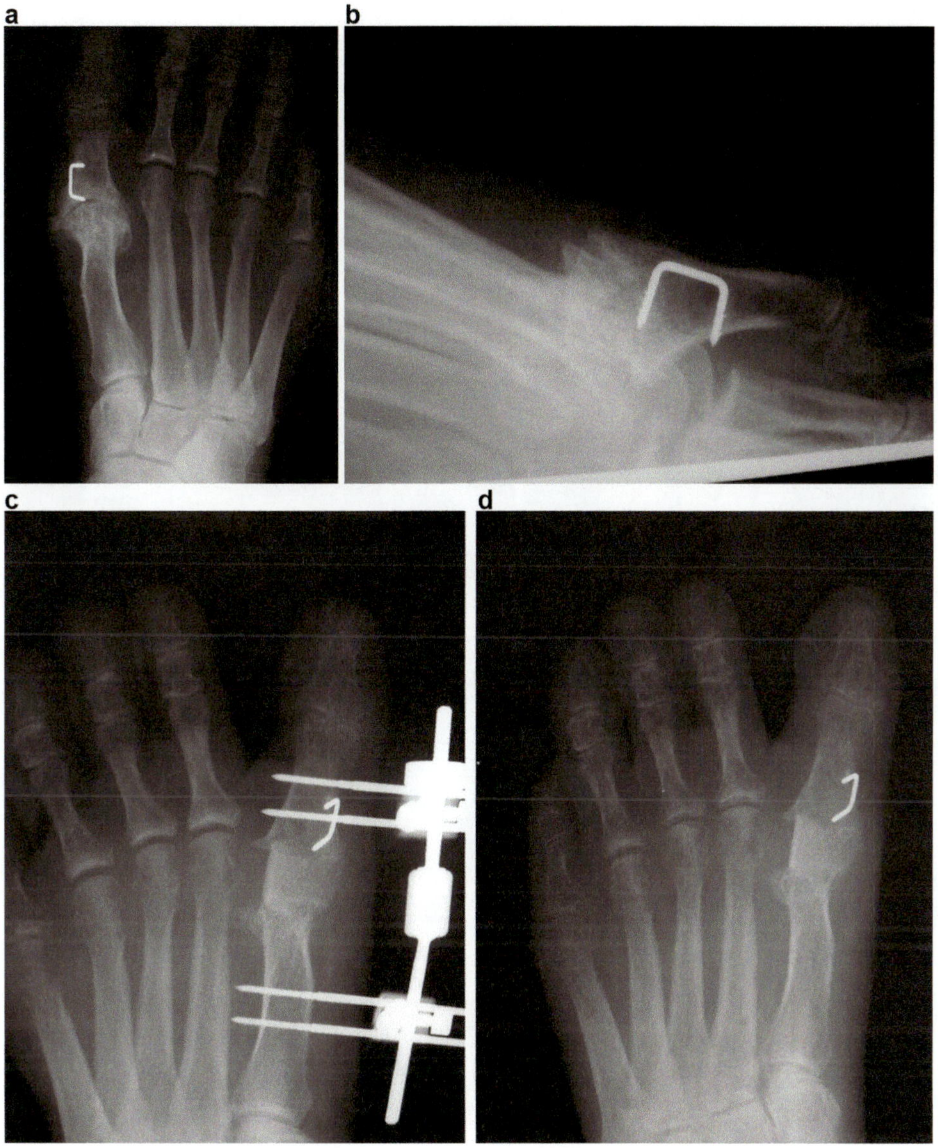

Fig. 13.27 (a–d) Preoperative and postoperative radiographs of an interpositional bone graft malunion as a result of utilizing a uniplanar external fixation

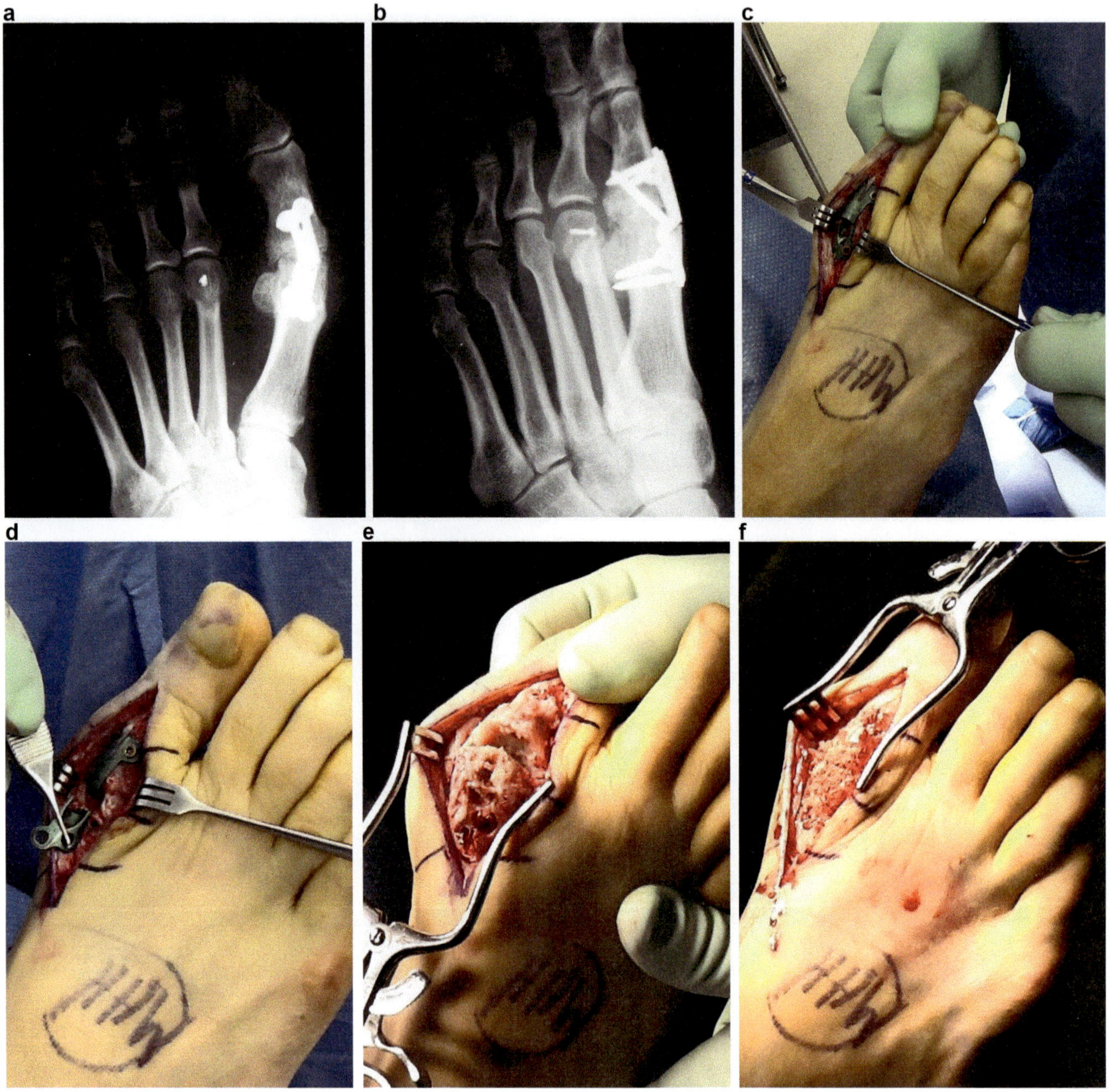

Fig. 13.28 (**a**, **b**) Ten weeks post-attempted first MTPJ arthrodesis with failed hardware, pain and motion. (**c**, **d**) Intraoperative view of broken plate. (**e**) Intraoperative view of bone destruction where length of the first ray was not compromised. (**f**, **g**) Joint debridement and packing with bone graft substitute and bone marrow aspirate. Spanning revisional locking plate. Note the plantarflexed bend in plate to allow for hallux purchase. (**h**, **i**) Ten weeks post-revision. (**j**, **k**) Clinical weight bearing position of hallux

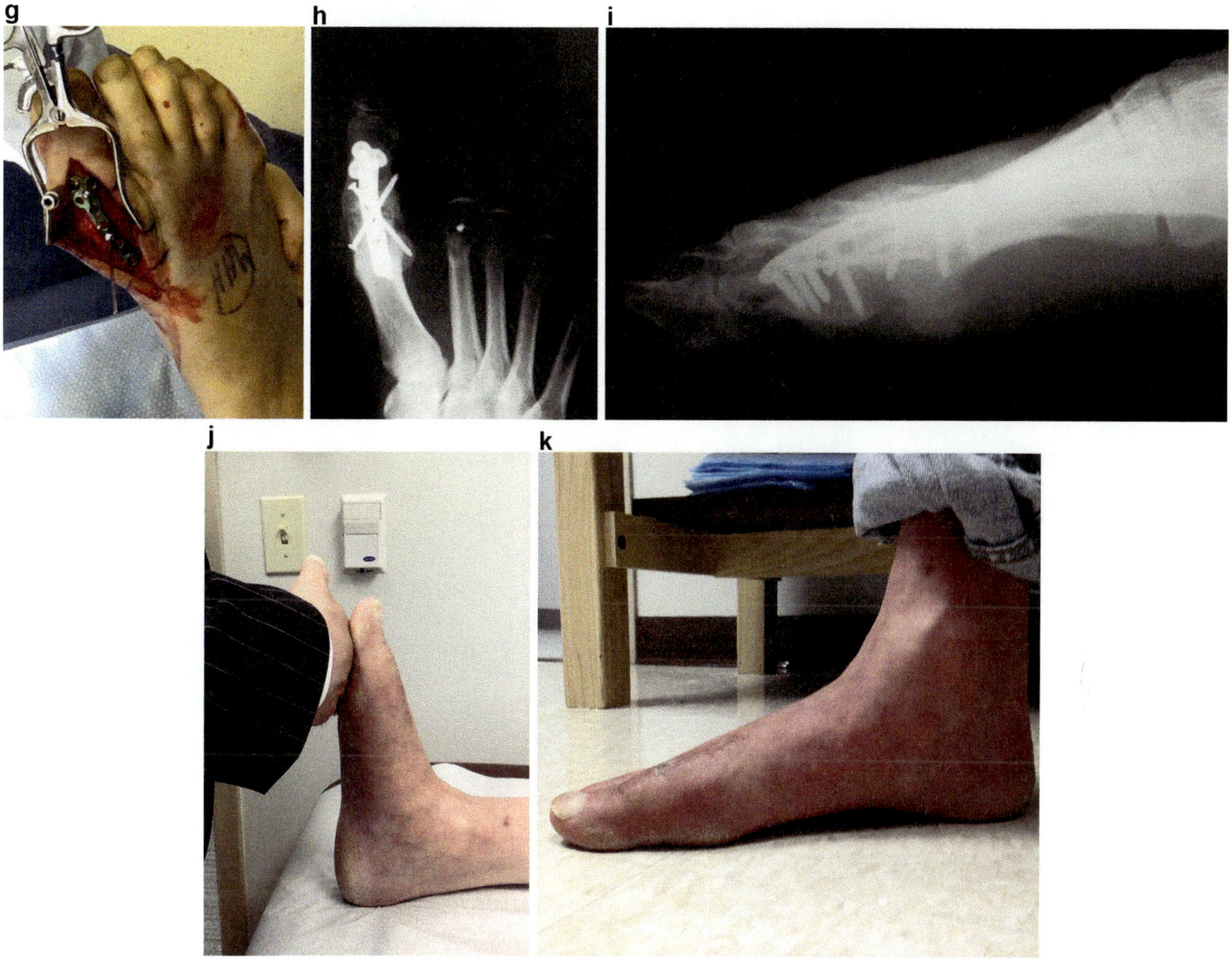

Fig. 13.28 (continued)

Fig. 13.29 (a, b) Bone marrow aspirate from the distal tibia and its use in revisional first MTPJ arthrodesis

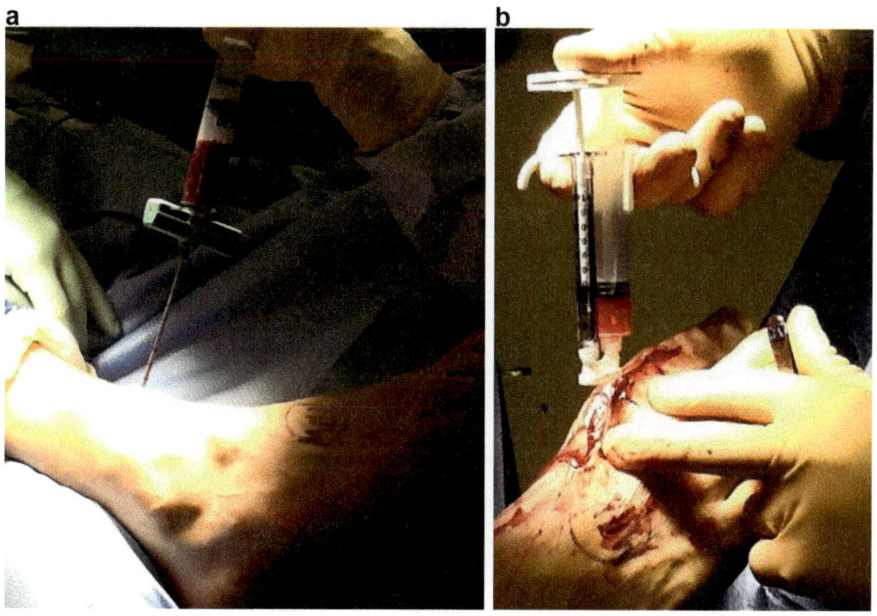

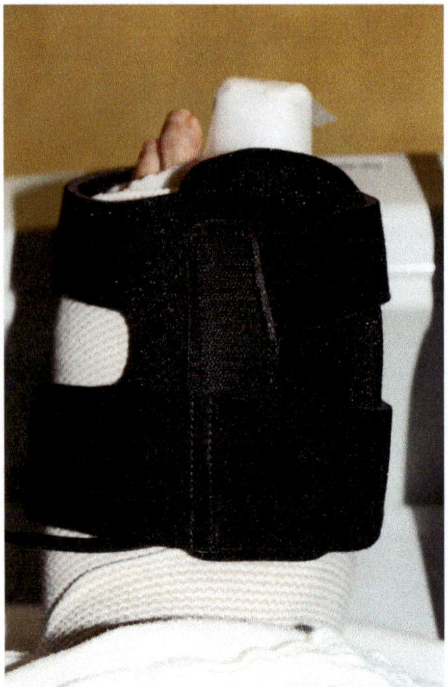

Fig. 13.30 Postoperative use of an external bone stimulator after revisional fusion

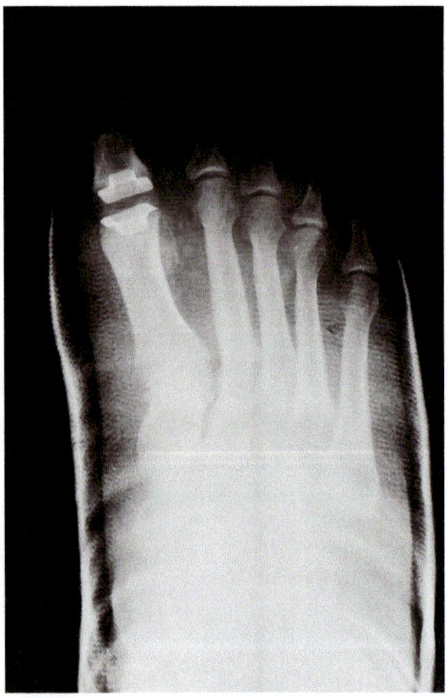

Fig. 13.31 Example of a silastic implant after a failed revisional nonunion

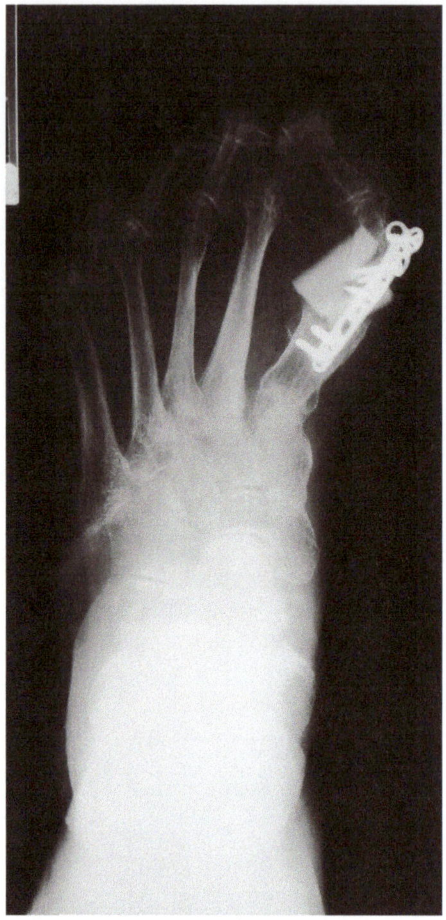

Fig. 13.32 Third attempt at repair in 8 days. Structural allograft strut with unstable fixation construct. Patient requested amputation of the first ray

Acknowledgments Special thanks to Dr. Michael C. Keller, DPM, and Dr. William T. DeCarbo for their photo contributions and insights on this chapter.

References

1. Bouche RT, Adad JM. Arthrodesis of the first metatarsophalangeal joint in active people. Clin Podiatr Med Surg. 1996;13(3):461–84.
2. Clutton HH. The treatment of hallux valgus. St Thomas Hosp Rep. 1894;22:1–12.
3. Coughlin MJ, Shurnas PS. Hallux rigidus: grading and long-term results of operative treatment. J Bone Joint Surg Am. 2003;85(11):2072–88.
4. Shereff MJ, Baumhauer JF. Hallux rigidus and osteoarthrosis of the first metatarsophalangeal joint. J Bone Joint Surg Am. 1998;80(6):898–908.
5. Lombardi CM, Silhanek AD, Connolly FG, Dennis LN, Keslonsky AJ. First metatarsophalangeal joint for treatment of hallux rigidus: a retrospective study. J Foot Ankle Surg. 2001;40(3):137–43.

6. Cronin JJ, Limbers JP, Kutty S, Stephens MM. Intermetatarsal angle after first metatarsophalangeal joint arthrodesis for hallux valgus. Foot Ankle Int. 2006;27(2):104–9.
7. Dayton P, LoPiccolo J, Kiley J. Reduction of the intermetatarsal angle after first metatarsophalangeal joint arthrodesis in patients with moderate to severe metatarsus primus adductus. J Foot Ankle Surg. 2002;41:316–9.
8. Coughlin MJ, Grebing BR, Jones CP. Arthrodesis of the first metatarsophalangeal joint for idiopathic hallux valgus: intermediate results. Foot Ankle Int. 2005;26(10):783–92.
9. Easley ME, Trnka H. Current concepts review: hallux valgus part II: operative treatment. Foot Ankle Int. 2007;6:748–58.
10. Paola LD, Carone A, Morisi C, Cardillo S, Pattavina M. Conservative surgical treatment of infected ulceration of the first metatarsophalangeal joint with osteomyelitis in diabetic patients. J Foot Ankle Surg. 2014;20:1–5. doi:10.1053/j.jfas.2014.08.004.
11. Castro MD, Klaue K. Revisiting an alternative method of fixation for first MTP joint arthrodesis. Foot Ankle Int. 2001;22:687–8.
12. Kumar S, Pradhan R, Rosenfeld PF. First metatarsophalangeal arthrodesis using a dorsal plate and a compression screw. Foot Ankle Int. 2010;31:797–801.
13. Bennett G, Sabatta J. First metatarsophalangeal joint arthrodesis: evaluation of plate and screw fixation. Foot Ankle Int. 2006;30: 752–7.
14. Roukis TS. Nonunion after arthrodesis of the first metatarsophalangeal joint: a systematic review. J Foot Ankle Surg. 2001;40: 136–13.
15. Sung W, Kluesner AJ, Irrgang J, Burns P, Wukich DK. Radiographic outcomes following primary arthrodesis of the first metatarsophalangeal joint in hallux abductovalgus deformity. J Foot Ankle Surg. 2010;49:446–51.
16. Dayton P, McCall A. Early weightbearing after first metatarsophalangeal joint arthrodesis: a retrospective observational case analysis. J Foot Ankle Surg. 2004;43:156–9.
17. Denning J, van Erve RHGP. Arthrodesis of the first metatarsophalangeal joint: a retrospective analysis of plate versus screw fixation. J Foot Ankle Surg. 2012;51:172–5.
18. Mah CD, Banks AS. Immediate weight bearing following first metatarsophalangeal joint fusion with Kirschner wire fixation. J Foot Ankle Surg. 2012;51:50–6.
19. Beeson P. The surgical treatment of hallux limitus/rigidus: a critical review of the literature. Foot. 2004;14:6–22.
20. Goucher NR, Coughlin MJ. Hallux metatarsophalangeal joint arthrodesis using dome-shaped reamers and dorsal plate fixation: a prospective study. Foot Ankle Int. 2006;27:869–76.
21. Hamalainen M, Raunio P. Long-term followup of rheumatoid forefoot surgery. Clin Orthop Relat Res. 1997;340:34–8.
22. Lipscomb PR. Arthrodesis of the first metatarsophalangeal joint for severe bunions and hallux rigidus. Clin Orthop Relat Res. 1979;142:48–54.
23. Mann RA, Schakel II ME. Surgical correction of rheumatoid forefoot deformities. Foot Ankle Int. 1995;16:1–6.
24. McKeever DC. Arthrodesis of the first metatarsophalangeal joint for hallux valgus, hallux rigidus, and metatarsus primus varus. J Bone Joint Surg. 1952;34A:129–34.
25. Sage RA, Lam AT, Taylor DT. Retrospective analysis of first metatarsal phalangeal joint arthrodesis. J Foot Ankle Surg. 1997; 36:425–9.
26. Machachek F, Easey ME, Gruber F, Ritschl P, Trnka HJ. Salvage of failed Keller resection arthroplasty. J Bone Joint Surg. 2004; 86:1754–64.
27. Mankovecky MR, Prissel MA, Roukis TS. Incidence of nonunion of first metatarsal-phalangeal joint arthrodesis with autogenous iliac crest bone graft after failed Keller-Brandes arthroplasty: a systematic review. J Foot Ankle Surg. 2013;52:53–5.
28. Wu KK. First metatarsophalangeal joint fusion in the salvage of failed hallux abducto valgus operations. J Foot Ankle Surg. 1994;33(4):383–95.
29. Vienne P, Sukthankar A, Farve P, Werner CM, Baumer A, Zingg PO. Metatarsophalangeal joint arthrodesis after failed Keller-Brandes procedure. Foot Ankle Int. 2006;27(11):894–901.
30. Grimes JS, Coughlin MJ. First metatarsophalangeal joint arthrodesis after failed Keller-Brandes procedure. Foot Ankle Int. 2006;27(11):887–93.
31. Myerson MS, Schon LC, McGuigan FX, Oznur A. Results of arthrodesis of the hallux metatarsophalangeal joint using bone graft for restoration of length. Foot Ankle Int. 2000;21(4): 297–306.
32. Coughlin MJ, Mann RA. Arthrodesis of the first metatarsophalangeal joint as salvage for the failed Keller procedure. J Bone Joint Surg. 1987;69A:68–75.
33. Hecht PJ, Gibbons MJ, Wapner KL, Cooke C, Hoisington SA. Arthrodesis of the first metatarsophalangeal joint to salvage failed silicone implant arthroplasty. Foot Ankle Int. 1997;18:383–90.
34. Myerson MS, Miller S, Saxby T, Henderson M. Staged arthrodesis for salvage of the septic hallux metatarsophalangeal joint. Clin Orthop Relat Res. 1994;307:174–81.
35. Garras DN, Durinka JB, Bercik M, Miller AG, Raikin SM. Conversion arthrodesis for failed first metatarsophalangeal joint hemiarthroplasty. Foot Ankle Int. 2013;34(9):1227–32.
36. Gross CE, Hsu AR, Lin J, Holmes GB, Lee S. Revision MTP arthrodesis for failed arthroplasty. Foot Ankle Spec. 2013;6(6): 471–8.
37. Schuh R, Trnka H. First metatarsophalangeal arthrodesis for severe bone loss. Foot Ankle Clin. 2011;16(1):13–20. doi:10.1016/j.fcl.2010.11.005.
38. Brodsky JW, Ptaskek A, Morris SG. Salvage first MTP arthrodesis utilizing ICBG: clinical evaluation and outcome. Foot Ankle Int. 2000;21(4):290–6.
39. Wassink S, van der Oever M. Arthrodesis of the first metatarsophalangeal joint using a single screw: retrospective analysis of 109 feet. J Foot Ankle Surg. 2009;48:675–81.
40. Beertema W, Draijer WR, van Os JJ, Pilot P. A retrospective analysis of surgical treatment in patients with symptomatic hallux rigidus: long-term follow-up. J Foot Ankle Surg. 2006;45:244–51.
41. Rajczy RM, McDonald PR, Shapiro HS, Boc SF. First metatarsophalangeal joint arthrodesis. Clin Podiatr Med Surg. 2012;29: 41–9.
42. Fadel GE, Rowley DI, Abboud RJ. Hallux metatarsophalangeal joint arthrodesis: various techniques. Foot. 2002;12:88–96.
43. DeOrio JK. Technique tip: arthrodesis of the first metatarsophalangeal joint-prevention of excessive dorsiflexsion. Foot Ankle Int. 2007;28:746–7.
44. Harisboure A, Joveniaux P, Madi K, Dehoux E. The Valenti technique in the treatment of hallux rigidus. Orthop Traumatol Surg Res. 2009;95:202–9.
45. Aas M, Johnsen TM, Finsen V. Arthrodesis of the first metatarsophalangeal joint for hallux rigidus-optimal position of fusion. Foot. 2008;18:131–5.
46. Fitzgerald JAW. A review of long-term results of arthrodesis of the first metatarsophalangeal joint. J None Joint Surg. 1969;51B: 488–93.
47. Alentorn-Geli E, Gil S, Bascuas I, Donaire MF, Boza R, Pidemunt G, Gines-Cespedosa A. Correlation of dorsiflexion angle and plantar pressure following arthrodesis of the first metatarsophalangeal joint. Foot Ankle Int. 2013;34(4):504–11.
48. Cullen NP, Angel J, Singh D, Smith J, Dudkiewicz I. Clinical tip: revision first metatarsophalangeal joint arthrodesis for sagittal plane malunion with an opening wedge osteotomy using a small fragment block plate. Foot Ankle Int. 2005;26(11):1001–3.

49. Curtis MJ, Myerson MS, Jinnah RH, Cox QG, Alexander I. Arthrodesis of the first metatarsophalangeal joint; a biomechanical study of internal fixation techniques. Foot Ankle. 1993;14(7): 395–9.
50. Coughlin MJ, Abdo RV. Arthrodesis of first metatarsophalangeal joint with Vitallium plate fixation. Foot Ankle Int. 1994;15: 18–28.
51. Riggs SA, Johnson EW. McKeever arthrodesis of the painful hallux. Foot Ankle. 1983;3(5):248–53.
52. Turan I, Lindgren U. Compression-screw arthrodesis of the first metatarsophalangeal joint of the foot. Clin Orthop Relat Res. 1987;221:292–5.
53. Gregory JL, Childers R, Higgins KR, Kyrch SM, Harkless LB. Arthrodesis of the first metatarsophalangeal joint: a review of the literature and long-term retrospective analysis. J Foot Surg. 1990;29:369–74.
54. Yu GV, Shook JE. Arthrodesis of the first metatarsophalangeal joint: current recommendations. J Am Podiatr Med Assoc. 1994; 84:266–80.
55. Smith RW, Joanis TL, Maxwell PD. Great toe metatarsophalangeal joint arthrodesis: a user friendly technique. Foot Ankle. 1992;13:367–77.
56. Hansen ST. Functional reconstruction of the foot and ankle. Philadelphia: Lippincott Williams & Wilkins; 2000. p. 343–7.
57. Bayomy AF, Aubin PM, Sangeorzan BJ, Ledoux WR. Arthrodesis of the first metatarsophalangeal joint: a robotic cadaver study of the dorsiflexion angle. J Bone Joint Surg. 2010;92:1754–64.
58. Hamilton GA, Ford LA, Patel S. First Metatarsophalangeal joint arthrodesis and revision arthrodesis. Clin Podiatr Med Surg. 2009;26:459–73.
59. Geppert MJ. Sagittal plane correction of a malunited first metatarsophalangeal arthrodesis utilizing a crescentic osteotomy. Foot Ankle Int. 1997;18(2):102.
60. Gipple K, Anspacher JC, Kopta JA. Metatarsophalangeal joint fusion of the great toe. Orthopedics. 1978;1:462–7.
61. Bingold AC. Arthrodesis of the great toe. Proc R Soc Med. 1958;51:425–7.
62. Coughlin MJ. Rheumatoid forefoot reconstruction: a long-term follow-up study. J Bone Joint Surg. 2000;82A:322–41.
63. Coughlin MJ. Arthrodesis of the first metatarsophalangeal joint. Orthop Rev. 1990;29:177–86.
64. Marks RM. Arthrodesis of the first metatarsophalangeal joint. Instr Course Lect. 2005;54:263–8.
65. Yee G, Lau J. Current concepts review: hallux rigidus. Foot Ankle Int. 2008;29:637–46.
66. Coughlin MJ. Arthrodesis of the first metatarsophalangeal joint with mini-fragment plate fixation. Orthopedics. 1990;13:1037–44.
67. Korim MT, Allen PE. Effect of pathology on union of first metatarsophalangeal joint arthrodesis. Foot Ankle Int. 2014;8:1–4. doi:10.1177/1071100714549046.
68. Berlet GC, Hyer CF, Glover JP. A retrospective review of immediate weightbearing after first metatarsophalangeal joint arthrodesis. Foot Ankle Spec. 2008;1(1):24–8.
69. Ellington JK, Jones CP, Cohen BE, Davis WH, Nickisch F, Anderson RB. Review of 107 hallux MTP joint arthrodesis using dome-shaped reamers and a stainless-steel dorsal plate. Foot Ankle Int. 2010;31(5):385–90.
70. Bennett GL, Kay DB, Sabatta J. First metatarsophalangeal joint arthrodesis : an evaluation of hardware failure. Foot Ankle Int. 2005;26:593–6.
71. Hyer CF, Glover JP, Berlet GC, Lee TH. Cost comparison of crossed screw versus dorsal plate construct for first metatarsophalangeal joint arthrodesis. J Foot Ankle Surg. 2008;47(1): 13–8.
72. Raikin SM, Ahmad J, Pour AE, Abidi M. Comparison of arthrodesis and metallic hemiarthroplasty of the hallux metatarsophalangeal joint. J Bone Joint Surg Am. 2007;89(9):1979–85.
73. Jarde O, Laya Z, Olory B, Basse G, Alovor G. Arthrodesis of the first metatarsophalangeal joint using convex and concave drills: a report on 50 cases. Acta Orthop Belg. 2005;71:76–82.
74. Johansson JE, Barrington TW. Cone arthrodesis of the first metatarsophalangeal joint. Foot Ankle. 1984;4:244–8.
75. Moore J, Berberian WS. Subaquatic reaming during arthrodesis of the first metatarsophalangeal joint to prevent thermal necrosis of bone. Orthopedics. 2014;37(6):389–91.
76. Pfeifer R, Sellei R, Pape HC. The biology of intramedullary reaming. Injury. 2010;41(2):S4–8.
77. Toksvig-Larsen S, Ryd L, Lindstrand A. On the problem of heat generation in bone cutting: studies on the effects on liquid cooling. J Bone Joint Surg Br. 1991;73(1):13–5.
78. Giannoudis PV, Snowden S, Matthews SJ, Smye SW, Smith RM. Temperature rise during reamed tibial nailing. Clin Orthop Relat Res. 2002;395:255–61.
79. Higgins TF, Casey V, Bachus K. Cortical heat generation using an irrigating/aspirating single-pass vs conventional stepwise reaming. J Orthop Trauma. 2007;21(3):192–7.
80. Kanakaris NK, Morell D, Gudipati S, Britten S, Giannoudis PV. Reaming irrigator aspirator system: early experience of its multipurpose use. Injury. 2011;42(4):S28–34.
81. Khanna A, Plessas SJ, Barrett P, Bainbridge LC. The thermal effects of Kirschner wire fixation on small bones. J Hand Surg Br. 1999;24B(3):355–7.
82. Franssen BBGM, Schuurman AH, Brouha PCR, Kon M. Hammering K-wires is superior to drilling with irrigation. Hand. 2009;4:108–12.
83. Franssen BBGM, Schuurman AH, Brouha PCR, Kon M. Drilling K-wires, what about the osteophytes? An experimental study in rabbits. Arch Orthop Trauma Surg. 2008;128:83–7.
84. Miskanen RO, Lehtimaki MY, Hamalainen MMJ, Tormala P, Rokkanen PU. Arthrodesis of the first metatarsophalangeal joint in rheumatoid arthritis biodegradable rods and Kirschner-wires in 39 cases. Acta Orthop Scand. 1993;64(1):100–2.
85. Yu GV, Gorby PO. First metatarsophalangeal joint arthrodesis. Clin Podiatr Med Surg. 2004;21:65–96.
86. Anderson JJ, Hansen M, Rowe GP, Swayzee Z. Complication rates in diabetics with first metatarsophalangeal joint arthrodesis. Diabet Foot Ankle. 2014;5. doi:10.3402/dfa.v5.24649.
87. Shibuya N, Humphers JM, Fluhman BL, Juniper DC. Factors associated with nonunion, delayed union, and malunion in foot and ankle surgery in diabetic patients. J Foot Ankle Surg. 2013; 52:53–5.
88. McCabe MP, Smyth MP, Richardson DR. Current concept review: vitamin D and stress fractures. Foot Ankle Int. 2012;33(36): 526–33.
89. Tenforde AS, Sayres LC, Sainani KL, Fredericson M. Evaluating the relationship of calcium and vitamin D in the prevention of stress fracture injuries in the young athlete: a review of the literature. PM R. 2010;2(10):945–9.
90. Groter EA, Hamdy NAT, Appelman-Dijkstra NM, Schipper IB. Bone. 2014;64:288–97.
91. Smith JT, Halim K, Palms DA, Okike K, Bluman EM, Chiodo CP. Prevalence of vitamin D deficiency in patients with foot and ankle injuries. Foot Ankle Int. 2014;35(1):8–13.
92. Brinker MR, O'Connor DP, Monla YT, Earthman TP. Metabolic and endocrine abnormalities in patients with nonunions. J Orthop Trauma. 2007;21(8):57–70.
93. Patel RA, Wilson RF, Patel PA, Palmer RM. The effect of smoking on bone healing: a systematic review. Bone Joint Res. 2013;2(6): 102–11.
94. Sorensen LT. The clinical impact of smoking and smoking cessation: a systematic review and meta-analysis. Arch Surg. 2012; 147(4):373–83.
95. Argintar E, Triantafillou K, Delahay J, Wiesel B. The musculoskeletal effects of perioperative smoking. J Am Acad Orthop Surg. 2012;20(6):359–63.

96. Lee JJ, Patel R, Beirmann S, Dougherty PJ. Current concepts review: the musculoskeletal effects of cigarette smoking. J Bone Joint Surg Am. 2013;95:850–9.
97. Wong J, Lam DP, Abrishami A, Chan MTV, Chung F. Short-term preoperative smoking cessation and postoperative complications: a systematic review and meta-analysis. Can J Anaesth. 2012;59:268–79.
98. Hope M, Savva N, Whitehouse S, Elliot R, Saxy TS. Is it necessary to re-fuse a non-union of a hallux metatarsophalangeal joint arthrodesis? Foot Ankle Int. 2010;31(8):662–9.
99. Thun JD, Keller MC, Longo D (2014) Nonunion of first metatarsophalangeal joint arthrodesis: a comparison of kirschner wire to modern osteosynthesis fixation. In: ACFAS annual scientific conference 2014, Orlando
100. Takacs IM, Swierstra BA. Pseudoarthrosis repair after failed metatarsophalangeal joint arthrodesis: turnaround inlay graft in 26 patients. Acta Orthop. 2011;82(1):114–5.
101. Baumhauer J, Pinsur MS, Donahue R, Beasley W, DiGiovanni C. Site selection and pain outcome after autologous bone graft harvest. Foot Ankle Int. 2014;35(2):104–7.
102. Fitzgibbons TC, Hawks MA, McMullen ST, Inda DJ. Bone grafting in surgery about the foot and ankle: indication and techniques. J Am Acad Orthop Surg. 2011;19(2):112–20.
103. Feeney S, Rees S, Tagoe M. Tricortical calcaneal bone graft and management of the donor site. J Foot Ankle Surg. 2007;46(2):80–5.
104. Roukis TS. A simple technique for harvesting autogenous bone grafts from the calcaneus. Foot Ankle Int. 2006;27(11):998–9.
105. DeOrio JK, Farber DC. Morbidity associated with anterior iliac crest bone grafting in foot and ankle surgery. Foot Ankle Int. 2004;25(7):451–5.
106. Mendicino RW, Leonheart E, Shromoff P. Techniques for harvesting autogenous bone graft of the lower extremity. J Foot Ankle Surg. 1996;35(5):428–35.
107. Hofbauer MH, Delmonte RJ, Scripps ML. Autogenous bone grafting. J Foot Ankle Surg. 1996;35(5):386–90.
108. Mahan KT. Calcaneal donor bone grafts. J Am Podiatr Med Assoc. 1994;84(1):1–9.
109. Qi L, Liu Y, Li H, Zhang Y. Results of 10-year follow-up of the iliac donor site of graft patients. J Int Med Res. 2014; doi:10.1177/0300060514550351.
110. Pirris SM, Nottmeier EW, Kimes S, O'Brien M, Rahmathulla G. A retrospective study of iliac crest bone grafting techniques with allograft reconstruction: do patients even know which iliac crest was harvested? J Neurosurg Spine. 2014;21(4):595–600.
111. Mahan KT, Hillstrom HJ. Bone grafting in foot and ankle surgery. A review of 300 cases. J Am Podiatr Med Assoc. 1998;88(3):109–18.
112. Nigro N, Grace D. Radiographic evaluation of bone grafts. J Foot Ankle Surg. 1996;35(5):378–85.
113. Freeman TA, Patel P, Pravizi J. Micro-CT analysis with multiple thresholds allows detection of bone formation and resorption during ultrasound-treated fracture healing. J Orthop Res. 2009;27(5):673–9.
114. Mukai S, Ito H, Nakagawa Y. Transforming growth factor-ß mediates the effects of low-intensity pulsed ultrasound in chondrocytes. Ultrasound Med Biol. 2005;31(12):1713–21.
115. Yang RS, Lin WL, Chen YZ, et al. Regulation by ultrasound treatment on the integrin expression and differentiation of osteoblasts. Bone. 2005;36:376–83.
116. Einhorn TA. Enhancement of fracture-healing. J Bone Joint Surg Am. 1995;77(6):940–56.
117. Schofer MD, Block JE, Aigner J, Schmelz A. Improved healing response in delayed unions of the tibia with low-intensity pulsed ultrasound: results of a randomized sham-controlled trial. BMC Musculoskelet Disord. 2010;11(1):229.
118. Roussignol X, Currey C, Duparc F, Dujardin F. Indications and results for the Exogen ultrasound system in the management of non-union: a 59-case pilot study. Orthop Traumatol Surg Res. 2012;98(2):206–13.
119. Gebauer D, Mayr E, Orthner E, Ryaby JP. Low-intensity pulsed ultrasound: effects on nonunions. Ultrasound Med Biol. 2005; 31(10):1391–402.
120. Cook SD, Ryaby JP, McCabe J, et al. Acceleration of tibia and distal radius fracture healing in patients who smoke. Clin Orthop Relat Res. 1997;337:198–207.
121. Leung KS, Cheung WH, Zhang C, et al. Low intensity pulsed ultrasound stimulates osteogenic activity of human periosteal cells. Clin Orthop Relat Res. 2004;418:253–9.
122. Coords M, Breitbart E, Paglia D, et al. The effects of low-intensity pulsed ultrasound upon diabetic fracture healing. J Orthop Res. 2011;29(2):181–8.
123. Kristiansen TK, Ryaby JP, McCabe J, et al. Accelerated healing of distal radial fractures with the use of specific, low-intensity ultrasound. A multicenter, prospective, randomized, double-blind, placebo-controlled study. J Bone Joint Surg Am. 1997;79(7):961–73.
124. Kumar V, Clough T. Silastic arthroplasty of the first metatarsophalangeal joint as salvage for failed revisional fusion with interpositional structural bone graft. BMJ Case Rep. 2013; doi:10.1136/bcr-2013-008993.
125. Godwin Y. Do they listen? A review of information retained by patients following consent for reduction mammoplasty. Br J Plast Surg. 2000;53(2):121–5.

14 Complications of First Metatarsal Phalangeal Joint Implants

Laurence G. Rubin and Michael Gentile

Introduction

Arthroplasty (joint replacement) of the first metatarsophalangeal joint (first MTPJ) is employed to address both deformity and arthritic conditions. Over the last 30 years, techniques and implants have evolved. Unfortunately there is a paucity of well-designed studies with adequate numbers and external validity from which to glean guidance on whether arthroplasty really is as valuable as one would like to believe [1, 2]. In fact, a recent review of the literature suggests the highest level of evidence for the treatment of hallux rigidus is around first MTPJ arthrodesis [3]. Gibson et al. present the only randomized controlled study of arthroplasty vs. arthrodesis. At 2 years follow-up, there was an overall 82% improvement with arthrodesis vs. 45% improvement with arthroplasty [1]. Nonetheless, certain trends can be appreciated and form the basis of this chapter.

Indications and Types of Implants

The goals of arthroplasty are to achieve pain relief, restore joint stability, and improve function. Further, the results should be durable and long lasting. Generally reserved for patients with lower functional demands, problems may arise when joint replacement is used in younger patients, those with greater functional expectations or demands and those with pronounced deformity. The quality of the surrounding soft tissues and bone also play a crucial role in the success or failure of these procedures [4]. Arthroplasty is a joint destructive procedure from which there is no going back and the implants themselves will have a finite life span.

The type of implant and the salvage upon failure should be taken into preoperative consideration. The implant should be convertible to a different implant or an arthrodesis. Because of the amount of the bone removed at the initial surgery, bipolar or total joint replacements will result in the greatest bone deficit and thus are more difficult to reconstruct.

Unipolar or hemi-arthroplasties have become more popular. Several case reports document the salvage of a failed phalangeal hemi-arthroplasty [5, 6]. Over the last 10 years, metatarsal head hemi-arthroplasties have been more widely used. Both of these options supposedly limit the amount of bone resection and thus the amount of bone loss to be replaced should failure occur, making salvage technically easier and potentially more successful.

Modes of Failure

Failure is defined by a loss of function due to pain, joint instability, or disturbance of the metatarsal weight-bearing parabola. There are times when surgeon bias or the impressive nature of radiographic changes may prompt the patient to believe there is a failure, although the three criteria above have not been met. This is an important point. Salvage of a failed first MTPJ arthroplasty is a challenging procedure and should be approached with sound judgement, advanced surgical skill, and realistic expectations [7].

The type of implant material plays a crucial role in the mode of failure. Silicone of the past presented with varying degrees of detritic synovitis and cystic changes in the bone due to shards of silicone breaking loose over time [8, 9] (Fig. 14.1). Contemporary silicone implants hold up better and reports of such failure have diminished. In addition, the introduction of titanium grommets also improved the situation [10, 11]. There can still be bone erosion secondary to the movement of the implant within the bone (Fig. 14.2).

Metallic implants may still present with a similar detritic reaction, but more often peri-implant lysis and secondary loosening of the implant. Subsidence of the implant can occur

L.G. Rubin (✉)
7016 Lee Park Road, Suite 105, Mechanicsville, VA 23111, USA
e-mail: Lgrubin@comcast.net

M.Gentile
Westside Foot and Ankle Specialists, 9900 SW Hall Boulevard Suite #100, Tigard, OR 97223

M.S. Lee, J.P. Grossman (eds.), *Complications in Foot and Ankle Surgery*, DOI 10.1007/978-3-319-53686-6_14

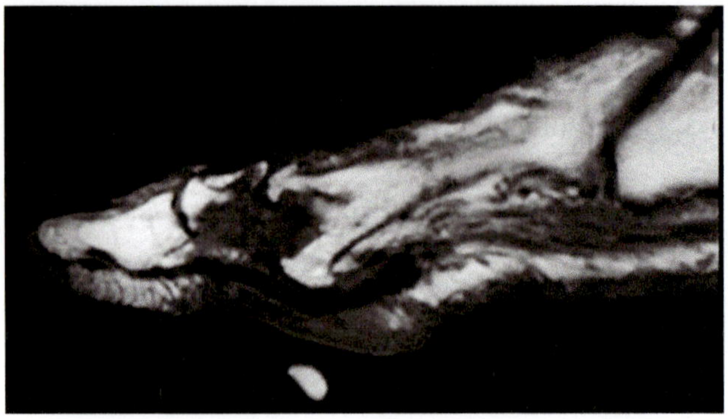

Fig. 14.1 Detritic synovitis from a silicone implant

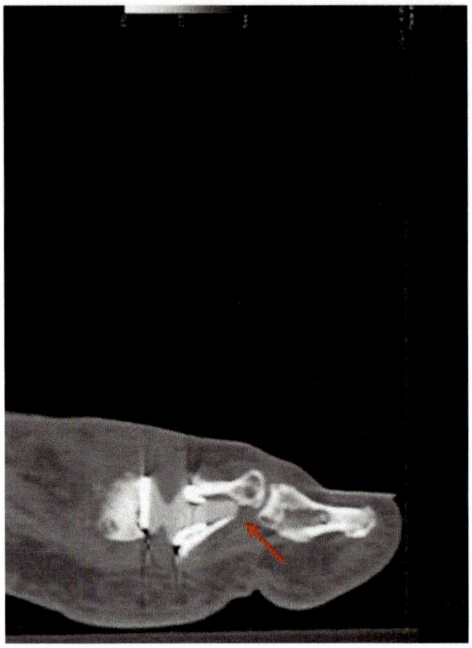

Fig. 14.2 Erosion of the plantar aspect of the proximal phalanx (*red arrow*)

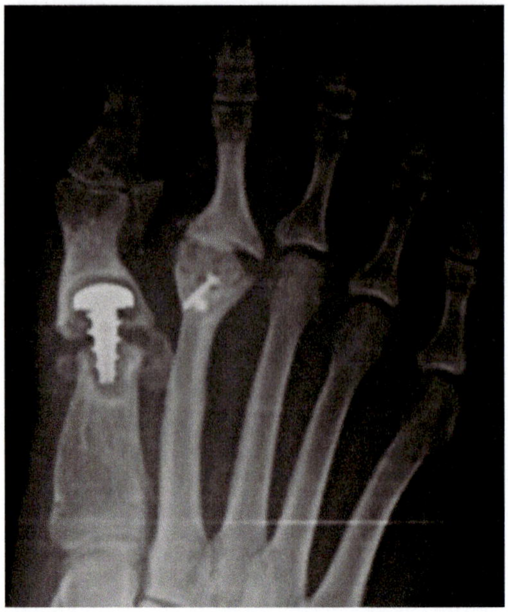

Fig. 14.3 Loosening and subsidence of a hemi-implant

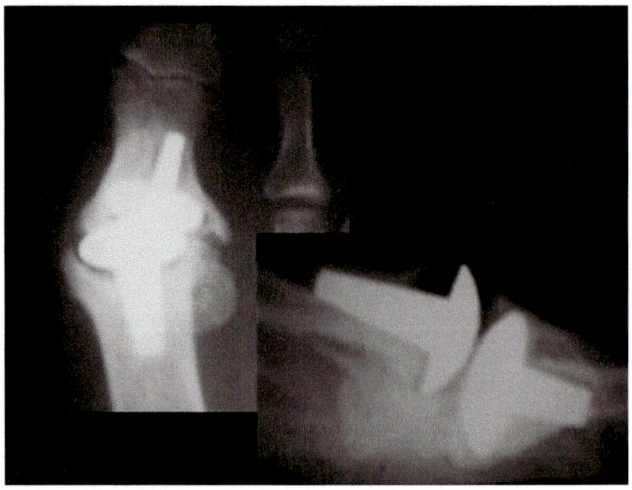

Fig. 14.4 Loosening of the implant in the head of the metatarsal and subsidence of the implant into the base of the proximal phalanx

in hemi- and total implants. This will often have significant bony destruction. Even in the case of a hemi-arthroplasty, bone loss can be significant enough that revision requires the use of a structural bone graft to restore normal metatarsal weight-bearing parabola [5, 12, 13] (Figs. 14.3 and 14.4).

As with any arthroplasty, the dreaded complication is infection. The literature specifically on the incidence of infection with first MTPJ arthroplasty is scant, but the percentages in the available case reports suggest it is quite low [14]. Furthermore, there is no evidence-based algorithmic approach to addressing infection, and protocols have been extrapolated from the hip and knee literature.

Workup

A thorough history will often guide the surgeon as to why the implant may have failed. Most patients will present with pain. This may be in the first MTPJ or elsewhere, for example, with sub-second metatarsal pain. A thorough understanding of the subjective issues must be complimented with an appreciation of the patient's expectations.

Signs and symptoms of infection (local and systemic) should be noted and addressed appropriately. History of a draining sinus tract over the joint is ominous and should heighten concerns that an infection, either fulminant or occult, is present.

Clinical Evaluation

The first step is to evaluate for signs of infection. The cardinal signs of inflammation may represent infection but may also be due simply to implant loosening or reactive synovitis or inflammation from the implant material. Any evidence of an open wound or draining sinus tract should be fully inspected and in and of itself is an indication for surgical exploration [15].

Once the likelihood of infection has been addressed, the next step is to assess for contributing proximal pathology. Ankle equinus and clinically significant hindfoot or midfoot deformity or instability may both contribute to the implant's failure. These should be fully evaluated and addressed at the time of revision [16].

Deformity and functional derangement of the first ray must be evaluated. First ray hypermobility should be taken into consideration and addressed. Deformity in the first MTPJ may present as hallux valgus and/or hallux malleus. Flexibility of these deformities will determine the optimal procedure(s).

Lesser MTPJ pain may be the chief complaint. Evaluation for MTPJ instability (plantar plate and/or collateral ligaments) and the existence of digital deformities should be considered and addressed appropriately.

Imaging

Weight-bearing plain films are evaluated for the presence of peri-implant lucency (Fig. 14.4). This likely suggests instability but should also be considered as a sign of infection if coupled with other clinical evidence. An inventory of bone loss and disturbance of the weight-bearing parabola is taken and severity determined. This is an essential component of the evaluation as this will have a profound impact on the reconstructive plan. With defects of >1 cm, serious consideration should be given for a staged reconstruction. Acute correction of defects of this size or larger may result in vascular and/or neural injury.

In the case of hallux valgus, standard radiographic evaluation is undertaken noting severity and apex of deformity. As first MTPJ arthrodesis is the most common salvage procedure, one can anticipate between 5 and 8° of IM correction [17]. The hallux interphalangeal joint (HIPJ) is evaluated for deformity in all three planes as well as for arthritis.

Laboratory Data

If an infection is suspected, an aspiration of the joint is recommended. The presence of purulence is not diagnostic of infection. In the case of metal on metal (MoM) implants, it may be indicative of a foreign body reaction. Fluid is evaluated for cultures (aerobic, anaerobic, fungal, AFB) and sensitivities. WBC and differential is evaluated as well. A synovial WBC >3000/mL and polymorphonuclear cells (PMNs) >80% have the highest accuracy and sensitivity for infection [18].

Evaluation of the erythrocyte sedimentation rate (ESR) and C-reactive protein (CRP) are also in order. ESR of >30 mm/h and CRP > 10 mg/dL are highly suggestive of infection. Taken together, the sensitivity for infection is estimated to be 93% and warrants further investigation [15]. In this instance, surgery is usually indicated to get synovial culture and biopsy. A negative culture doesn't rule out infection. In addition, an elevated synovial CRP has been reported to have an accuracy of 91% [15]. In addition to a positive culture, this can be the impetus to start an infected implant treatment protocol.

Procedures

There are four options for treatment for failed implants of the first metatarsal phalangeal joint: maintain the implant, removal of the implant and reimplantation at a later date, removal of implant, or arthrodesis. The decision of which option to choose will be determined by the diagnosis, quality of the soft tissues and bone, and whether there is an infection. An arthrodesis is the most definitive of these procedures but can be a challenging surgery. Hecht et al. [19] showed that arthrodesis of a failed silicone implant improved patient's average walking tolerance, ability to wear shoes, and overall level of satisfaction. Garras et al. [5] followed 18 patients that were converted from a failed hemi-arthroplasty to a fusion. They showed that the VAS pain score went from 0.75 to 7.8 out of 10.

The surgeon should attain adequate intraoperative range of motion during implant surgery of the first metatarsal phalangeal joint. It is essential to make sure that enough bone has been removed, the implant is well placed, and the sesamoids are gliding. There are times when the postoperative motion is significantly reduced even when good surgical technique has been followed. Patients should be educated on range of motion exercises preoperatively and instructed to do range of motion exercises in the immediate postoperative period to prevent arthrofibrosis and limitation of joint range of motion. Conservative measures should be attempted as soon as loss of motion becomes evident. Physical therapy for range of motion exercises combined with ultrasound may be used in conjunction with cortisone injections. When cortisone injections are used, injectables that do not contain crystals are recommended; crystals can be destructive to the implant. When there is no improvement in the range of motion or continued loss of motion, closed manipulation of the joint under anesthesia can be attempted. Doing a local block and attempting this in the office are not advised as this can be painful and the patient will guard preventing the motion from being attained. An open arthrotomy with debridement of the fibrosis can be used, but the authors have not found this to be very successful. There are times when inadequate bone resection is preventing motion (Fig. 14.5).

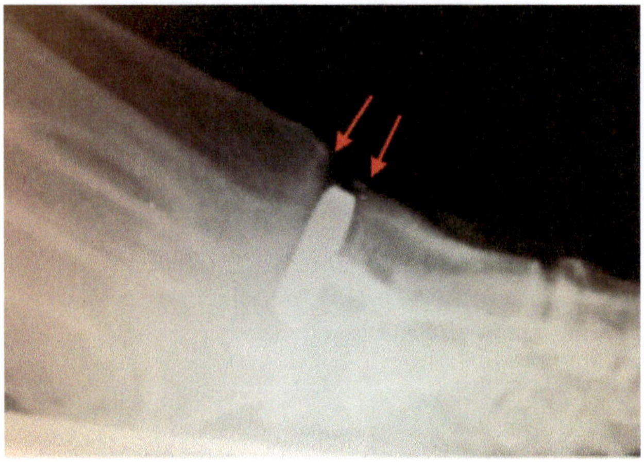

Fig. 14.5 Arrows demonstrating inadequate bone resection, preventing range of motion

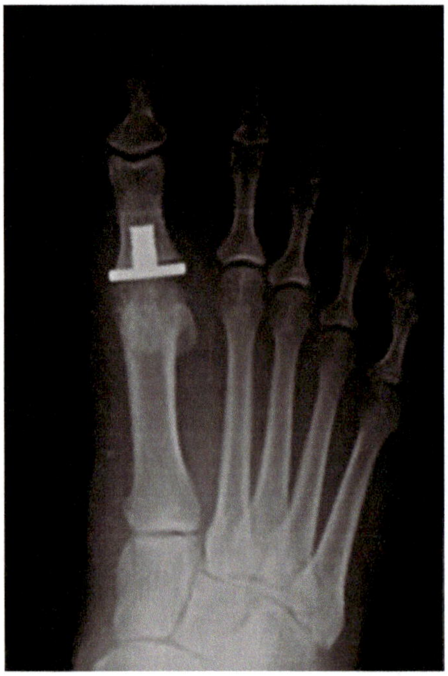

Fig. 14.6 There is no joint space after insertion of hemi-implant

These cases will require revision surgery with adequate debridement to allow for improved range of motion. If there is continued loss of motion, but no pain, the patient may opt to live with the implant and limited range of motion. For those patients that have pain along with the loss of motion, arthrodesis is usually the best option. Patients that have had a hemi-implant can be converted to a total implant. The authors have found that there is often a significant loss of joint space in failed hemi-implants (Figs. 14.6 and 14.7). This may prevent successful conversion to a total implant and necessitate an arthrodesis.

Postoperative hematoma can occur in implant surgery and should be addressed sooner than later. The hematoma can lead

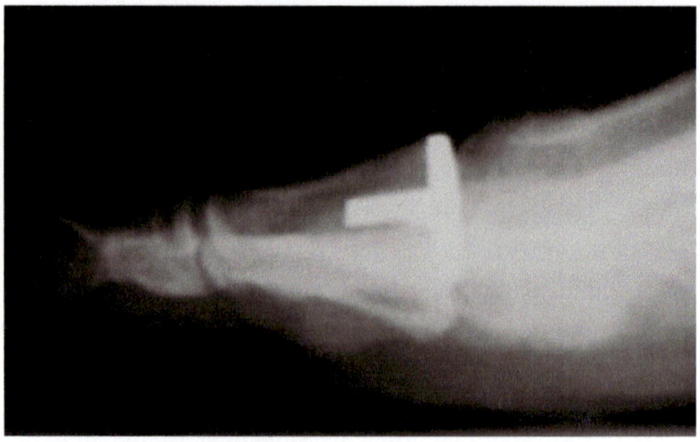

Fig. 14.7 Loss of joint space after insertion of hemi-implant

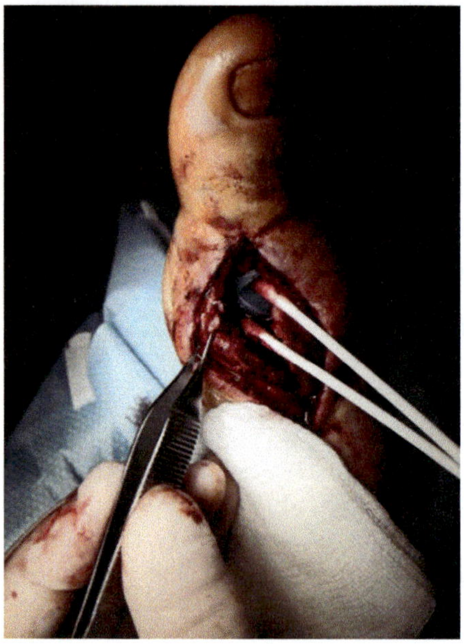

Fig. 14.8 Postoperative hematoma

to dehiscence, fibrosis with limited range of motion, and infection. It is advisable to perform an incision and drainage if the hematoma does not resolve quickly. During the procedure a thorough lavage along with a culture and sensitivity should be performed (Fig. 14.8). If there is no infection, the implant can be left in place. In cases where there is a postoperative infection, the implant should be removed.

Postoperative infection is another complication that can occur and will need to be treated by thorough debridement and lavage along with appropriate antibiotic coverage. Consideration should be given to a prolonged course of antibiotics. The infection will need to be completely eliminated prior to doing the revision surgery. It is recommended to wait for several weeks before proceeding with the revision whether it is reimplantation or arthrodesis to ensure there is no recurrence of infection. A spacer made of antibiotic-loaded bone cement should be used to help maintain the position and joint space between the metatarsal head and the base of the proximal phalanx especially if reim-

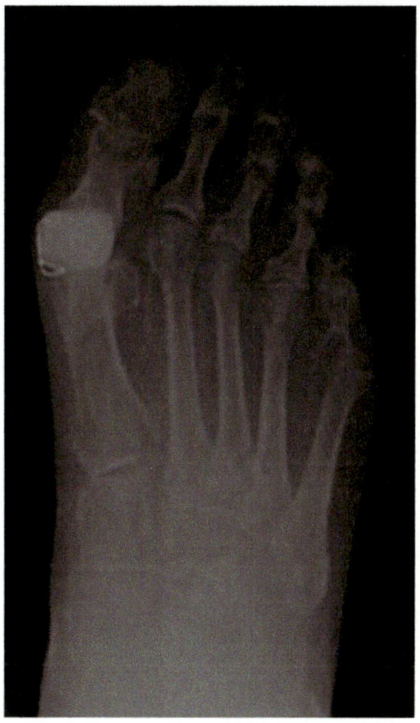

Fig. 14.9 Antibiotic cement spacer after removal of an infected total implant in the first metatarsal phalangeal joint

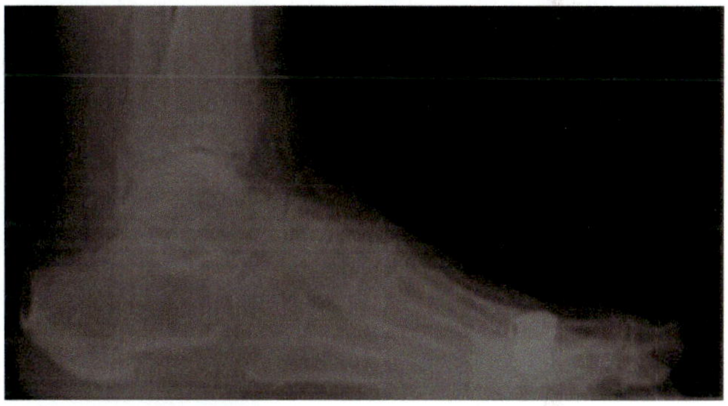

Fig. 14.10 Antibiotic cement spacer after removal of an infected total implant in the first metatarsal phalangeal joint

plantation is being considered (Figs. 14.9 and 14.10). This will also provide increased local antibiotic delivery.

Subsidence, bone over growth, or implant failure can occur over time. These can be handled by either excisional implant arthroplasty or conversion to an arthrodesis. Excisional implant arthroplasty will give the patient a short toe and will most likely not be a stable platform for propulsion (Figs. 14.11 and 14.12).

Arthrodesis can be a technically challenging procedure but will allow the surgeon to maintain length and provide stability to the hallux, which will aid in propulsion. Once the decision to remove the implant and convert to an arthrodesis has been made, the surgeon will need to decide whether the patient will need a bone block graft to maintain length or whether an end to end fusion is possible. Even if an end-to-end fusion is planned, it is advised to be prepared to have grafting material available to fill in the bone defects from the implant removal. Garras et al. [5] required bone graft in all 18 fusions. Both Garras [5] and Gross [20] showed there was a longer time to fusion than a primary arthrodesis. Gross [20] also had a 58% reoperation rate in their study. Fusions, after implant failure, should follow the same basic surgical principles as any other fusion. The surgeon must debride to healthy bleeding bone and fixate the fusion. The debridement will often remove more bone than anticipated. In cases where a bone block graft is used, the fusion should be fixated with a plate (Figs. 14.13, 14.14, 14.15, 14.16, and 14.17).

In conclusion complications of implants in the first metatarsal phalangeal joint can and do occur. It is important to get the appropriate testing to make the correct diagnoses and be sure the surgeon understands the extent of the bone damage. The surgeon will have several choices on what procedure to perform. Revision surgery of a failed first metatarsal phalan-

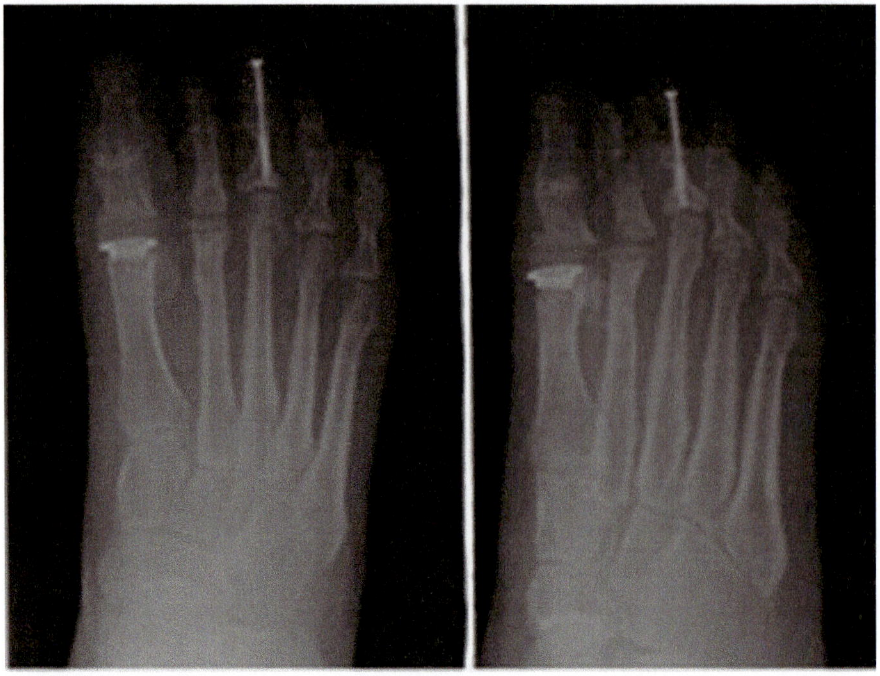

Fig. 14.11 Failed implant of the first metatarsal phalangeal joint

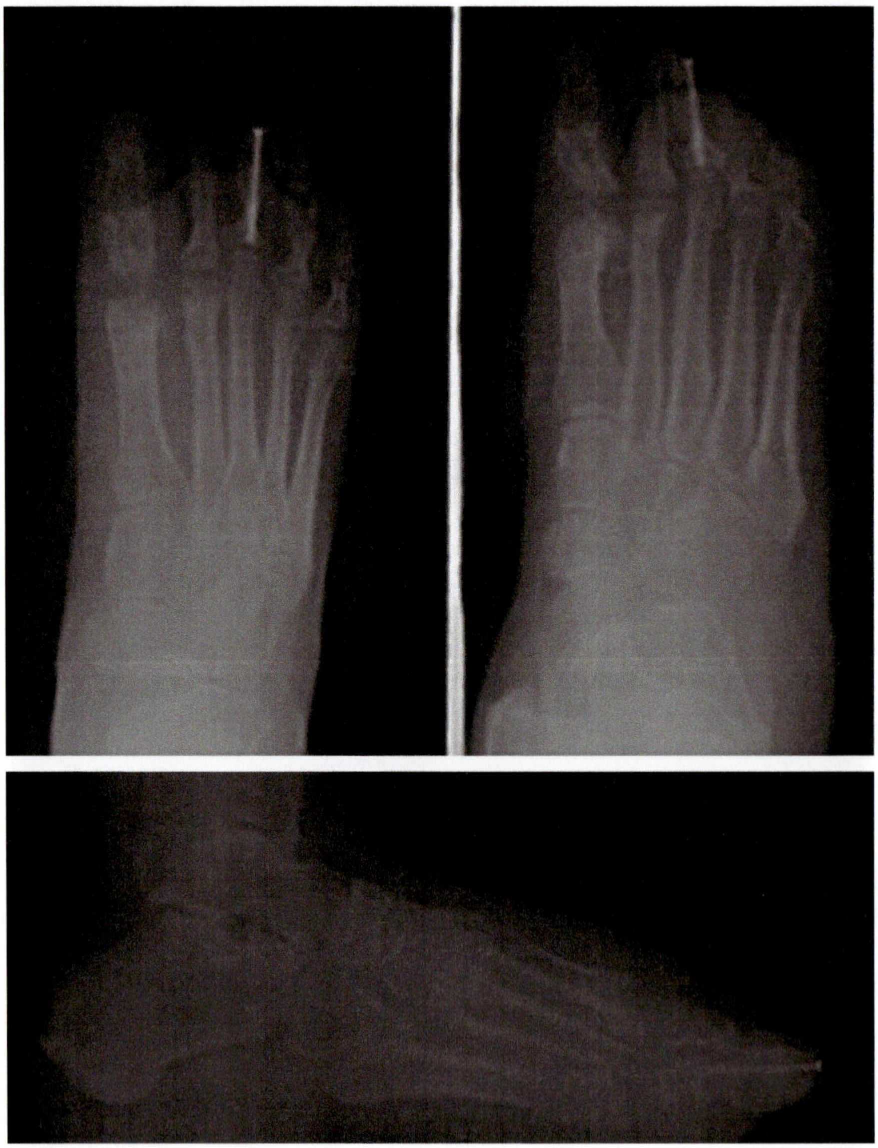

Fig. 14.12 Resection implant arthroplasty

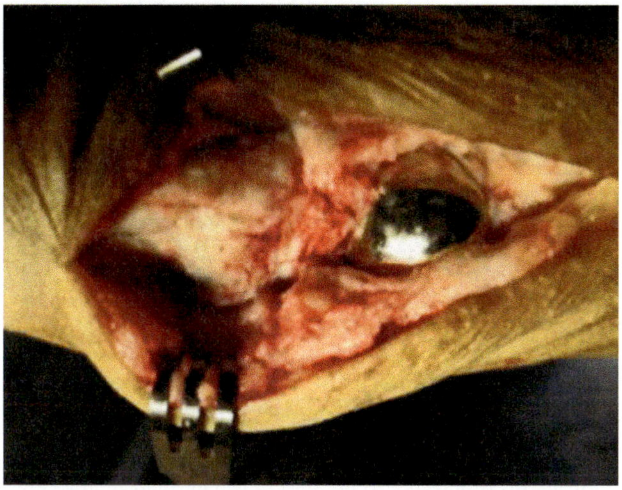

Fig. 14.13 Subsidence of implant

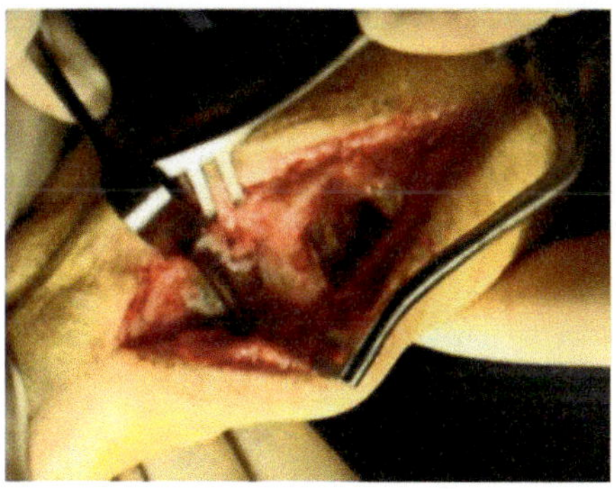

Fig. 14.14 Removal of the proximal part of the implant. Notice the distal aspect is still in place

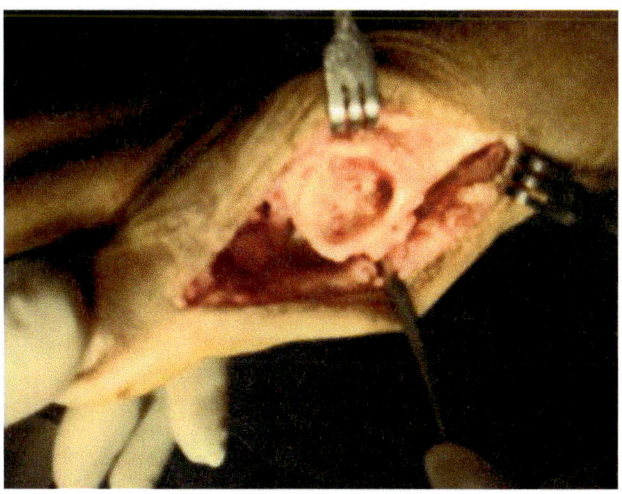

Fig. 14.15 Debridement of the bone after the implant is totally removed

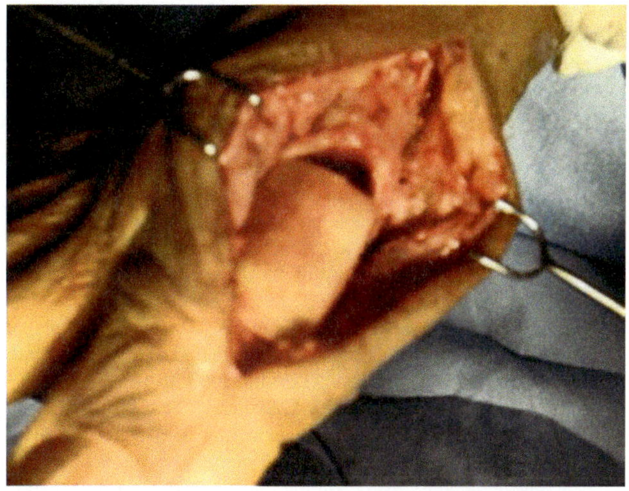

Fig. 14.16 Bone block in place, filling in the defect created by the implant removal

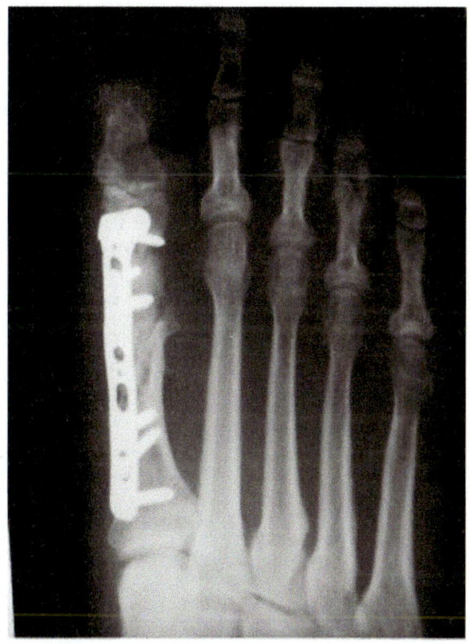

Fig. 14.17 X-ray of final result

geal implant can be a challenging procedure; careful preoperative planning is essential to the outcome.

References

1. Gibson JN, Thomson CE. Arthrodesis or total replacement arthroplasty for hallux rigidus: a randomized controlled trial. Foot Ankle Int. 2005;26(9):680–90.
2. Cook E, Cook J, Rosenblum B, Landsman A, Giurini J, Basile P. Meta-analysis of first metatarsophalangeal joint implant arthroplasty. J Foot Ankle Surg. 2009;48(2):180–90.

3. McNeil DS, Baumhauer JF, Glazebrook MA. Evidence-based analysis of the efficacy for operative treatment of hallux rigidus. Foot Ankle Int. 2013;34(1):15–32.
4. Fuhrmann RA, Wagner A, Anders JO. First metatarsophalangeal joint replacement: the method of choice for end stage hallux rigidus? Foot Ankle Clin. 2003;8:711–21.
5. Garras DN, Durinka JB, Bercik M, Miller AG, Raikin SM. Conversion arthrodesis for failed first metatarsophalangeal joint hemiarthroplasty. Foot Ankle Int. 2013;34(9):1227–32.
6. Raikin SM, Ahmad J, Pour AE, Abidi N. Comparison of arthrodesis and metallic hemiarthroplasty of the hallux metatarsophalangeal joint. J Bone Joint Surg Am. 2007;899:1979–85.
7. Myerson MS, Schon LC, Mcguigan FX, Oznur A. Results of arthrodesis of the hallux metatarsophalangeal joint using bone graft for restoration of length. Foot Ankle Int. 2000;21(4):297–306.
8. Patel DC, Frascone ST, DeLuca A. Synovitis secondary to silicone elastomeric joint implant. J Foot Ankle Surg. 1994;33(6):628–32.
9. Pugliese D, Bush D, Harrington T. Silicone synovitis: longer term outcome data and review of the literature. J Clin Rheumatol. 2009;15(1):8–11.
10. Schmidt K, Willburger R, Ossowski A, Miehlke RK. The effect of the additional use of grommets in silicone implant arthroplasty of the metatacarpophalangeal joints. J Hand Surg Br. 1999;24(5):561–4.
11. Sebold EJ, Cracchiolo A. Use of titanium grommets in silicone implant arthroplasty of the hallux metatarsophalangeal joint. Foot Ankle Int. 1996;17(3):145–51.
12. Anakwe RE, Middleton SD, Thomson CE, McKinley JC. Hemiarthroplasty augmented with bone graft for the failed hallux metatarsophalangeal silastic implant. Foot Ankle Int. 2011;17(3):e43–6.
13. Hopson M, Stone P, Paden M. First metatarsal head osteoarticular transfer system for salvage of a failed hemicap-implant: a case report. J Foot Ankle Surg. 2009;48:483–7.
14. Stone PA, Barnes ES, Savage T, Paden M. Late hematogenous infection of first metatarsophalangeal joint replacement: a case presentation. J Foot Ankle Surg. 2010;49:489.e1–4.
15. Parvizi J, Adeli B, Zmistowski B, Restrepo C, Greenwald AS. Management of periprosthetic joint infection: the current knowledge: AAOS exhibit selection. JBJS Am. 2012;94(14):e104.
16. Greisberg J. The failed first metatarsophalangeal joint arthroplasty. Foot Ankle Clin. 2014;19(3):343–8.
17. Pydah SK, Toh EM, Sirikonda SP, Walker CR. Intermetatarsal angular change following fusion of the first metatarsophalangeal joint. Foot Ankle Int. 2009;30(5):415–8.
18. Spangehl MJ, Masri BA, O'Connell JX, Duncan CP. Prospective analysis of preoperative and intraoperative investigations for the diagnosis of infection at the sites of two hundred and two revision total hip arthroplasties. J Bone Joint Surg Am. 1999;81(5):672–83.
19. Hecht PJ, Gibbons MJ, Wapner KL, Cooke C, Hoisington SA. Arthrodesis of the first metatarsophalangeal joint to salvage failed silicone implant arthroplasty. Foot Ankle Int. 1997;18(7):383–90.
20. Gross CE, Hsu AR, Lin J, Holmes GB, Lee S. Revision MTP arthrodesis for failed MTP arthroplasty. Foot Ankle Spec. 2013;6(6):471–8.

15 The Lapidus

Byron Hutchinson

Introduction

The Lapidus procedure was first described in 1911 by Dr. Albrecht and then popularized by Paul Lapidus in 1934 [1, 2]. From 1934 to 1976, there were a number of authors that advocated this procedure in extreme cases, but the procedure was not a "mainstream" technique until it became repopularized by Clark, Veith, and Hansen in Seattle in 1987 [3]. They reported on a long-term retrospective review of 32 ft. They had a high recurrence rate, which led to some modifications in the technique [3]. In 1989, Sangeorzan and Hansen reported retrospectively on 40 ft with additional technique modifications. They felt that this procedure was indicated for revision and when there was significant "hypermobility" of the first ray [4]. In the past decade or two, the Lapidus has become a popular revisional as well as an index procedure for hallux valgus surgery because of its versatility and low complication profile [5–8]. Nevertheless, complications do occur when performing a Lapidus, and this chapter will emphasize how to manage the most common complications attributed to this procedure.

Complications when performing the Lapidus procedure are generally not considered catastrophic, and revision techniques can be extremely successful. The most common complication is nonunion, which has been reported at 3–12% [5–8]. Elevation and shortening of the first ray has also been described as complications of the Lapidus procedure [4–6]. Undercorrection and overcorrection can also be problematic when performing the Lapidus or any hallux valgus procedure [9–11].

B. Hutchinson (✉)
Department of Ortho, CHI/Fransiscan Health System, Spine and Foot and Ankle, Saint Francis Hospital, Federal Way, WA 98003, USA
e-mail: byronhutchinson@chifranciscan.org

Indications

The primary indication for performing a Lapidus is first ray insufficiency (hypermobility). There is no specific way to measure or quantify first ray insufficiency, and the surgeon must rely on a continuum of clinical and radiographic parameters to assess a patient for this condition (Table 15.1).

This has been described best as a syndrome and is a collection of signs and symptoms that occur clinically and are caused by dynamic imbalance between the first and second metatarsal segments to transmit body weight [12–15]. Failure to recognize the importance of first ray function can result in postoperative complications or recurrence. Probably the most reliable clinical indicator to test first ray insufficiency is the windlass activation test [16] (Figs. 15.1, 15.2, 15.3, and 15.4). The windlass mechanism has been shown to directly affect stability of the first ray, and this dynamic test can elucidate the presence of insufficiency of the first ray [17, 18].

Patients who have benign hypermobile joint syndrome or any mixed connective tissue disease are also prime candidates for this procedure (Figs. 15.5 and 15.6). Juvenile hallux valgus patients with physeal plate closure do well with this technique. In addition, patients with hallux valgus and residual metatarsus adductus do extremely well with a Lapidus procedure (Figs. 15.7 and 15.8).

Contraindications/Limitations

The foot and ankle surgeon today cannot consider any fusion procedure without a high index of suspicion for metabolic bone disorders or in the management and cessation of smoking. The effects of nicotine on bone healing have been well established, and in recent years greater attention has been placed on vitamin D deficiency, thyroid problems, and the effect of medications on bone healing. Correction of these disorders prior to performing the index Lapidus procedure is

M.S. Lee, J.P. Grossman (eds.), *Complications in Foot and Ankle Surgery*, DOI 10.1007/978-3-319-53686-6_15

Table 15.1 Clinical and radiographic parameters for hypermobility

Clinical findings	Radiographic findings
Hypermobility first ray (benign hypermobile joint syndrome)	Increased obliquity of the first metatarsal cuneiform joint
Diffuse callus sub-second	Intercuneiform split
Metatarsalgia	Thickening of cortex second metatarsal
Plantar plate insufficiency (Lachman test positive)	Plantar gapping at the first metatarsal cuneiform joint
Second digital deformity (sagittal or frontal plane)	Second metatarsal stress fracture

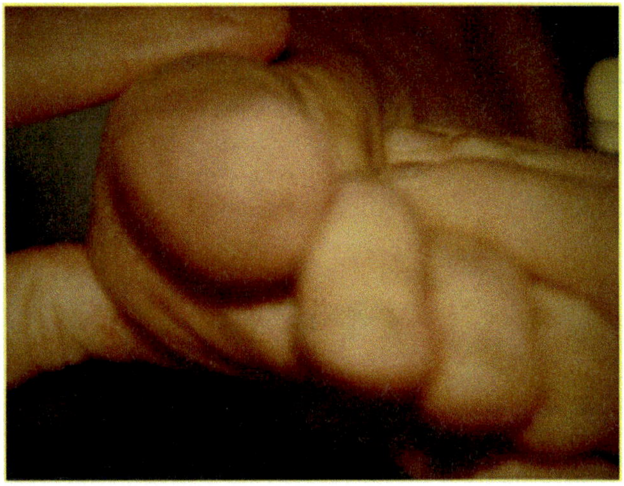

Fig. 15.1 Windlass activation test. Traditional first ray examination showing elevation of the first ray

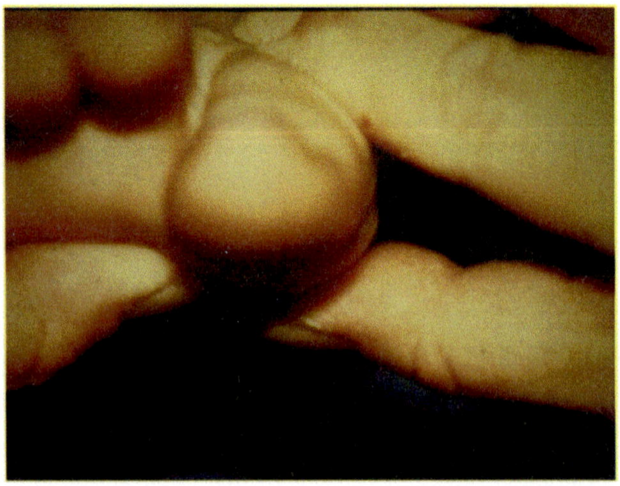

Fig. 15.2 Windlass activation test. Traditional first ray examination showing plantarflexion

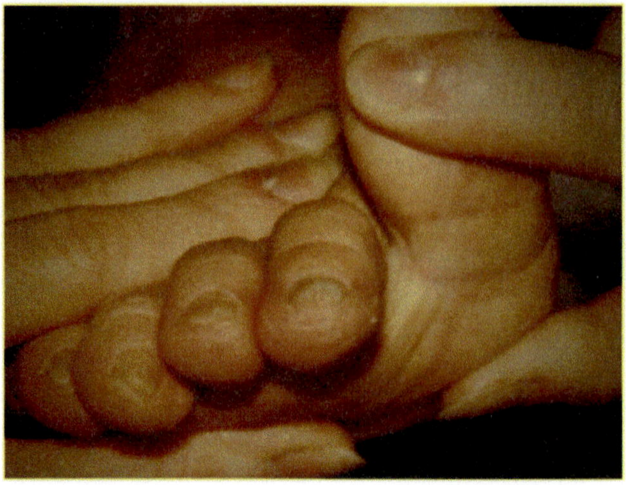

Fig. 15.3 Windlass activation test showing elevation of the first ray with the hallux dorsiflexed to engage the windlass mechanism

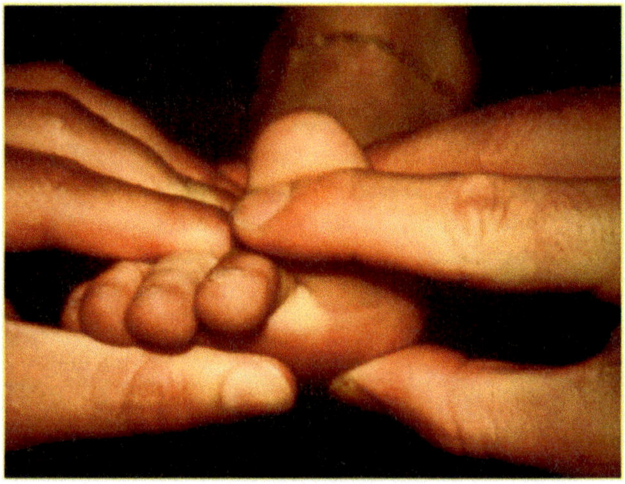

Fig. 15.4 Windlass activation test showing plantarflexion of the first ray with dorsiflexion of the hallux to engage the windlass mechanism

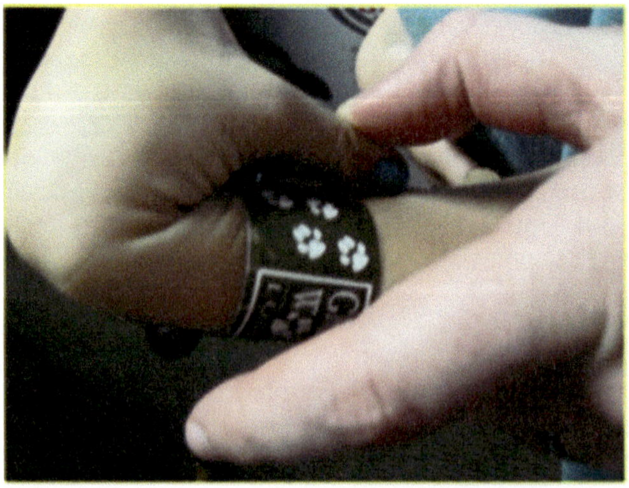

Fig. 15.5 Testing for Benign hypermobile joint syndrome

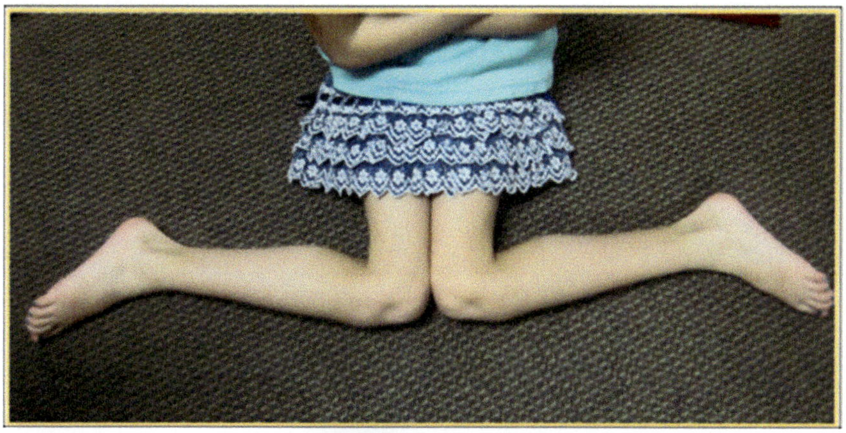

Fig. 15.6 Testing for Benign hypermobile joint syndrome

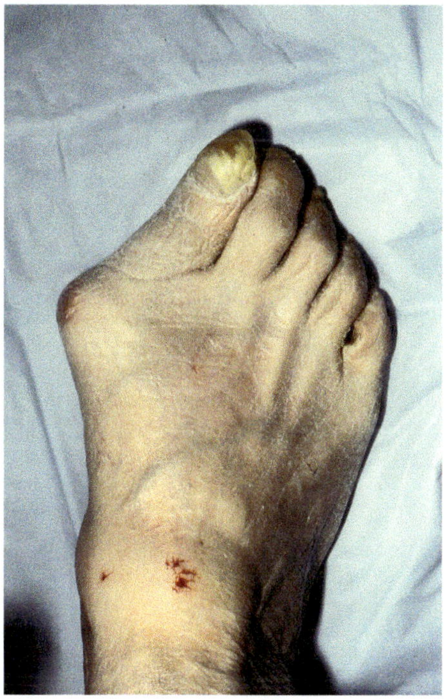

Fig. 15.7 Hallux valgus with metatarsus adductus

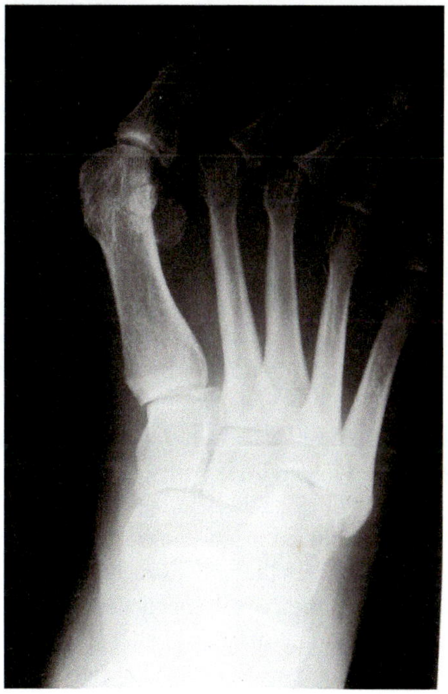

Fig. 15.8 Hallux valgus with Metatarsus adductus

critical to avoid some of the complications that will be discussed in this chapter.

Technique Pearls and Pitfalls

Although there is regional variation in the performance of the Lapidus arthrodesis, there are some universal technique pearls that can help to minimize complications and pitfalls in performing the procedure. Placement of the incision more dorsal medial can help to avoid nerve entrapment and can increase visualization of the entire dorsal to plantar dimensions of the joint (Fig. 15.9). This can help in resection of bone along the long axis of the metatarsal so as not to elevate the first metatarsal by not resecting enough bone from the plantar aspect of the joint. Adequate joint exposure and mobility are extremely important to be able to reduce the deformity in all three planes, and utilization of a small osteotome to free the plantar ligament structures can assist in obtaining this exposure and mobility of the bony segments for reduction.

Bony resection needs to be perpendicular to the long axis of the first metatarsal and the cuneiform to avoid excessive shortening and elevation of the first metatarsal, which are frequent complications reported with this procedure [20, 27]. In addition, nonunion of the Lapidus can occur because of poor joint preparation. Often, there is sclerosis of the subchondral plate, and poor preparation of the fusion site can be

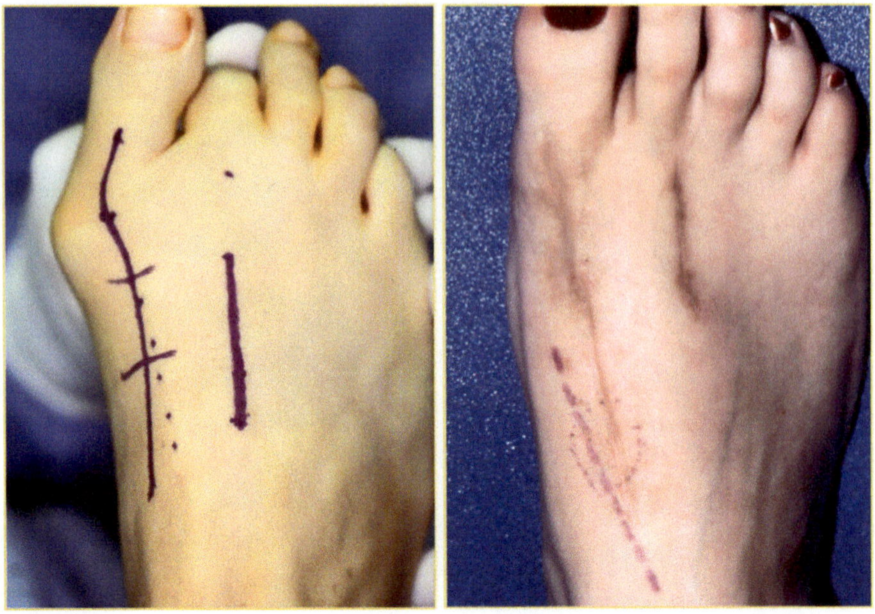

Fig. 15.9 The dorsal medial incision on the left helps to avoid nerve entrapments that are more common with the traditional dorsal approach shown on the right

a major factor in the development of a nonunion. Resection of this sclerotic subchondral plate is key in helping to prevent nonunion of the fusion site [19, 20] (Figs. 15.10 and 15.11). Curettage techniques for joint preparation are still popular, but the author prefers bony resection in most cases to ensure good bleeding surfaces instead of the risk that a sclerotic subchondral plate has been "fish scaled" or fenestrated with lack of adequate blood supply for bony union. Some have argued that by leaving the subchondral plate intact, it provides more stability at the fusion site. This may be true with the crossed screw technique, but with recent advancements in plate fixation constructs, stability is excellent without preservation of the subchondral plate.

Correction of the intermetatarsal angle is usually accomplished by removing more bone on the lateral aspect of the articular surface of the cuneiform (Fig. 15.12). When there is difficulty with reduction of the IM angle, one easy technique is to resect a small portion of bone off of the lateral flare of the first metatarsal base to help "morits" the arthrodesis site (Fig. 15.13).

There are a couple of key points regarding alignment of the fusion site to consider. Certainly reduction of the intermetatarsal angle is the primary consideration, but rotation and translation of the metatarsal head are equally important and often overlooked. Using a small *K*-wire as a "joystick" can help in relocation of the sesamoids underneath the first metatarsal head by rotating the metatarsal out of valgus malalignment [21, 22] (Fig. 15.14). In addition, the entire metatarsal segment can be translated in a plantar direction a few millimeters to make up for some shortening of the metatarsal during the cartilage resection. Small *K*-wires can be used on either side of the first metatarsal base to temporarily stabilize the fusion and to check under fluoroscopy prior to final fixation (Fig. 15.14).

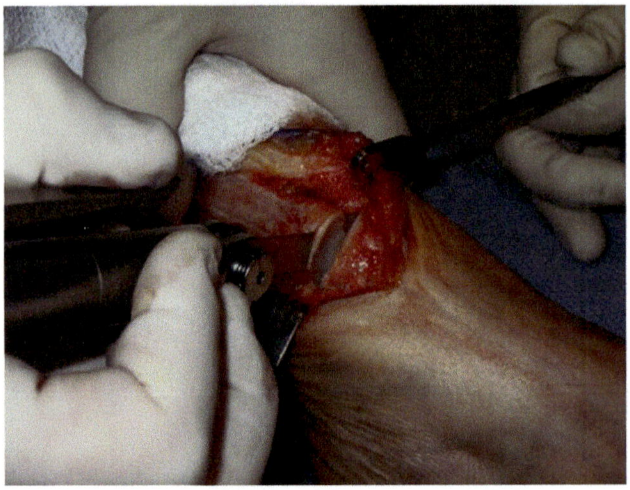

Fig. 15.10 Demonstrating the resection of the subchondral bone plate with excellent dorsal to plantar exposure. Minimal bone resection is performed on the metatarsal side of the joint

Traditional stacked screw fixation is still widely utilized, but interfragmentary screw and plate fixation has gained popularity in recent years [23, 24]. Delivery of one interfragmentary screw and plate supplementation on the plantar medial aspect of the fusion is an extremely stable construct and allows for early loading of the extremity [25, 26] (Fig. 15.15). The anterior tibial tendon attachment is extremely broad in this area, and the plate can be put just under the attachment by elevating a small flap and in some cases directly over the tendon attachment without compromise to the tendon.

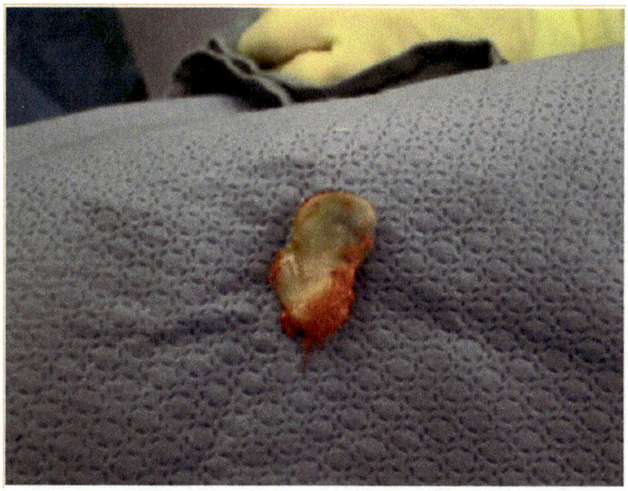

Fig. 15.11 The entire cartilaginous surface has been removed from the first metatarsal base with a small amount of subchondral bone especially at the periphery of the saddle-shaped joint

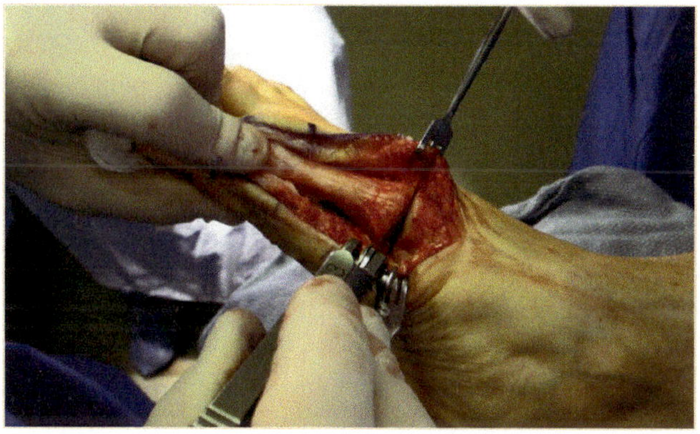

Fig. 15.12 The resection of the cuneiform involves taking more bone laterally to correct the IM angle and reduce the deformity. Note that some of the medial cartilage is left so as not to remove too much subchondral bone. This medial cartilage can then be removed with a small curette

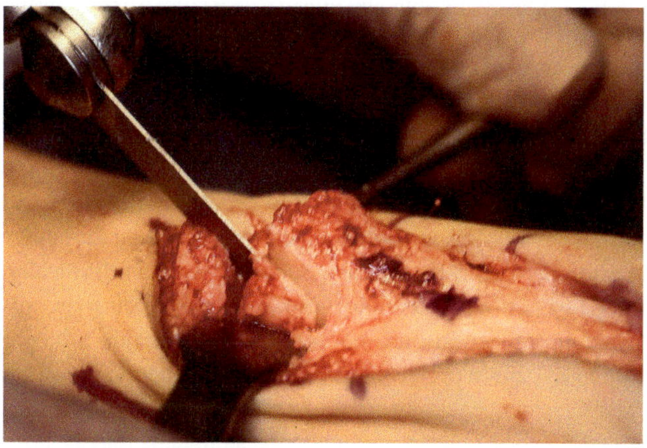

Fig. 15.13 Resection of a small amount of the lateral flare at the base of the metatarsal can help to reduce the IM angle and to "mortis" the medial cuneiform, first metatarsal and second metatarsal base

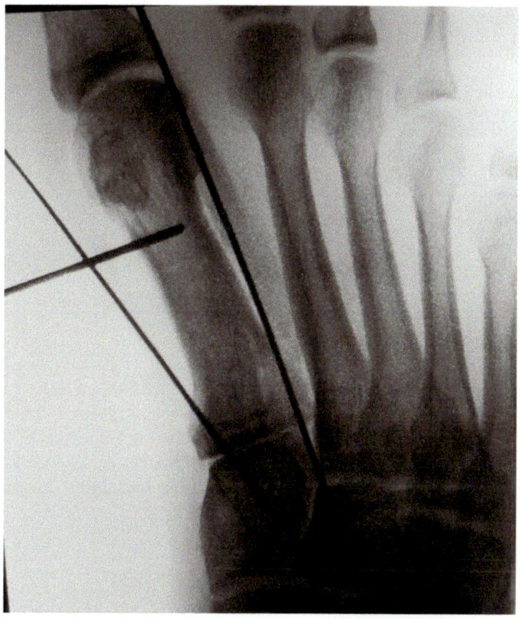

Fig. 15.14 The *K*-wire traversing the metatarsal is used to derotate the first metatarsal. The *K*-wire is moved in a cephalad direction until the metatarsal is brought directly under the sesamoids. The other *K*-wires are used to temporarily maintain this position prior to definitive fixation

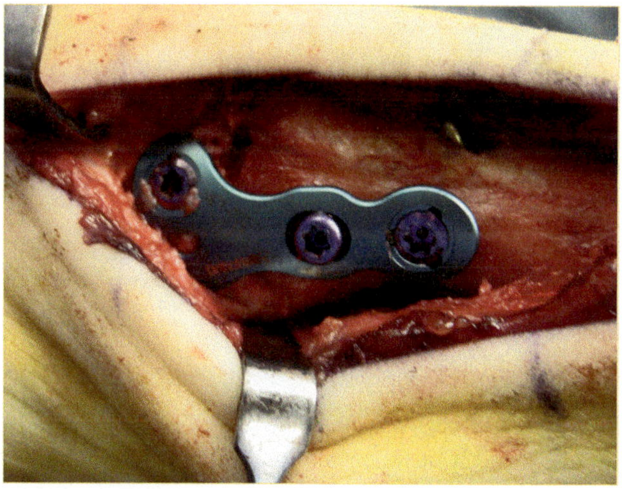

Fig. 15.15 This figure demonstrates the typical construct with one interfragmentary screw from dorsal distal to plantar proximal across the fusion site and then placement of a plate along the plantar medial aspect of the fusion site. Note that this is placed under the expansions of the anterior tibial tendon

Nonunion

Nonunion is the most frequent complication reported in the performance of a Lapidus arthrodesis [4–7, 27]. The nonunion rate has been estimated to be between 5.3 and 12% [4–7, 27]. As was previously outlined, this particular complication has a number of etiological factors that can contribute to its occurrence. Correction of any metabolic causes prior to

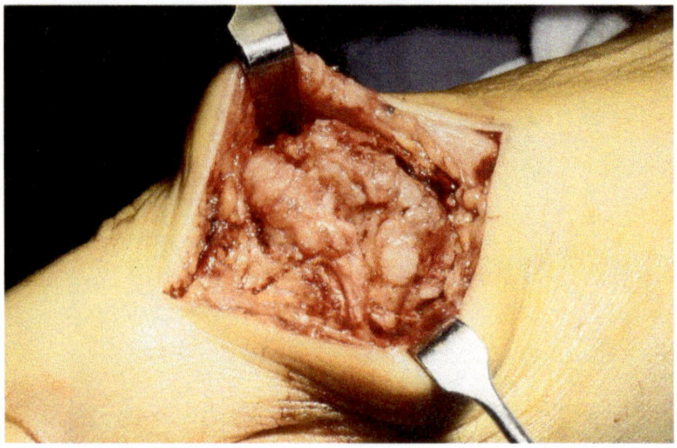

Fig. 15.16 This demonstrates the typical appearance of a hypervascular Lapidus nonunion. Note the ectopic bone formation around the arthrodesis site

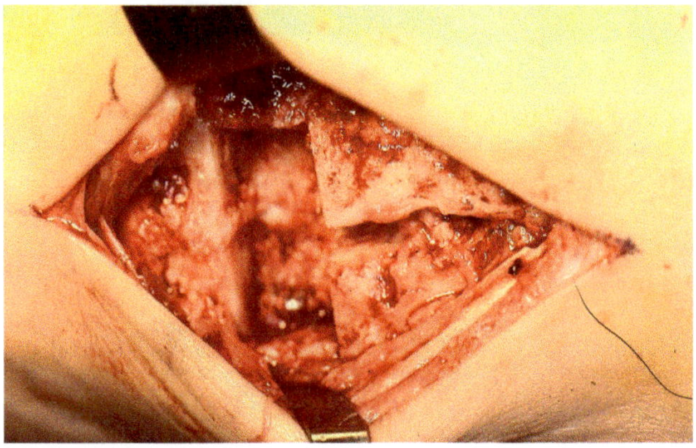

Fig. 15.17 This demonstrates the removal of the fibrous tissue in the center of the nonunion preserving the peripheral soft tissues, which provide vascularity to the bony segments. There was good correction of the deformity in this patient, but the patient developed a hypervascular nonunion

surgery is recommended. There are several considerations in the management of a nonunion of the Lapidus procedure. Determination of the type of nonunion is extremely important. Certain characteristics surrounding the nonunion have to be considered as well.

Typically, there will be a specific pattern of swelling around the midfoot that generally is persistent with increased weight bearing. Pain is consistent on a daily basis with any loading activities and can be described as constant, throbbing, and aching. Plain radiographs will show loose or broken hardware most of the time, and an area of radiolucency will be seen with some ectopic bone formation surrounding the fusion site. In the presence of a hypovascular nonunion, there will be a space between the bony segments indicating a poor biologic response for healing.

Advanced imaging is helpful to identify the type of nonunion and the quality of the bone. The circumstances will

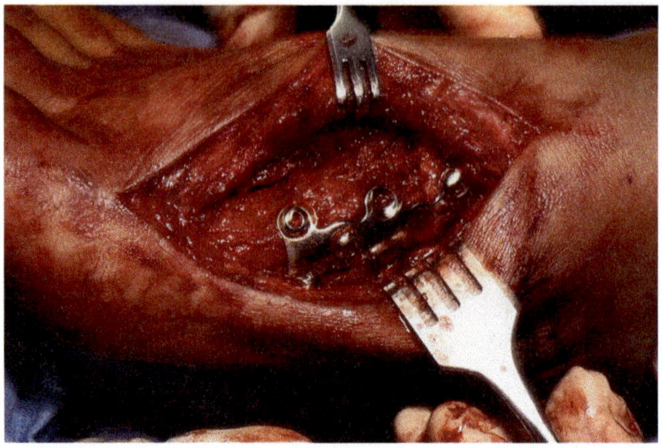

Fig. 15.18 An autogenous calcaneal bone graft was placed in the resection area, and then a medial plate was used to stabilize the graft and the nonunion repair

dictate which imaging study is the best for that particular situation. The author has found that utilization of a CT scan tends to be the best study for most situations. Certainly if there are concerns about the quality of the surrounding tissues or the potential for an infected nonunion, then there are more appropriate studies to help in preoperative planning in those situations followed by a bone biopsy if indicated.

Nonunion Without Deformity

The majority of nonunions at this location are primarily hypervascular. This can generally be determined with plane radiographs. As previously mentioned, advanced imaging such as a CT scan, SPECT CT, or MRI can help in diagnosis and planning [28–30]. When deformity is not present, then the goal of the revisional surgery is to improve the biological response at the nonunion site. This typically involves removing the previous fixation and preserving as much viable tissue around the bone to preserve vascularity and then removing the fibrous elements within the nonunion to replace this interface with healthy bone graft and matrix to mount a biologic response toward solid bony fusion (Figs. 15.16, 15.17, and 15.18). All too often, surgeons dissect periarticular tissues to "mobilize" the corresponding bony structures that results in further devascularization of the area compromising the ability of the soft tissue to aid in a successful fusion. Typically, osteoconduction, osteoinduction, and in certain circumstances osteogenesis are necessary to aid in this biologic response. In elderly patients or immunocompromised patients, osteogenesis becomes a critical component in fusion success, and the use of mesenchymal stem cells may be considered. The osteoinductive and conductive properties in a cancellous bone graft is usually enough to obtain success in most cases. Both allograft and autograft have been recom-

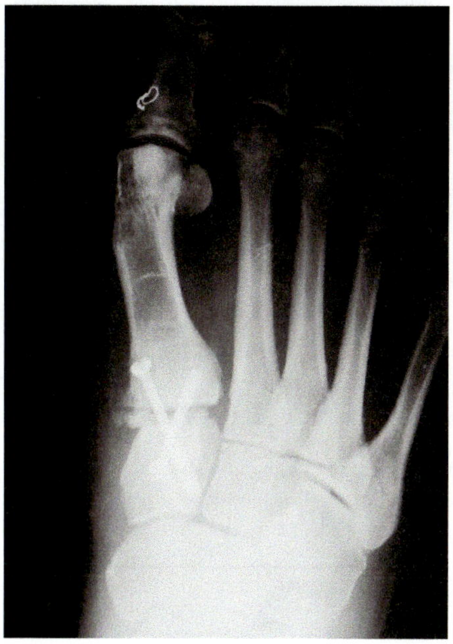

Fig. 15.19 Anteroposterior radiograph of bone graft dissolution and development of a hypovascular nonunion

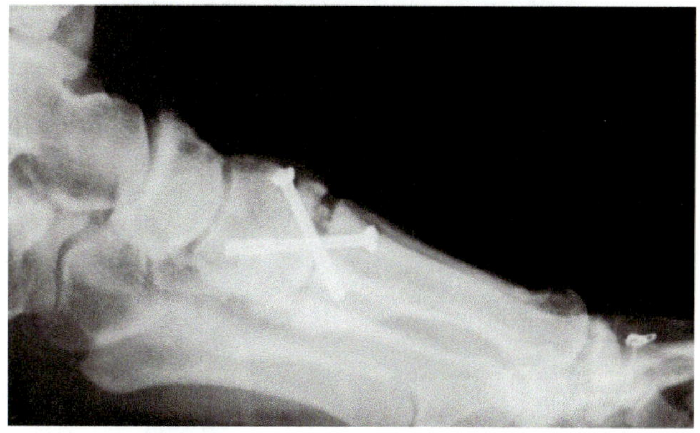

Fig. 15.20 Lateral radiograph demonstrating dissolution of previous bone graft and development of a hypovascular nonunion

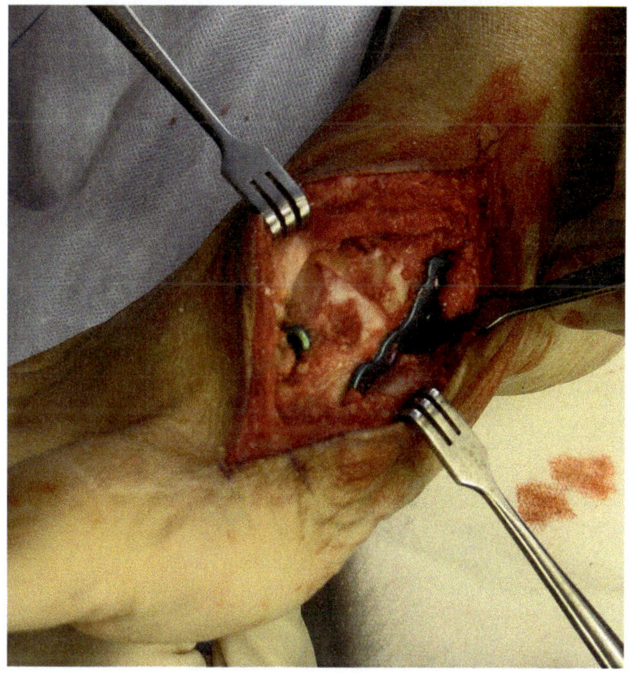

Fig. 15.21 Intraoperative photograph of the autogenous bone graft in the nonunion site and employment of a different fixation construct

mended with success [31–34]. The author prefers autograft in these revisional situations because it provides all three properties previously outlined osteoconduction, osteoinduction, and osteogenesis. The most popular donor sites are the calcaneus or tibia. Both of these sites have a low complication profile and provide the necessary volume needed in revisional situations involving the Lapidus procedure.

Fixation is typically designed to stabilize and prevent excessive motion at the fusion site instead of an emphasis on compression. Changing fixation is sometimes necessary to achieve solid fusion, and this is usually a surgeon preference. This may require redirection of screws or application of specific plates and/or external fixation in some circumstances. Attempting to place the same exact fixation should be discouraged.

In rare situations, hypovascular nonunions or infected nonunions can occur with the Lapidus procedure. Again, advanced imaging will help define the existence of these rare types of nonunion. When a hypovascular nonunion exists, the surgeon has to consider increasing the biologic response with the use of intercalary autogenous bone grafts in combination with other orthobiologics to improve success rates (Figs. 15.19, 15.20, 15.21, 15.22, and 15.23). The need for incorporation of the graft extends the rehabilitation time for the patient. When an infected nonunion exists, then infection management principles become a priority. Removal of implants and adequate resection of involved bone and tissues is paramount. Initially obtaining definitive cultures, placement of antibiotic spacers, IV antibiotics, and segmental stabilization with external fixation are vital to eradicate the infection. Reconstructive options can then be discussed. Septic fusion, Masquelet grafting, or amputation are all viable options depending on the clinical situation [35, 36].

Nonunion with Deformity

This is a more complicated situation because it involves having to correct the deformity, which can only be done by mobilizing the bony segments, and this will compromise some of the vascularity around the fusion site. There is a greater emphasis placed on providing some structural support with this type of nonunion than when deformity is absent. Structural bone grafts are more important to maintain

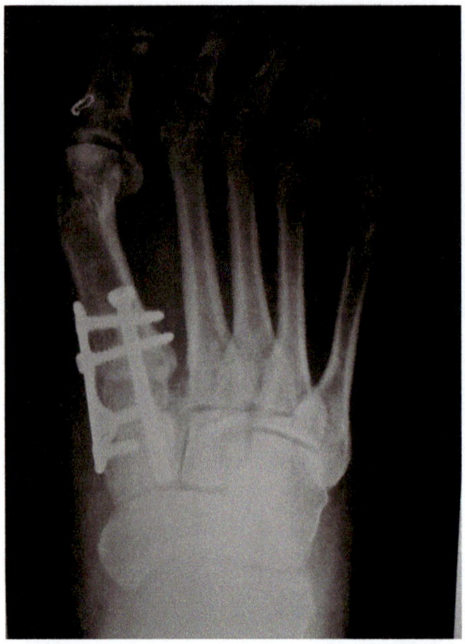

Fig. 15.22 Anteroposterior radiograph showing incorporation of the revisional bone graft for the hypovascular nonunion

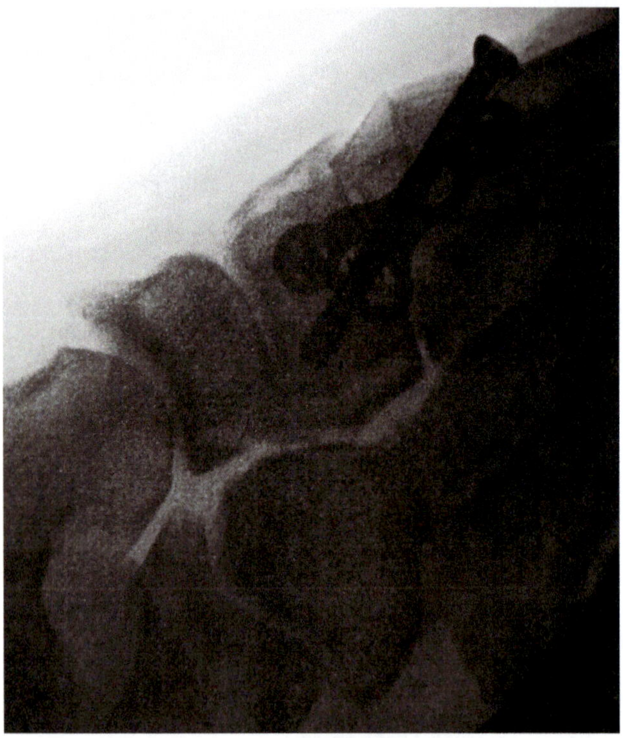

Fig. 15.23 Lateral radiograph demonstrating the interposition autogenous bone graft and fixation construct for hypovascular nonunion

correction and provide the support needed in these scenarios. Autogenous corticocancellous bone grafts can provide support, osteoinduction, osteoconduction, and osteogenesis. Supplementation may again be needed in the elderly and immunocompromised patients.

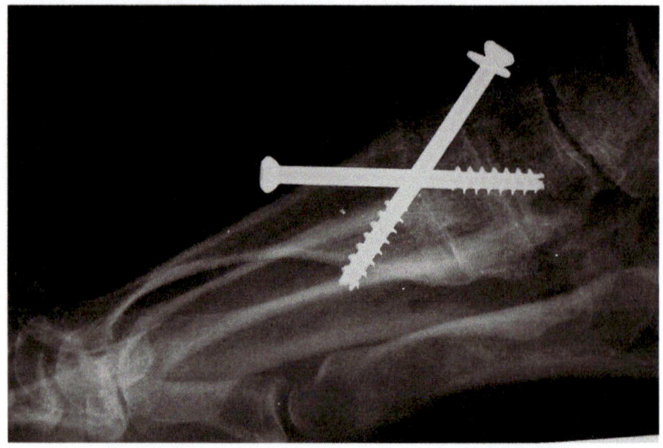

Fig. 15.24 Preoperative radiograph showing crossed screw fixation with a dorsally malunited first metatarsal segment following a Lapidus procedure

Elevated First Ray

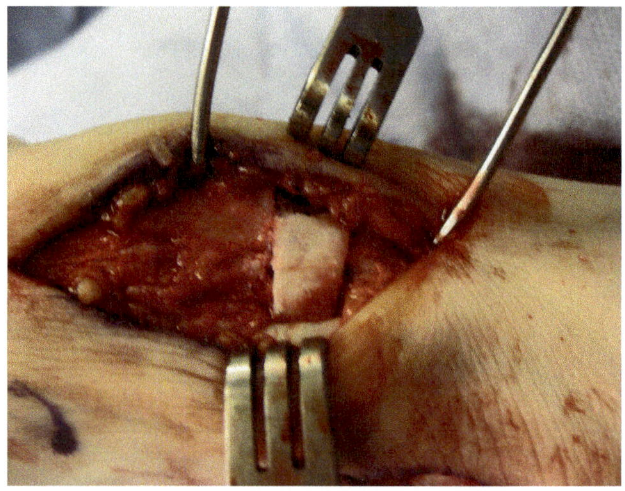

Fig. 15.25 Intraoperative photograph, demonstrating a dorsally positioned bone graft to plantarflex the first metatarsal segment

Elevation of the first ray needs to be corrected in a timely fashion to prevent fairly rapid degeneration of the first metatarsal phalangeal joint. Fortunately, this is a fairly benign complication in terms of surgical correction if addressed early on after recognition. When this is not addressed or recognized, then invariably it involves joint destructive procedures at the first metatarsal phalangeal joint to alleviate symptoms. If there is a solid union in the presence of elevation, then procedures designed to plantarflex the first ray are extremely powerful. The surgeon can remove existing hardware and perform an opening wedge procedure on either side of the fusion site making sure this is as close as possible to the fusion site since that is the apex of the deformity (Figs. 15.24 and 15.25). The cancellous nature of the bone within the cuneiform makes it an ideal place for this type of osteotomy and is performed routinely as a cotton procedure in many other reconstructive scenarios.

Short First Ray

It has been the author's experience that this complication may or may not need to be addressed depending on whether or not these patients develop lateral overload to the second metatarsal. Development of pain under the second metatarsal does not always occur and can simply be monitored over time and treated with orthotics. If the patients develop pre-dislocation syndrome or frank plantar plate insufficiency, then in my opinion this is a more immediate situation for surgical management.

Surgical management of a short first ray provides another complex challenge for the foot and ankle surgeon. Lengthening of the bony segment will tend to jamb the first metatarsal phalangeal joint depending on the length needed to restore a functional parabola. The additional problem is the incorporation of the bone graft over time. Although interpositional bone grafts are widely used for segmental defects, they are not without problems [37, 38].

When the segmental defect is small (0.5 cm), then it is reasonable to use an interpositional bone graft with no distraction of the first MPJ. When the length necessary is upward of a centimeter or more, then consideration should be given to distraction osteogenesis. When a large bone graft is used or distraction osteogenesis is performed, distraction of the first MPJ should be done at the same time to prevent jamming of the joint (Figs. 15.26 and 15.27).

Undercorrected First Ray

Undercorrection can occur with any hallux valgus procedure, but with the Lapidus there are some specific causes. Failure to take into account the amount of medial cuneiform obliquity is probably the most common reason for undercorrection. The lateral flare of the first metatarsal base can prevent reduction when there is a severe increase in the intermetatarsal angle. Failure to recognize an intercuneiform split can also lead to undercorrection and recurrence especially in a supple hypermobile foot. Finally, inadequate reduction of the sesamoids can cause undercorrection or recurrence of a hallux valgus deformity especially in severe cases.

First metatarsal cuneiform obliquity is a common finding in moderate to severe hallux valgus deformities and, when present, can lead to inadequate reduction of the first metatarsal during surgery (Figs. 15.28, 15.29, 15.30, 15.31, 15.32, 15.33, and 15.34). When the joint does not have this obliquity, reduction of the intermetatarsal angle is less difficult, and manipulation is easier without much bony resection. The presence of this obliquity requires some resection of bone on the lateral aspect of the medial cuneiform to accomplish reduction of the intermetatarsal angle.

The lateral flare at the base of the first metatarsal can also make it difficult to reduce the intermetatarsal angle because of abutment of the flare against the intermediate cuneiform during reduction. This occurs commonly after resection of the medial cuneiform previously described. Resection of the lateral flare of the first metatarsal creates a "mortis" between the medial cuneiform and the second cuneiform to aid in reduction of the intermetatarsal angle.

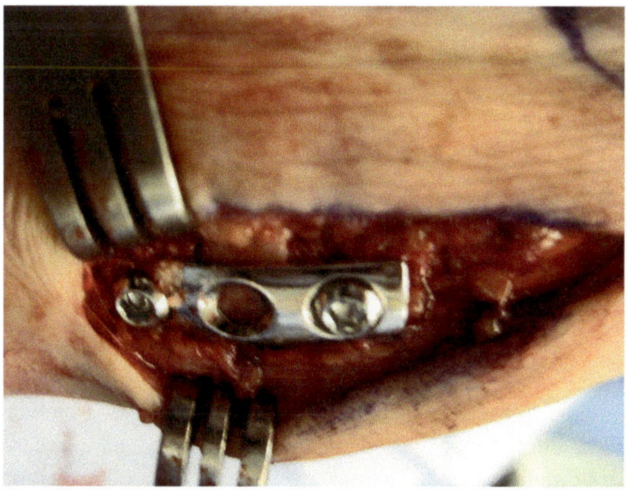

Fig. 15.26 Intraoperative photograph, showing dorsal plate fixation over the interpositional bone graft

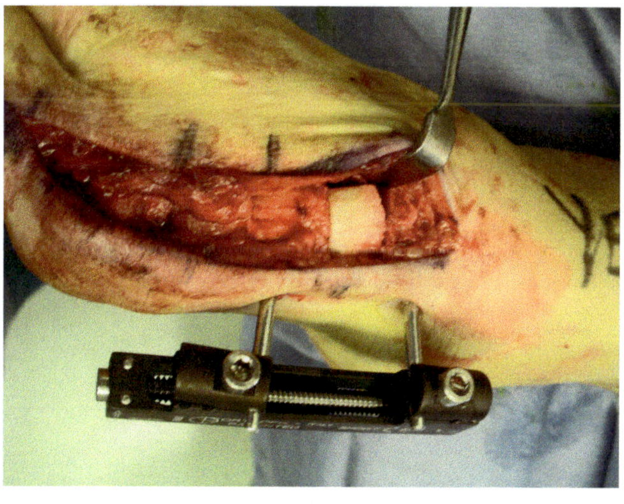

Fig. 15.27 Intraoperative photograph of the placement of an interpositional bone graft after bone resection for a hypovascular nonunion. In this case, a monolateral mini-external fixator was used instead of a plate

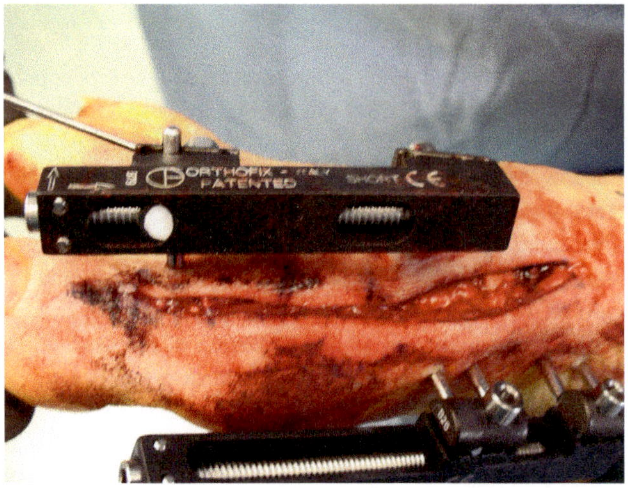

Fig. 15.28 Radiographic representation of first metatarsal obliquity

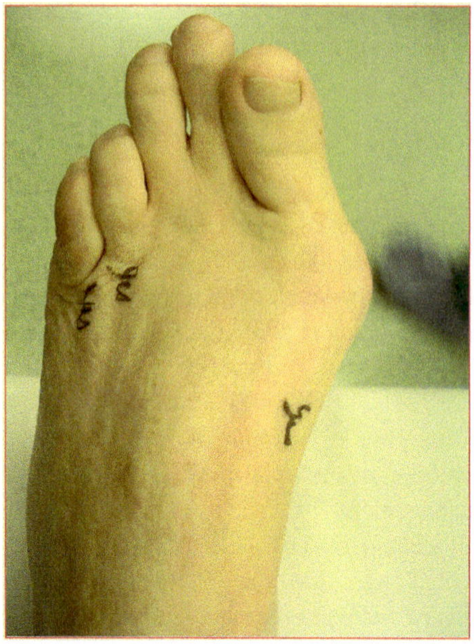

Fig. 15.30 Preoperative appearance of the foot showing the recurrence and undercorrection of the hallux valgus condition

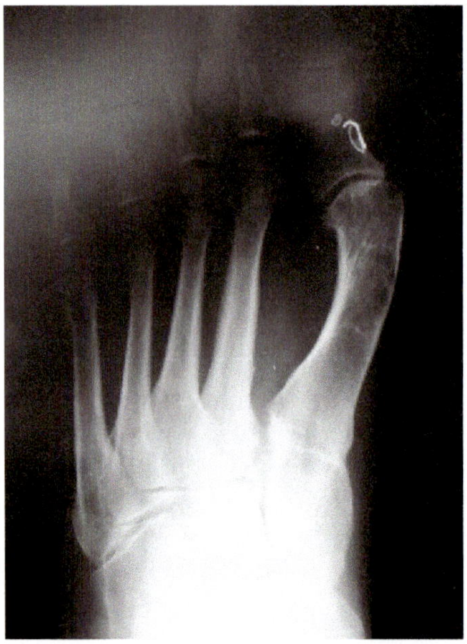

Fig. 15.29 Preoperative radiograph, demonstrating the healed Lapidus procedure with shortening and undercorrection of the deformity. Note the adaptive changes at the first metatarsal phalangeal joint

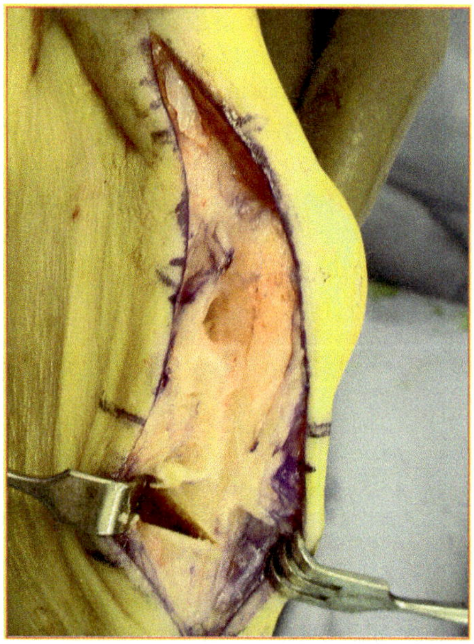

Fig. 15.31 Acute correction of the intermetatarsal angle, at the proximal corticotomy site. The gradual correction will be for lengthening of the metatarsal

Recurrence

The most common factor in recurrence of a hallux valgus deformity when a Lapidus procedure has been performed is failure to recognize an "intercuneiform split" between the medial and intermediate cuneiforms (Fig. 15.35). This is not to suggest that every intercuneiform split leads to a recurrent hallux valgus, but when this intercuneiform split is mobile under fluoroscopy intraoperatively, then it can lead to recurrence unless one addresses this in the operating room. Preparation of the corresponding surfaces by denuding cartilage and then applying one or two interfragmentary compression screws across the split can help to prevent this complication from occurring.

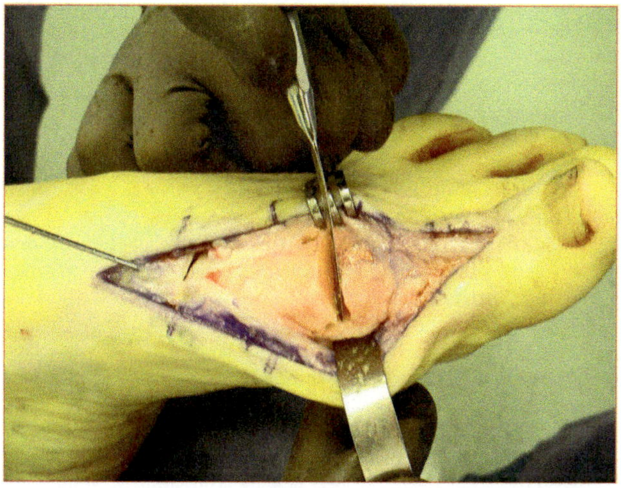

Fig. 15.32 Intraoperative photograph of proximal corticotomy and distal metatarsal osteotomy to correct the articular cartilage of the first metatarsal

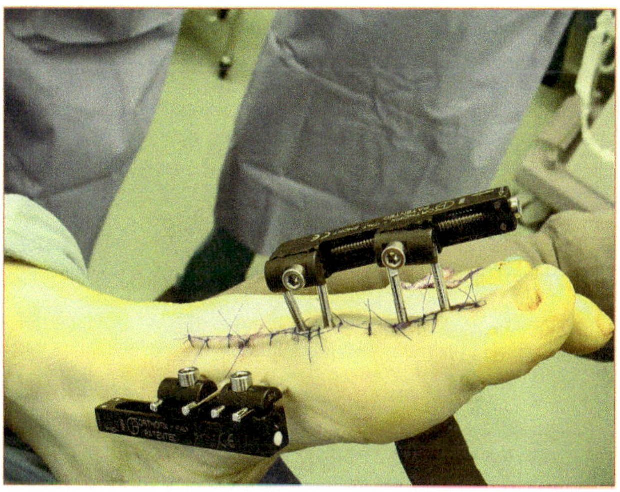

Fig. 15.33 Closure of the surgical site, with placement of the two mini-rail external fixators, for first metatarsal distraction osteogenesis and first MPJ joint distraction. Note that the second half pin proximally was used to fixate the distal metatarsal osteotomy

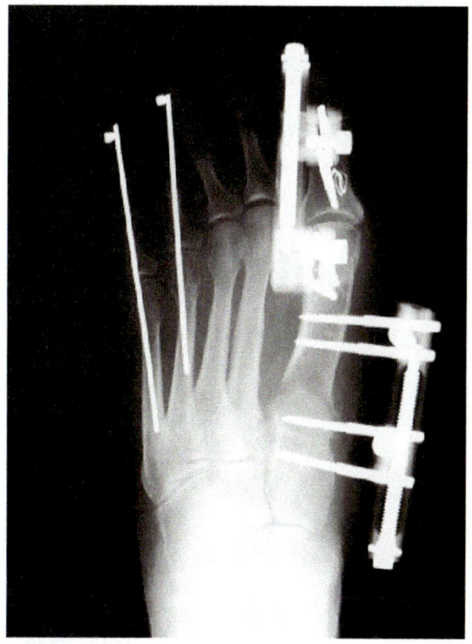

Fig. 15.34 Radiograph demonstrating distraction osteogenesis at the first metatarsal base and an additional fixator to provide joint distraction during the lengthening process

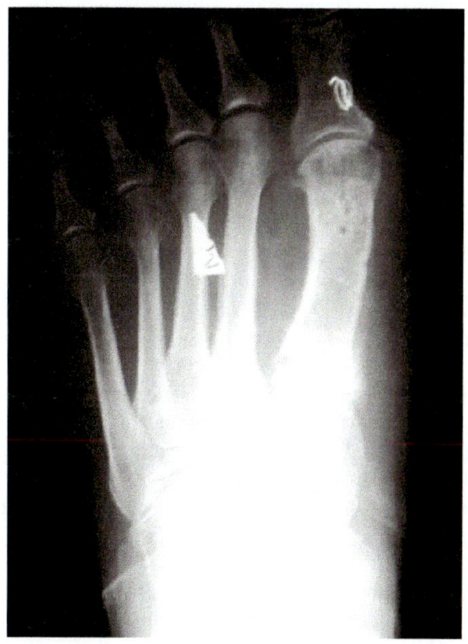

Fig. 15.35 Final X-ray of correction, showing restoration of metatarsal length through distraction osteogenesis and maintenance of first MPJ joint space with joint distraction

References

1. Albrecht GH. The pathology and treatment of hallux valgus. Russ Vrach. 1911;10:14.
2. Lapidus PW. The operative correction of the metatarsus varus primus in hallux valgus. Surg Gynecol Obstet. 1934;58:183.
3. Clark MR, Veith RG, Hansen ST. Adolescent bunion treated by modified lapidus procedure. Bull Hosp Jt Dis. 1987;47:109.
4. Sangeorzan BJ, Hansen ST. Modified lapidus procedure for hallux valgus. Foot Ankle Inst. 1989;9:262.
5. Catanzariti AR, Mendicino RW, Lee MS, Gallina MR. The modified lapidus arthrodesis: a retrospective analysis. J Foot Ankle Surg. 1999;38:322–32.
6. McInnes BD, Bouche RT. Critical evaluation of the modified lapidus procedure. J Foot Ankle Surg. 2001;40:71–90.
7. Patel S, Ford LA, Etcheverry J, Rush SM, Hamilton GA. Modified lapidus arthrodesis: rate of nonunion in 227 cases. J Foot Ankle Surg. 2004;431:37–42.
8. Coetzee JC, Resig SG, Kuskowski M, Saleh KJ. The lapidus procedure as a salvage after failed surgical treatment of hallux valgus: a prospective cohort study. J Bone Joint Surg Am. 2003;85:60–5.
9. Faber FM, Mulder PH, Vehaar JN. Role of first ray hypermobility in the outcome of the hohmann and the lapidus procedure. A prospective, randomized trial involving one hundred and one feet. J Bone Joint Surg. 2004;86:486–95.
10. Sammarco GJ, Idusuyi OB. Complications after surgery of the hallux. Clin Orthop Rel Res. 2001;391:59–71.
11. Kilmartin TE. Revision of failed foot surgery: a critical analysis. J Foot Ankle Surg. 2002;41:309–15.
12. Christensen JC, Jennings MM. Normal and abnormal function of the first ray. Clin Podiatr Med Surg. 2009;26(3):255–71.
13. Khaw FM, Mak P, Johnson GR, et al. Distal ligamentous restraints of the first metatarsal. An in vitro biomechanical study. Clin Biomech (Bristo, Avon). 2005;20:653–8.
14. Sarrafian SK. Functional characteristics of the foot and plantar aponeurosis under tibiotalar loading. Foot Ankle. 1987;8:4–18.
15. Thordason DB, Schmotzer H, Chon J, et al. Dynamic support of the human longitudinal arch. A biomechanical evaluation. Clin Orthop. 1995;316:165–72.
16. Rush SM, Christensen JC, Johnson CH. Biomechanics of the first ray. Part II: metatarsus primus varus as a cause of hypermobility. A three-dimensional kinematic analysis in a cadaveric model. J Foot Ankle Surg. 2000;39:68077.
17. Rolling BA, Christensen JC, Johnson CH. Biomechanics of the first ray. Part IV: the effect of selected medial column arthrodesis. A three-dimensional kinematic analysis in a cadaver model. J Foot Ankle Surg. 2002;41:278–85.
18. Lungren P, Nester C, Liu A, et al. Invasive in vivo measurements of rear-mid-forefoot motion during walking. Gait Posture. 2008;28:93–100.
19. Johnson JT, Schuberth JM, Thornton SD, Christensen JC. Joint curettage arthrodesis technique in the foot. A histological analysis. J Foot Ankle Surg. 2009;48(5):558.
20. Donnenwerth MP, Borkosky SL, Abicht BP, Plovanich EJ, Roukis TS. Rate of nonunion after first metatarsal-cuneiform arthrodesis using joint curettage and two crossed compression screw fixation: a systematic review. J Foot Ankle Surg. 2011;50:707.
21. Dayton P, Feilmeier M, Kauwe M, Hirschi J. Relationship of frontal plane rotation of first metatarsal to proximal articular set angle and hallux alignment in patients undergoing tarsal metatarsal arthrodesis for hallux abducto valgus: a case series and critical review of the literature. J Foot Ankle Surg. 2013;52:348–54.
22. Dayton P, Feilmeier M, Hirchi J, Kauwe M, Kauwe JS. Observed changes in radiographic measurements of the first ray after frontal plane rotation of the first metatarsal in a cadaveric foot model. J Foot Ankle Surg. 2014;53:274–8.
23. Gruber F, Sinkov VS, Bae SY, Parks BG, Schon LC. Crossed screws versus dorsomedial locking plate with compression screw for first metatarsocuneiform arthrodesis: a cadaver study. Foot Ankle Int. 2008;29(9):927–30.
24. Klos K, Gueorguiev B, Muckley T, Frober R, Hofmann GO, Schwieger K, Windolf M. Stability of medial locking plate and compression screw versus two crossed screws for lapidus arthrodesis. Foot Ankle Int. 2010;31(2):158–63.
25. Blitz NM, Lee T, Williams K, Barkan H, DiDimenico LA. Early weight bearing after modified lapidus arthrodesis: a multicenter review of 80 cases. J Foot Ankle Surg. 2010;49(4):357–62.
26. Nwokolo IO Podiatry Institute Chapter 4
27. Thompson IM, Bohay DR, Anderson JG. Fusion rate of first tarsometatarsal arthrodesis in the modified lapidus procedure and flatfoot reconstruction. Foot Ankle Int. 2005;26(9):698–703.
28. Bhattacharyya T, Bouchard KA, Phadke A, Meigs JB, Kassarjian A, Salamipour H. The accuracy of computed tomography for diagnosis of tibial nonunion. JBJS A. 2006;88(4):672–97.
29. Schnarkowski P, Ridei J, Peterfly CG, et al. Tibial shaft fractures: Assessment of fracture healing with computed tomography. J Comp Assisted Tomogr. 1995;19(5):777–81.
30. Ianni M, Kaicker J, Choudur H. Efficacy of high resolution CT for detection of early healing of scaphoid fractures. Open J Clin Diagn. 2012;2:51–5.
31. Singleton TJ, Schuberth JM. Bone graft from the distal medial tibia in foot and ankle surgery. Foot Ankle Spec. 2012;5(3):168–74.
32. Fitzgibbons TC, Hawks MA, McMullen ST, Inda DJ. Bone grafting in surgery about the foot and ankle: indications and techniques. J Am Acad Orthop Surg. 2011;19(2):112–20.
33. Soohoo NF, Cracchiolo A. The results of utilizing proximal tibial bone graft in reconstructive procedures of the foot and ankle. Foot Ankle Surg. 2008;14(2):62–6.
34. Luk PC, Johnson JE, McCormick JJ, Klein SE. First metatarsal joint arthrodesis technique with interpositional allograft bone block. Foot Ankle Int. 2015;36:936.
35. Ronga M, Ferraro S, Fagetti A, Cherubino M, Valdatta L, Cherubino P. Masquelet technique for the treatment of a severe acute tibial bone loss. Injury. 2014;45(suppl 6):S111–5.
36. Makridis KG, Theocharakis S, Fragkakis EM, Giannoudis PV. Reconstruction of an extensive soft tissue and bone defect of the first metatarsal with the Masquelet technique: a case report. Foot Ankle Surg. 2014;20(2):19–22.
37. Gross CE, Hsu AR, Lin J, Holmes GB, Lee S. Revision MTP arthrodesis for failed MTP arthroplasty. Foot Ankle Spec. 2013;6(6):471–8.
38. Coughlin MJ, Mann RA. Arthrodesis of the first metatarsophalangeal joint as salvage for the failed Keller procedure. J Bone Joint Surg Am. 1987;69(1):68–75.

Part IV

Midfoot/Hindfoot

16 Lisfranc Fracture-Dislocation/ Arthrodesis

Lawrence A. Di Domenico and Frank A. Luckino

Introduction

The term "Lisfranc" was coined by Jacques Lisfranc, a field surgeon of Napoleon's army, whose original description referred to an amputation at the tarsometatarsal joint (TMTJ) level secondary to vascular injury. Today, this term is used mainly in reference to a ligamentous or frank, fracture dislocation at the Lisfranc joint. These injuries can result from low- to high-energy incidents [1]. Low-energy injuries may occur indirectly with bending stress or twisting motion [2]. Higher-energy injuries occur more directly from crush injuries [3] or motor vehicle accidents. Lisfranc injuries are said to occur in 1 per 55,000 people in the United States annually which represents about 0.2% of all fractures. Due to the subtle nature of some injury patterns, a missed or delayed diagnosis is not uncommon. Reports show this may occur up to 20% of the time [4]. Because of a delayed diagnosis, misdiagnosis, or complications of a treated Lisfranc injury, arthritis of the midtarsal and tarsometatarsal joints (midfoot) has emerged as a challenging problem leading to high potential for chronic foot pain and functional disability. To truly understand the injury patterns, one must have a thorough knowledge of the anatomy. The joint complex consists of articulations between the bases of the metatarsals with the cuneiforms and cuboid as well as the intermetatarsal articulations. The medial column articulation consists of the first metatarsal and medial cuneiform; the central column consists of the second and third metatarsals and their articulation with the intermediate and lateral cuneiforms, respectively; and the lateral column consists of the fourth and fifth metatarsal articulations with the cuboid [5]. The joint configuration forms an arch, sometimes referred to as a "Roman" arch, which is inherently stable (Fig. 16.1). Tarsometatarsal (TMT) pathologic change is a debilitating condition characterized by midfoot malalignment, severe functional impairment, and pain. When faced with this challenging problem, the primary aim of treatment is to balance the foot and provide pain relief by enhancing midfoot stability. Treatment should be attempted initially through non-operative management such as orthoses and bracing followed by surgery.

L.A. Di Domenico (✉)
Ankle and Foot Care Centers, Youngstown, OH, USA

Kent State University, College of Podiatric Medicine, Cleveland, OH, USA
e-mail: LD5353@aol.com

F.A. Luckino
Ankle and Foot Care Centers, Youngstown, OH, USA

Functional Midfoot Pathomechanics

A neglected and/or a poorly treated Lisfranc injury can lead to midfoot instability and significant secondary malalignment. A lack of midfoot stability during mid stance phase of gait will have an impact on the patient's lower extremity structurally and functionally. Based on the extent of the primary injury and the time of the revision surgery, the extent of involvement can vary significantly. The lack of stability in the midfoot often results in excessive motion at the Lisfranc joint leading to degenerative joints to varying degrees. The forefoot is often affected by the changes with forefoot overload and secondary contractors at the metatarsal phalangeal joints. If severe enough, the lack of stability can lead to severe disabling soft tissue changes secondary to the bony malalignment. In addition arthritic conditions of the diseased joints may develop. Osteophytes can progress and create increased pressure on the tendons and soft tissues that are worsened with shoes and/or weight bearing. The loss of the midfoot stability eventually will have a consequence of secondary functional changes which may lead to the inability to position the foot effectively during mid stance or for push-off in the gait cycle. The loss of midfoot stability is indicative in patient's complaints and symptoms during stance, ambulation, and activities. Also, as the midfoot loses stability, the foot develops an abnormal foot posture. These changes are consistent with the collapsing of the arch and

M.S. Lee, J.P. Grossman (eds.), *Complications in Foot and Ankle Surgery*, DOI 10.1007/978-3-319-53686-6_16

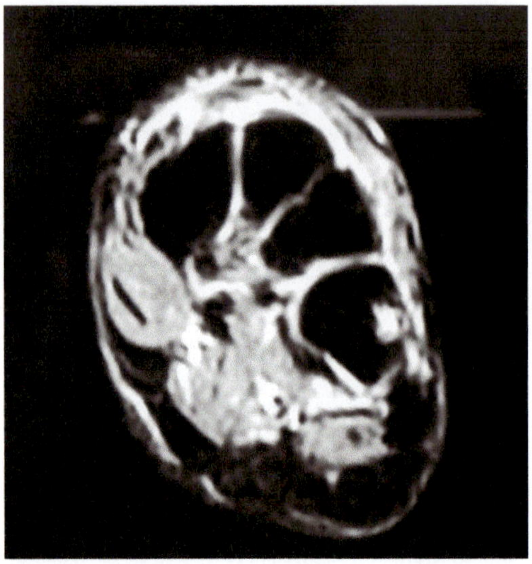

Fig. 16.1 A cross section of the cuneiforms and cuboid similar to a "Roman Arch." Note the natural occurring arch and how the cuneiforms and cuboid are anatomically wedged together. The middle cuneiform is most superiorly positioned relative to the medial and lateral cuneiform. The base of the cuneiforms are situated dorsally and the apex is planetary, which provides for the naturally occurring support in the frontal plane

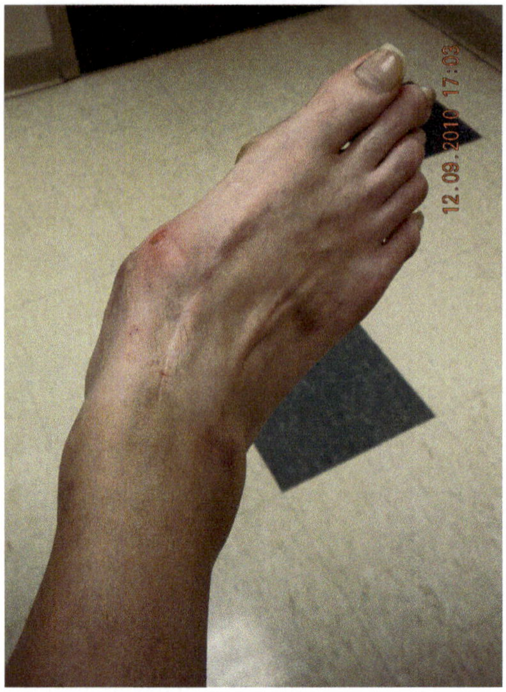

Fig. 16.2 A patient who underwent an unsuccessful open reduction and internal fixation of a Lisfranc injury. Subsequently the patient experienced failed pathomechanics of the midfoot leading to abnormal alignment and pain with a deformity. Note the abduction of the forefoot, the prominent medial bone, and significant alignment relative to the tibia

increased stress to the plantar soft tissue and osseous structures as the foot is loaded, resulting in foot and ankle pain (Fig. 16.2) [6]. These architectural changes of the foot typically lead to greater demands on muscular and ligamentous structures, resulting in fatigue and pain in the foot and ankle. It has been the author's experience that degenerative arthritis along with abnormal foot postures and/or gait patterns makes the foot more susceptible to foot and ankle pain due to mechanical overloading. The changes in alignment lead to abnormal mechanical forces which in turn have a direct effect causing an increase of stress on the soft tissues. As a consequence of the injury, patients with a compromised sensory system may experience a breakdown in their soft tissues with the focused abnormal pressures (Fig. 16.3).

Indications of Procedure

Following complex trauma in the foot, oftentimes there is a loss of mechanical integrity that leads to structural breakdown and secondary soft tissue changes. Injuries that may cause the pain and breakdown of the Lisfranc joint consist of unsuccessful ligamentous repair, severe articular fractures, failed open reductions and internal fixation, chronic neglected/misdiagnosed Lisfranc injury, deformity at the tarsal metatarsal joint, posttraumatic osteoarthritis, and Charcot arthropathy/neuropathic midfoot. These injuries may cause pain, malalignment, atrophy, impairment of the soft tissue envelope, contractures, soft tissue loss, joint adhesions, malunion,

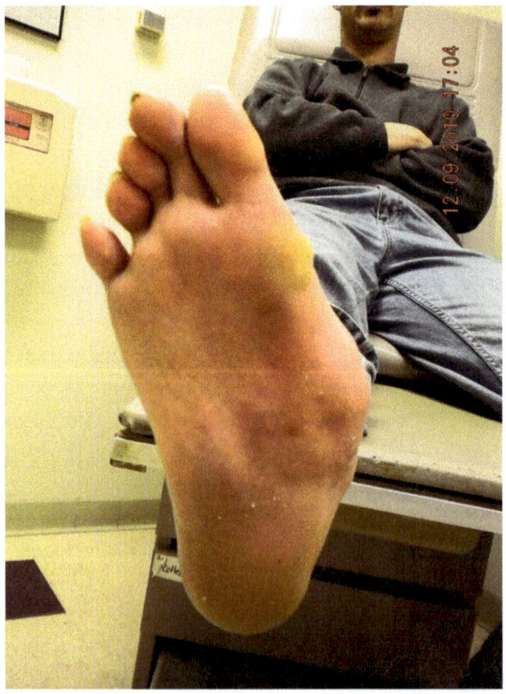

Fig. 16.3 A plantar view of a patient with a previously attempted Lisfranc repair with malalignment. Note the large callus tissue at the first metatarsal phalangeal joint because of the pathomechanics

nonunion, dystrophic changes, and neurologic and/or vascular injury. When the index procedure has been misdiagnosed, mistreated, or ineffective, the proposed revision procedure must take into consideration the length of time since the original disability and the quality of the soft tissue envelop. Expectations on functional activities following a revision procedure are directly related to the individual patient's given condition. In patients with residual deformity, the extent of the arthrodesis depended on the number of affected joints and the severity of deformity. Selecting the appropriate procedures is key to providing realignment and stability to the foot.

In Situ Arthrodesis

Patients that present with a failed or mistreated Lisfranc injury and are in need of a revision Lisfranc arthrodesis without significant malalignment can proceed with an in situ arthrodesis. An in situ arthrodesis is indicated for those patients with a condition that is limited to the medial or middle column and/or both and without malalignment. The surgeon needs to evaluate the entire lower extremity with a focus at the Lisfranc joint. The patient should be evaluated weight bearing and nonweight bearing. A Silfverskiold test should be performed to assess if there is a contracture of the posterior muscle group [7]. It has been the experience of the authors with revision surgery at the Lisfranc joint that the adaptive changes in this patient population typically exhibit a tight posterior muscle group and are in most instances in need of lengthening the posterior muscle group. The results of the Silfverskiold test will dictate the indication of an Achilles tendon lengthening or a gastrocnemius recession. When indicated, it has been the author's choice to perform the Achilles tendon lengthening percutaneous or the gastrocnemius release through endoscopic technique [8, 9].

A single curvilinear incision is made over between the first and second tarsal metatarsal joint. The incision is made with care to identify and protect the superficial and deep peroneal nerves, dorsalis pedis artery, and vein. A full-thickness flap is created exposing the deformity. All soft tissue retraction is performed with either double-pronged skin hooks or mini Hohmann retractors in best efforts to protect the soft tissue envelop. If previous hardware is present, it is removed. If the hardware is fractured and can be easily obtainable, it is removed. Attention is directed to the involved joints and is exposed and checked under fluoroscopy. Typically there is a great deal of fibrous and capsular tissue in the involved joints. An extended period of time should be spent resecting this tissue and mobilizing the joints. This will expose the involved joints very well, will allow for mobilization, and also by removing this fibrous tissue and debris will prevent an unsatisfactory reduction in attempt to prevent a failed bony union. Next, manipulation of the forefoot from

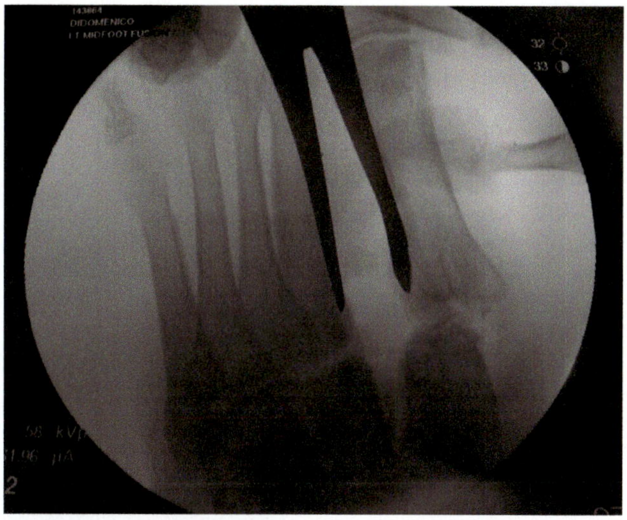

Fig. 16.4 An intraoperative AP view demonstrating a lamina spreader being utilized to help enable the surgeon to view the joints

the midfoot is done with an osteotome and mallet and insertion of a laminar spreader (Fig. 16.4). The adjacent joints are checked for instability or malalignment. If the adjacent joints are involved, then attention is directed to the necessary joints, and debridement with joint preparation is performed. The cartilage and subchondral bone are removed with an osteotome and mallet to the intended joints. It is important to resect the plantar aspect of the joint in order to prevent dorsal angulation and malunion. A significant amount of time should be spent debriding and preparing the necessary joints. The authors typically utilize an osteotome, mallet, 2.0 drill bits, pics, and curettage technique to be sure extensive subchondral bone is debrided while maintaining the osseous integrity. Once all the required joints are adequately prepared for arthrodesis, a laminar spreader is inserted to each joint to inspect for loose fragments, and to be certain, the joint is prepared adequately.

The Lisfranc joint is deep and has a large surface area, and special attention is focused plantarly. In reducing the deformity, the aim is to restore alignment of the medial aspect of the base of the first metatarsal with the medial edge of the first cuneiform. Next, restoring alignment of the medial aspect of the base of the second metatarsal with the medial edge of the second cuneiform in the transverse plane is necessary. Alignment of the long axis of the talus with the long axis of the first metatarsal in both the sagittal and transverse planes is required to restore anatomical alignment (Fig. 16.5).

This is facilitated by initially correcting the position of the first metatarsal. This is performed by grasping the great toe, dorsiflexing the great toe joint, and rotating the first metatarsal into a neutral position (varus direction-out of valgus), while the base of the first metatarsal is pushed firmly against a stable well-aligned midfoot [10]. If there is noted

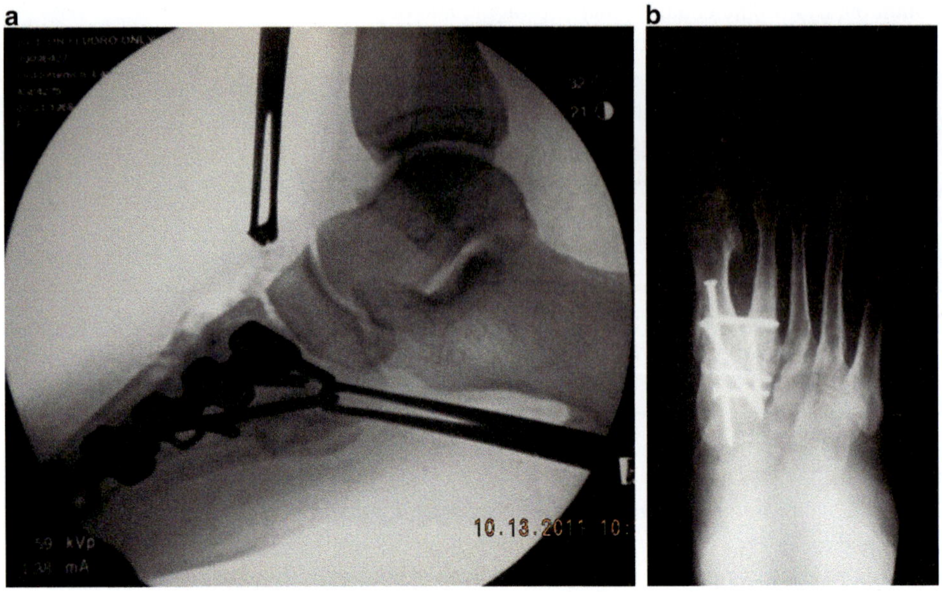

Fig. 16.5 (a) An intraoperative view demonstrating appropriate alignment of the talus with the long axis of the first metatarsal in the sagittal plane. (b) A postoperative AP radiograph demonstrating appropriate alignment of the talus with the first metatarsal in the transverse plane

instability of the proximal tarsal bones, medial, and/or lateral cuneiforms of the midfoot, these joints are debrided, aligned, and temporary stabilized prior to reducing the first tarsal metatarsal joint. Stabilization should occur from proximal to distal. Following reduction of the first metatarsal to a stable proximal midfoot, it is temporarily secured with a 2.0 Kirschner wire and is inserted from the first metatarsal proximally into the medial cuneiform while maintaining alignment. Next, the base of the second metatarsal is positioned appropriately followed by the third tarsal metatarsal. A large bone-reduction Weber clamp and/or Kirschner wire is placed obliquely to close the gap between the base of the second metatarsal and the medial cuneiform. A Kirschner wire is inserted from the proximal medial cuneiform aiming distally toward the base of the second metatarsal. If the third tarsal metatarsal joint is involved, this is reduced, and a 2.0 Kirschner wire is inserted from the proximal shaft of the third metatarsal into the respected cuneiform. If the fourth and fifth metatarsal tarsal joints are involved, it has been the author's experience that once the first three tarsal metatarsal joints are positioned, the fourth and fifth metatarsal tarsal joints will be reduced anatomically [11]. The second and the third metatarsal are secured with additional Kirschner wires used in multiple planes stabilizing the metatarsals into the respective cuneiforms. Anteroposterior, medial oblique, and lateral fluoroscopic images are made to confirm the corrected alignment (Figs. 16.6 and 16.7).

Fixation is achieved using a lag technique involving solid 3.5 or 4.0 solid cortical screws and/or plating techniques. If there is noted proximal joint involvement, the proximal joints need to be fixated first to provide a stable midfoot in order to successfully align and fixate the Lisfranc joint [11]. A screw hole technique as described by Manoli and Hansen [12] allows for a difficult angulation, and the first screw is inserted from the first metatarsal to the medial cuneiform creating inter-fragmentary compression. The next screw is inserted from the stable superior proximal medial cuneiform obliquely oriented into the second metatarsal base. It is important that the surgeon understands the anatomy as the base of the second metatarsal is elevated or is at the peak of the "Roman Arch." When inserting this screw, the surgeon should be aiming slightly superior so that the base of the second metatarsal is fixated adequately. This screw also employs inter-fragmentary compression. Additional screws can be inserted from the proximal metatarsal base into the cuneiform and from the base of the first metatarsal into the base of the second and/or third metatarsal. A high-speed burr is then used to debride the edges of the involved joints, and bone voids are then packed with autogenous or allogenic cancellous bone graft for a shear strain relief graft as described by Perren [13]. The gaps are filled with local bone graft which can be harvested from the calcaneus, and if additional bone graft is needed, allogenic bone or a bone graft substitute can be utilized [14]. Typical soft tissue and skin closure is performed.

Postoperatively, the patient is placed in a dorsally slotted non-weight-bearing plaster cast for 2 weeks [15]. Provided there are no wound problems and the reduction and construct is stable, a fiberglass below the knee cast is applied for an additional 4–6 weeks and until radiographic consolidation is evident. Full weight bearing in a fracture boot with physical therapy is then prescribed for 4 weeks.

Realignment Arthrodesis

Patients who present with malalignment and deformity of the forefoot require a realignment arthrodesis of the Lisfranc joint. Oftentimes, a severe or progressed failed Lisfranc

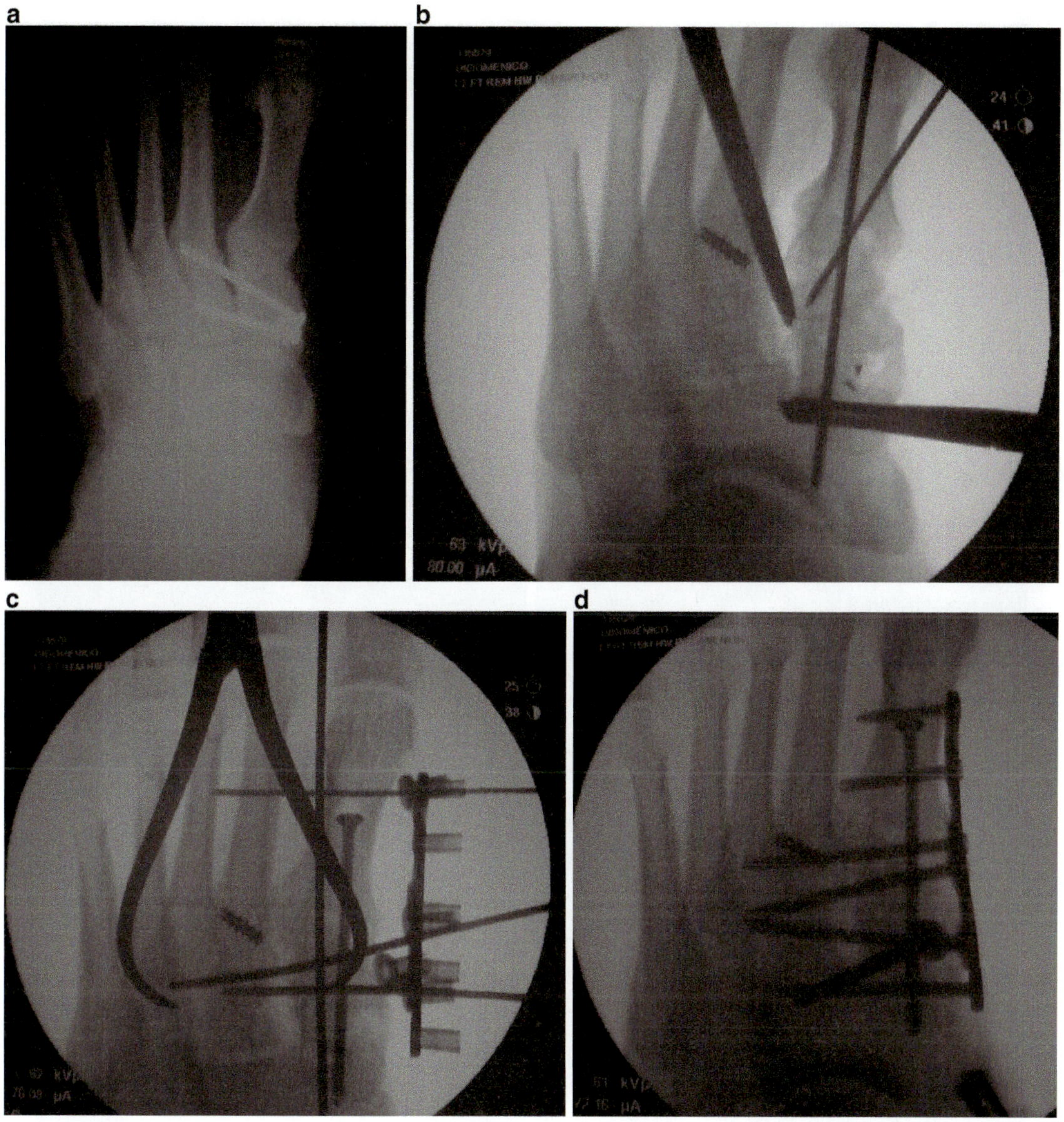

Fig. 16.6 (**a**) A preoperative AP radiograph with fractured hardware. Note the fracture of the screw is at the run out portion of the cannulated screw. This patient presented with continued pain following the index procedure which consisted of an open reduction and internal fixation and of Lisfranc injury. (**b**) An intraoperative view during a revision in situ Lisfranc arthrodesis. The original injury consisted of an open reduction and internal fixation. While preparing for an in situ arthrodesis, an osteotome and mallet were used preparing the intercuneiform joint in preparation for arthrodesis and the use of autogenous bone graft for an in situ arthrodesis revision arthrodesis. (**c**) An intraoperative AP fluoroscopic image while performing a revision surgery for a Lisfranc injury. A long 3.5 mm fully threaded "home run screw" is inserted from the distal first metatarsal into the plantar most proximal cuneiform. A large Weber clamp is used to assist with temporary intercuneiform compression while preparing to apply a medial base locking plate. (**d**) An intraoperative AP fluoroscopic image of an in situ revision arthrodesis with a stable rigid internal fixation construct for an intercuneiform and Lisfranc arthrodesis prior to inserting a shear strain relief graft

joint will require additional procedures in order to reduce the foot into an anatomical position. There are varying degrees of deformity based on the initial injury, the original treatment, the type of treatment, and the secondary bony and soft tissue pathological changes to the adjacent joints. The medial and middle column arthrodesis requires fixation of the first, second, and sometimes the third tarsal metatarsal joints along with their intercuneiform joints. The naviculocuneiform and other adjacent joints may need to be included in this fusion if found to be unstable. In addition, the summation of time from the index injury and original treatment will have a secondary effect on the pathological bone and soft tissue changes. Patients needing a realignment arthrodesis typically present with an abduction of the forefoot and lateral translation and dorsiflexion of the metatarsals (Fig. 16.8).

A valgus deformity may present with medial soft tissues that may be stressed and the lateral soft tissues maybe contracted.

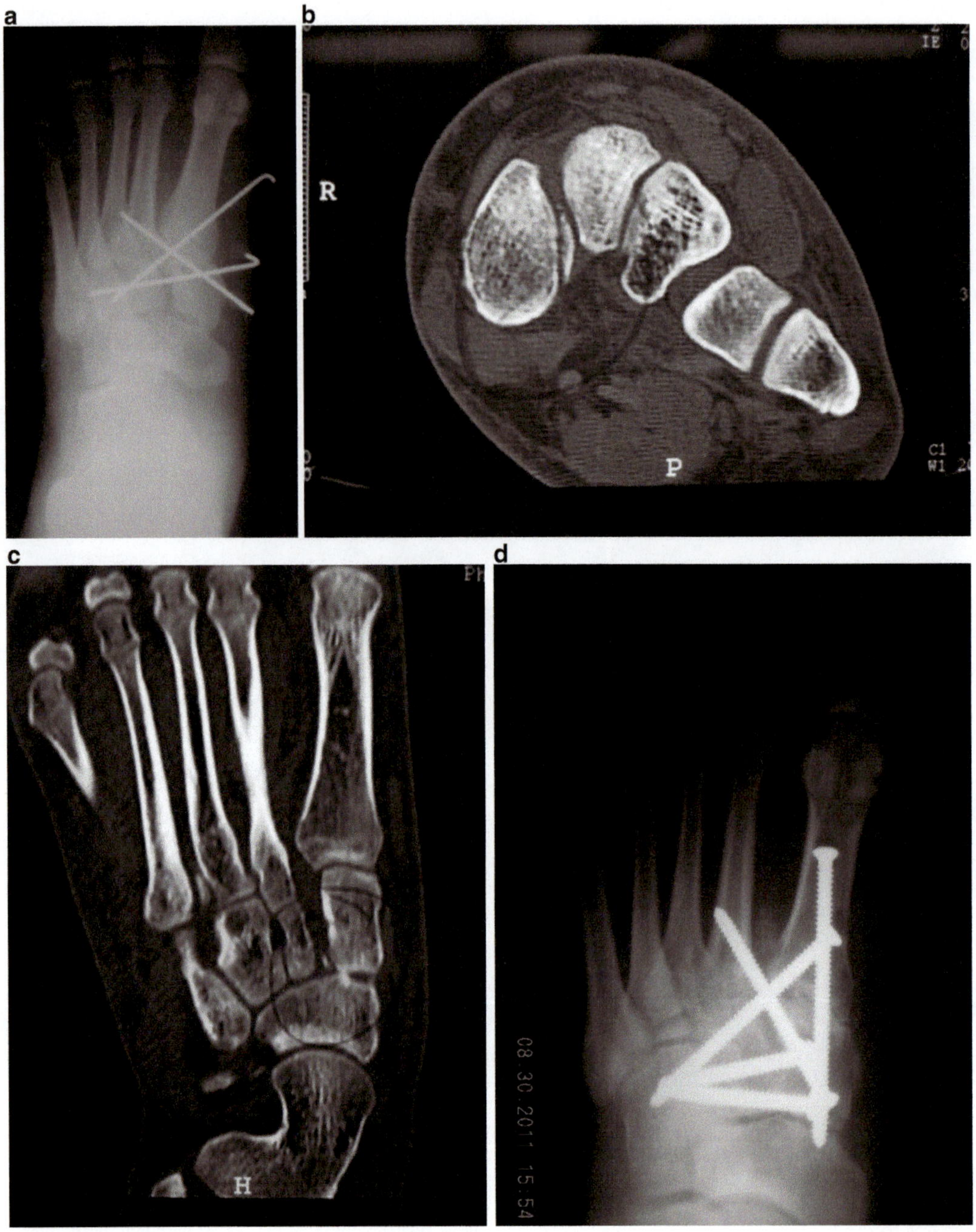

Fig. 16.7 (**a**) An attempted open reduction with K-wire fixation for an original Lisfranc injury. (**b** and **c**) Advanced imaging demonstrating failure of adequate reduction and malalignment following open reduction with K-wire fixation from the original Lisfranc injury. (**d**) An in situ arthrodesis was performed with long fully threaded solid cortical screws repairing the failed K-wire reduction at the Lisfranc joint

In most cases, these patients present with a differing degree a flatfoot deformity along with a collapsing arch in association with abduction of the forefoot, lateral translation and dorsiflexion of the metatarsals, and a potentially progressed hindfoot valgus. The surgeon needs to evaluate the entire lower extremity. The patient should be evaluated weight bearing and nonweight bearing. A Silfverskiold test needs to be performed to assess if there is a contracture of the posterior muscle group [7]. It has been the experience of the authors that this patient population exhibits a tight posterior muscle group and is in need of lengthening the Achilles tendon or gastrocnemius. It is the author's choice to most commonly perform the indicated Achilles tendon lengthening percutaneous or the gastrocnemius release through endoscopic technique [8, 9].

Incision planning is based on the quality of the soft tissue, the extent and the degree of deformity, and the previous history of the injury and treatment (Fig. 16.9).

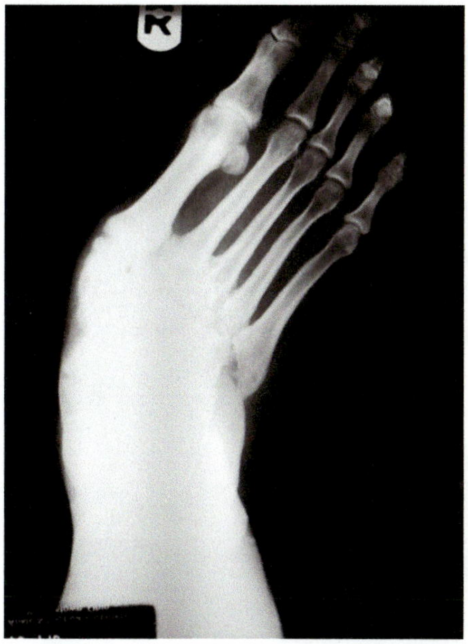

Fig. 16.8 A patient who presents following a failed Lisfranc treatment who now is experiencing an abducted forefoot and dorsiflexion of the metatarsals

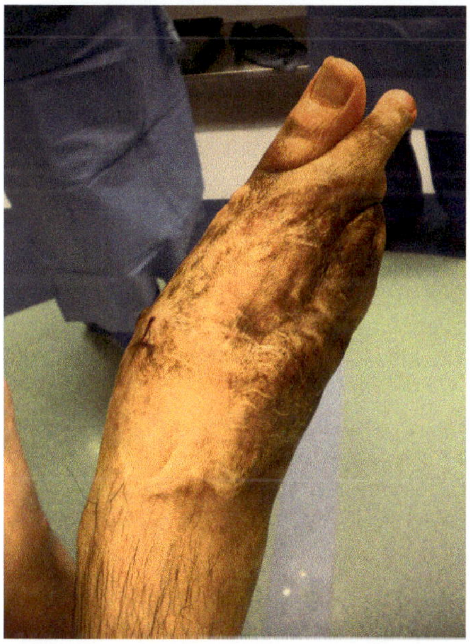

Fig. 16.9 This patient was a poly trauma patient who experienced a failed reduction of the Lisfranc joint and experienced soft tissue injuries from the initial trauma

The soft tissue envelope needs to be taken in to consideration. In some instances, there may have been previous incisions, there may be soft tissue changes as a result of the initial trauma, and/or the attenuation of the soft tissues changes from malalignment. The incisions are planned according to the deformity. For a severe deformity, two longer incisions are made: one dorsal medial over the first metatarsal and one over the third metatarsal. In some instances, the authors have been able to utilize one large curvilinear incision over the second tarsal metatarsal joint. If planned appropriately, the first, second, and third tarsal metatarsal joints as well as adjacent joints can be exposed appropriately. Regardless of the incision, the incision needs to be full thickness, and care must be taken to avoid the neuromuscular bundles of the dorsal aspect of the Lisfranc joint (Figs. 16.10, 16.11, and 16.12).

In reducing the deformity, the aim is to restore alignment of the medial aspect of the base of the first metatarsal with the medial edge of the first cuneiform. Next, restoring alignment of the medial aspect of the base of the second metatarsal with the medial edge of the second cuneiform in the transverse plane is needed. Next, alignment of the long axis of the talus with the long axis of the first metatarsal in both the sagittal and transverse planes is needed to restore anatomical alignment.

In patients who present with significant abduction of the forefoot, the surgeon must assess the stability or lack of stability of the lesser tarsal metatarsal joints and the lateral column and investigate the hindfoot for malalignment. Based on Lisfranc reduction, as well as clinical and radiographic findings, the surgeon may need to supplement the lateral column and hindfoot for stability. It is possible that the peroneus brevis tendon and other lateral soft tissues are contracted and may need to be lengthened. If the contracture is severe, an external fixator may need to be used intraoperatively to assist with the reduction [16].

An osteotome and a mallet are used to identify and determine which joints are pathologic. These joints are mobilized, and aggressive resection of scar tissue, fibrous tissue, and debris is removed allowing mobilization of the pathologic joints into a more normal alignment. Once the extent of the joint involvement is identified, the osteotome is utilized to denude the cartilage of the joint with little bone resection attempting to maintain the osseous integrity. A significant amount of time is spent at this junction of the surgery ensuring that the joints are appropriately prepared and plantar ossicles are removed. It is important to remove the plantar aspect of the joint in order to prevent dorsal angulation and malunion. This is facilitated by initial correction of the position of the first metatarsal. In most instances, the forefoot is adducted, plantar flexed, and de-rotated into a varus direction. When dealing with a large deformity, the surgeon must be cautious not to overcorrect or realign in adduction, in plantar flexion, or in the frontal plane. This is performed by grasping the great toe, dorsiflexing the great toe joint, and rotating the first metatarsal into a neutral position (varus direction), while the base of the first metatarsal is pushed against a stable aligned midfoot [10, 11]. If there is noted instability of the proximal tarsals of the midfoot, these joints are debrided, aligned, and temporary stabilized prior to

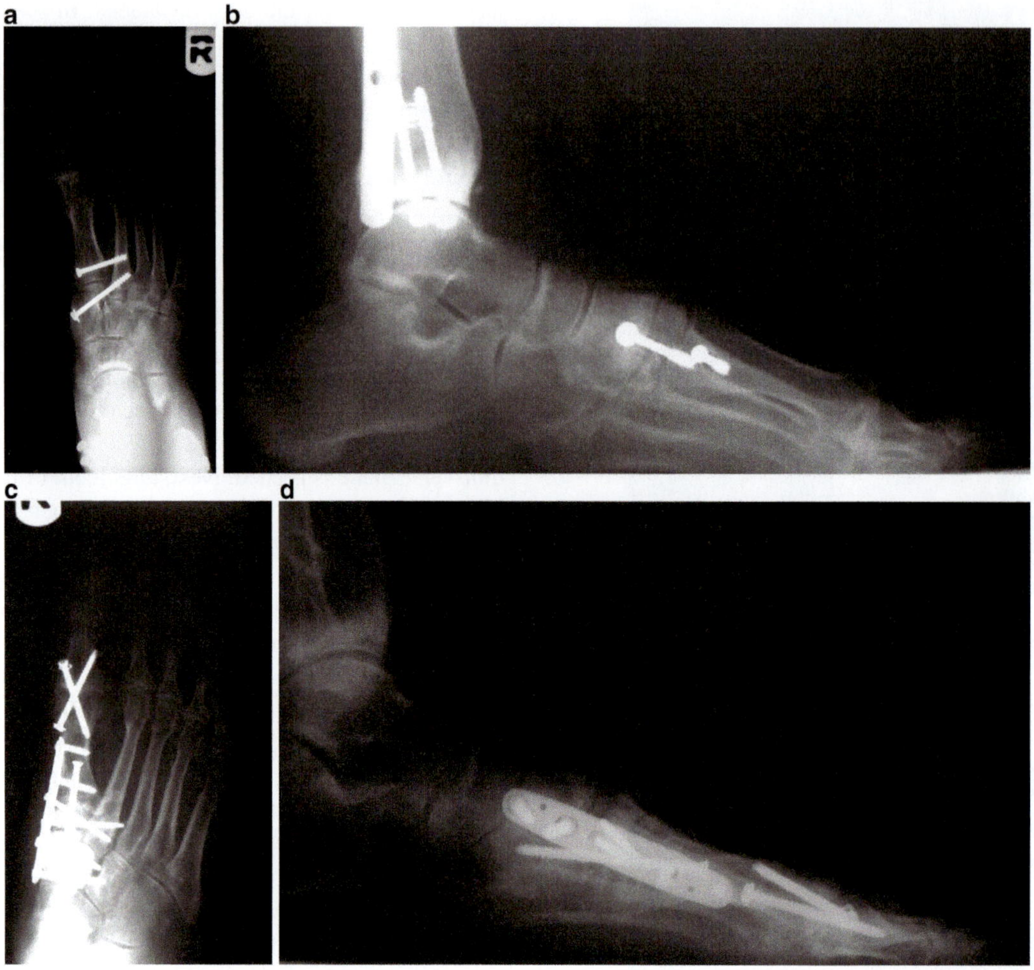

Fig. 16.10 (**a** and **b**) A anterior-posterior and lateral radiograph projection demonstrating a failed open reduction and internal fixation of a Lisfranc injury. Note that the failed reduction in the sagittal plane resulting in an elevatus, subsequently resulting in significant malalignment and pathological changes at the tarsal metatarsal joint, first metatarsal phalangeal joint, and the interphalangeal joint. (**c** and **d**) Postoperative radiograph following an realignment arthrodesis of the Lisfranc joint and arthrodesis of the first metatarsal phalangeal joint and percutaneous K-wire fixation (and removal) of the interphalangeal joint

reducing the first tarsal metatarsal joint. The first metatarsal is then temporary fixated with a 2.0 Kirchner wire and is inserted from the dorsal surface of the metatarsal proximally into the medial cuneiform while maintaining alignment. Next, the base of the second metatarsal is positioned appropriately followed by the third tarsal metatarsal. If the fourth and fifth metatarsal tarsal joints are involved, it has been the author's experience that once the first three tarsal metatarsal joints are positioned anatomically, the fourth and fifth metatarsal tarsal joints will be reduced anatomically similar to the vassal principle of an ankle fracture reduction [11]. A large bone-reduction clamp is placed obliquely to close the gap between the base of the second metatarsal and the medial cuneiform. Both the second and the third metatarsal are secured with multiple 2.0 Kirschner fixation through their respective cuneiforms in multiple planes. A 2.0 Kirschner wire is inserted from the medial cuneiform proximally toward the base of the second metatarsal. Anteroposterior, medial oblique and lateral fluoroscopic images are made to confirm the corrected alignment.

The reduction is held temporarily with multiple Kirschner wires, and radiographs are made to confirm the anatomical reduction. The authors prefer the use of 3.5 or 4.0 long, fully threaded solid cortical screws in a lag fashion with or without plating. In cases that involved extended proximal joints and significant deformity, the authors have employed interfragmentary screw compression, screw fixation, and an application of a plantar plate to the tension side of the foot [17]. The initial lag screw is inserted from the distal first metatarsal into the medial cuneiform. To avoid splitting of the dorsal cortex of the first metatarsal, the hole must be burred so that the screw can be countersunk carefully. A screw hole technique as described by Manoli and Hansen [12] allows for a difficult angulation, and the first screw is inserted from the

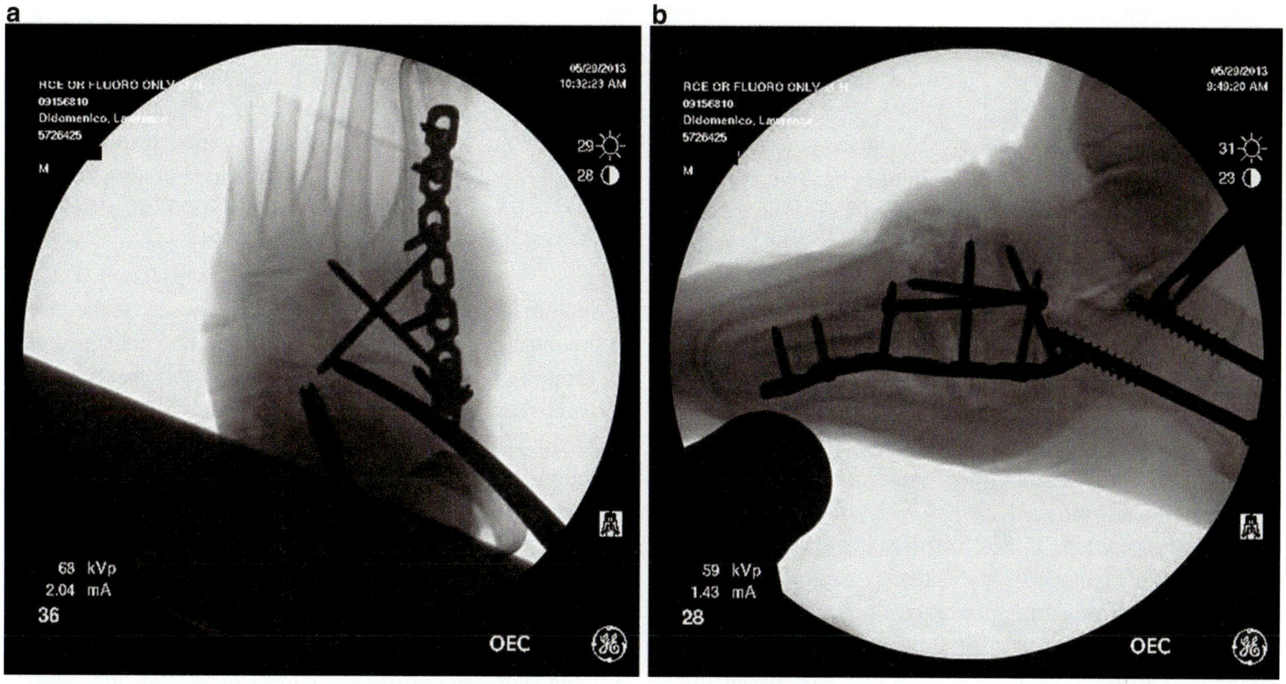

Fig. 16.11 (**a** and **b**) Intraoperative AP and lateral fluoroscopic images following a endoscopic gastrocnemius recession, a percutaneous medial calcaneal slide osteotomy, and a realignment arthrodesis with a large wedge resection at the Lisfranc joint. The base of the wedge resection was medial and plantar, and the apex was lateral and dorsal allowing for adduction, plantar flexion, and derotation in the frontal plane placing the Lisfranc joint into anatomic alignment. Fixation consisted of a 3.5 recon plate with independent long fully threaded solid cortical screws. This anatomically reduced the significant forefoot abduction, dorsally translated metatarsals and the forefoot values deformity, and realigned the hindfoot under the long axis of the tibia. Adjacent joint arthrodesis was additionally needed to control and realign the foot. Note the alignment of the talus first metatarsal alignment on the lateral and AP radiographs

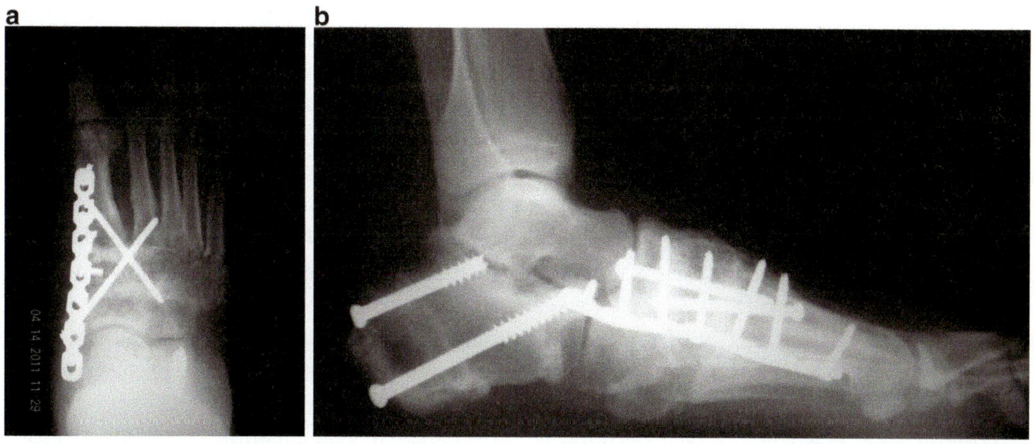

Fig. 16.12 (**a** and **b**) AP and lateral X-rays demonstrating an interfragmentary compression fixation coupled by a plantar plate on the tension side of the Lisfranc joint. Preoperatively the patient suffered a failed Lisfranc reduction and had an abducted forefoot, hindfoot values, and an unstable midfoot. The surgery consisted of an endoscopic gastrocnemius recession to address the equinus contracture, the percutaneous calcaneal slide osteotomy addressed the hind foot valgus, an Evans lateral column lengthening addressed the unstable mid foot, and a Lisfranc arthrodesis with adjacent joint fusions addressed the pathologic midfoot

first metatarsal to the medial cuneiform creating inter fragmentary compression. If there is noted proximal joint involvement, the proximal joints need to be fixated first to provide a stable midfoot in order to successfully align and fixate the Lisfranc joint. The next screw is an inter-fragmentary compression screw inserted from the stable superior proximal medial cuneiform obliquely oriented into the second metatarsal base. Understanding the anatomy of the Lisfranc joint in the frontal plane is required in order to successfully fixate the lesser metatarsal and lateral cuneiforms. Additional screws can be inserted from the proximal metatarsal base into the respected cuneiform and from the base of the first metatarsal into the base of the lesser metatarsals and/or lesser cuneiforms. A high-speed burr and rongeur is then used to debride the edges of the involved joints, and all bone voids are packed with autogenous or allogenic cancellous bone graft for a shear strain relief graft as described by Perren [13]. The gaps are preferably filled with local bone graft which can be harvested from the calcaneus [14], and if additional bone graft is needed, allogenic bone or a bone graft substitute can be utilized. It has been our experience that despite substantial radiographic changes, usually there is no symptomatic clinical pain in the joints between the fourth and fifth metatarsals and the tarsal bones, postoperatively, provided that the alignment has been corrected. If the fourth and fifth metatarsals are displaced, once anatomically reduced, 2.0 K-wire fixation can be used to maintain the position. Typical soft tissue and skin closure is performed. Postoperatively, the patient is placed in a dorsally slotted non-weight-bearing plaster cast for 2 weeks and is to keep the extremity elevated [15]. Provided there are no wound problems and the reduction and construct is stable, a fiberglass below the knee cast is applied for an additional 4–6 weeks and until radiographic consolidation is evident. Full weight bearing in a fracture boot with physical therapy is then prescribed for 4 weeks [11].

Neuropathic Arthrodesis

Lisfranc joint dislocation secondary to injury and/or Charcot arthropathy is a debilitating condition that can result with an ulceration and/or infection. After conservative care fails, treatment may be limited to realignment arthrodesis of the Lisfranc joint or amputation. Charcot neuroarthropathy is characterized by episodes of active and inactive periods. In the active phase, an edematous, erythematous, warm foot can show progressive destruction and dislocation. In the chronic phase, the foot can reveal a stiff malaligned, rocker bottom foot with soft tissue contractures and compromised skin integrity.

In a patient with a neuropathic Lisfranc joint, attention is directed to the posterior muscle where a Silfverskiold test is performed [7]. Based on the results, an Achilles tendon lengthening or a gastrocnemius recession is performed. Next, a straight incision is made, beginning at the talonavicular joint and extending to the distal one-third of the first metatarsal shaft. The incision is deepened, and a full-thickness flap is retracted superiorly and inferiorly off the tarsometatarsal joints. If previous hardware was utilized, it is removed. Attention is directed toward the base of the tarsal metatarsal articulation. Typically there is significant subluxation/dislocation with significant bony changes. An osteotome is used to resect this bone in order to identify the first tarsal metatarsal joint. Intraoperative fluoroscopic imaging is needed to assist in identifying the first tarsal metatarsal joint. Evaluation of the extent of the fracture/subluxation/dislocation proximal and lateral is necessary. The authors often utilize a 2.0 Kirschner wire inserted from medial to lateral for the most distal portion of the healthy tarsal bones and to the most proximal portion of the healthiest bone at base of the metatarsals. This acts as a rail system for the surgeon and provides a guide for an aggressive bone resection that can correct the deformity in all three planes. Based on the extent of involvement, the bone across the Lisfranc joint is resected to good, healthy, bleeding bone. The resection is typically performed as a wedge resection which allows for a tri-planar correction. The base of the wedge is medial and the apex lateral in the transverse plane. In the sagittal plane, the base is plantar, and the apex is dorsal. This allows the forefoot to be corrected by adducting and plantar flexing and rotated into a neutral position. Based on the extent of the lateral involvement of the Lisfranc joint, a second incision can be made on the lateral aspect of the foot between the fourth and fifth metatarsals; however, in most scenarios, the authors have been able to perform this through one large medial utility incision. If a lateral incision needed, it is deepened down to the base of the fourth and fifth metatarsals and cuboid. All diseased bone from medial to the lateral is removed. Depending on the extension of the Charcot destruction, bone resection may need to be performed through the naviculocuneiform, talonavicular joints, or other adjacent joint in order to restore the medial arch of the foot. If the more proximal joints are destabilized, they must be realigned and stabilized first starting proximally. The Lisfranc joint is adducted, rotated, and held in a plantar-flexed position with multiple 2.0 Kirschner wires. The first metatarsal, fifth metatarsal, and calcaneus must be on the same plane creating a tripod effect with the foot loaded. With the foot loaded, the ankle joint motion is checked to demonstrate that the equinus contracture is no longer present allowing the ankle to get into a neutral position. Alignment is checked using fluoroscopic imaging to ensure the talus first metatarsal angle in the transverse and sagittal plane is aligned. Next, a plate is eccentrically loaded plate is applied to the plantar aspect of the first metatarsal, medial cuneiform, and navicular.

A 3.5 cm or 4.0 solid cortical screw is placed outside the plate in an oblique fashion, beginning on the medial wall of the first metatarsal and aiming at the lateral edge of the navicular. A second cortical screw is inserted from the medial cuneiform or navicular into the second or third metatarsal base. The fourth and fifth metatarsals reduce to an anatomic position as the soft tissue and muscular attachments maintain consistency with anatomic reduction of the first and second tarsal metatarsals. Again, typically no fixation is used on the fourth and fifth rays. Autogenous or allogenic cancellous bone is used to back fill any voids at the arthrodesis site [11].

Typical soft tissue and skin closure is performed. Postoperatively, the patient is placed in a dorsally slotted non-weight-bearing plaster cast for 2 weeks and is to keep the extremity elevated [15]. Provided there are no wound problems and the reduction and construct is stable, a fiberglass below the knee cast is applied for an additional 6–8 weeks and/or until radiographic consolidation is evident. Partial weight bearing in a fracture boot with physical therapy is then prescribed for four additional weeks followed by full protective weight bearing. The postoperative course included serial radiographs every 3 weeks until radiographic evidence of consolidation is noted.

Contraindications/Limitations

An absolute contraindication for correcting a Lisfranc deformity is a dysvascular limb or a patient who is afflicted with a medical conditions prohibiting surgery. Also if a patient has an open wound and an active infection, the infection and wound management must be treated and stabilized prior to attempt at surgical corrections. Relative contraindications included altered bone quality, advanced age, tobacco use, patients who suffer from chronic regional pain syndrome, wound problems, ischemia due to peripheral vascular disease, osteomyelitis, and infections.

Prior to embarking on a revision reconstruction surgery, consideration must be given to the soft tissue envelop and assessing the vascular status of the patient. Given the history of the index injury and the previous failed treatment, the soft tissues must be closely examined. It is imperative that the soft tissue have the ability to respond to the proposed surgery. Obtaining vascular studies is often needed to predict the healing ability.

Due to the extent of the presenting deformity, some patients may present with chronic open wounds. It is essential for the surgeon to evaluate these patients thoroughly, use appropriate testing, and consult with the proper and needed specialties to manage these complex problems to determine if and when the best time is to address the deformity. Patients with a diagnosis of osteomyelitis from a previous infection or secondary to an ulcer deformity must be managed appropriately before, during, and after the surgery. If an active osteomyelitis is present, then the infection must be addressed first. In cases of a chronic osteomyelitis, a bony resection to clean margins and arthrodesis can be performed along with the appropriate comanagement of the chronic osteomyelitis. The bony resection serves as a function of a surgical treatment by removing the infected bone. The bony resection of infected bone to clean, heathy margins coupled with treatment of intravenous antibiotics has been a successful combination for the authors. Fixation provisions may be impacted based on the circumstances. In cases with a chronic osteomyelitis, resection of the infected bone serves as a surgical treatment; however, this may affect the quantity of bone and alter the fixation needed to reduce the deformity.

Given the magnitude of the deformity, in some cases, the foot may be shortened (medial column). The patient should understand that the operative foot may change the size of the foot compared to the preoperation size and compared to the contralateral side. As described earlier, if the hindfoot is unstable, the surgeon must be prepared to perform additional surgical procedures that most likely will need additional hardware and/or bone graft. With large deformities, the surgeon needs to be prepared to employ the use of an external fixator to assist in the reduction of the deformity.

Technique Pearls and Pitfalls to Avoid Complications

The recommended incision should be curvilinear over the first tarsometatarsal. This provides excellent exposure to the first, second, and third tarsometatarsal joints while avoiding the deep peroneal nerve and dorsalis pedis artery. Additionally, this prevents unnecessary traction on the skin and neurovascular structures. If a second incision is needed, it should be over the fourth metatarsal shaft. It should be noted that the soft tissue island between the incisions needs to be adequate in size to prevent tissue necrosis. If only the medial tarsometatarsal joints are involved, it has been the experience of the authors to make a large dorsal curvilinear incision starting at the dorsal lateral first metatarsal and extending to the naviculocuneiform joint. Care should be taken not to undermine/separate the tissues in order to prevent soft tissue injury. The exposure must be adequate once the incision is made; the tissues should be reflected off the bony structures as a full-thickness flap. Preferred retraction is accomplished with small fine tooth double prong retractors and/or mini Hohmann retractors to reduce trauma to the tissues and to avoid trauma to the neuromuscular structures [11].

The goal of the treatment is a stable, painless, plantigrade foot. The goal is achieved by anatomical reduction, alignment, and stable fixation. Preparation of the joints to ensure adequate consolidation is essential. Joint distraction can be achieved with tarsal distractors or a laminar spreader. The use of drills, osteotomes, picks, curettes, and rongeurs is utilized to prepare the joint(s) for arthrodesis. Debridement is performed down the level of healthy, bleeding bone with the goal of maintaining normal articular surfaces as much as possible. Specific attention should be made to the plantar tarsal metatarsal joints during preparation to confirm there is no residual bone/cartilage remaining which could predispose the reduction to dorsal angulation and malunion. Excellent reduction must be accomplished. An AO (Arbeitsgemeinschaft für Osteosynthesefragen) pointed reduction forcep may be used to aid in reduction. The use of intraoperative fluoroscopic imaging is extremely helpful in ensuring appropriate and anatomic alignment.

Prior to fixation of the Lisfranc joint, the surgeon needs to assess the proximal and adjacent joints. If the nearby joints are unstable and overlooked, the surgery may result with complications.

The fixation construct is extremely important to the success of the surgery. Solid fully threaded screws are recommended. A stable solid fixation construct is necessary and should be designed specifically for each particular case with a great deal of thought. When inserting the fixation specifically from the metatarsal into the cuneiforms, a burr hole technique as described by Manoli and Hansen [12] is extremely helpful for drilling the difficult angles and inserting the screws from distal to proximal. Additionally, the burr hole allows the screw to be recessed so it is not proud and palpable. Lastly it prevents stress risers in the cortical bone of the metatarsals and prevents fracturing of the bone.

To avoid inefficient fixation, while inserting screws from the medial cuneiform or first metatarsal into the base of the respective second metatarsal and intermediate cuneiform, the screw should be directed more superiorly to successfully obtain a good purchase. The anatomy of the midfoot in the frontal plane mimics a "Roman Arch"; thus, the base of the second metatarsal and intermediate cuneiform is positioned more superiorly than the base of the first metatarsal and the medial cuneiform.

Bone to bone contact while maintaining anatomic alignment is a key to a successful outcome and bony union when attempting an arthrodesis at the Lisfranc joint. Due to the challenges of Lisfranc joint configuration, preoperative malalignment, the given number of joints involved following articular cartilage, and bone debridement, it can be difficult to appropriately anatomically align multiple aspects of each joint while trying to maintain as much bone to bone contact. Because anatomic alignment is paramount, in situations where dorsal gaps are noted in order to preserve anatomic alignment while attempting to have as much bone to bone contact (usually the plantar edges of the joints), a shear strain relief bone graft is used to backfill the voided areas of the joints [11]. For example, when revising the first tarsal metatarsal joint, it is critical to align the first metatarsal appropriately with the long axis of the talus in the sagittal plane. In order to appropriately align the joint with bone to bone contact, the first metatarsal may need to be plantar flexed relative to the cuneiform in order to maintain the talus first metatarsal angle in the sagittal plane. The result oftentimes will leave the first metatarsal cuneiform joint with nice bone to bone contact at the plantar edges of the joint and gapped at the dorsal surface. This is a perfect scenario where tightly backfilling of a joint with bone graft while maintaining alignment without sacrificing position.

Lastly in order to prevent increased stress across the tarsal metatarsal joint, equinus contractures should be appropriately managed intraoperatively. This is important to reducing load and weight-bearing forces through the forefoot and midfoot, thus, increasing the rate of union and chance for a successful outcome.

Management of Specific Complications

Malunion

Anatomic reduction is the goal of any Lisfranc injury. However, the type and extent of the injury as well as the previous treatment may prove to make revision surgery difficult. Patient comorbidities may also play a role. A malunion may ensue leading to arch collapse, arthritis, and lesser metatarsalgia. Malunion of the second TMTJ has been reported to be the most common with displacement in a dorsolateral direction [27]. Typically, Lisfranc injuries involve multidirectional instability so all planes need to be addressed and reduced appropriately. For example, if the first ray is inadequately reduced, particularly in the sagittal plane, an elevatus may ensue. This could alter the joint mechanics of the hallux at the more distal metatarsophalangeal and interphalangeal joint (see Fig. 8a, b) and predispose the patient to lesser metatarsal overload. Gross malalignment or the neuropathic foot may require a medial- and plantar-based wedge arthrodesis at the Lisfranc joint [17, 18].

Brunet reported on the long-term sequela of Lisfranc fracture dislocations at an average follow-up of 15 years for 33 patients. The purpose of their paper was to determine the anatomical, functional, and radiographic results at over a 10-year follow-up. Even though the large majority of patients had Hardcastle type B injuries, most patients were treated with closed reduction and immobilization, closed reduction with immobilization and pinning, or no reduction with a cast. Open reduction was performed in only one patient. Foot pain was attributed to malunion of metatarsal fractures in three patients, sesamoiditis in four patients, and adjacent joint arthritis in six patients. Hallux rigidus was common in three patients. Posttraumatic arthritis on radiographs did not correlate to functional outcomes as most patients returned to full work-and non-work-related activities despite the presence of severe to mild arthritis. This study stresses the importance of anatomic reduction as malalignment will alter mechanics through the forefoot [19].

Basic principles consisting of excellent joint debridement, precise anatomic alignment, and a stable, solid fixation construct are essential in order to avoid a malunion. Most of the time spent during the surgical procedure should be identifying the appropriate joints involved, joint preparation in cases requiring arthrodesis, and building the fixation construct. Attention to detail with these principles will help prevent malunion.

Revising a malunion of the Lisfranc joint typically consists of hardware removal and aggressive joint resection to healthy bleeding bone. Wedge resection is often needed in order to align the malunion joint, and bone graft is often needed in gapped areas in order to retain anatomic alignment.

Lesser Metatarsalgia

Lesser metatarsalgia can develop in case where malalignment exist and the foot is not balanced appropriately. If there is gross angulation of the lesser metatarsals particularly in the sagittal plane, the patient may present with pain and/or calluses of the adjacent lesser metatarsals. When performing revision arthrodesis, the key suggestions to prevent lesser metatarsalgia from developing is to be sure the talar first metatarsal angle in both the transverse and sagittal plane are aligned well. Focused attention to the medial tarsal metatarsal joint ensures the joints are aligned appropriately and that weight bearing will be restored through the first ray. Once reduction of the medial (dominant segment) tarsal metatarsal is successfully reduced, the remaining lesser tarsal metatarsal joint will become anatomically aligned. It has been the author's experience that once the first three tarsometatarsal joints are positioned, the fourth and fifth metatarsal tarsal joints will be reduced anatomically [11]. The fixation utilized should be long and begin as far distal in the metatarsals to provide a cantilever effect which in turn will help to prevent ground reactive forces from causing dorsal drifting of the metatarsals. Also the forefoot pressures are reduced by addressing the tight posterior muscle group through an Achilles tendon lengthening or a gastrocnemius recession. In unfortunate cases which an isolated metatarsal is maligned, an isolated lesser metatarsal osteotomy can be performed to address the malalignment. Lesser metatarsal osteotomies should be limited to cases of only isolated metatarsal deformity or isolated malalignment. Lesser osteotomies applied to cases of global metatarsal deformity or malalignment often will not resolve the issue and can provide transfer lesions and metatarsal pathology.

Komenda et al. reported on 32 patients who underwent arthrodesis following traumatic Lisfranc injuries. Metatarsalgia was a complaint postoperatively in two patients secondary to malunion. Both patients were treated with a dorsal-based wedge osteotomy [20]. Mann et al. reported on five patients with prominent metatarsal heads following tarsometatarsal arthrodesis.

Arthrosis of the Fourth and Fifth Tarsometatarsal Joints

Based on the author's experience, fusion of the fourth and fifth tarsal metatarsal joints in the non-neuropathic patient is rarely indicated if appropriate alignment is maintained. When arthritis is present in the fourth and fifth tarsal metatarsal joints, it has been the experience of the authors that excellent reduction and anatomic alignment with stable fixation of the medial column coupled with anatomic alignment of the fourth and fifth tarsal metatarsal joints creates a predictable satisfactory outcome. In the neuropathic patient population, arthrodesis of the fourth and fifth tarsal metatarsal is well tolerated and provides stability provided it is well aligned. Management strategies for lateral column arthritis are varied and controversial. Because the lateral column is more mobile compared with the other columns, attempt is made to preserve the motion. Despite the fact that arthritis may be present, it is usually asymptomatic [18, 20]. There is a concern that fusing the lateral column could cause stiffness and increase the chances for a stress fracture [21]. As discussed previously, the motion through the lateral column is the greatest as compared to the medial and central columns [22], and therefore these joints should typically be preserved. With this increased motion, there is also a greater risk for nonunion [21] if an arthrodesis is attempted.

Raikin and Shon in 2003 retrospectively reviewed 23 patients (28 feet) who had undergone a complete midfoot arthrodesis. The large majority had neuroarthropathy, 22 patients, with the other six patients being sensate. Clinical and radiographic fusion was achieved in 26/28 patients. The overall AOFAS scores improved from 35.3 points preoperatively to 77.7 points postoperatively. Average pain scores overall also decreased from 5.1 points preoperatively to 1.3 points postoperatively. Lateral column stiffness was reported postoperatively in 13 patients; however, it did appear to alter their function according to the study. They concluded that lateral column arthrodesis may be indicated for patients with lateral column collapse, a rocker bottom deformity, or significant arthritis not amenable to conservative care [23].

Berlet et al. in 2002 retrospectively reviewed 12 patients who underwent tendon, interpositional arthroplasty for arthritis of the fourth and/or fifth tarsometatarsal joints. At an average of 25 months of follow-up, the mean AOFAS midfoot rating scale was 64.5. They noted that patients that scored higher postoperatively typically had preoperative pain relief with a diagnostic, intra-articular injection. They recommended an injection preoperatively as both a therapeutic and prognostic indicator for patients one may consider for surgical intervention [24].

Viens et al. reported on five patients who underwent ceramic interpositional arthroplasty for fourth and fifth TMTJ arthritis. The mean clinical and radiographic follow-up was 18 months. All patients reported subjective improvement in pain. There was complete resolution of pain in three patients. Two patients experienced complications postoperatively consisting of wound dehiscence and delayed healing, respectively. No scoring systems were evaluated before or after the surgery [25].

Shawen et al. also reported on interpositional arthroplasty via a ceramic implant in 2007. They reported on 13 patients who underwent this procedure after failing non-operative care. Eleven patients were available for follow-up at an average of 34 months. Their results showed an average midfoot AOFAS score of 52.5 which was an 87% overall increase compared to preoperative values. The VAS pain scores improved on average by 42%. A large majority of patients (11/13) reported that they would have the procedure performed again [26].

References

1. Stavlas P, Roberts CS, Xypnitos FN, Giannoudis PV. The role of reduction and internal fixation of Lisfranc fracture-dislocations: a systematic review of the literature. Int Orthop. 2010;34:1083–91.
2. Elefttheriou KI, Rosenfeld PF. Lisfranc injury in the athlete. Foot Ankle Clin N Am. 2013;18:219–36.
3. DiDomenico LA, Thomas ZM. Midfoot crush injuries. Clin Podiatr Med Surg. 2014;31:493–508.
4. Watson TS, Shurnas PS, Denker J. Treatment of Lisfranc joint injury: Current Concepts. J Am Acad Orthop Surg. 2010;18:718–28.
5. DiDomenico LA, Cross D. Tarsometatarsal/Lisfranc joint. Clin Podiatr Med Surg. 2012;29:221–42.
6. Gazdag AR, Cracchiolo A, 3rd. Rupture of the posterior tibial tendon. Evaluation of injury of the spring ligament and clinical assessment of tendon transfer and ligament repair. J Bone Joint Surg Am 1997;79:675–681.
7. Silfverskiod N. Reduction of the uncrossed two joint muscles of the leg to one joint muscle in spastic conditions. Acta Chir Scand. 1924;56:315–30.
8. Haro AA, DiDomenico LA. Frontal plane—guided percutaneous tendo achilles lengthening. J Foot Ankle Surg. 2007;46:55–61.
9. DiDomenico LA, Groner TW, et al. Endoscopic gastrocnemiues recession. In: Saxena A, editor. International advances in foot and ankle surgery. London: Springer; 2012. p. 431–8.
10. DiDomenico LA, Fahim R, et al. Correction of frontal plane rotation of sesamoid apparatus during the lapidus procedure: a novel approach. J Foot Ankle Surg. 2014;53(6):248–51.
11. DiDomenico LA, Stein DY. Tarsal metatarsal (Lisfranc) dislocation. In: McGlamry's comprehensive textbook of foot and ankle surgery, 4th ed. p. 1677–84 [Chapter 106].
12. Manoli II A, Hansen Jr ST. Screw hole preparation in foot surgery. Foot Ankle Int. 1990;11:105–6.
13. Perren SM. Physical and biological aspects of fracture healing with special reference to internal fixation. Clin Orthop Relat Res. 1979;138:175–96.
14. Di Domenico LA, Haro AA. Percutaneous harvest of calcanea bone graft. JFAS. 2006;45(2):131–3.
15. DiDomenico LA, Sann P. Univalve split plaster cast for postoperative immobilization in foot and ankle surgery. JFAS. 2013;52:260–2.
16. Sangeorzan BJ, Veith RG, et al. Salvage of lisfranc's tarsometatarsal joint by arthrodesis. Foot Ankle Int. 1990;10(4):193–200.
17. Garchar D, Di Domenico LA. Reconstruction of isfrnac joint dislocations secondary to charcot neuroarthropathy using a plantar plate. J Foot Ankle Surg. 2013;52(3):295–7.
18. Aranow MS. Treatment of the missed Lisfranc Injury. Foot Ankle Clin N Am. 2006;11:127–42.
19. Brunet JA, Wiley JJ. The late results of tarsometatarsal joint injuries. JBJS. 1987;69-B(3):437–40.
20. Komenda GA, Myerson MS, Biddinger KR. Results of arthrodesis of the tarsometatarsal joints after traumatic injury. JBJS. 1996;78-A(11):1665–76.
21. Patel A, Rao S, Nawoczenski D, et al. Midfoot arthritis. J Am Acad Orthop Surg. 2010;18:417–25.
22. Ouzounian TJ, Shereff MJ. In vitro determination of midfoot motion. Foot Ankle. 1989;10(3):140–6.
23. Raikin SM, Schon LC. Arthrodesis of the fourth and fifth tarsometatarsal joints of the midfoot. Foot Ankle Int. 2003;24(8):584–90.
24. Berlet GC, Anderson R. Tendon arthroplasty for basal fourth and fifth metatarsal arthritis. Foot Ankle Int. 2002;23(5):440–6.
25. Viens NA, Adams SB, Nunley JA. Ceramic interpositional arthroplasty for fourth and fifth tarsometatarsal joint arthritis. J Surg Orthop Adv. 2012;21(3):126–31.
26. Shawen SB, Anderson RB, Cohen BE, et al. Spherical ceramic interpositional arthroplasty for basal fourth and fifth metatarsal arthritis. Foot Ankle Int. 2007;28(8):896–901.
27. Bellabarba C, Barei DP, Sanders RW. Dislocaitons of the foot. In: Coughlin MJ, Mann RA, Saltzman CL, editors. Surgery of the foot and ankle. Philadelphia: Elsevier; 2007. p. 2175.

Calcaneal Fractures

17

James Thomas

Introduction

Treatment of calcaneal fractures has evolved over the last 25 years from primarily nonoperative care to a more aggressive approach involving open reduction and internal fixation, with a recent rejuvenation of limited exposure and percutaneous fixation in select fractures. Many of the treatment recommendations have evolved from the type and rate of complications that have been seen as the result of various treatments of calcaneal fractures, both operative and nonoperative. Complications range from wound problems to malunion, whether treated open or closed [1–3], (Tables 17.1 and 17.2).

Anatomy certainly plays a significant role in predisposing the patient with a calcaneal fracture to possible complication. When the complex and variable arrangement of the articular facets of the subtalar joint is combined with the limited soft tissue envelope of the hind foot and ankle, as well as the surrounding tendon and neurovascular structures coursing medially and laterally along the calcaneus, it is easy to appreciate why an array of complications can occur regarding the treatment of calcaneal fractures (Fig. 17.1a, b). Fractures of the calcaneus may also involve the calcaneocuboid joint, and post-traumatic arthritis of this joint may also be seen. Resultant gait abnormalities are not uncommon.

Possibly the most frequent and significant complication of calcaneal fractures is malunion, which can lead to its own subset of problems. Wound complications, primarily from open treatment of calcaneal fractures, present unique challenges of their own. Advanced diagnostic imaging, in addition to plain radiographs, is necessary for proper fracture evaluation especially in the case of intra-articular fractures [4, 5]. Complications from calcaneal fractures can be arbitrarily divided into nonoperative and operative complications, although certainly some overlap does occur.

J. Thomas (✉)
The Orthopaedic Clinic, Auburn, AL, USA
e-mail: jthomas@theorthoclinic.com

Nonoperative Complications

Nonoperative complications primarily are a result of malunion of displaced calcaneal fractures. Fracture malunion may produce an array of problems. Non-union, although extremely rare, can occur, but if present, it is usually associated with a degree of malunion. Direct complications from malunion may include heel shortening, loss of heel height, varus deformity of the hind foot, and displacement of the lateral calcaneal wall which can produce peroneal tendon impingement, sural neuritis, fibular impingement, and increased heel width with resultant shoe fit problems [4]. Chronic edema, tendinopathy (including peroneal, flexor hallucis, and flexor digitorum longus), peroneal subluxation/dislocation, posterior heel pain (especially with tongue or avulsion fractures), Achilles tendon dysfunction, and even compartment syndrome with resultant toe flexion deformities may occur [6–8]. Intra-articular step-off may lead to both subtalar and calcaneocuboid joint arthritis [1]. Failure to recognize and timely reduce displaced tongue-type or avulsion fractures with tenting of the posterior soft tissues can result in significant skin necrosis and breakdown [9, 10], (Fig. 17.2a, b). Neurovascular injury may occur from displaced sharp osseous fragments and, if left untreated, may result in permanent nerve impairment. The sustentaculum tali area is of most concern regarding displaced fracture fragments due to its close proximity to the medial neurovascular bundle [11] (Fig. 17.3).

Operative Complications

One of the most frequent complications following operative treatment of calcaneal fractures is wound healing problems involving the incisional approach. These may result from ill timing of surgical intervention, inappropriate placement or performance of lateral flap development if using a lateral extensile approach, or other patient issues such as a history of smoking [12–15]. Wound breakdown runs the full

M.S. Lee, J.P. Grossman (eds.), *Complications in Foot and Ankle Surgery*, DOI 10.1007/978-3-319-53686-6_17

spectrum from superficial only to deep wounds with hardware exposure and possible associated infection, including calcaneal osteomyelitis (Figs. 17.4, 17.5). Fracture blisters and their sequelae should be allowed to resolve and skin wrinkles observed before surgical intervention is undertaken to help in prevention of postoperative wound breakdown (Fig. 17.6a, b). Placing hardware along and under incision lines or subtalar joint penetration of hardware (so-called in-out-in of the posterior facet) must be avoided (Fig. 17.7). Medial neurovascular and tendon injury can also result from inappropriately long screws or drill bit penetration into the medial soft tissues during internal fixation maneuvers [16]. Mal-reduction of operatively treated calcaneal fractures can lead to all of the same issues as described for malunion of nonoperatively treated calcaneal fractures, including post-traumatic arthritis. Sural nerve injury, including neuroma, paresthesia, and permanent impairment, as well as peroneal tendon injury can occur during surgical exposure of the lateral calcaneal wall [17–20]. Side to side plantar pressure mismatch has been reported 2 years after open reduction of calcaneal fractures, even with improvement of Bohler's angle [21].

Table 17.1 Potential complications of non-operative treatment of calcaneal fractures

Malunion	Chronic edema
Non-union	Tendonopathy (peroneal and flexor tendons)
Heel shortening	Peroneal dislocation
Decreased heel height	Posterior heel pain
Varus deformity	Achilles tendon dysfunction
Lateral calcaneal displacement	Compartment syndrome
Peroneal tendon impingement	Toe flexion deformities
Sural nerve neuritis	Arthritis
Fibular impingement	Anterior ankle impingement
Increased heel width	Wound complications (open and tongue/avulsion fractures)
Shoe fit problems	Neurovascular damage

Table 17.2 Potential complications of operatively treated calcaneal fractures

Wound (incision) complications	Mal-reduction (may result in all of the problems listed in Table 17.1)
Osteomyelitis	
Hardware complications (loosening, soft tissue/joint impingement, soft tissue injury from drill bits, etc.)	
Sural nerve injury	
Peroneal tendon injury	
Medial neurovascular/tendon injury	

Management of Complications

Management of complications stemming from calcaneal fractures ranges from fairly straightforward treatments to more complex surgical procedures. In the acute setting, one must be observant for compartment syndrome which has been reported in up to 10% of cases [22–24]. If fasciotomy is indicated, release should be performed emergently of the affected compartments to prevent permanent neuromuscular impairment and its resultant toe contractures as well as possible resultant chronic pain issues. Post-traumatic arthritis and its subsequent symptom complex is often an end result of calcaneal fractures [1]. If the fracture is well reduced, and little to no deformity is present, bracing, orthotic control, shoe modifications, corticosteroid injections, and medical management may be sufficient to control symptoms associated with arthritis. If nonoperative treatment is unsuccessful, in situ arthrodesis of the subtalar joint in the well-aligned

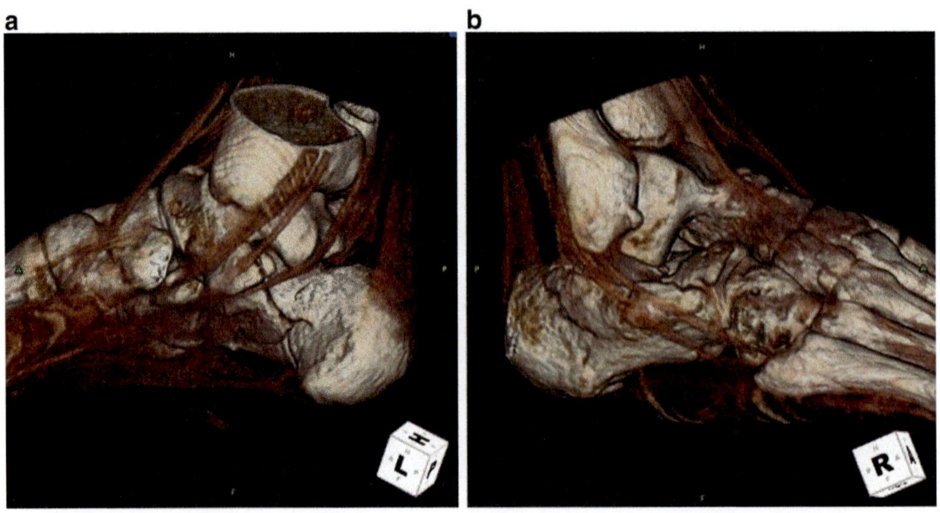

Fig. 17.1 (**a**) Medial view of CT reconstruction of a calcaneal fracture with tendon outline overlay demonstrating close proximity of flexor tendons to fracture lines and subsequent vulnerability to injury. (**b**) Lateral view of same demonstrating vulnerability of peroneal tendons to injury, especially in the area of the peroneal tubercle

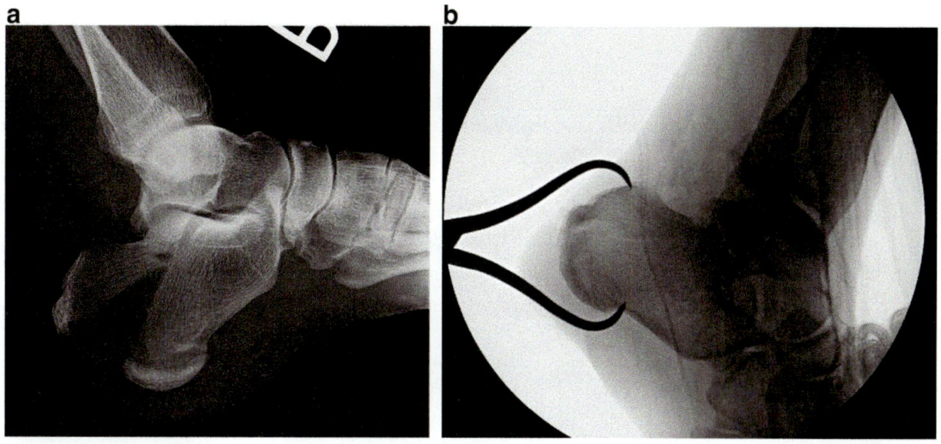

Fig. 17.2 (**a**) Radiograph of avulsion-type calcaneal fracture producing impingement of the posterior soft tissues. Emergent reduction of this fracture type may be necessary to prevent tissue breakdown secondary to skin tenting. (**b**) Intraoperative image of reduction of the same fracture before fixation. Note decompression of posterior soft tissues

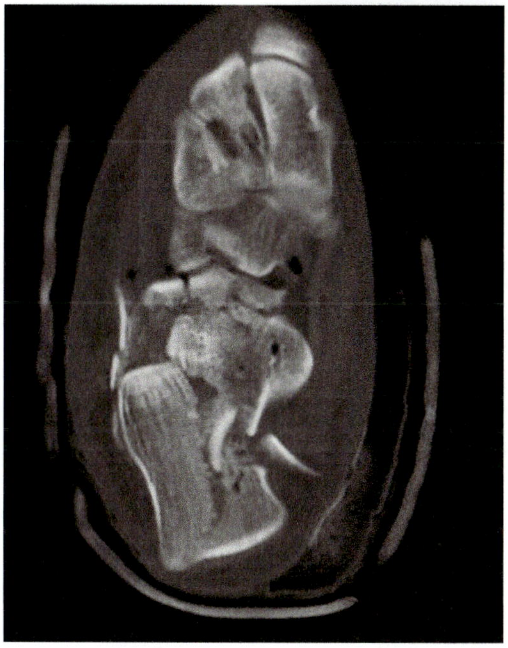

Fig. 17.3 CT scan example of sharp, osseous bone fragment in the area of the medial neurovascular bundle which may result in vascular injury and/or nerve impingement

fracture may be performed (Fig. 17.8a, b). If peroneal tendon or sural nerve pathology is present, this may be addressed simultaneously. If calcaneocuboid joint arthritis is also present, extended hind foot arthrodesis may be required. However, in many cases of post-traumatic arthritis following intra-articular fractures of the calcaneus, alignment is less than satisfactory and varying degrees of malunion may be present making in situ arthrodesis not an option. Malunion can be found both in the nonoperatively unreduced fracture and with mal-reduction in the operatively treated fracture (Figs. 17.9 and 17.10). Malunion results in a variety of problems that may produce symptoms. Some of the most disabling of these problems include arthritis, loss of heel height, increased heel width, shortening, varus deformity, peroneal tendon/fibular impingement, and anterior ankle impingement

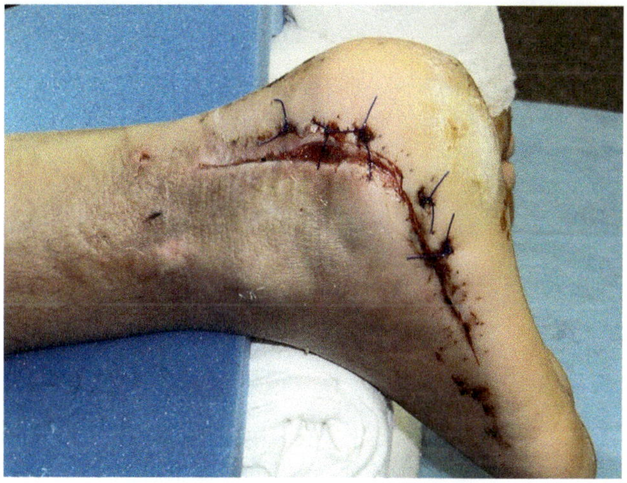

Fig. 17.4 Early postoperative superficial breakdown of the posterior vertical arm of the lateral extensile approach. Appropriate wound treatment is indicated to prevent deeper wound breakdown

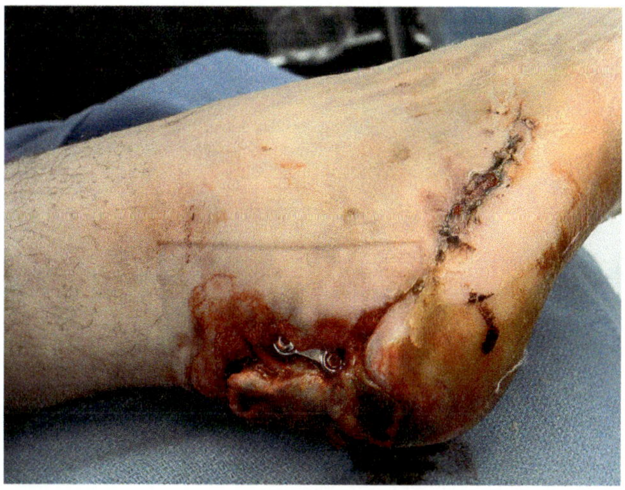

Fig. 17.5 Breakdown of the vertical arm of the lateral extensile approach with exposed hardware and Achilles tendon involvement. Deep wound breakdown may be associated with calcaneal osteomyelitis, and aggressive wound treatment is indicated. Partial or complete hardware removal may be required (Photo courtesy of Randy Clements, DPM)

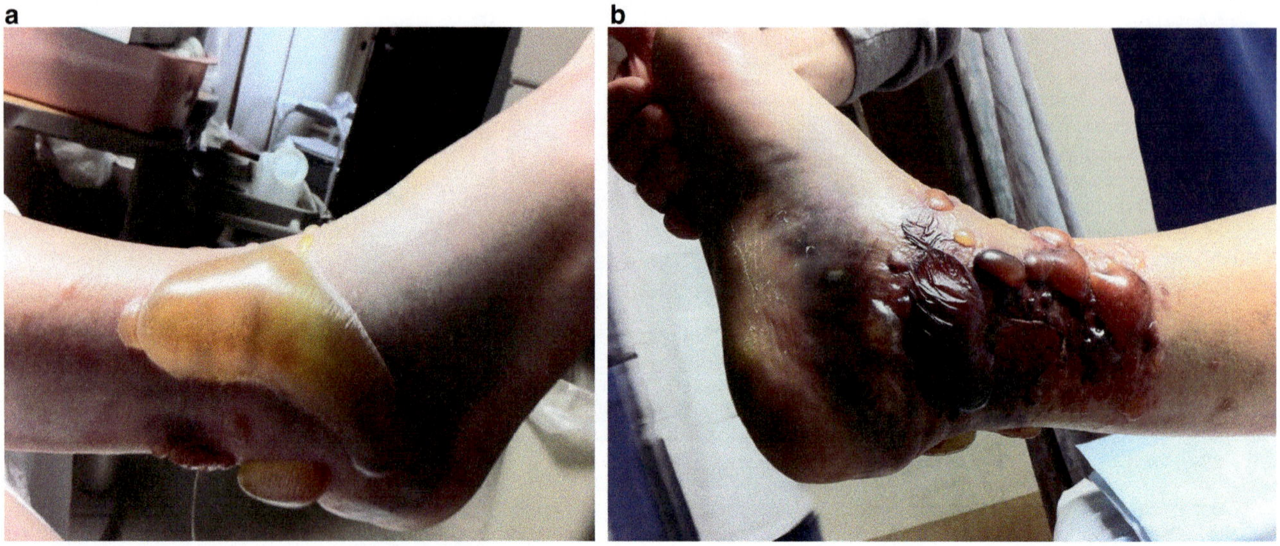

Fig. 17.6 (**a**) Lateral fracture blisters following closed calcaneal fracture. (**b**) Medial fracture blisters in the same patient. These must be addressed, edema reduced, and allowance for soft tissue recovery accomplished before surgical intervention is under taken

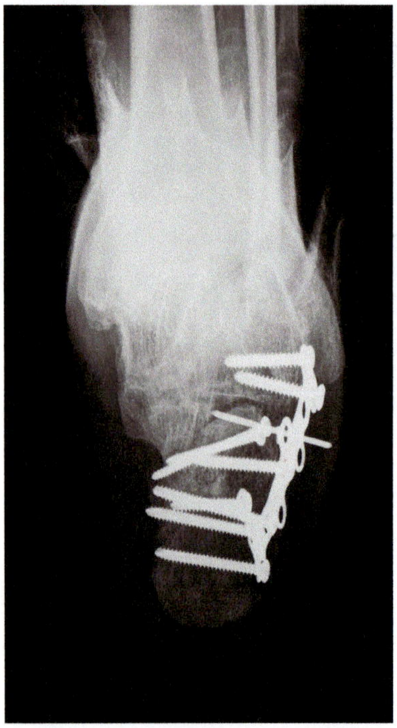

Fig. 17.7 Example of intra-articular penetration of the subtalar joint by Kirschner wire fixation. Note mal-reduction of posterior facet also

[25] (Fig. 17.11a, b). Diagnostic imaging workup is absolutely necessary in determining type and degree of deformity and condition of the articular surfaces. Bohler's angle is determined from standard lateral views and comparison views to the uninjured contralateral side help establish the normal value for the patient and assist in preoperative planning to determine the amount of correction which may be necessary [26]. In addition to standard radiographic views and CT imaging of the hind foot and ankle, calcaneal axial and long leg axial as well as hind foot alignment views may be beneficial in evaluating the patient with late complications of calcaneal fractures [4]. MRI may be helpful in cases of suspected associated soft tissue pathology.

In cases of fracture malunion, posterior bone block arthrodesis is a very effective way of addressing all of the abovementioned pathology, as it can restore height; resolve impingement of the fibula, peroneal tendons, and anterior ankle; and treat the symptoms associated with post-traumatic osteoarthritis [25, 27–29]. The lateral extensile incision commonly employed in open reduction of calcaneal fractures may be utilized for posterior bone block arthrodesis, although this incision may at times be difficult to close at the posterior apex if significant correction is required and if the deformity is long-standing in nature (Fig. 17.12). After incision placement, a full-thickness flap can then be developed off of the lateral calcaneal wall and a thorough debulking of the lateral calcaneus can then be undertaken (Fig. 17.13). Care must be taken to protect the sural nerve and peroneal tendons. Bone removed can be saved for use as bone graft in the arthrodesis site if needed. Debulking of the lateral calcaneal wall should effectively decompress the peroneal tendons and sural nerve and its branches. However the peroneal tendons should still be inspected for tears or subluxation with appropriate repair of any pathology present, and neurolysis of the sural nerve can be performed if entrapment is found. Alternatively the incision may be modified by elongating the vertical posterior arm and making the distal horizontal arm somewhat more oblique and shorter (Fig. 17.14a, b). This modification results in a more posterior approach to the

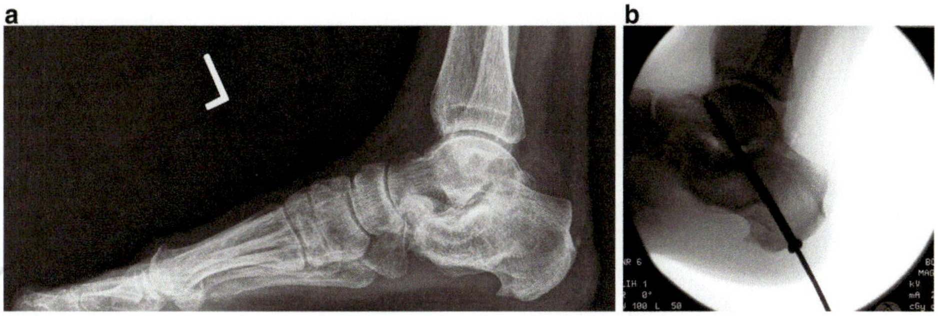

Fig. 17.8 (**a**) Preoperative radiograph of old intra-articular calcaneal fracture with subtalar arthritis but normal height and alignment of the calcaneus. (**b**) Intra-operative fluoroscopic image of the same patient after in situ subtalar joint arthrodesis. Bone graft is usually not necessary as calcaneal height is maintained

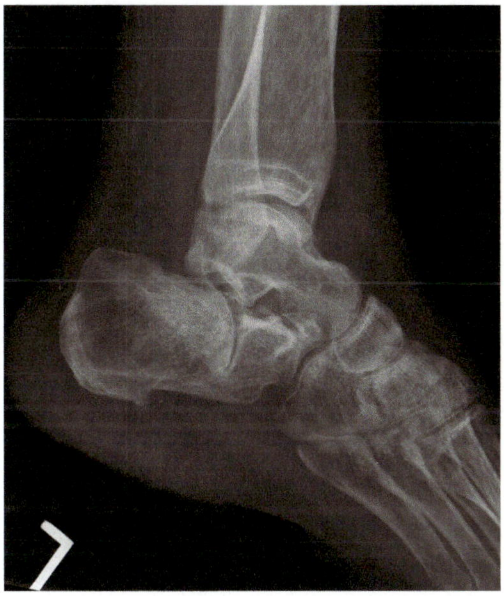

Fig. 17.9 Lateral radiograph of 8-month-old joint depression-type calcaneal fracture with subsequent malunion, but prior to complete collapse of the talus into the calcaneus

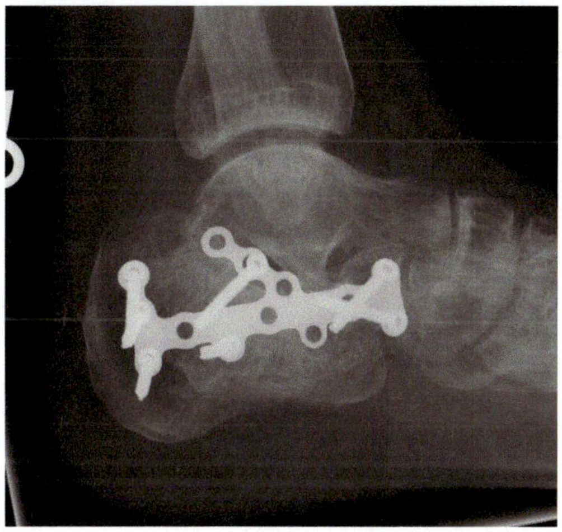

Fig. 17.10 Lateral radiograph of a mal-reduced, operatively treated joint depression calcaneal fracture. Note loss of calcaneal height, subsidence of the talus into the calcaneus, and hardware impingement along the lateral subtalar joint

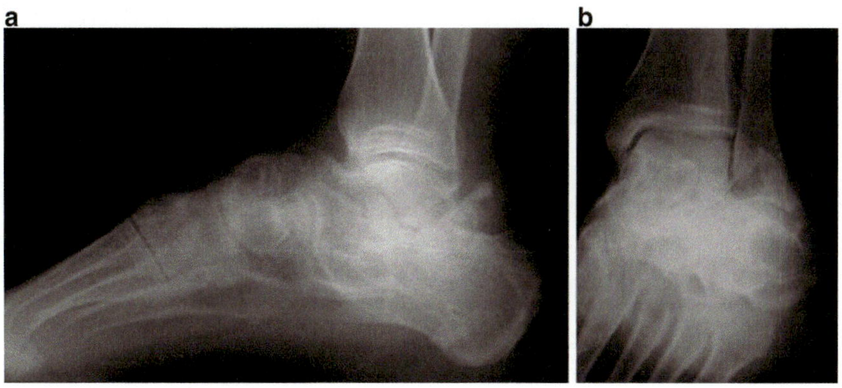

Fig. 17.11 (**a**) Preoperative lateral radiograph of nonoperatively treated joint depression calcaneal fracture. Note significant anterior ankle impingement and loss of height of the calcaneus with subsidence of the talus into the calcaneus. (**b**) Ankle mortise radiograph of the same patient demonstrating sub-fibular impingement of displaced lateral calcaneal wall

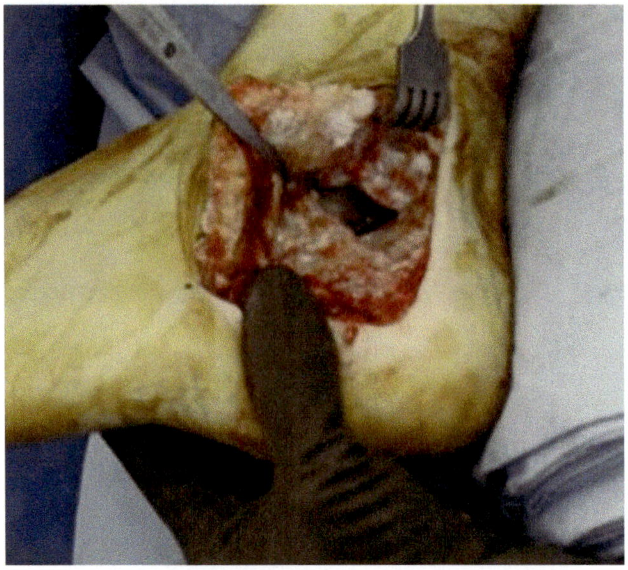

Fig. 17.12 Intraoperative exposure using lateral extensile incisional approach of the same patient as seen in Fig. 17.11a, b. Note excellent exposure of the displaced lateral calcaneal wall, the fibular impingement that is present, and the significant joint depression and subsidence of the talus into the calcaneus

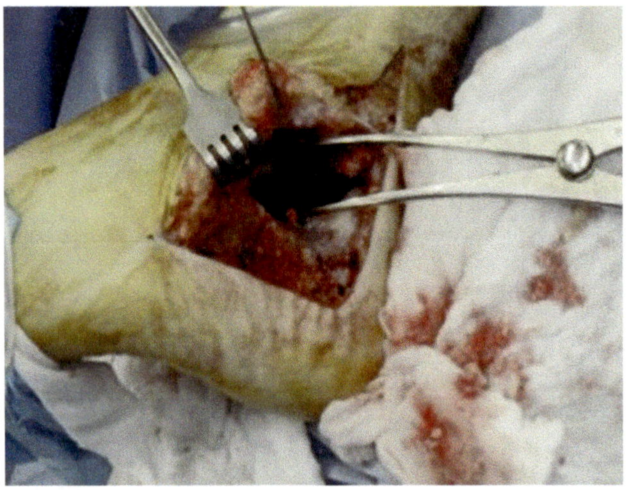

Fig. 17.13 Demonstration of complete debulking of the lateral calcaneal wall of the same patient seen in Fig. 17.12, with resolution of fibular impingement and good access to the subtalar joint. Lamina spreader allows for distraction

subtalar joint. A straight vertical posterior incisional approach (either just lateral to or through the Achilles tendon) may also be utilized, but if lateral calcaneal wall debulking is required, access to this area may be difficult with this approach. After debulking of the lateral calcaneal wall, the subtalar joint can then be addressed and its respective surfaces are then denuded to bleeding cancellous bone surfaces in preparation for arthrodesis. At times, fluoroscopic imaging may be necessary before joint debridement to properly identify the location of the subtalar joint, especially in cases of long-standing deformity and significant subsidence of the talus into the calcaneus. To restore height and relieve anterior ankle impingement, distraction of the subtalar joint is necessary. This can be accomplished by a lamina spreader inserted into the joint or by other distraction devices (Fig. 17.15). Distraction is performed under fluoroscopic guidance to confirm restoration of calcaneal height and normalization of the lateral talo-first metatarsal angle (Fig. 17.16). Care must be taken not to over-distract or to produce a varus deformity. The void created by distraction is then filled by allograft or autograft. Femoral head allograft provides more than adequate bone graft volume as well as strong cortical struts to maintain height [28, 29] (Figs.17.17 and 17.18a, b). Release of distraction should allow for a "press fit" of the graft. Fixation can then be obtained by either Steinmann pins, fully threaded screws, or partially threaded screws with threads crossing the calcaneus, graft, and talus to minimize compression across the graft site to prevent graft collapse (Figs. 17.19a–c and 17.20). If pin fixation is utilized, they may be left percutaneous for easy future removal. This can be beneficial to eliminate artifact if advanced diagnostic imaging (CT or MRI) is employed postoperatively for monitoring of healing and union at the host/graft interface areas. A period of 8–10 weeks of non-weight bearing is employed postoperatively.

Occasionally, osteotomy of the calcaneal body may be necessary if significant shortening or varus malunion is present. Various osteotomies have been described, from simple oblique osteotomies to multiplane osteotomies, with and without subtalar arthrodesis, to assist in deformity correction [30–32] (Fig. 17.21). Distraction osteogenesis may also be employed and can be helpful in deformity correction in case's of malunion or in previous failed reconstructions of malunited calcaneal fractures [33] (Figs. 17.22 and 17.23a–d). Achilles tendon lengthening may also be necessary as an adjunct in both osteotomy and arthrodesis procedures.

Wound healing problems with the lateral extensile approach to calcaneal fractures have been reported [12–15] (Figs. 17.4 and 17.5). Proper reduction of the deformity, avoiding placing hardware under incision lines (placing the vertical arm of the lateral extensile incision more posterior helps in avoiding this), and proper tissue handling including a "no touch" technique in handling the soft tissue flap all help in minimizing wound complications. Dynamic flap retraction as opposed to static wire retraction and preoperative Doppler ultrasound evaluation of arterial supply to the flap may be beneficial in avoiding wound breakdown [34]. A more limited sinus tarsi approach when performing open reduction and internal fixation of calcaneal fractures, with or without arthroscopic assistance, combined with percutaneous reduction and screw and/or pin fixation only, may be an

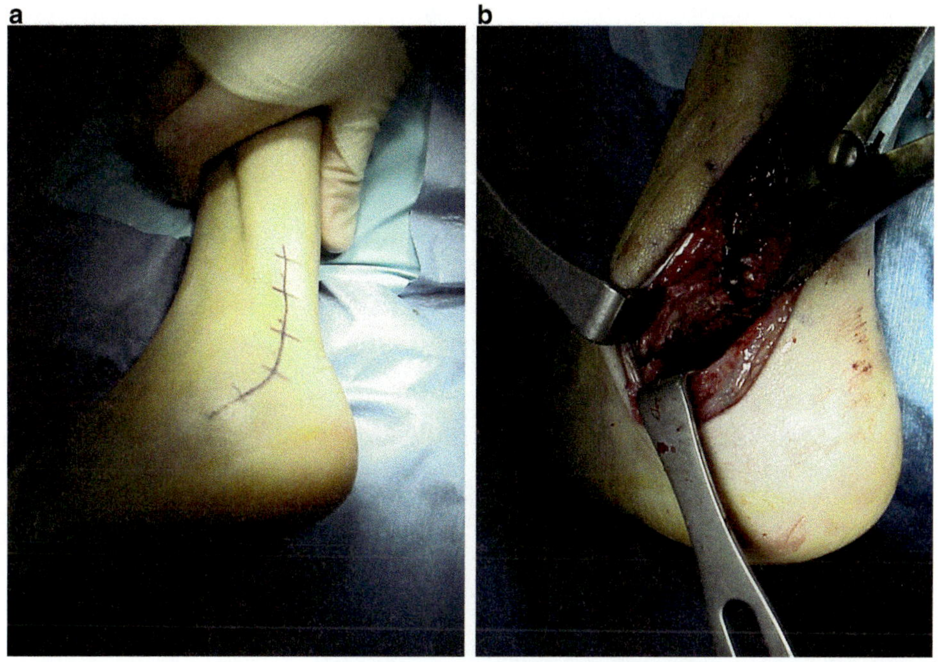

Fig. 17.14 (**a**) Alternative incision to conventional lateral extensile approach. The vertical arm is elongated and the horizontal portion is shorter and more oblique (photo courtesy of Michael S. Lee, DPM). (**b**) Exposure afforded by more vertical incisional approach (Photo courtesy of Michael S. Lee, DPM)

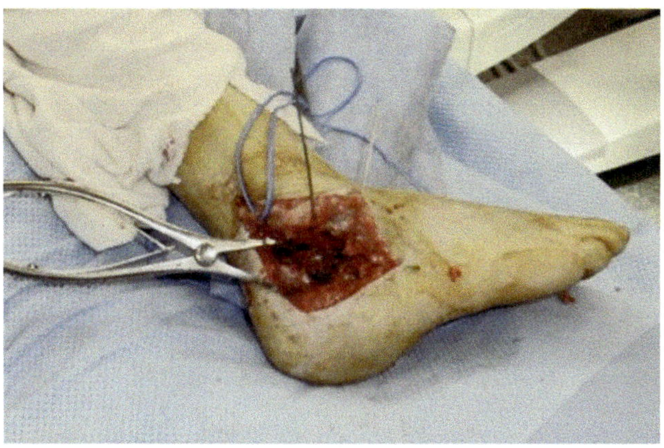

Fig. 17.15 Another example of distraction of the subtalar joint accomplished by lamina spreader insertion between talus and calcaneus after joint preparation has been performed. This allows for restoration of height and resolution of anterior ankle impingement. Note small vessel loop around sural nerve after neurolysis was performed

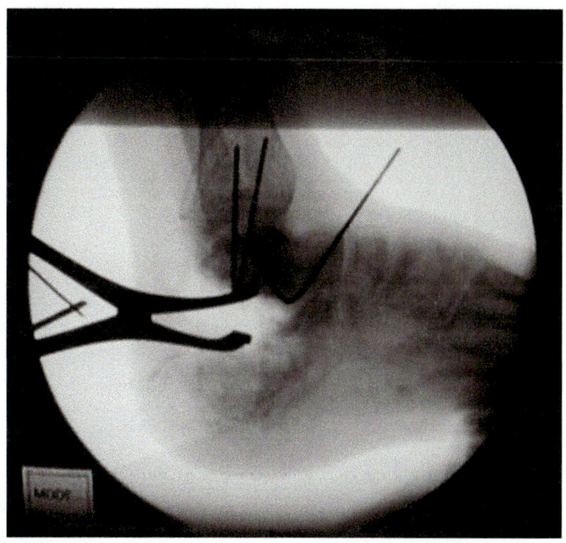

Fig. 17.16 Fluoroscopic imaging is utilized to determine proper amount of distraction required for deformity correction

alternative in some cases in an attempt to avoid the wound healing problems reported with the extended lateral approach [35, 36] (Fig. 17.24). If wound complications occur, one must monitor for possible osteomyelitis and consideration should be given to hardware removal if necessary (partial or complete). Superficial or deep infection should be aggressively treated to minimize post-infection sequelae. Large soft tissue defects, which may occur in cases of significant wound breakdown, may require flap rotation for coverage [37] (Figs. 17.25 and 17.26a–c).

Various hardware problems may be encountered after open reduction and internal fixation of calcaneal fractures. Plate irritation of soft tissue, loosening of screws, as well as improper length of screws may be encountered (Fig. 17.26). In particular, screw length must be exact in the area of the sustentaculum tali to prevent inadvertent damage to medial neurovascular and tendon structures. As well as the proper placement and length of screw fixation constructs, inadvertent damage to medial soft tissue structures can be avoided by the judicious use of drills during hardware insertion.

Even hardware removal after open reduction and internal fixation of intra- articular calcaneal fractures using an lateral extensile approach has been reported to result in a 10% wound complication rate [16]. Screws which do not purchase well during initial open reduction and internal fixation should not be allowed to remain as these will lead to later loosening and soft tissue irritation. As described earlier, if at all possible, hardware should not be placed under incision lines.

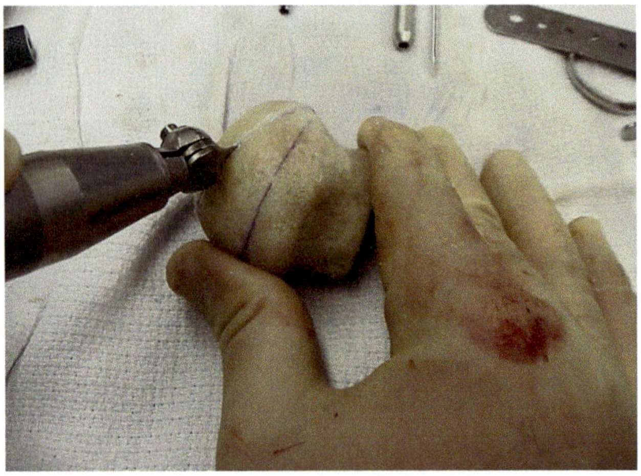

Fig. 17.17 Example of typical size of femoral head allograft utilized for posterior bone block distraction arthrodesis (Photo courtesy of Michael S. Lee, DPM)

Summary

Complications following fractures of the calcaneus are not uncommon. One must assure minimal to no displacement of any intra-articular component, normal calcaneal height and varus alignment, and no soft tissue impingement if one is to avoid complications in the nonoperative treatment of calcaneal fractures.

In regard to operative treatment of calcaneal fractures, proper timing of surgery is the first factor to consider. Allowance for soft tissue recovery (resolution of fracture blisters, edema, etc.) must be accomplished to avoid unnecessary wound complications. Soft tissue flaps may be required in cases of significant would breakdown following open reduction and internal fixation of calcaneal fractures. All components of fracture deformity (joint displacement, shortening, varus malalignment, etc.) must be addressed to prevent malunion and minimize post-traumatic arthritis of the subtalar and calcaneocuboid joints. Posterior bone block arthrodesis is an especially useful procedure in addressing the late complications of calcaneal fractures.

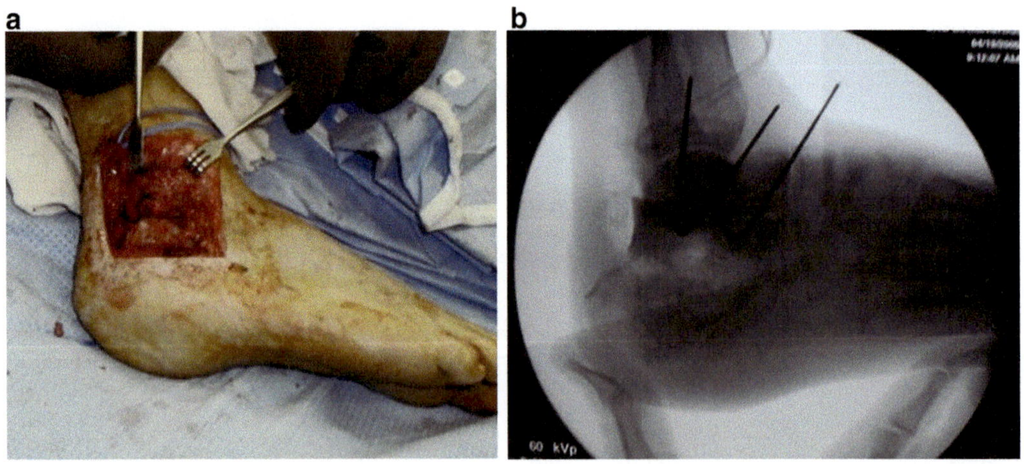

Fig. 17.18 (**a**) Intraoperative view of femoral head allograft in place with "press fit." (**b**) Intraoperative fluoroscopic view of the same patient with allograft in place before fixation

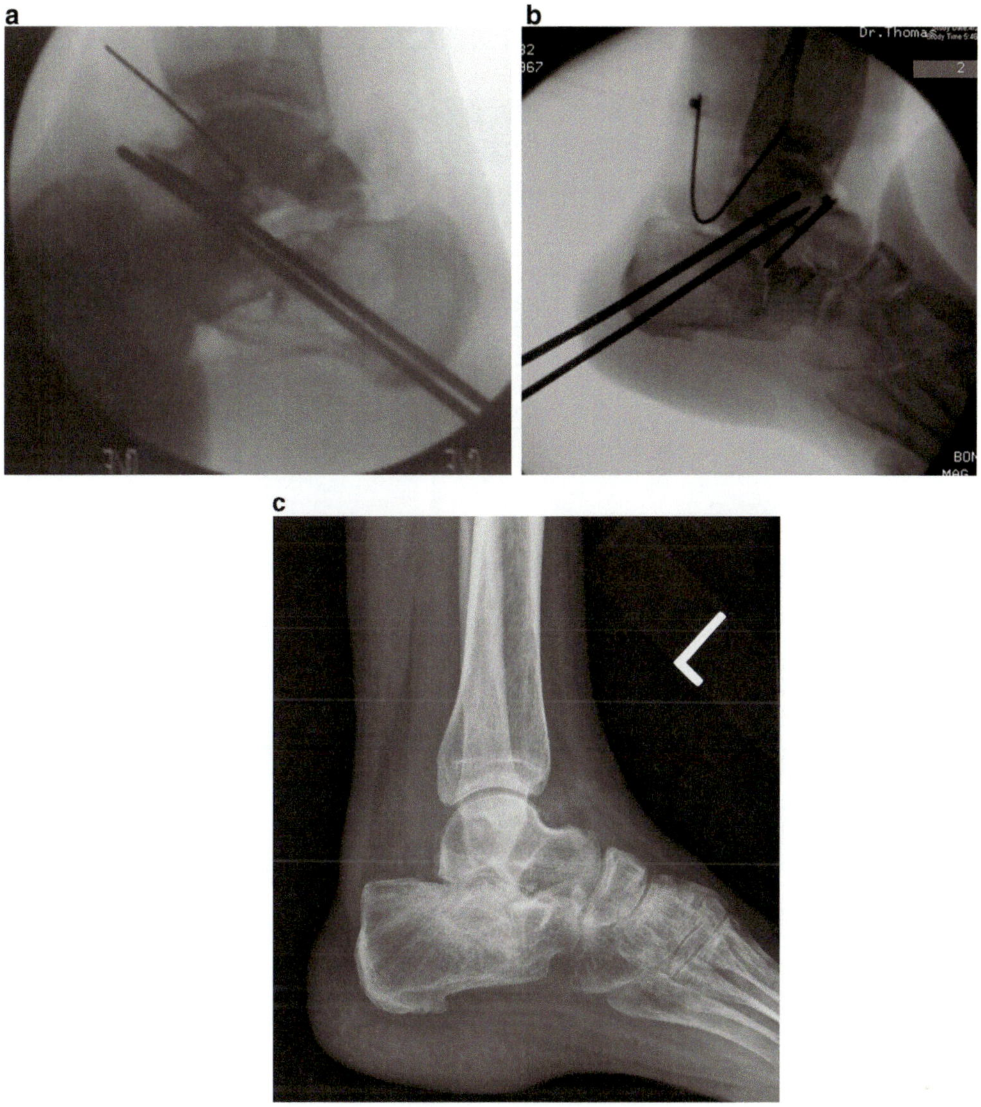

Fig. 17.19 (**a**) Intraoperative view of Steinmann pin fixation of posterior bone block arthrodesis of the same patient as seen in Fig. 17.13. Note restoration of height and correction of anterior ankle impingement. (**b**) Intraoperative fluoroscopic imaging of the same patient seen in Fig. 17.9 demonstrating Steinmann pin fixation for posterior bone block distraction arthrodesis. (**c**) Eight weeks post-op of the same patient following pin removal in clinic. Leaving pins superficial allows for easy post-op removal and unencumbered CT or MRI monitoring for host/graft interface union

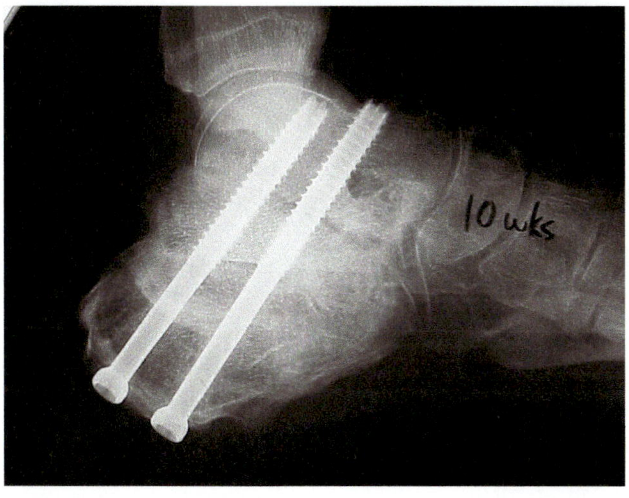

Fig. 17.20 Alternatively screw fixation with threads crossing the calcaneus, graft, and talus to minimize compression forces across the graft site to reduce risk of graft collapse may also be used for fixation (Photo courtesy of Michael S. Lee, DPM)

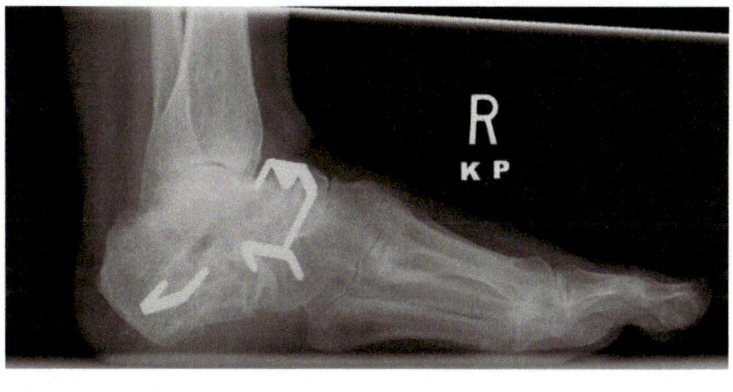

Fig. 17.21 Lateral view of old joint depression calcaneal fracture treated with triple arthrodesis and Dwyer-type calcaneal osteotomy. Note severe shortening of the calcaneal body and residual hind foot varus with resultant forefoot varus. Achilles tendon was quite dysfunctional secondary to shortened fulcrum

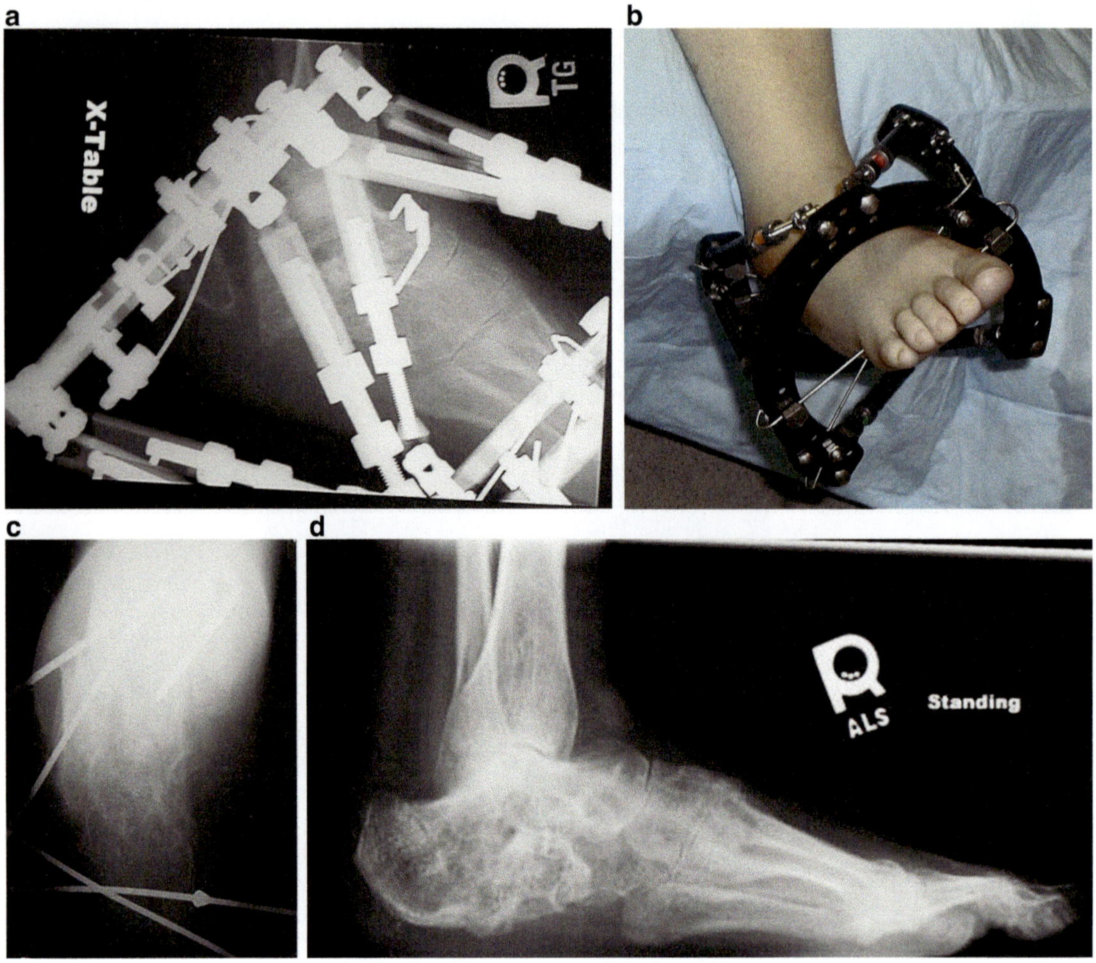

Fig. 17.22 a) Lateral view demonstrating calcaneal osteotomy with Taylor Spatial Frame application and distraction osteogenesis process started, to restore calcaneal length and bring hind foot out of varus. (**b**) Clinical photo of frame placement prior to deformity correction. Note varus deformity. (**c**) Calcaneal axial following osteotomy and frame placement. Note placement of olive wire medially to assist with varus correction. (**d**) Lateral view after correction. Note restoration of calcaneal length to restore normal Achilles tendon function, as well as varus correction of the hind foot and forefoot. This patient later required posterior bone block graft through old subtalar arthrodesis site to restore height and relieve anterior ankle impingement

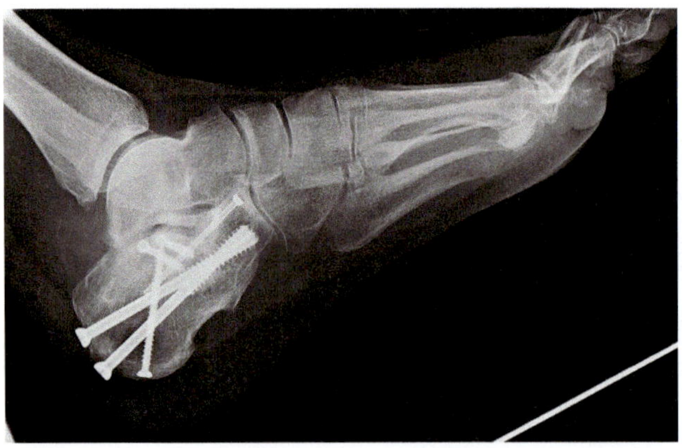

Fig. 17.23 Lateral radiograph of screw fixation only of joint depression calcaneal fracture delivered through limited sinus tarsi approach and percutaneous screw delivery in attempt to limit wound complication

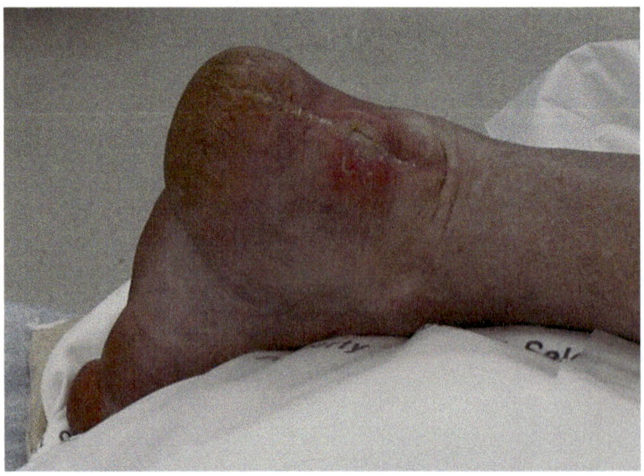

Fig. 17.24 Chronic non-healing, draining wound involving posterior incision line from surgically treated tongue-type fracture

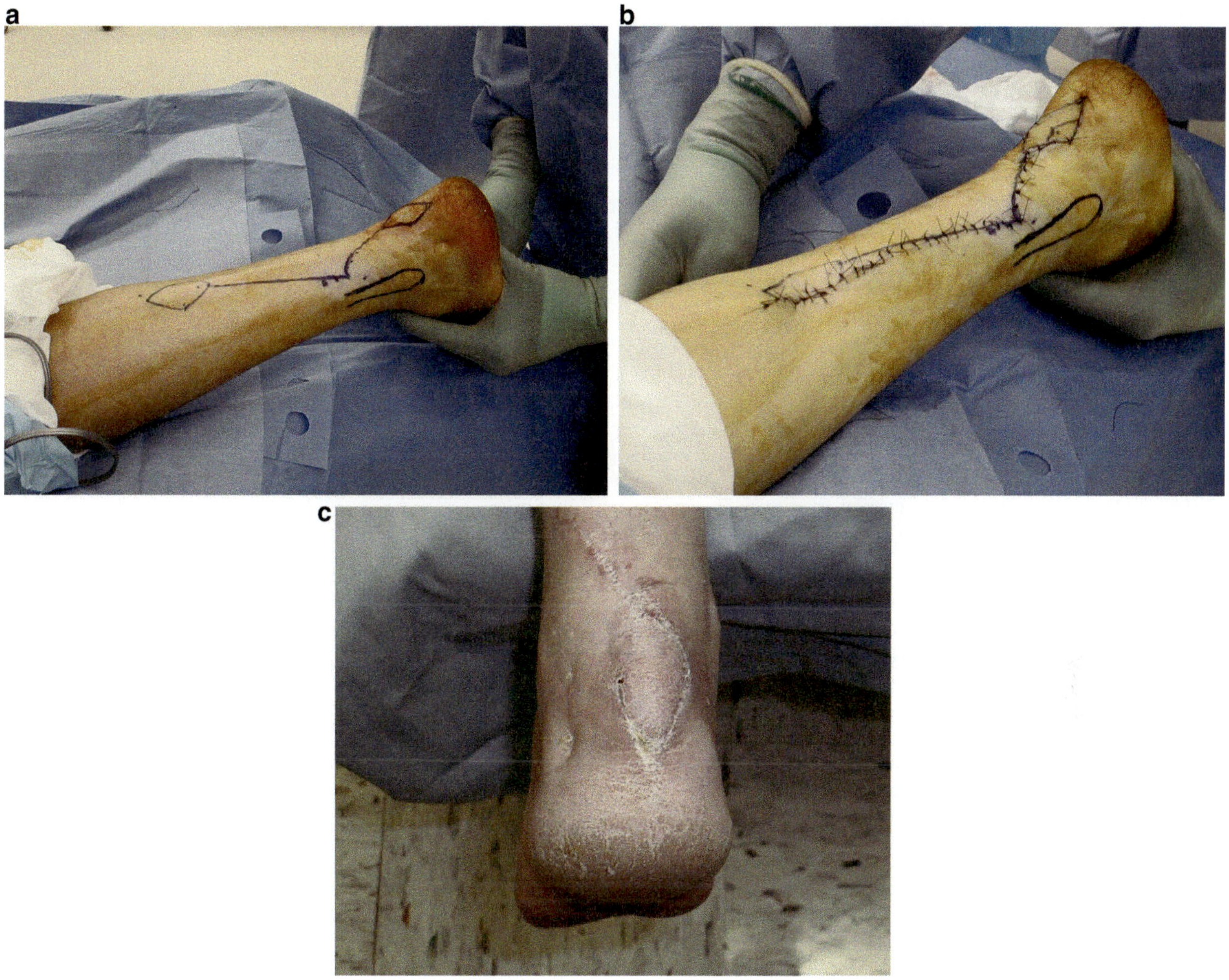

Fig. 17.25 (**a**) The same patient as seen in Fig. 17.24. Planned reverse sural artery flap for wound closure after debridement of chronic wound. (**b**) Completed rotation of reverse sural artery flap. (**c**) Three months postoperative with successful wound coverage

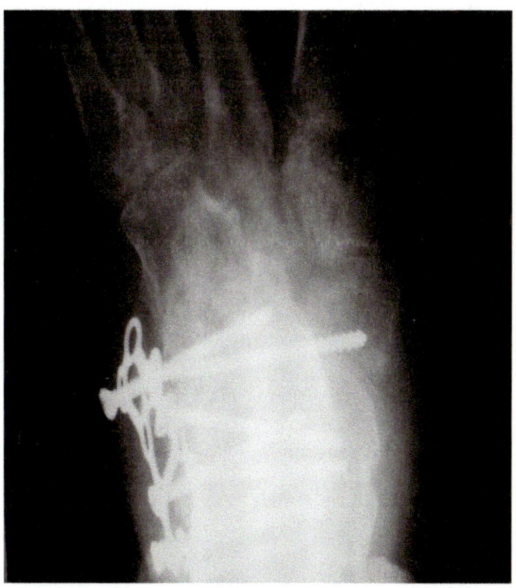

Fig. 17.26 Example of poor hardware placement resulting in postoperative hardware problems. Note improper screw length with medial soft tissue penetration, loosening of screws laterally, and improper juxtaposition of the plate to the lateral calcaneal wall (Photo courtesy of Randy Clements DPM)

References

1. Myerson M, Quill GE. Late complications of fractures of the calcaneus. J Bone Jt Surg AM. 1993;75(3):331–41.
2. Spranger M, Rubenseifuer L. Late sequelae of calcaneal fractures. Orthop Ihren Grenzgeb. 1975;113(4):686–8.
3. Clare MP, Lee WE, Saunders RW. Intermediate to long term results of a treatment protocol for calcaneal fracture malunions. J Bone Jt Surg AM. 2005;87(5):963–7.
4. Stapleton JJ, Balczyk R, Zgonis T. Surgical treatment of calcaneal fracture malunions and post traumatic deformities. Clin Podiatr Med Surg. 2009;26(1):79–90.
5. Sanders R, Vaupel ZM, Erdogan M, et al. Operative treatment of displaced intraarticular calcaneal fractures: long-term (10–20 years) results in 108 fractures using a prognostic CT classification. J Orthop Trauma. 2014;28(10):551–63.
6. Romash MM. Fracture of the calcaneus: an unusual fracture pattern with subtalar joint interposition of the flexor hallucis longus. A report of two cases. Foot Ankle. 1992;13(1):32–41.
7. Wright DG, Sangeorzan BJ. Calcaneal fracture with peroneal impingement and tendon dysfunction. Foot Anke Int. 1996;17(10): 650.
8. Walter JH, Rockett MS, Goss LR. Complications of intra articular fractures of the calcaneus. J Am Podiatr Med Assoc. 2004;94(4):382–8.
9. Chhabra N, Sherman SC, Szatkowski JP. Tongue-type calcaneus fractures: a threat to skin. Am J Emerg Med. 2013;31(7):1151.
10. Yu GR, Pang QJ, Yu X, et al. Surgical management for avulsion fracture of the calcaneal tuberosity. Orthop Surg. 2013;5(3):196–202.
11. Edwards P, Kurth L. Posterior tibial pseudoaneurysm after calcaneus fracture: a case report. Foot Ankle. 14:411–3.
12. Wu K, Wang C, Wang Q, et al. Regression analysis of controllable factors of surgical incision complication in closed calcaneal fractures. J Res Med Sci. 2014;19(6):495–501.
13. Soni A, Vollans S, Malhotra K, Mann C. Association between smoking and wound infection rates following calcaneal fracture fixation. Foot Ankle. 2014;7(4):266–70.
14. Benirschke SK, Kramer PA. Wound healing complications in closed and open calcaneal fractures. J Orthop Trauma. 2004;18(1): 1–6.
15. Gupta A, Ghalambor N, Nihal A, Trepman E. The modified Palmer lateral approach for calcaneal fractures: wound healing and postoperative computed tomographic evaluation of fracture reduction. Foot Ankle Int. 2003;24(10):744–53.
16. Backes M, Schep NWL, Luitse JSK, Goslings JC, Schepers T. Indications for implant removal following intra-articular calcaneal fractures and subsequent complications. Foot Ankle Int. 2013; 34(11):1521–5.
17. Haugsdal J, Dawson J, Phisitkul P. Nerve injury and pain after operative repair of calcaneal fractures: a literature review. Iowa Orthop J. 2013;33:202–7.
18. Bahari Kashani M, Kachooei AR, Ebrahimi H, Peivandi MT, Amelfarzad S, Bekhradianpoor N, Azami M, Fatehi A, Bahari Kashani G. Comparative study of peroneal tenosynovitis as the complication of intraarticular calcaneal fracture in surgically and non-surgically treated patients. Iran Red Crescent Med J. 2013; 15(10):1–3.15.
19. Sanders R.. Radiological evaluation and CT classification of calcaneal fractures. In: Jahss M editor. Disorders of the foot and ankle. Philadelphia: WB Saunders; 1990.
20. Benirschke SK, Sangeorzan BJ. Extensive intraarticular fractures of the foot: surgical management of calcaneal fractures. Clin Orthop. 1993;291:128–34.
21. Hetsroni I, Ben-Sira D, Nyska M, Ayalon M. Plantar pressure anomalies after open reduction with internal fixation of high-grade calcaneal fractures. Foot Ankle Int. 2014;35(7):712–8.
22. Mittlmeier T, Machler G, Lob G. Compartment syndrome of the foot after intraarticular calcaneal fracture. Clin Orthop. 1991;269: 241–8.
23. Myerson M, Manoli A. Compartment syndrome of the foot after calcaneal fractures. Clin Orthop. 1993;290:142–50.
24. Saxby T, Myerson M, Schon L. Compartment syndrome of the foot following calcaneal fracture. Foot. 1992;2:157–61.
25. Carr J, Hansen S, Benirschke S. Subtalar distraction bone block fusion for late complications of os calcis fractures. Foot Ankle. 1988;9:81–6.
26. Thomas JL, Kunkel MW, Lopez R, Sparks D. Radiographic values of the adult foot in a standardized population. J Foot Ankle Surg. 2006;45(1):3–12.
27. Chung HJ, Bae SY, Choo JW. Mid-term follow up results of subtalar distraction arthrodesis using a double bone-block for calcaneal malunion. Yonsei Med J. 2014;55(4):1087–94.
28. Lee MS, Tallerico V. Distraction arthrodesis of the subtalar joint using allogenic bone graft. A review of 15 cases. J Foot Ankle Surg. 2010;49(4):369–74.
29. Schepers T. The subtalar distraction bone block arthrodesis following the late complications of calcaneal fractures: a systematic review. Foot (Edinib). 2013;23(1):39–44.
30. Romash MM. Reconstructive osteotomy of the calcaneous with subtalar arthrodesis for malunited calcaneal fractures. Clin Orthop Relat Res. 1993;290:157–67.
31. Yu GR, Hu SJ, Yang HM, Zhang SM. Reconstruction of calcaneal fracture malunion with osteotomy and subtalar joint salvage: technique and outcomes. Foot Ankle Int. 2013;34(5):726–33.
32. Young KW, Lee KT, Lee YK, Jang MK, Yoon JH, Kim JH. Calcaneal reconstruction for the late complication of calcaneus fracture. Orthopedics. 2011;34(10):634–8.
33. Fan WL, Sun HZ, Wu SY, Wang AM. Subtalar distraction osteogenesis for posttraumatic arthritis following intra-articular calcaneal fractures. Foot Ankle Int. 2013;34(3):398–402.
34. Bibbo C, Ehrlich DA, Nguyen HM, et al. Low wound complication rates for the lateral extensile approach for calcaneal ORIF when the lateral calcaneal artery is patent. Foot Ankle Int. 2014;35(7): 650–6.
35. Popescu ER, Panaitescu C, Circota G, Cirstoiu M, Cirstoiu C. Low complications after minimally invasive fixation of calcaneus fracture. J Med Life. 2013;6(1):80–3.
36. DeWall M, Henderson CE, McKinley TO, Phelps T, Dolan L, Marsh JL. Percutaneous reduction and fixation of displaced intra-articular calcaneus fractures. J Orthop Trauma. 2010;24(8): 466–72.
37. Kose R, Mordeniz C, Sanli C. Use of expanded reverse sural artery flap in lower extremity reconstruction. J Foot Ankle Surg. 2011; 50(6):695–8.

Talar Fractures: The Injury, the Management, and the Aftermath

18

Justin J. Fleming, Kwasi Y. Kwaadu, and Michael W. Downey

Osseous Anatomy

The talus is a complex bone with multiple articulations. Approximately 60 % of its surface is articular. As a result, fractures of the talus are rarely extra-articular. The implication of this concept lends additional credence to the morbidity associated with this injury. The talus articulates with the tibia superiorly, the fibula laterally, the calcaneus inferiorly, and the navicular distally. Sagittal plane motion at the tibiotalar articulation is converted by the talus into pronatory and supinatory motion at the talocalcaneal articulation and the subtalar and talonavicular joints [1].

The talus is composed of a head, a neck, and a body (Fig. 18.1). The head of the talus, which is convex in all directions and almost entirely articular, articulates with the concave navicular distally, the acetabular pedis. The head of the talus also rests on the anterior and middle facets of the calcaneus proximally and inferiorly. Directly inferiorly, the talar head rests on the calcaneonavicular (spring) ligaments [2].

The talar neck, unlike the head, is conversely entirely nonarticular. It courses anteromedially from the body. It is bordered anteriorly by the articular head and posteriorly by the articular body. The superior surface of the talar neck serves as the insertion for the respective capsules of the tibiotalar and talonavicular joints and as the entry point for the nutrient branches of the anterior tibial and dorsalis pedal arteries. The inferior aspect of the neck forms the roof of the tarsal canal. The lateral surface of the neck serves as part of the insertion of the anterior talofibular ligament [2] (Fig. 18.1).

The talar body boasting a highly complex architecture is almost entirely articular. On its *superior surface*, or the *trochlea*, it is convex in the both the frontal plane and sagittal planes, with a central groove in the sagittal plane that corresponds to an articulating but subtle protrusion of the distal tibial plafond. The trochlea is wider anteriorly than posteriorly. The lateral aspect of this trochlea is larger and has a wider radius of curvature in the sagittal plane than the medial aspect. The triangular *lateral surface* of the body extending from the lateral trochlea articulates with the fibular. The lateral surface continues inferiorly and laterally into a projection named the *lateral talar process*. The *medial surface* of the trochlea superiorly boasts a comma-shaped facet that articulates with the medial malleolus (Fig. 18.1). The inferior aspect of the medial surface is nonarticular and serves as the insertion for the deep deltoid ligament. This ligament serves as the entrance site for the deltoid artery. The *inferior surface* of the trochlea serves as the superior half of the posterior subtalar joint, articulating with the posterior calcaneal facet (Fig. 18.1). This facet is concave in both the sagittal and frontal planes. The distal extent of the facet lies just posterior to the tarsal canal. Just anterior to this facet are the cervical and interosseous talocalcaneal ligaments through which branches that supply the body from the arteries within the tarsal canal course. The *posterior aspect* of the talar body is characterized by a smaller posteromedial tubercle and a larger posterolateral tubercle. The flexor halluces longus tendon courses between these two tubercles. The larger posterolateral tubercle may ossify independently, articulating separately to the talar body through a fibrous articulation. This accessory ossicle is called an *os trigonum* [2].

The original version of this chapter was revised. An erratum to this chapter can be found at DOI 10.1007/978-3-319-53686-6_31

J.J. Fleming (✉)
Aria 3B Orthopaedics, 3110 Grant Ave, Philadelphia, PA 19114, USA
e-mail: flemingjmak@gmail.com

K.Y. Kwaadu
Temple University School of Podiatric Medicine, 148 N 8th Street, Philadelphia, PA 19107, USA

M.W. Downey
Fellowship Trained Trauma and Reconstruction Foot/Ankle Surgeon, Trinity Foot and Ankle Specialists, Texas Health Harris Southwest Hospital, Fort Worth, TX, USA
e-mail: michael.w.downey@gmail.com

M.S. Lee, J.P. Grossman (eds.), *Complications in Foot and Ankle Surgery*, DOI 10.1007/978-3-319-53686-6_18

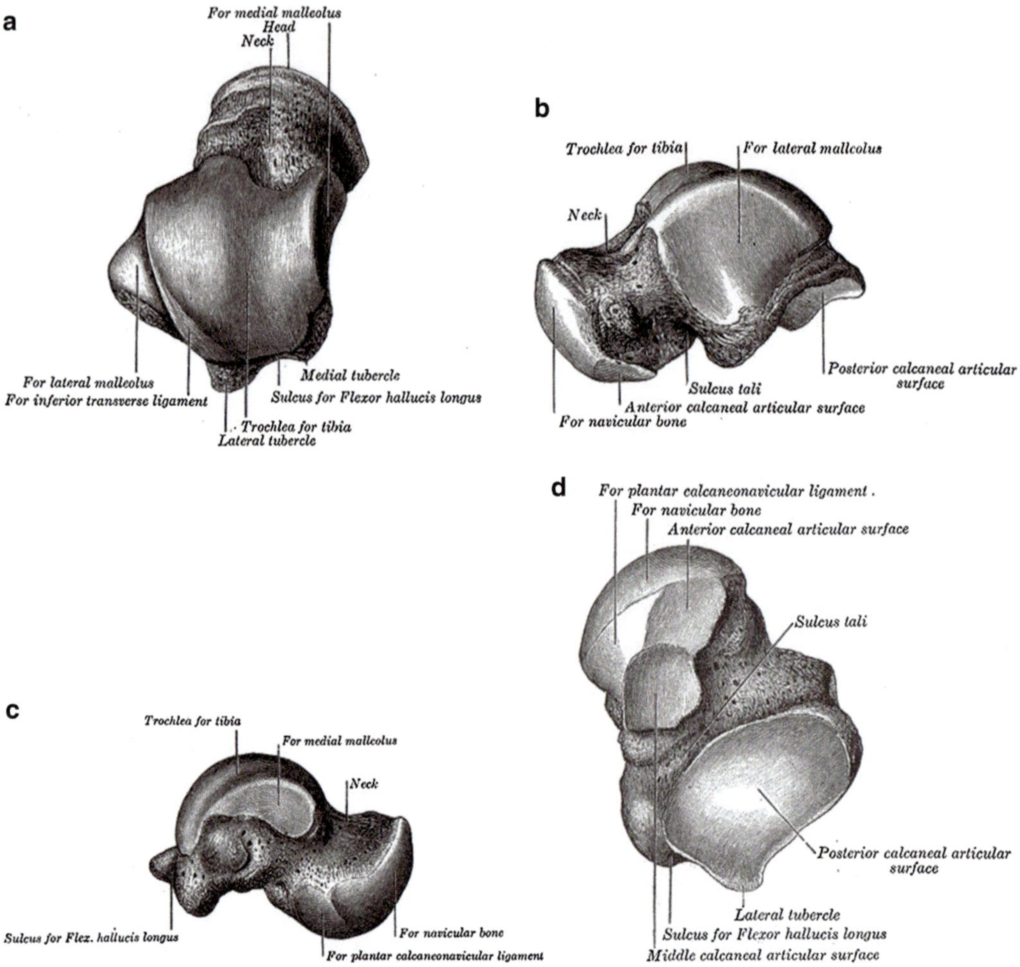

Fig. 18.1 (**a**) Dorsal view of the talus. (**b**) Lateral view of the talus. (**c**) Medial view of the talus. (**d**) Plantar view of the talus

Arterial Supply

The blood supply to the talus is rich and extensive, but delicate (Fig. 18.2). It has been studied extensively as a result of the incidence of avascular necrosis that may occur with varying degrees of vascular disruption associated with certain fracture types [3–6]. Different cadaveric studies have described some differences in the arterial supply resulting in perhaps a lower incidence of avascular necrosis that have been described in earlier studies [6–8]. The main sources are the *posterior tibial artery* and the *dorsalis pedal arteries* (Fig. 18.2). The *peroneal artery* provides some arterial supply but to a much lesser degree than the aforementioned arteries [8, 9].

The *posterior tubercle branches* from the posterior tibial artery branch to supply the posterior tubercle before the posterior tibial artery enters the flexor retinaculum. After entering the flexor retinaculum, the posterior tibial artery gives off the *artery of the tarsal canal* approximately a centimeter proximal to the distal bifurcation of the posterior tibial artery [9, 10] (Fig. 18.2). The *deltoid artery* originates from the artery of the tarsal canal or at times directly from the posterior tibial artery at the level inferior to the medial malleolus. The deltoid artery at this level supplies the medial 1/3 of the talar body [9] (Fig. 18.2).

The artery of the tarsal canal courses distally and laterally into the tarsal canal. Within the tarsal canal, it anastomosis with the *artery of the sinus tarsi*, which itself originates either from the anterior lateral malleolar branches of the perforating peroneal artery, from the lateral tarsal artery of the dorsalis pedis, or from an anastomosis of both. The artery of the sinus tarsi supplies the lateral aspect of the talar body and the lateral talar process [7].

The anastomosis of the arteries of the sinus tarsi and the tarsal canal within the tarsal canal has been described to provide retrograde perfusion to the majority of the talar body [7].

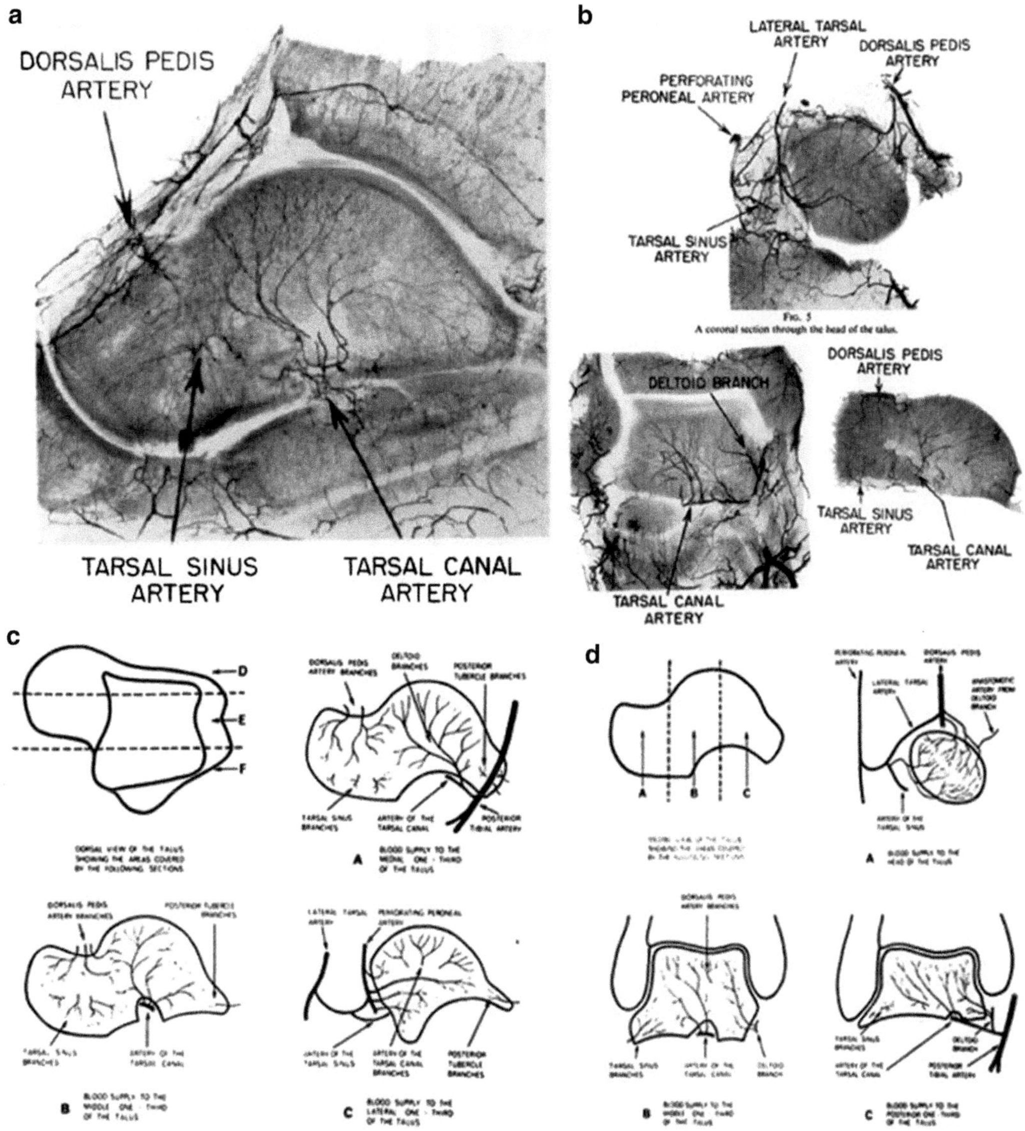

Fig. 18.2 From Mulfinger GL, Trueta J. The blood supply of the talus. J Bone Joint Surg Br. 2011 Feb;52(1): 160–167. (**a**) Sagittal plane arteriography of the talar blood supply. (**b**) Coronal plane arteriography of the talar blood supply. (**c**) Sagittal plane schematic of the talar blood supply. (**d**) Coronal plane schematic of the talar blood supply

As a result, fracture/dislocations of the neck of the talus have historically been associated with varying degrees of avascular necrosis depending on the severity and initial fracture displacement [10]. Recent studies however have describe anterograde vascularity into the talar body entering posteriorly, potentially explaining the relatively lower incidence of talar body avascular necrosis than expected following fracture/dislocations of the neck [8].

The *dorsalis pedis* provides branches directly into the superior aspect of the neck of the talus through small nutrient foramina, providing anterograde perfusion for the neck and head. The lateral head receives perfusion from the artery of the sinus tarsi. The medial head is supplied to a degree by distal extensions of the deltoid branch. A portion of the inferior head is supplied by the branches from the anastomosis within the tarsal canal [7].

Fractures of the Talus

Head Fractures

Intra-articular fractures of the head are uncommon, due to its inherent anatomy. Nestled snuggly within the acetabular pedis, it is protected by the navicular and the strong surrounding capsular and ligamentous structures [11]. However, ankle sprains and shearing injuries can result in periarticular avulsions by these same ligaments and strong capsular insertions. These avulsion injuries respond well to immobilization and protected weight bearing and rarely require radiographic follow-up. When intra-articular, direct reduction via open means is important to reduce disability from late posttraumatic arthrosis. As seen with most midfoot and hindfoot fractures because of the complex architecture, computed tomography can yield significant information in fracture geography facilitating decision making [12].

Articular realignment is the goal, so displaced fractures should be anatomically reduced because these missed injuries and subtle malalignments can result in accelerated posttraumatic arthritis [13]. If discovered prior to symptomatic arthritis, realignment osteotomies are recommended. A misaligned and healed head fracture, which usually is malaligned in varus and adduction, may be approached through a medial incision extending toward the naviculocuneiform joint between the tibialis anterior and tibialis posterior tendons (Fig. 18.3). A sagittal saw is then used to osteotomize the head just proximal to the cartilage [14]. A lamina spreader is inserted into the osteotomy site and opened until the first metatarsal talar head angle is parallel on the dorsoplantar fluoroscopic projection. The defect can be filled with autogenous corticocancellous structural graft. The iliac crest serves as an excellent donor site, but typically the defects are small, and in lieu of the iliac crest, proximal or distal tibia, or even a calcaneal graft, can be harvested. The length of the bone graft should match the maximum length of the defect. The remaining defect can be filled with autogenous cancellous bone from the donor site. The lamina spreader is removed, and the osteotomy site is fixated with a small minifragment buttress plate with positional screw fixation within the plate on either side of the osteotomy site. Care must be employed to confirm that the distal screw orientation is not within the talonavicular joint. Acute or missed compression fractures of the head should be disimpacted and backfilled with bone graft as described above. Temporary augmented external fixation helps to allow consolidation of the head by neutralizing compressive forces to the site. A delta frame con-

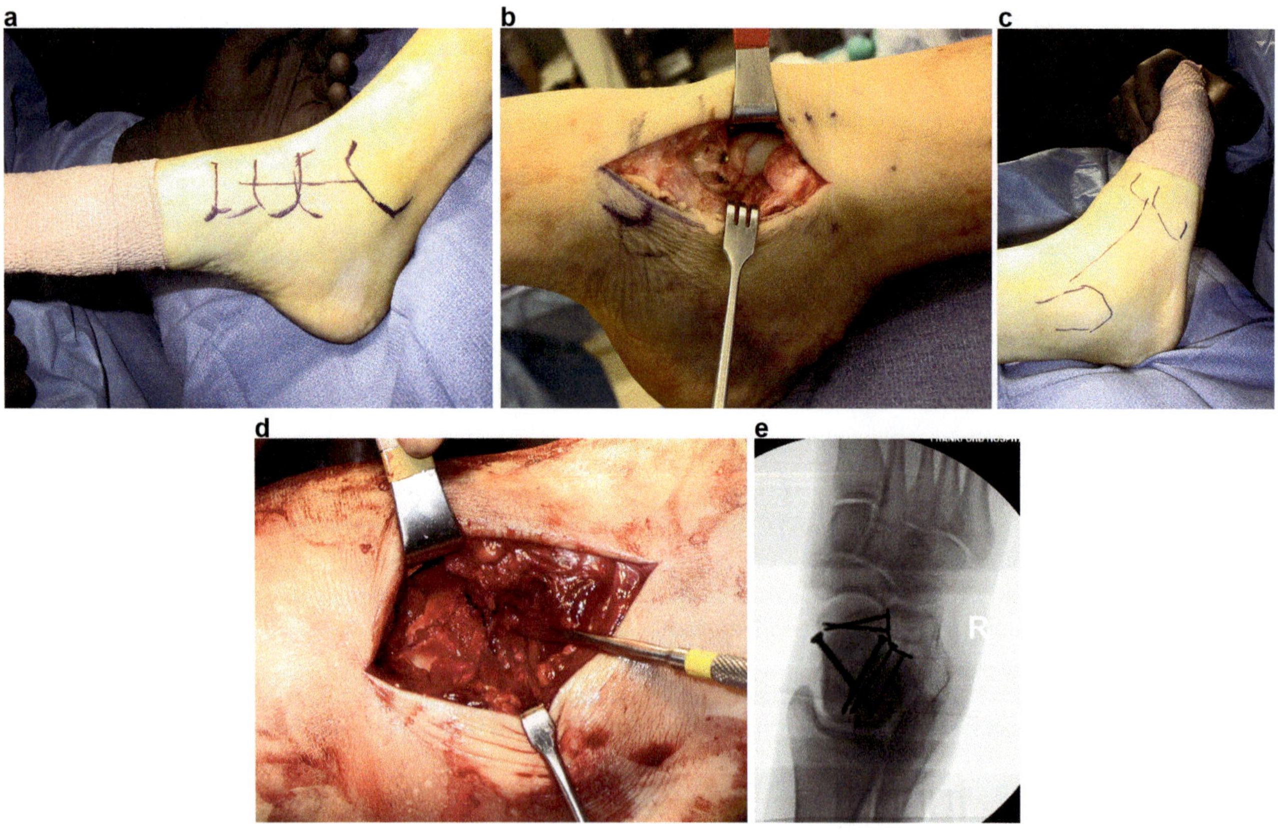

Fig. 18.3 (**a** and **b**) Medial incisional approach to the neck bounded by the tibialis anterior tendon superiorly and the posterior tibial tendon inferiorly. (**c** and **d**). Lateral incisional approach to the neck. (**e**) Dorsoplantar fluoroscopy of lateral plate

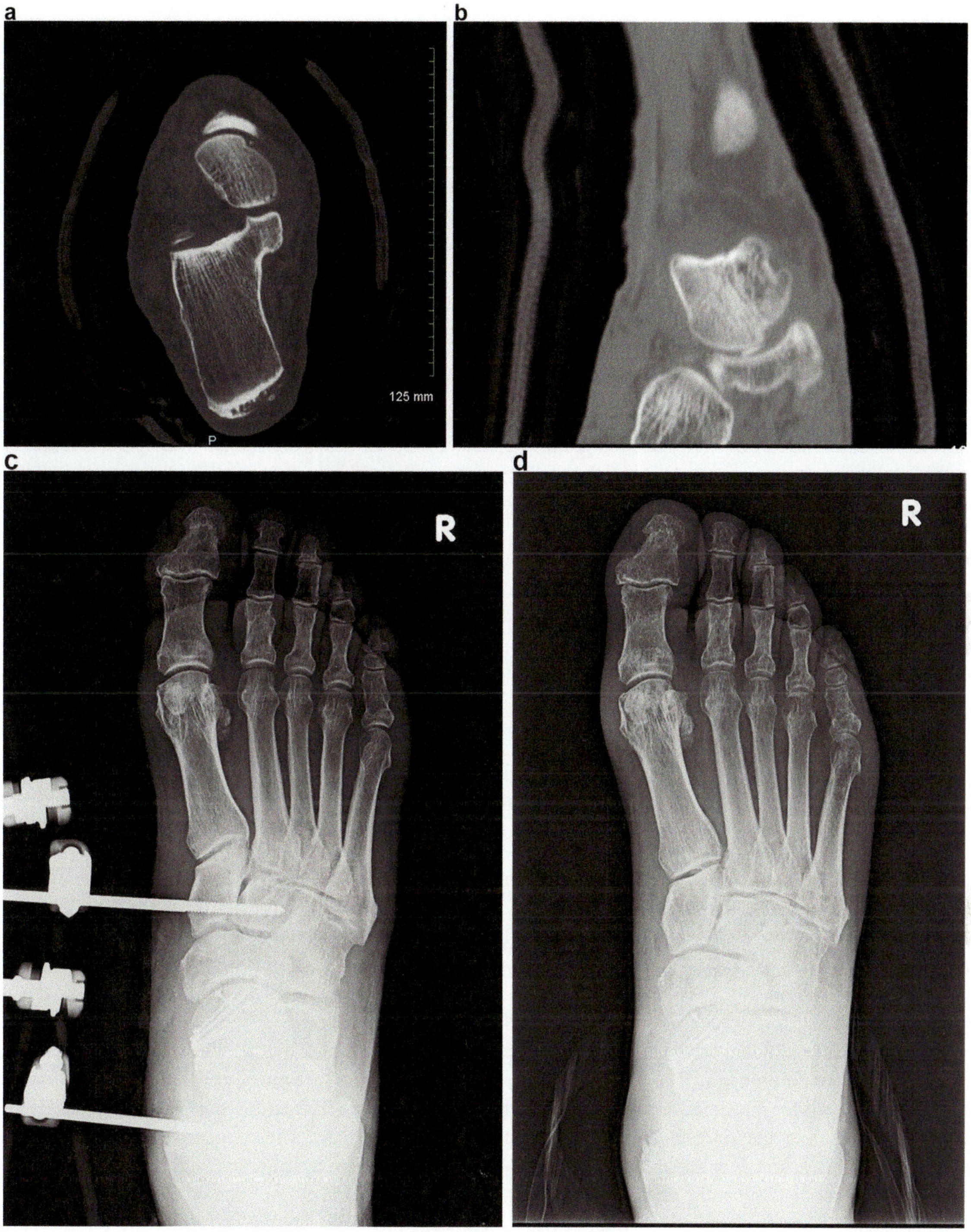

Fig. 18.4 (**a** and **b**) Coronal- and axial-oriented computed tomographic image demonstrating impaction of the medial talar head. (**c** and **d**) Postoperative dorsoplantar radiographic projection of head disimpaction with plate fixation before and after external fixator removal

struct can be placed with Schanz pins within the distal tibia metaphysis, the calcaneus, and the cuneiforms (Fig. 18.4).

Hindfoot stiffness can be debilitating, and as a result early mobilization with passive range of motion exercises postoperatively may reduce the incidence of postoperative arthrofibrosis and are initiated immediately after suture removal. The duration of non-weight bearing nonetheless remains 12 weeks or until clinical and radiographic union is confirmed. These reconstructions are last ditch efforts, and as such early weight bearing can potentially compromise the reconstruction leading to delayed or nonunion.

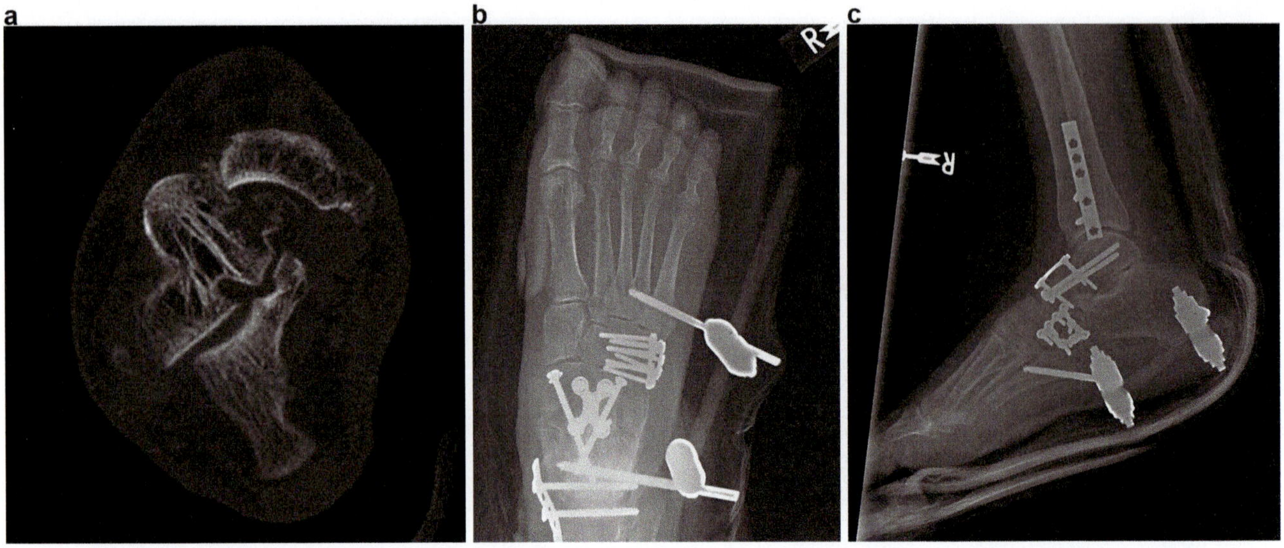

Fig. 18.5 (**a**) Preoperative CT of a severe fracture dislocation with lost inherent soft tissue stability. (**b**) Postoperative dorsoplantar radiographic projection of primary talonavicular arthrodesis, with concurrent cuboid reconstruction, medial malleolar ORIF, and temporary external fixation. (**c**) Lateral radiographic projection

Primary talonavicular arthrodesis should be reserved for severe fractures of the head that are not reconstructible and are approached with standard arthrodesis techniques [15, 16] (Fig. 18.5).

Neck Fractures

Fractures of the talar neck have been the subject of extensive discussion and scientific publications. The mechanism has historically been described as a hyperdorsiflexion injury where the hard talar neck is cleaved on impact by the distal tibial plafond. The absence of routine distal tibial injury with this injury calls into question the legitimacy of this proposed mechanism [11]. A reproducible mechanism was described as sudden and significant vertically oriented force directed caudally at the forefoot on a locked and stable hindfoot. At injury, while the talar body compressed between the calcaneus and the tibia, a dorsally directed force applied to the plantar forefoot distal to the tibial plafond results in cantilever bending at the talar neck, cleaving off the neck resulting in the fracture. Immediately following the fracture, with continued application of force, the posterior ankle capsule is opened and the talar body is pinched outward and posteriorly as seen in Hawkins II and III fractures [17]. Describing this injury as a hyperdorsiflexion injury may not be entirely incorrect but may inaccurately presume that the ankle goes through range of motion during the injury.

Hawkins in 1970 provided the current classification system most commonly relied upon to describe these injuries [18]. Hawkins further sought to correlate the rate of avascular necrosis with associated periarticular dislocation in addition to the neck fracture. The Hawkins *type I* injury describes an isolated talar neck fracture with absent to minimal fracture displacement without periarticular subluxation/dislocation. The *type II* fracture involves concomitant neck fracture with subtalar joint subluxation/dislocation with posterior and medial dislocation of the body on the intact deltoid ligament. The *type III* fracture involves subluxation/dislocation of both the subtalar and tibiotalar articulation in the presence of the neck fracture. In this injury, the deltoid ligament along with the deltoid artery is disrupted. Kelly and Canale described the *type IV* fracture which describes pantalar subluxation/dislocation with the neck fracture [19]. This injury is even more rare and not necessarily the final progression of the Hawkins classification.

Hawkins classically described avascular necrosis rates in zero of six type I fractures, in 10 of 24 type II fractures, and in 25 of 27 type III fractures corresponding to 0 %, 42 %, and 91 %, respectively. The cumulative vascular disruption with each progressive articular discontinuity he theorized was the reason behind the progression of AVN rates with each respective fracture/dislocation type.

Talar neck fractures are typically high-energy injuries, and as a result there is little diagnostic ambiguity [10, 20]. Patients routinely report catastrophic mechanisms with severe and generalized ankle and hindfoot pain. The physical exam and the lateral radiographic foot or ankle projection are useful. The anteroposterior ankle radiographic projection is helpful when isolating the type II form the type III injury. Because they are high-energy injuries, concomitant injuries are not uncommon and computed tomographic evaluation is critical [4, 10].

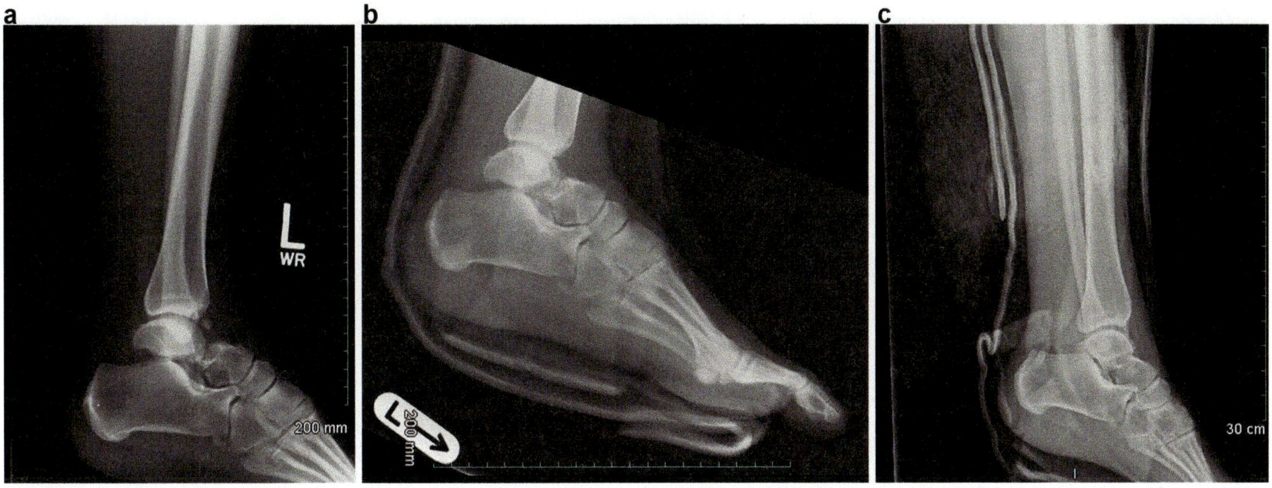

Fig. 18.6 (**a**) Hawkins II fracture. (**b**) Closed reduction with foot incorrectly splinted in neutral. (**c**) Closed reduction with foot correctly splinted in plantarflexion

Initial closed reduction is crucial to relieve stress on intact vascular supply. This typically involves longitudinal distraction in line with the longitudinal orientation of the native talus and casting/splinting with the foot plantarflexion. Casting with the ankle in neutral is intuitive but unfortunately with these injuries will result in re-displacement of the neck fracture (Fig. 18.6). If closed reduction is unsuccessful, urgent operative reduction is critical and must not be delayed. Repeated attempts at closed reduction should be avoided unless in rare cases when the operating room staff are preoccupied with other life-threatening emergencies. Operative reduction may involve reduction via small open approaches with temporary external fixation. Definitive open reduction with internal fixation may be performed at a later date following meticulous computed tomographic evaluation after the surrounding soft tissue is supportive for the iatrogenic insult of surgery. Urgent open reduction of these injuries has been reported to reduce the incidence of avascular necrosis; not only has this been unsubstantiated, but recent literature report that this may actually be an incorrect belief [10].

Nondisplaced type I injuries may be treated nonoperatively with non-weight-bearing immobilization. If displaced, open reduction with internal fixation is indicated. Unlike most fractures, even minimal displacement with these injuries may have profound effects on late arthrosis and hindfoot stiffness [21]. Thus, the threshold for open reduction should be low. The surgical approaches and fixation concepts for type I–III fractures are virtually identical. Because type IV injuries are inherently unique, the same approaches may not fully support the fracture orientation, and as such, these should be approached on a case by case basis following extensive computed tomographic evaluation and preoperative surgical planning.

The postoperative course for operatively treated type I–IV injuries typically involves non-weight bearing for 12 weeks or until radiographic union occurs. However, non-weight-bearing passive range of motion exercises is initiated as soon as the incisions are healed in 2 weeks. Full cast immobilization of operatively treated fractures should be avoided to limit postoperative stiffness.

For operative type I–III fractures, dual anteromedial and anterolateral approaches are recommended to reduce varus malalignment in the frontal plane that may occur with the isolate anteromedial incisional approach [6, 22]. The concern for the additional soft tissue dissection of the dual approach has been theorized to further compromise vascular supply but has not been substantiated to further disrupt vascular supply significantly enough to increase risk of avascular necrosis [6]. Both incisions are centered along the bisection of the neck. The lateral incision runs adjacent the lateral branch of the intermediate dorsocutaneous nerve and the extensor digitorum longus (Fig. 18.3). The medial incision runs just medial and inferior to the course of the tibialis anterior tendon and superior to the posterior tibial tendon (Fig. 18.3). This allows for excellent visualization of both the fracture and the subtalar joint where evacuation of fracture debris may help reduce posttraumatic of the subtalar joint, a common postoperative complication (Fig. 18.7). The medial incision may course proximally, turning upward in line with the central orientation of the medial malleolus, in instances where a medial malleolar osteotomy is needed to facilitate reduction. A small transversely oriented Schanz pin placed into the head of the talus is helpful in controlling frontal plane rotation and fracture reduction. Small wire fixation helps to temporarily maintain the reduction prior to delivery of definitive fixation. These wires are placed from both surgi-

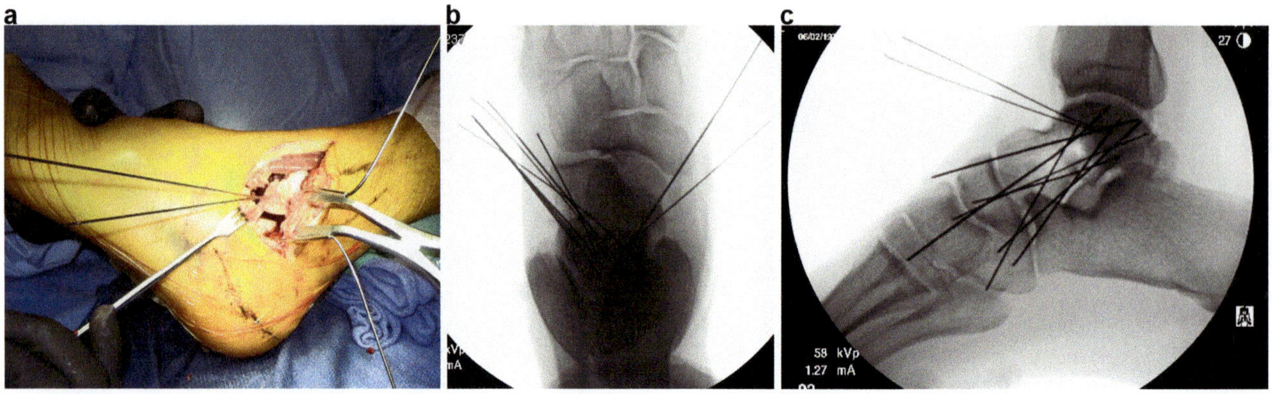

Fig. 18.7 (**a**) Exposure of the subtalar joint with the Weinraub retractor to facilitate extraction of fracture debris. (**b** and **c**) Temporary fracture fixation with Kirschner wires on the dorsoplantar and lateral fluoroscopic projection

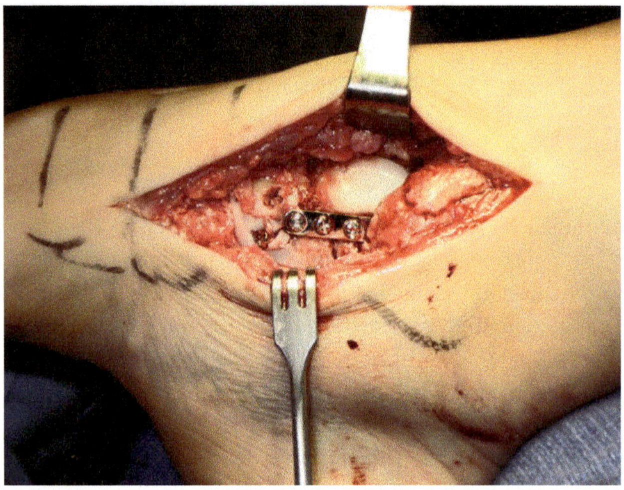

Fig. 18.8 Intraoperative placement of a medial plate for talar neck fracture

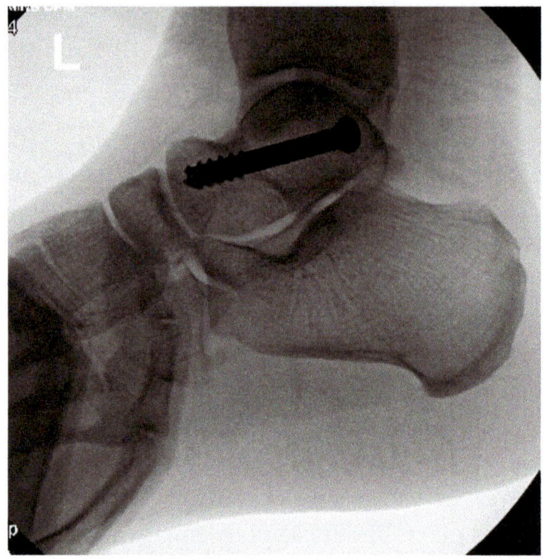

Fig. 18.9 Anterograde cannulated partially threaded screw countersunk into the body of the talus

cal sites oriented into the body from entry points distal to the neck fracture, adjacent to the talar head (Fig. 18.7). When possible, mini fragment plate fixation contoured adjacent to the lateral neck near the insertion of the anterior talofibular ligament facilitates delivery of stable fixation in a fan-like orientation with two screws on either side of the fracture (Fig. 18.3). Along the medial aspect of the talus, the area for plate fixation is further limited and is located just inferior to the comma-shaped facet and just distal to the deep deltoid ligament (Fig. 18.8). In lieu of plate fixation medially, mini or small fragment screws may be delivered with the same retrograde orientation as the temporary wires countersunk below the articular cartilage of the medial talar head. In the absence of significant comminution and good cortical fracture interdigitation, lag screw fixation may be employed (Fig. 18.3). In the presence of comminution, lag screw fixation may promote varus malreduction, and as such, bridge plating and positional screw fixation are preferred. Anterograde screw fixation may also be employed but requires significant skill (Fig. 18.9). The heads of these screws may also be prominent at the posterior aspect of the tibiotalar articulation, blocking normal sagittal plane ankle kinematics. Countersinking the screws below the chondral surface may avoid this. Following fracture reduction intraoperatively and postoperatively, standard anteroposterior and lateral ankle radiographic projection, standard dorsoplantar and medial oblique foot radiographic projections, and the Canale radiographic projection are helpful in confirming anatomic reduction [23]. This radiographic projection is also helpful in assessing radiographic avascular necrosis because the lateral ankle radiographic projection superimposes the medial and lateral talar domes and the medial and lateral malleoli, potentially resulting in a falsely positive diagnosis. Utilization of titanium fixation may be useful in cases where evaluation of avascular necrosis may warrant magnetic resonance imaging.

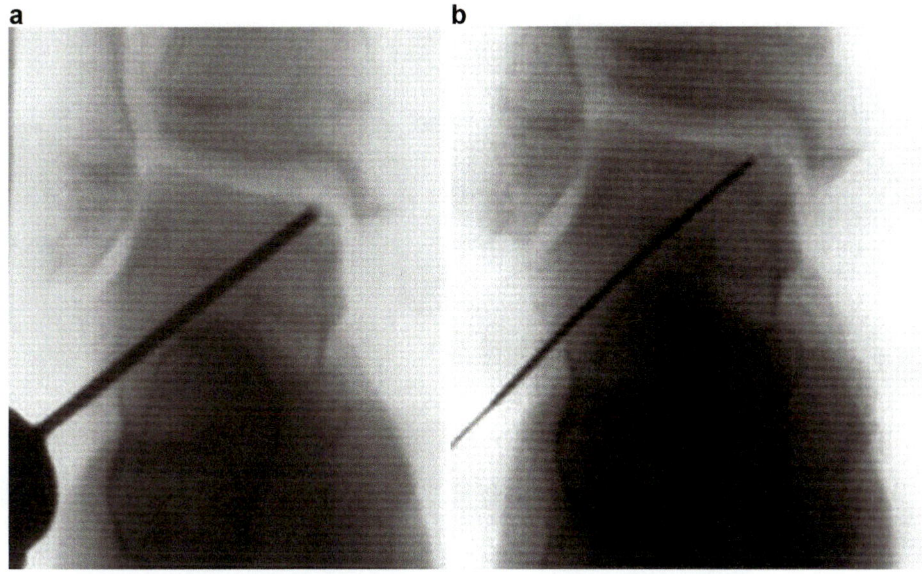

Fig. 18.10 (**a** and **b**) Talar body retrograde guide wire insertion with cannulated drilling from a lateral approach

The dual incisional approach may also be employed for the type IV fracture. These incisions may require further distal extension to incorporate talonavicular reconstruction or arthrodesis when indicated.

Though avascular necrosis is an extensively described and devastating complication, posttraumatic arthritis of the subtalar joint is the most common postoperative complication [24, 25]. Overall, the complication rate correlates with the initial fracture severity and anatomic reduction. As one would imply from Wolfe's law, the disuse osteopenia that occurs during the non-weight-bearing period of recovery with an intact vascular architecture in bone may be visible in the talus just below the subchondral plate of the talar trochlea. This disuse osteopenia described as the *Hawkins' sign* foretells intact vasculature and is classically described as an excellent prognostic finding seen approximately 6–8 weeks following injury but may be visualized even later at 12 weeks [4]. The presence of this sign usually precludes impending avascular necrosis and collapse. However, its absence may not always result in catastrophe [4]. Not all patients with avascular necrosis ultimately experience collapse of the talar body. More importantly avascular necrosis may not always affect the entire talar body; thus, collapse may not always be global. Collapse may occur subtly deforming the talar body without further collapse. Even in light of avascular necrosis, late revascularization has been reported occurring at different rates in different patients [26].

The entire process and exact mechanism and physiology governing avascular necrosis are unknown [27]. Nevertheless, when avascular necrosis is suspected, offloading devices like patellar tendon-bearing braces may be employed to the patient's tolerance. This again is not a global recommendation as not all patients with avascular necrosis undergo collapse [4]. Furthermore, collapse has been reported even with the utilization with these offloading devices.

Core decompression has been described with surgical management of avascular necrosis [28]. This involves retrograde drilling of the area of concern and removal of necrotic bone with the hope that revascularization will more likely occur in less dense bone (Fig. 18.10). Most lesions can be approached from and area just anterior to the lateral talar process. An appropriately sized guide wire be inserted in retrograde fashion. The cannulated drill bit is then passed over the guide wire. Ankle arthroscopy may be of assistance to confirm that the overlying cartilage is not violated by the guide wire or drill. Though outcomes are less than uniform, this is a procedure that burns few bridges in case a more complex reconstruction is warranted.

Rates of nonunion of talar neck fractures following open reduction and internal fixation have been reported from 5 % to 12% [10, 29]. Fracture nonunions are typically treated symptomatically; however, because they are uncommon, nonunions of the talar neck should be investigated to rule out a septic origin because of its proximity to the ankle joint and the relatively limited interventions available for treatment of fulminant talar osteomyelitis. Bone biopsy, computed tomographic evaluation, complete blood count, inflammatory markers, and adjunctive laboratory studies may yield useful information. In the presence of a confirmed symptomatic aseptic nonunion, we recommend revision with autogenous structural bone grafting through the same anteromedial and anterolateral incisional approaches, solid minifragment fixation, and bone stimulation with non-weight bearing for 12 weeks or until radiographic and clinical union is confirmed. In the presence of a suspected septic nonunion, bone biopsies and bone cultures should be sent for microscopic

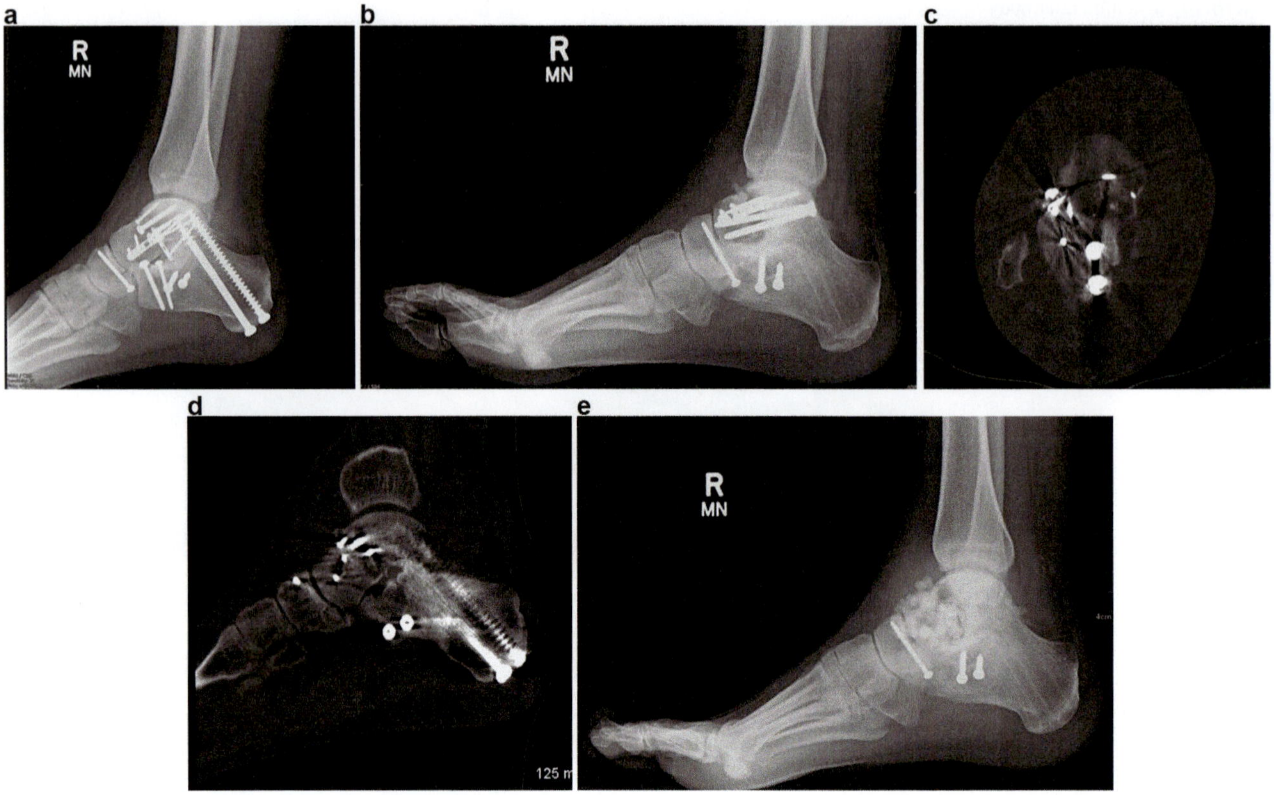

Fig. 18.11 (**a**) Lateral radiograph following initial fracture ORIF with concomitant navicular ORIF and primary subtalar joint arthrodesis. (**b**) Lateral radiograph demonstrating nonunion of the talar neck fracture. (**c**) Axial CT demonstrating nonunion. (**d**) Sagittal CT demonstrating nonunion. (**e**) Lateral radiograph following interval hardware removal with debridement of the talar nonunion with placement of antibiotic cement beads

analysis. If positive, staged debridement and sterilization with local and intravenous antibiotics tailored to the cultured organism or empiric to the most likely organisms according to the recommendations of the consulted infectious disease specialist are indicated. After 6–8 weeks of the intravenous antibiotic and normalized laboratory findings, we recommend aggressive debridement and revision in the same manner as the aseptic nonunion following removal of the antibiotic beads (Fig. 18.11). If this fails and the patient remains symptomatic, a formal talectomy with tibiocalcaneal arthrodesis may be indicated.

Malunion of the talar neck fracture usually occurs intraoperatively and relates directly to visualization and the difficulty in obtaining anatomic reduction [22]. Malunion and malalignment reported at 32 % in some cases have been associated with nonoperatively treated injuries, suboptimal visualization specifically with fractures approached through a single medial incision, and initial fracture comminution or displacement reducing the surgeon's ability to utilize cortical interdigitation to facilitate reduction [29]. Inadvertent impaction of the medial neck through this isolated approach with lag screw fixation adducts the forefoot, placing the longitudinal bisection of the talus lateral to the longitudinal bisection of the first metatarsal, as well as reduces the talocalcaneal angle on the dorsoplantar radiographic projections. The effects of varus malunion and malalignment have been documented and associated with hindfoot varus, forefoot varus, and adduction, resulting in rigidly locked and unadaptable hindfoot. This malposition has also been associated with altered contact mechanics and accelerated rates of adjacent articular degeneration particularly of the subtalar joint [13, 21]. When confirmed clinically and on plain films and computed tomography, realignment osteotomies with bone grafting and internal fixation are indicated [30, 31]. The same surgical approach as described earlier with the malaligned head fracture may be employed. Distal screw fixation in this case has a lower chance of violating the talonavicular joint.

Posttraumatic arthritis, when symptomatic, is treated with bracing and injections as dictated by the patient's clinical findings. When indicated, arthrodesis of affected joints is preferred via techniques no different from arthrosis of any etiology, with the caveat that areas of avascular necrosis may benefit from aggressive debridement and autogenous bone grafting [28]. Primary utilization of bone stimulation may demonstrate utility as an adjunct to the procedure.

In the setting of a largely avascular body, total excision of the body with tibiocalcaneal arthrodesis and arthrodesis of the talar head to the decorticated anterior distal tibia may be a salvage even in light of the significant loss in limb length and height. External braces with built-in height fillers may help compensate for this. This procedure may be approached through a lateral incision centered over the lateral aspect of the ankle over the fibula. The fibula is resected just superior to the tibiotalar articulation and even further depending on the proposed fixation method of choice. The resected distal fibula may be utilized for autogenous structural graft or morselized to backfill any defects. The talar neck is cut with a sagittal saw. Extraction of the body may be facilitated by drilling a 5 or 6 mm Schanz pin into the body to use as a joystick while releasing the soft tissue structures about the body. Removal of the talar body in a single total piece is difficult and is at times easier to extract in multiple pieces. A large sagittal saw is utilized to decorticate the tibial plafond, the superior calcaneus, and the anterior distal tibial cortex. The foot and the posterior aspect of the talar head is then posteriorly translated onto the tibia then the plantar foot, and calcaneus is axially compressed manually to the tibia and provisionally pinned with large Steinman pins. Any defects may be backfilled with the autogenous fibula bone graft. Fixation may be employed with large fragment lag screws augmented with plates. The tibiocalcaneal arthrodesis instead can be fixated with a retrograde intramedullary nail.

Symptomatic partial avascular necrosis with or without collapse can be treated in the same fashion as the large and cystic osteochondral lesions described by Raikin with large bulk allograft cutdown and replacement [32] (Fig. 18.12).

Isolated talectomy as a treatment for primary fracture or for delayed treatment has yielded unpredictable results. Outcomes have involved a relatively unstable hindfoot that at best, but rarely, is pain free. As a result, even in the setting of a talectomy, stabilization via arthrodesis of the tibial to the hindfoot is preferentially performed. Blair originally described a fusion technique in which the talar body was resected and a sliding anterior cortical tibial graft was docked

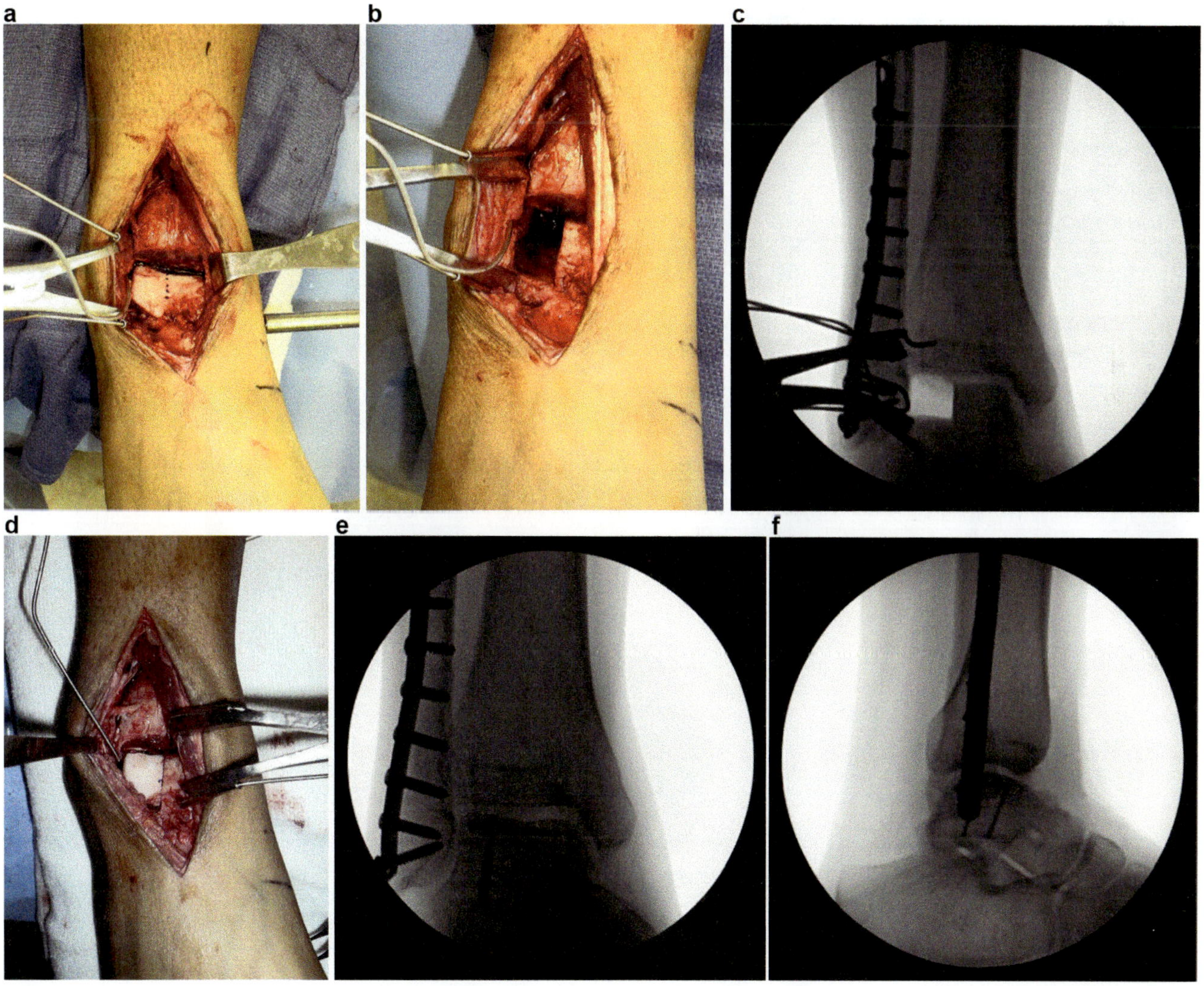

Fig. 18.12 (**a**) Intraoperative approach to talar en bloc resection. (**b**) Intraoperative view after resection. (**c**) Fluoroscopy after resection. (**d**) Intraoperative view after replacement with donor allograft cut to size. (**e**) Postoperative anteroposterior view. (**f**). Postoperative lateral

into the remaining talar head and allowed to heal. This served primarily to maintain limb length while maintaining some hindfoot motion. Because of the size of the inlay graft, fracture of the graft can be of concern [11].

Body Fractures

Because of the innate strength of the talus, fractures of the body are, like neck fractures, the result of high-energy mechanisms [1]. The true mechanisms however are unknown and not reproducible, but there is speculation that because of the frontal or sagittal plane foot position at the time of injury, the large compressive axial force results in fracture of the body of the talus in lieu of the more common joint depression calcaneal fracture or the tibial plafond fracture. Nonetheless, concurrent ipsilateral fractures of these areas have been described [4]. As with neck fractures, these are not occult injuries and not easily missed. Standard anteroposterior, mortise, and lateral projections of ankle radiographs are helpful [23]. Computed tomography is routinely indicated for fracture planning.

Violation of the body occurs either with extensive comminution with very high-energy injuries or with dislocation and larger fracture fragments with comparably lower-energy injuries [4, 33]. Because these fractures are universally intraarticular, nonoperative treatment is rarely indicated. Reducing the incidence of tibiotalar arthrosis is crucial and takes priority over the subtalar joint if the fracture involves both joints. As with the neck fracture, closed reduction may be attempted, but the threshold for operative reduction should be low even if temporary. Urgent and full open operative reduction should be deferred to allow soft tissue resuscitation and to reduce postoperative wound complications (Fig. 18.13).

Total extrusion of the talar body has been described without operative fractures. Initial relocation is indicated with percutaneous pinning or external fixation (Fig. 18.14).

a b c d e

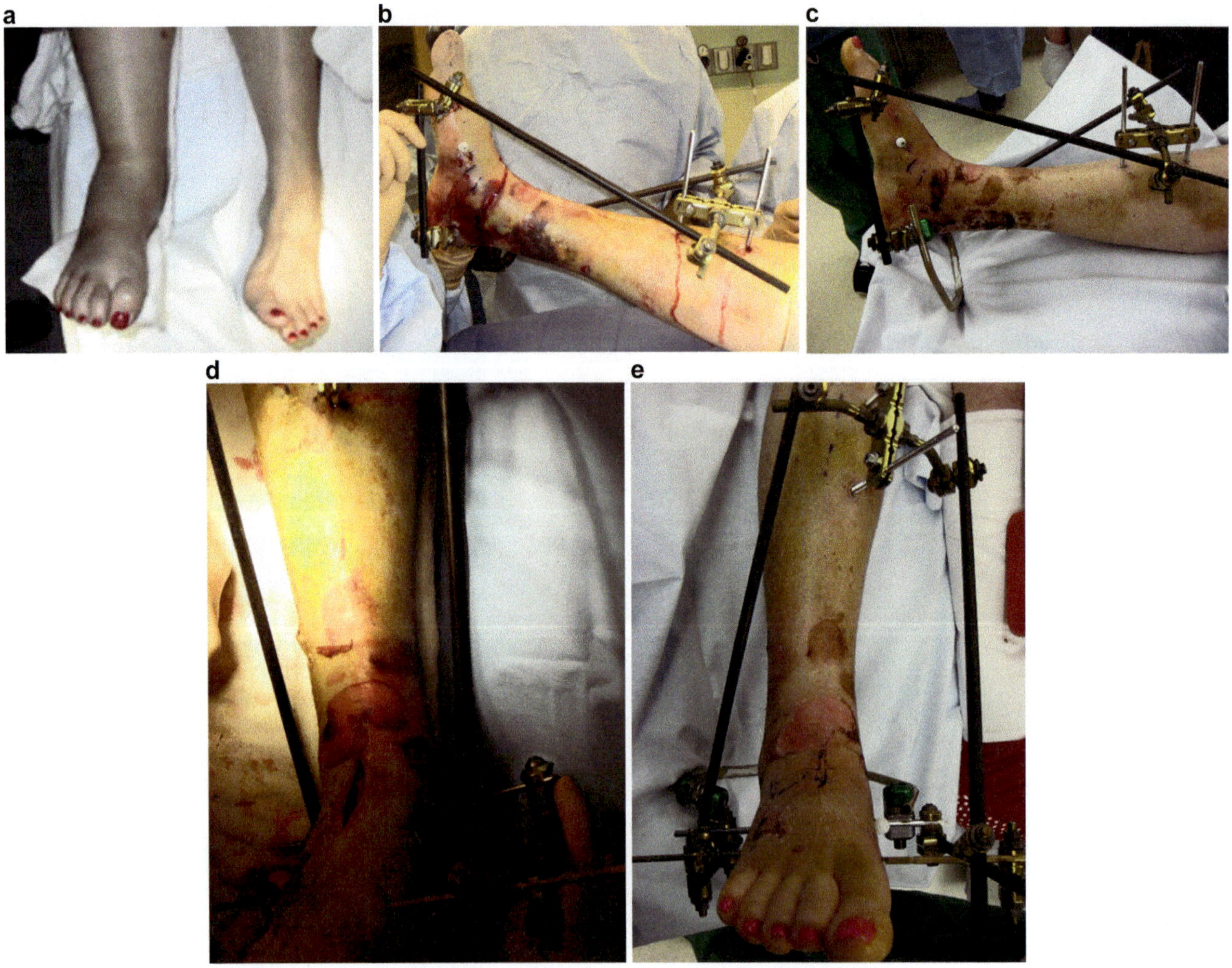

Fig. 18.13 (**a**) Soft tissue edema following talar fracture. (**b** and **c**) Lateral clinical view of soft tissue edema following talar fracture after temporary fixation and soft tissue resuscitation 10 days after external fixation. (**d** and **e**). Anterior clinical view of soft tissue edema following talar fracture after temporary fixation and soft tissue resuscitation 10 days after external fixation. A small dorsal foot incision was initially performed to facilitate reduction of concurrent talonavicular fracture/dislocation

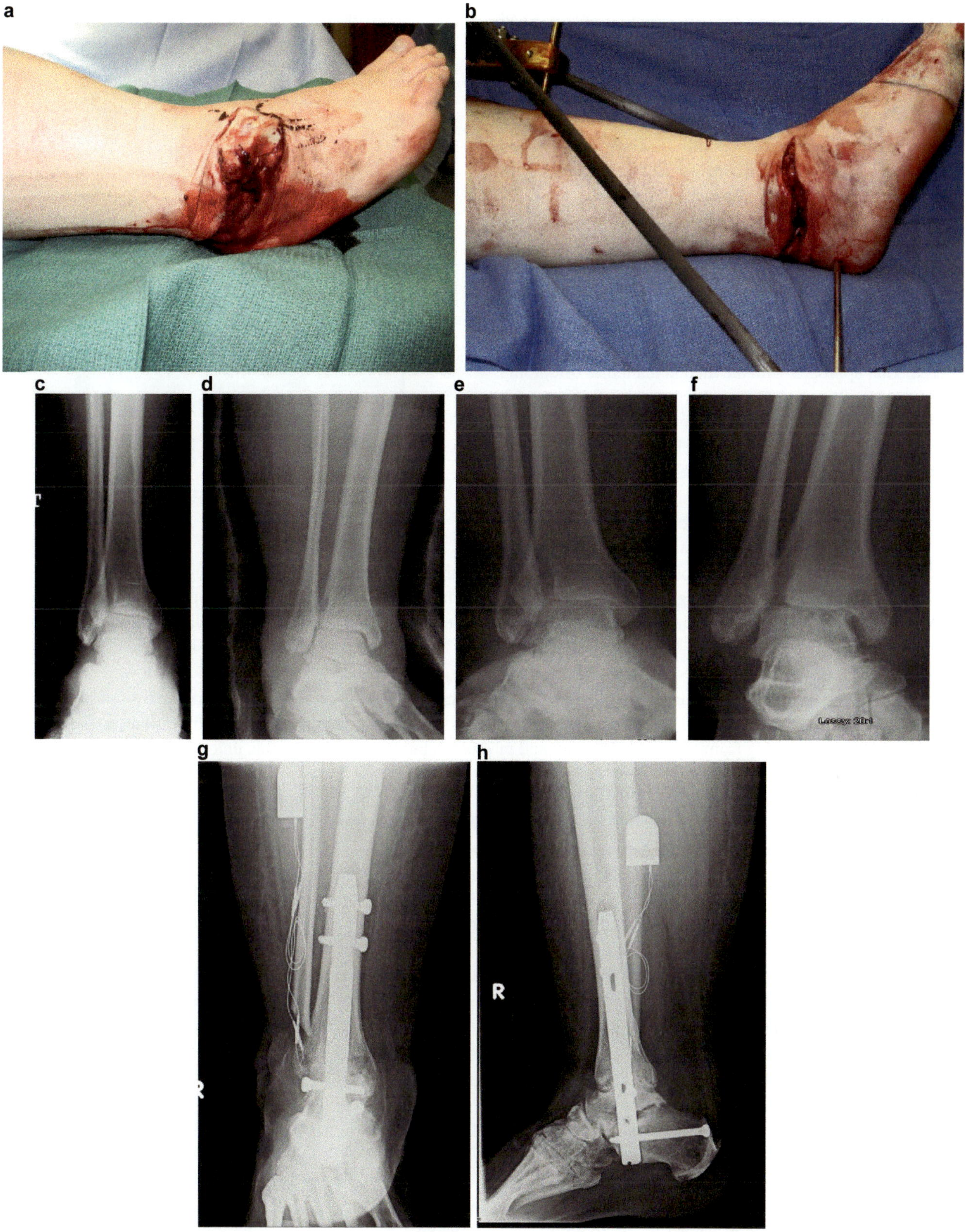

Fig. 18.14 (**a**) Total talar extrusion. (**b**) Closed reduction with external fixator application. (**c**) Postoperative AP ankle radiograph following external fixator removal. (**d**) Postoperative AP ankle radiograph 30 weeks following external fixator removal. (**e**) Postoperative AP ankle radiograph 1 year following external fixator removal. (**f**) Postoperative AP ankle radiograph 2 years following external fixator removal. (**g** and **h**). Postoperative AP and lateral ankle radiograph following trans-fibular tibiotalar calcaneal arthrodesis with intramedullary fixation with implantable bone stimulator

These cases are at particular risk for avascular necrosis and posttraumatic arthritis [34, 35]. The treatment strategies and goals of these even rarer injuries in light of late complications like avascular necrosis and posttraumatic arthritis are treated with traditional arthrodesis techniques [36]. Avascular necrosis in these injuries along with the body fractures has not been described as extensively as neck fractures but has been reported and should be monitored for during the postoperative period [4].

Because the trochlea when anatomic is intimately congruent within the ankle mortise, surgical access can be difficult and malleolar osteotomies or temporary lateral ligamentous releases may facilitate visualization. Traditional incisional approaches are not as uniform as with neck fractures, but the anteromedial approach with the medial malleolar osteotomy is useful. A dry 2.7 mm 30 % wrist arthroscopic instrumentation may assist with reduction of the articular surface. Temporary small wire fixation is helpful prior to hardware delivery. As these fractures are whole articular, plate fixation is never indicated even with comminuted fractures. Small mini fragment screws countersunk below the chondral surface are preferred. Stable fixation is preferred, but absorbable wires may be useful in stabilizing small chondral fractures without attached underlying bone.

Depending on the extent of comminution, definitive reconstruction may not always be feasible. Under these conditions, initial morphological reconstruction with symptomatic treatment of posttraumatic arthritis at a later date should be the goal. Primary ankle arthrodesis should be avoided if possible for a host of reasons ranging from logistical difficulty and in candidates where total ankle replacement may be a more viable procedure than ankle arthrodesis. Under these conditions, reconstructing the overall talar morphology should be the priority. Indications of primary ankle arthrodesis are non reconstructible fractures with severe and irreparable chondral injury where concern for postoperative noncompliance, the medical facts, and the patient's body habitus may preclude staged arthroplasty. If the incisional approach incorporated a medial malleolar osteotomy, a supplementary anterior or anterolateral pilon fracture incision may facilitate visualization of the lateral talar trochlea and joint preparation. Joint preparation and fixation may be performed in standard technique. Intramedullary fixation for primary tibiotalocalcaneal arthrodesis in light of the severely comminuted talar body fracture may result in fracture scattering during nail insertion and should be deferred for screw and plate fixation.

Isolated subtalar arthrodesis either in the primary setting or for late treatment of arthrosis is approached via a sinus tarsi incision from the inferior aspect of the fibula headed toward the fourth metatarsal base. Joint preparation and fixation may be performed in standard technique. Tibiotalocalcaneal arthrodesis may be approached with a single isolated lateral transfibular approach. Alternatively, a sinus tarsi approach may be employed for the sinus tarsi with an anterior ankle incision for the tibiotalar joint. An isolated posterior trans-Achilles approach allows for visualization of both the ankle and subtalar joints (Fig. 18.15).

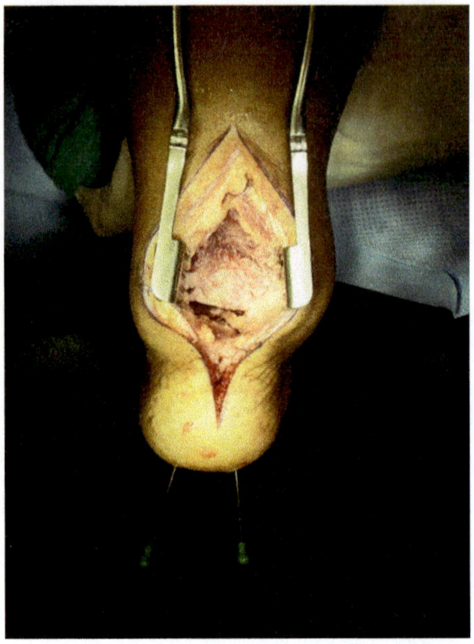

Fig. 18.15 Tibiotalocalcaneal arthrodesis through posterior incisional approach

The postoperative course for revisional reconstruction is the same as described for malaligned head. However, if primary arthrodesis is undertaken, the postoperative course involves full and circumferential cast immobilization for 8–12 weeks until clinical and radiographic union is confirmed.

Posterior Tubercle Fractures

Fractures or rather injury of the posterior tubercles is not uncommon. Because of their anatomic location and surrounding and attaching soft tissue structures, these tubercles are at particular risk during extreme dorsiflexion and plantarflexion position of the ankle. This is commonly seen with sporting activities with a high incidence of ankle sprains but has been specifically associated with ballet dancers and the *en pointe* position [37].

The *os trigonum* is a secondary ossicle that is sometimes found in association to the posterolateral tubercle. When present it may be attached to the posterolateral process through fibrous connections. These connections may become injured during the same extreme sagittal plane mechanisms, resulting in acute symptoms. This is generally treated with protected weight-bearing immobilization for 4–6 weeks. On the lateral radiographic projection, a smooth or sclerotic interface between the suspected os trigonum and the remaining posterolateral process may rule out a true fracture. Alternatively, a radiolucent jagged line may be more indicative of an acute fracture. Computed tomography can better assess fracture extent and when indicated, reduced under direct visualization through a posterolateral incision adjacent to the Achilles tendon. In some instances, hallux dorsiflexion may exacerbate the symptoms clinically as the flexor hallucis longus tendon courses adjacent to the fracture. The posteromedial tubercle is rarely injured due to its size compared to the posterolateral tubercle, but the same qualifications apply pertaining to treatment depending on size and computed tomographic findings [25].

CeDell first described the fracture of the posteromedial tubercle of the talus [38]. Because of its location, this injury can be easily missed even on standard lateral radiographic projection. The true mechanism is unknown and may present occultly. Computed tomography may be of assistance when suspicious, but because of the occult presentation, it is not routinely ordered. This may result in delayed diagnosis and protracted convalescence.

If small and nondisplaced, nonoperative cast immobilization is indicated for 4–6 weeks. But because of its intraarticular extent, operative treatment is indicated even with mild displacement. This involves a posteromedial incision over the tarsal tunnel. The landmarks here are the posterior aspect of tibial nerve and the flexor hallucis longus tendon as it courses deep to the posteromedial tubercle. Direct visualization with mini fragment compression screw fixation is preferred with the screw head countersunk below the chondral surface. In the setting of a delayed diagnosis, smaller fractures may be preferentially excised through the same incisional approach.

Managing malunions or delayed diagnosis of either tubercle has received little attention in the literature. Thus, management takes on a more practical approach. Large symptomatic malunions and delayed unions involving a significant portion of the subtalar joint confirmed with computed tomography are treated with subtalar arthrodesis [11]. Small symptomatic malunions or delayed unions may be excised. Unfortunately outcomes are not uniform and some authors defer to primary subtalar joint arthrodesis [11]. A subtalar joint diagnostic injection and computed tomographic study may help with discerning the clinical picture.

Excision is approached through the same incisional approaches for the initial respective fractures. An ancillary lateral sinus tarsi incision may be used to address the subtalar joint arthrodesis. If the patient's body habitus does not preclude the prone operative position, excision of the posterolateral fragment and concurrent subtalar arthrodesis can be approached through a single posterior longitudinal incision lateral to the Achilles tendon like the posterior approach for the tibiotalocalcaneal arthrodesis. Following subcutaneous dissection, the Achilles is retracted laterally. Kager's fat pad is dissected in the same linear orientation as the original skin incision. A similarly oriented longitudinal incision is made within the posterior crural fascia. The anatomic landmark here is the muscle belly and tendon of the flexor hallucis longus. The posterolateral tubercle lies just lateral to the tendon. With medial retraction and plantar flexion, the posterior subtalar joint is easily visualized and prepared. Two large fragment lag screws are delivered from the calcaneal tuber into the talar body and the talar neck for fixation of either arthrodesis approaches.

The postoperative course for simple fracture excision involves immobilization until wound healing. Following this, protected weight bearing and physical therapy are aggressively initiated for 4 weeks to reduce arthrosis. When subtalar arthrodesis is performed, the patient is cast immobilized for 6–8 weeks until clinical and radiographic union is confirmed.

Lateral Talar Process Fractures

Fractures of the lateral talar process, though rare, can result from various mechanism but have historically and classically been described in snowboarders. These fractures have thus earned the moniker, *snowboarders fracture* [39]. It has been described as a hyperdorsiflexion injury on an inverted foot [40]. Patients sometimes describe what sounds like an ankle sprain, and as a result, these fractures can be easily missed. Ankle anteroposterior and mortise radiographic projection with the foot in neutral may isolate the lateral process enough to visualize the presence of fracture. If suspicious and plain radiographs are inconclusive, computed tomography is indicated and will provide crucial information relating to the true size and articular extent. Fractures when larger and extending into the subtalar joint are initially treated with direct visual open reduction with internal fixation through a lateral subtalar arthrotomy (Fig. 18.16). Smaller fractures can be treated nonoperatively or with excision.

Management principles of lateral process malunions, nonunions, or late and missed injuries are approached in the same practical manner as the posterior tubercle injuries. Small fragments are excised [41]. Larger fragments are osteotomized and reconstructed. Minifragment lag screw fixation is employed. If the subtalar joint is arthritic, and confirmed with diagnostic injected and computed tomography, arthrodesis is indicated. The sinus tarsi incision provides excellent visualization in both settings.

Postoperatively, simple fracture excision is immobilization until suture removal. Following this, protected weight bearing and physical therapy are aggressively initiated for 4 weeks to reduce arthrosis. If the fracture is osteotomized and reconstruction is performed, the patient is immobilized until suture removal. Aggressive passive range of motion exercises is initiated for 4 weeks while the patient remains non-weight bearing and immobilized. Following clinical and radiographic union, protected weight bearing is initiated. When subtalar arthrodesis is performed, the patient is cast immobilized for 6–8 weeks until clinical and radiographic union is confirmed.

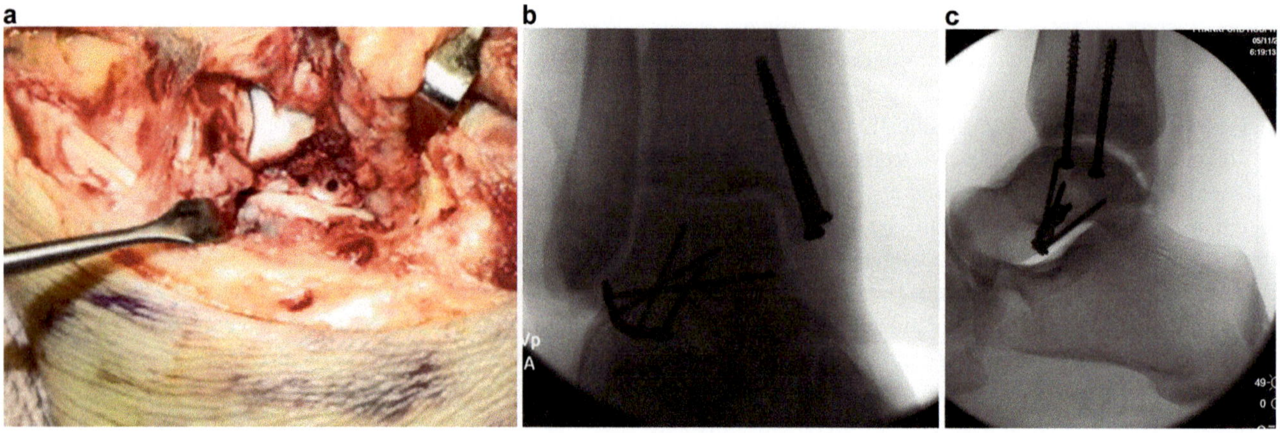

Fig. 18.16 (**a**) Intraoperative approach to lateral process fracture and revision. (**b** and **c**) Postoperative anteroposterior and lateral fluoroscopic images

References

1. Kleiger B. Injuries of the talus and its joints. Clin Orthop Relat Res. 1976;121:243–62.
2. Sarrafian SK. Anatomy of the foot and ankle. 2nd ed. Philadelphia: Lippincott; 1993.
3. Halvorson JJ, Winter SB, Teasdall RD, Scott AT. Talar neck fractures: a systematic review of the literature. J Foot Ankle Surg. 2013;52(1):56–61.
4. Metzger MJ, Levin JS, Clancy JT. Talar neck fractures and rates of avascular necrosis. J Foot Ankle Surg. 1999;38(2):154–62.
5. Adelaar RS, Madrian JR. Avascular necrosis of the talus. Orthop Clin North Am. 2004;35(3):383–95.
6. Vallier HA, Nork SE, Barei DP, Benirschke SK, Sangeorzan BJ. Talar neck fractures: results and outcomes. J Bone Jt Surg Am. 2004;86(8):1616–24.
7. Mulfinger GL, Trueta J. The blood supply of the talus. J Bone Jt Surg Br. 1970;52(1):160–7.
8. Miller AN, Prasarn ML, Dyke JP, Helfet DL, Lorich DG. Quantitative assessment of the vascularity of the talus with gadolinium-enhanced magnetic resonance imaging. J Bone Jt Surg Am. 2011;93(12):1116–21.
9. Prasarn ML, Miller AN, Dyke JP, Helfet DL, Lorich DG. Arterial anatomy of the talus: a cadaver and gadolinium-enhanced MRI study. Foot Ankle Int. 2010;31(11):987–93.
10. Vallier HA, Reichard SG, Boyd AJ, Moore TA. A new look at the Hawkins classification for talar neck fractures: which features of injury and treatment are predictive of osteonecrosis? J Bone Jt Surg Am. 2014;96(3):192–7.
11. Sanders R, Lindvall E. Fractures and fracture-dislocations of the talus. In: Coughlin MJ, Mann RA, Saltzman CL, editors. Surgery of the foot and ankle, 8th ed. Philadelphia: Mosby; 2007. p. 2075–2136.
12. Rush SM, Hamilton GA. Talus fractures: surgical principles. Clin Podiatr Med Surg. 2009;26(1):91–103.
13. Daniels TR, Smith JW, Ross TI. Varus malalignment of the talar neck. Its effect on the position of the foot and on subtalar motion. J Bone Jt Surg Am. 1996;78(10):1559–67.
14. Matsumura T, Sekiya H, Hoshino Y. Correction osteotomy for malunion of the talar head: a case report. J Orthop Surg (Hong Kong). 2008;16(1):96–8.
15. Fishco WD. Talonavicular fusions. In: Southerland JT, Boberg JS, Downey MS, Nakra A, Rabjohn LV, editors. McGlamry's comprehensive textbook of foot and ankle surgery, 4th ed. Philadelphia: Lippincott Williams & Wilkins; 2013. p. 851–854.
16. Mann RA. Arthrodesis of the foot and ankle. In: Coughlin MJ, Mann RA, Saltzman CL, editors. Surgery of the foot and ankle, 8th ed. Philadelphiae: Mosbey; 2007: p. 1087–1123.
17. Peterson L, Romanus B, Dahlberg E. Fracture of the collum tali--an experimental study. J Biomech. 1976;9(4):277–9.
18. Hawkins LG. Fractures of the neck of the talus. J Bone Jt Surg Am. 1970;52(5):991–1002.
19. Canale ST, Kelly Jr FB. Fractures of the neck of the talus. Long-term evaluation of seventy-one cases. J Bone Jt Surg Am. 1978;60(2):143–56.
20. Inokuchi S, Ogawa K, Usami N. Classification of fractures of the talus: clear differentiation between neck and body fractures. Foot Ankle Int. 1996;17(12):748–50.
21. Sangeorzan BJ, Wagner UA, Harrington RM, Tencer AF. Contact characteristics of the subtalar joint: the effect of talar neck misalignment. J Orthop Res. 1992;10(4):544–51.
22. Lindvall E, Haidukewych G, Dipasquale T, Herscovici Jr D, Sanders R. Open reduction and stable fixation of isolated, displaced talar neck and body fractures. J Bone Jt Surg Am. 2004; 86(10):2229–34.
23. Furlong J, Morrison WB, Carrino JA. Imaging of the talus. Foot Ankle Clin. 2004;9(4):685–701.
24. Early JS. Talus fracture management. Foot Ankle Clin. 2008;13(4): 635–57.
25. Summers NJ, Murdoch MM. Fractures of the talus: a comprehensive review. Clin Podiatr Med Surg. 2012;29(2):187–203.
26. Schuberth JM, Rush SM, Jennings MM. Talar fractures. In: Southerland JT, Boberg JS, Downey MS, Nakra A, Rabjohn LV, editors. McGlamry's comprehensive textbook of foot and ankle surgery, 4th ed. Philadelphia: Lippincott Williams & Wilkins; 2013: p. 1707–1738.
27. Léduc S, Clare MP, Laflamme GY, Walling AK. Posttraumatic avascular necrosis of the talus. Foot Ankle Clin. 2008;13(4):753–65.
28. Hyer CF, Decarbo WT. Talar avascular necrosis. In: Southerland JT, Boberg JS, Downey MS, Nakra A, Rabjohn LV, editors. McGlamry's comprehensive textbook of foot and ankle surgery, 4th ed. Philadelphia: Lippincott Williams & Wilkins; 2013: p. 1890–1913.
29. Rammelt S, Zwipp H. Talar neck and body fractures. Injury. 2009;40(2):120–35.
30. Monroe MT, Manoli A, 2nd. Osteotomy for malunion of a talar neck fracture: a case report. Foot Ankle Int. 1999;20(3): 192–195.
31. Huang PJ, Cheng YM. Delayed surgical treatment for neglected or mal-reduced talar fractures. Int Orthop. 2005;29(5):326–9.

32. Raikin SM. Fresh Osteochondral allografts for large-volume cystic osteochondral defects of the talus. J Bone Jt Surg Am. 2009;91(12):2818–26.
33. Sneppen O, Christensen SB, Krogsøe O, Lorentzen J. Fractures of the body of the talus. Acta Orthop Scand. 1977;48(3):317–24.
34. Early JS. Management of fractures of the talus: body and head regions. Foot Ankle Clin. 2004;9(4):709–22.
35. Fournier A, Barba N, Steiger V, Lourdais A, Frin JM, Williams T, et al. Total talar fracture—long-term results of internal fixation of talar fractures. A multicentric study of 114 cases. Orthop Traumatol Surg Res. 2012;98(4 Suppl):s48–55.
36. Fleming JJ, Hurley KK. Total talar extrusion: a case report. J Foot Ankle Surg. 2009;48(6):690.e19–23.
37. Nault ML, Kocher MS, Micheli LJ. Os trigonum syndrome. J Am Acad Orthop Surg. 2014;22(9):545–53.
38. Cedell CA. Rupture of the posterior talotibial ligament with the avulsion of a bone fragment from the talus. Acta Orthop Scand. 1974;45(3):454–61.
39. Kirkpatrick DP, Hunter RE, Janes PC, Mastrangelo J, Nicholas RA. The snowboarder's foot and ankle. Am J Sports Med. 1998;26(2):271–7.
40. Hawkins LG. Fractures of the lateral process of the talus. A review of thirteen cases. J Bone Jt Surg Am. 1965;47(6):1170–5.
41. Funasaki H, Kato S, Hayashi H, Marumo K. Arthroscopic excision of bone fragments in a neglected fracture of the lateral process of the talus in a junior soccer player. Arthrosc Tech. 2014;3(3):e331–4.

Posterior Heel Complications

19

Eric A. Barp and Rachael Poore

Introduction

Surgical treatment of the posterior heel has become a mainstay of foot and ankle surgery due to its highly successful outcomes. Pathology of the posterior heel remains narrow, typically with an origin rooted in inflammation or structural deformity. Differential diagnoses include Haglund's deformity, Achilles tendinosis/insertional calcification, and retrocalcaneal bursitis. Many patients develop symptoms as their activity increases or when donning new shoes that irritate the deformity.

When evaluating the patient population with Haglund's triad [1], those most affected by it are athletes, specifically those who participate in middle- and long-distance running, orienteering, track and field, tennis, badminton, volleyball, and soccer [2]. The pain associated worsens with activity, and in a population that relies on the Achilles tendon for performance, this can be a debilitating condition. Older athletes are affected more often than younger and they are predominantly male [2]. When considering the nonathletic population, the insertional Achilles tendinopathy presents more often in females who are middle aged, sedentary, and overweight and will often times have other medical conditions [3].

In addition to pursuing surgical options in the patient with posterior heel pathology, it is important to enlist a team of therapist to evaluate and treat any training errors in the athletic patient. Correction of these errors preoperatively and guided therapy postoperatively will ensure an optimal outcome. In all patients, lower extremity malalignment and/or limb length discrepancies should be assessed.

E.A. Barp (✉)
Foot and Ankle Surgery, The Iowa Clinic,
5950 University Ave Ste 160, West Des Moines, IA 50266, USA
e-mail: ebarp@iowaclinic.com

R. Poore
Podiatric Medicine and Surgery, Unity Point Health-Des Moines,
1415 Woodland Avenue, Des Moines, IA, USA

Procedures

A variety of surgical procedures have been described as treatment for posterior heel pathology. They all serve to accomplish the same goal: to eliminate strain on the posterior calcaneus caused by a tightened and partially diseased Achilles tendon. Haglund's resection involves exostectomy of the posterior superior calcaneal tuber with or without Achilles tendon detachment. The Keck and Kelly is a dorsal closing wedge of posterior superior calcaneus. A simple bursectomy involves removal of inflamed bursal sac; however, this is rarely performed as an isolated procedure, except when infected. An Achilles tendon debridement involves detachment and reattachment with bone anchor(s) and in cases of extensive debridement is accompanied by an FHL transfer to adjunct the remaining Achilles tendon. FHL transfer can also be used in cases of a partial Achilles tendon rupture to restore strength. Finally, arthroscopic posterior heel surgery is known as endoscopic calcaneoplasty. This is an arthroscopic debridement of inflamed retrocalcaneal bursa and the posterior superior calcaneal tuber.

Indications of Procedure

Haglund's Deformity/Retrocalcaneal Exostosis

Also known as the "pump bump," Haglund's deformity is defined as a posterolateral prominence of the superior calcaneal tuberosity (Fig. 19.1). Its presence will cause pain when compressed by shoe gear resulting in "sandwiching" of the Achilles tendon and its bursal sac. Irritation of the bursal sac can lead to retrocalcaneal bursitis as well. Due to its posterolateral location, this can be difficult to visualize on radiographs and is best documented clinically.

M.S. Lee, J.P. Grossman (eds.), *Complications in Foot and Ankle Surgery*, DOI 10.1007/978-3-319-53686-6_19

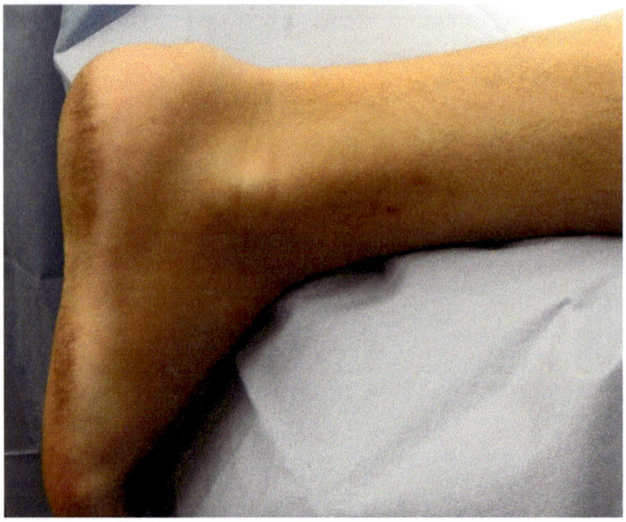

Fig. 19.1 The subtle posterior heel bump can be visualized. In this particular patient, the bump was present directly posterior to the Achilles tendon insertion due to calcification here and bursitis which can be seen in Fig. 19.2

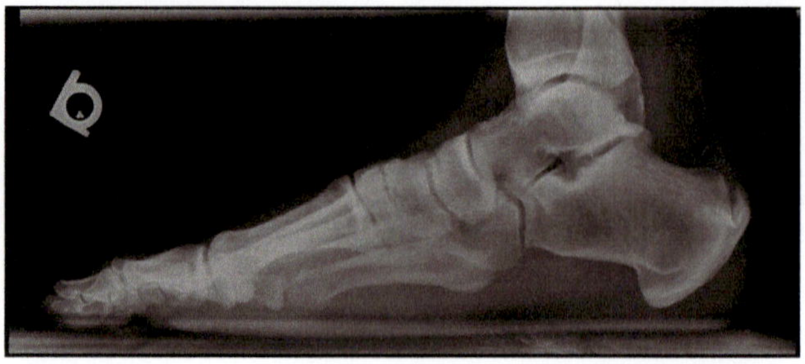

Fig. 19.2 Insertional Achilles calcification. Calcification appearing as spurring is present along this patient's posterior heel. As the calcifications worsen and become larger, the bump on the posterior heel becomes more prominent. This leads to rubbing on shoes and inflammation of the bursal sac all while the Achilles tendon is remodeling and becoming tighter

Insertional Achilles Tendinopathy

Pain at the insertion of the Achilles tendon is indicative of insertional tendinopathy. As the disease progresses, the Achilles tendon will attempt to remodel. The remodeling however is inadequate and results in unequal and irregular crimping of collagen which can eventually be replaced by calcification. This intratendinous calcification is easily visualized on routine radiographs (Fig. 19.2). The calcification can appear as one or many spurs off the posterior heel; however, it is important to remember that this is intratendinous. Any swelling or convex changes to the posterior heel will be located directly posterior (as opposed to the lateral and more superior Haglund's deformity). On occasion, swelling of the tendon may be present due to the intratendinous inflammation and remodeling.

Bursitis

There are two bursa in the posterior heel which act to protect the Achilles tendon from external forces (i.e., shoe gear) and internal forces (i.e., calcaneal tuberosity). The deeper of the two is named the bursa tendinis calcanei (or retrocalcaneal bursa) and the superficial bursa named bursa subcutanea calcanea (superficial calcaneal bursa) [4]. It is common for bursitis to present in conjunction to insertional Achilles tendinopathy and Haglund's deformity (i.e., Haglund's triad) [2]. If primarily involved, likely causes include infection or inflammation due to an arthropathy, both of which are best treated conservatively with oral medications.

Failed Conservative Therapies

Prior to performing surgery on any patient with posterior heel pain, a conservative treatment algorithm should be in place. In no specific order, the patient should fail conservative options with use of heel lifts/pads, stretching, NSAIDs, immobilization, and physical therapy. Physical therapy intervention is especially useful preoperatively as it can help retrain poor mechanics in athletes. Physical therapists are also a valuable member of the treatment postoperatively for recovery and return to activities.

Contraindications/Limitations

Elective surgery should be performed through the skin that has been thoroughly cleaned, is free of infection, and is well perfused. The amount of soft tissue coverage available over the Achilles tendon in the posterior heel is minimal, and any local infection must be treated and resolved prior to surgical intervention to avoid infection of the Achilles tendon. In addition, the presence of peripheral vascular disease warrants an appropriate workup and optimization before performing surgery. The skin to the posterior heel is supplied by calcaneal branches of the posterior tibial and peroneal arteries [5]. If either vessel is diseased, this can lead to poor wound healing or wound dehiscence, infection of soft tissue, and potentially infection of the calcaneus.

Technique Pearls and Pitfalls to Avoid Complications

Incision Placement and Tissue Handling

Many incisional approaches have been reported for posterior heel surgery with some studies specifically observing outcomes related to this alone. To better understand placement

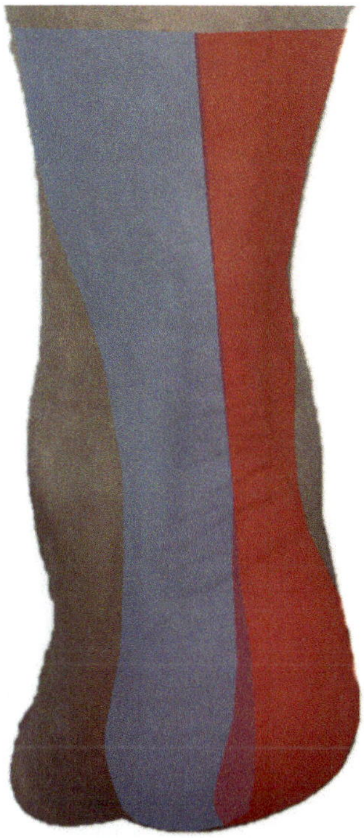

Fig. 19.3 Angiosomes of the posterior heel. The *blue area*, laterally, is supplied by the calcaneal arteries from the peroneal artery. The *red area* is supplied by the calcaneal arteries from the posterior tibial artery. There exists some overlap between these two distally; however, they predominantly meet exactly midline over the Achilles tendon

of the incision, one must understand the angiosomes of the posterior heel.

There are two angiosomes to consider on the posterior heel. The division between these two lies directly central on the heel with each supplying 50 % and significant overlap exists between the two. On the medial side, calcaneal branches of the posterior tibial artery provide perfusion and calcaneal branches of the peroneal artery perfuse the lateral side. The plantar heel is also supplied by the calcaneal branches peroneal artery. With this in mind, incisions are best made midline over the Achilles tendon [5] (Figs. 19.3 and 19.4). This will fulfill the four principles set forth by Attinger [5] when considering incision placement:

1. Incision must provide adequate exposure for the planned procedure.
2. There must be adequate blood supply on either side to optimize healing.
3. Incision should spare sensory and motor nerves.
4. Incision should not be perpendicular to a joint.

In the event that exposure is needed to continue into the heel pad, it is suggested that the incision curve laterally to follow the distal angiosome boundary and avoid damage to the medial calcaneal neurovascular structures [6]. In a systematic review performed in 2011 by Highlander and Greenhagen, the incidence of wound complications related to incision placement was recorded [7]. Their findings revealed an overall complication rate of 7 % for posterior

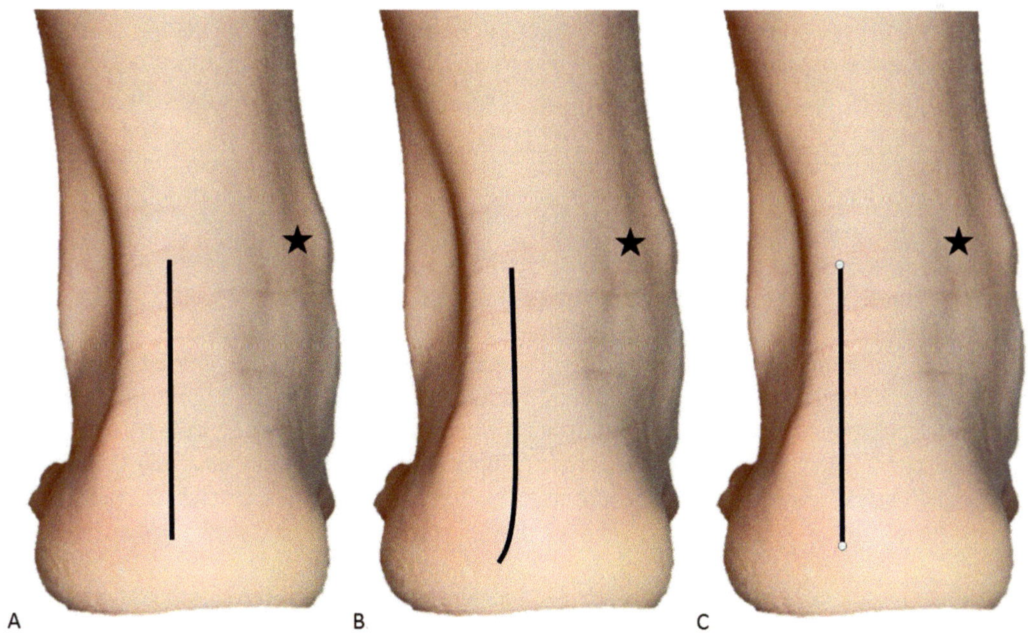

Fig. 19.4 Incision placement: (**a**) Incisions on the posterior heel should be precisely midline. (**b**) Past the glabrous junction, incision lateral to the Achilles tendon (**c**) is better tolerated with fewer healing complications. Incisions medial to the Achilles tendon should be avoided. The *star* indicates the medial malleolus

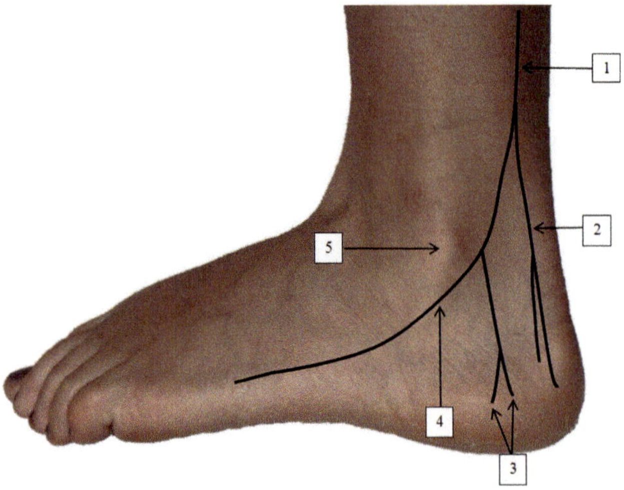

Fig. 19.5 Note the lateral neurovascular structures

midline incisions and 8.3 % for posterior medial incisions, concluding they have similar complication rates. Interestingly, they did report there were no incidences of painful scar or skin necrosis in the midline incision group; there was 1.2% incidence for the former and 0.6% for the latter in the medial incision group.

In procedures such as the retrocalcaneal exostectomy, arthroscopy, and the Keck and Kelly osteotomy, the incision placement can also be made on the lateral posterior ankle. The greater concern in this region is the sural nerve and its calcaneal branches. The sural nerve typically lays 17.5 mm lateral to the Achilles tendon insertion and gives off an average of three branches to the lateral heel as lateral calcaneal branches in the retromalleolar region [7]. An overall incidence of sensory deficits has not been reported in the literature aside from individual case studies. The anatomy of this region affords patient education of the risk of sensory alterations postoperatively. The few cases that have been reported have either gone on to resolve spontaneously or were treated with gabapentin, corticosteroid injections, or additional surgery [8–11] (Fig. 19.5).

With any incision that is at an increased risk of delayed wound healing, a "no-touch" technique is advocated for handling the skin edges throughout the procedure. Full thickness flaps should be created and secured using suture (Fig. 19.6). This technique will minimize accidental aggressive retraction by assistant or retraction device. Minimal tissue handling and soft tissue trauma will result in improved healing results.

Patient Positioning

The patient should be positioned prone when performing posterior heel surgery through a posterior incision. In the event that a lateral approach will be utilized, a prone/lazy lateral can be used. It is important to maintain access for exposure of the Achilles tendon or medial structures in the event that further exposure is needed or adjunct procedures must be performed. When positioning the patient in the prone position, the foot should hang over the end of the table on a pillow. This positioning will allow natural plantar flexion of the foot by elevating the leg and flexing the knee to remove tension on the Achilles tendon and allow ease of exposure of the calcaneal tuberosity. When positioning the patient in the lateral position, the foot should be elevated off the table to allow assessment of ROM with the leg, knee, and hip in appropriate alignment (Fig. 19.7).

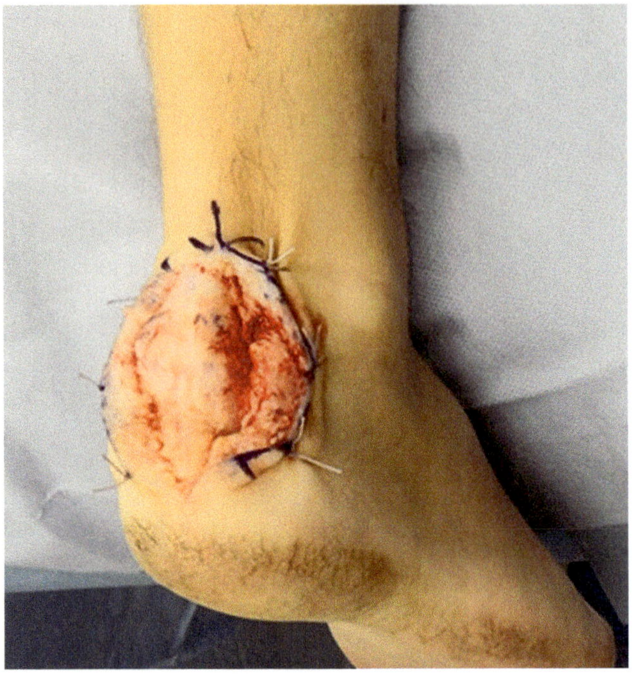

Fig. 19.6 No-touch technique: After creating a full thickness flap incision, the skin edges are sutured back to facilitate surgical exposure and minimize skin trauma/handling

Tourniquet

A thigh tourniquet should be utilized for posterior heel surgery to allow full ROM of the ankle during surgery. For ease of application, we have found it best to apply this while the patient is supine just prior to positioning into the prone position. The application of a calf tourniquet will compress and restrict motion within the gastro soleus complex. It may be surgeon preference to use no tourniquet, but this may lead to longer operative times and increased anesthesia requirements for the patient.

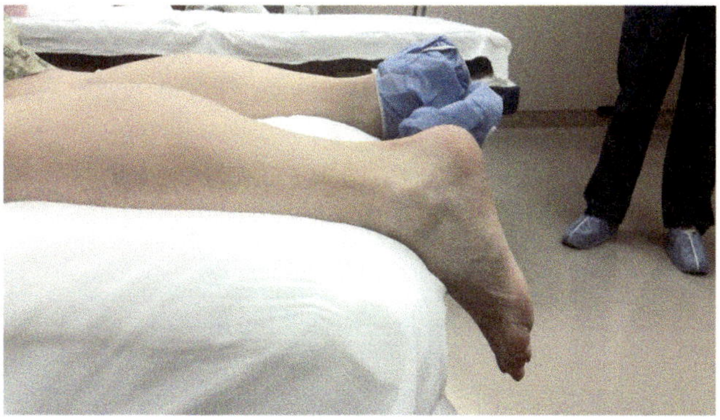

Fig. 19.7 Patient positioning. A patient positioned in prone and a pillow under the ankles. This allows a gentle flexion of the knees and eliminates tension on the gastro-soleal complex. In addition, this position provides superior visualization

Anesthesia

General anesthesia is absolutely necessary for optimal surgical outcomes in posterior heel surgery, especially when positioned in the prone position. Complete paralysis is necessary throughout the procedure for ROM assessment and repair. General anesthesia will also prevent movements due to pain/stimulation of a thigh tourniquet. Nerve blocks can be administered prior to the induction of general anesthesia to provide postoperative analgesia. Either femoral popliteal or popliteal saphenous can be administered with the aid of a nerve stimulator to ensure adequate placement.

Management of Specific Complications

The operative strategy for insertional Achilles tendinopathy is removal of the degenerative tendon and associated calcification, excision of the inflamed retrocalcaneal bursa, and resection of the prominent posterior calcaneal prominence [10]. With respect to the soft tissues, postoperative complications can be avoided. Patient education prior to surgical intervention is a key to success. Patients should be educated that full recovery may take up to 12 months postoperatively. Full recovery is defined as return to full activity without pain or discomfort [12, 13]. This also could vary with the choice of fixation techniques [14].

Over Correction

Proper intraoperative assessment is necessary to ensure that lengthening will allow the ankle dorsiflex to neutral position. Often times, the Achilles tendon insertion is advanced proximally to relieve some of the insertional strain [15]. If this is over-advanced or combined with a lengthening, weakness of the triceps surae can ensue and potentially result in a calcaneal gait (although this complication has never been recorded in the literature). Calcaneal gait is defined as increased ankle dorsiflexion during midstance which places the heel under a longer weight-bearing phase. It has only been reported in studies where heel cord lengthening was utilized in spastic neurologic disorders. In a healthy adult with normal biomechanics, the calcaneal gait will be temporary and will resolve as strength and weight bearing with push off are increased during the postoperative phase. In the event that a patient develops pain due to increased heel weight bearing that their equinus deformity did not previously allow, conservative therapies such as physical therapy to strengthen the posterior muscle group and orthotics with a padded heel cup have been anecdotally beneficial. Gastrocnemius recessions are not typically done in adjunct to these procedures as we feel that this could lead to overcorrection.

Patients may experience continued postoperative pain from overaggressive resection of the insertional spur or the retrocalcaneal exostosis. Patients may also develop pain due to absorption of bone anchors when used to reattach the Achilles tendon. This will typically resolve with postoperative physical therapy and nonsteroidal anti-inflammatories (NSAIDS).

Achilles Tendinosis/Rupture

Rupture of an Achilles tendon after surgical correction of insertional pathology is rare [16]. We commonly obtain MRIs of our patients with both posterior heel pathology and Achilles tendon pathology to ensure they are adequately treated with conservative and surgical measures. If tendon pathology is seen in the watershed zone (2–6 cm proximal to the Achilles tendon insertion), we recommend resecting all pathologic tendon intraoperatively and lengthening their postoperative recovery period to allow complete healing [17]. In regard to ruptures due to anchor pullout after repair, it is the tendon that will tear and rupture or the suture used to attach the tendon to the anchor that will give way before anchor fixation fails [18, 19]. This most commonly occurs at the point where the tendon twists, a location that is anatomically at risk for rupture despite surgical treatment [20]. Increased risks for tendon rupture include aggressive post-op therapy, falls, and increasing activity too quickly. If re-rupture does occur, revision of the surgical procedure is warranted.

Infections

The overall incidence of postoperative infections reported in the literature over the past 14 years after posterior heel surgery is 2.6 % (total of 18 out of 702 cases) [21]. Infections in the posterior heel area need to be treated aggressively due to the lack of subcutaneous tissue interface between the tendon and skin. We recommend treating with oral antibiotics if possible and local wound care. In the event that the wound worsens or deepens, suture material should be removed as it can serve as a nidus for deeper infection. Plans for secondary closure should be made if primary closure cannot be obtained after debridement.

Delayed Wound Healing

The overall incidence of wound complications reported in the literature over the past 14 years after posterior heel surgery is 3.56% (total of 25 out of 702) [21]. These account for skin edge necrosis, delayed healing, and painful/hypertrophic scars.

To avoid complications, we recommend several intraoperative protocols. Skin incision placement should follow angiosome intersection either equally midline or slightly lateral. A medially deviated incision should be avoided. Maintain full-thickness skin flaps and avoid over dissection of deep tissue layers (from skin to bone). Too much dissection will disrupt the delicate vascular network intact to the soft tissues and Achilles tendon. Separation of the layers can also increase the risk of seroma. Additionally, careful skin handling intraoperatively utilizing a self-retaining retractor or the no-touch suturing technique should be utilized. Both will minimize human error of overly aggressive retraction.

In the event that wound complications are encountered, it is most commonly marked by dehiscence of the distal incision at the transition of supple skin to more glabrous skin [22–27]. Aggressive wound therapy will typically warrant success. We typically start within office wound care utilizing a wound specialist and close follow-up. Plans should be arranged for secondary wound closure or a plastic surgery and/or vascular surgery consult if the wound does not appear to be improving.

Deep Venous Thrombosis

We routinely prescribe deep venous thrombosis (DVT) prophylactic medications to patients undergoing posterior heel surgery. Postoperatively, the patient is immobilized in a posterior splint to eliminate ankle motion and hold correction in ankle neutral. The incidence of DVT after posterior heel surgery has been poorly reported in the literature, and prophylaxis guidelines do not recommend prophylaxis for routine surgery of the foot and ankle [28]. However, an observational study in 2013 found that without thromboprophylaxis, the highest incidence of DVT in foot and ankle surgery occurred after repair of Achilles tendon ruptures [29]. Given the morbidity, potential long-term complications of a DVT, and possibly fatal outcomes if the DVT progressed to a pulmonary embolism, we have elected to provide thromboprophylaxis to our patients until they can begin physical therapy.

Neural Symptoms

The sural nerve provides branches to the posterior calcaneus that lie in close proximity to the incision. Excessive retraction, lateral dissection, and posterior lateral ankle incisions can result in neurologic symptoms. Resolution is patient specific, and care should be taken when dissecting in these areas to prevent permanent nerve damage. With a lateral approach, altered sensation postoperatively has been reported as high as 40 % [9]. Since the sural nerve and its branches are responsible for sensory and not motor functions, injury here has been well tolerated by individuals. Many reported cases have gone on to resolve spontaneously over time. In the event that neurosensory alteration results in pain, we recommend treating with desensitization therapy, massaging the skin, and corticosteroid injections.

References

1. Sella EJ, Caminear DS, McLarney EA. Haglund's syndrome. J Foot Ankle Surg. 1998;37(2):110–4.
2. Paavola M, Kannus P, Järvinen TA, Khan K, Józsa L, Järvinen M. Achilles tendinopathy. J Bone Joint Surg. 2002;84(11):2062–76.
3. Nunley JA, Ruskin G, Horst F. Long-term clinical outcomes following the central incision technique for insertional Achilles tendinopathy. Foot Ankle Int. 2011;32(9):850–5.
4. Van Dijk CN, Van Sterkenburg MN, Wiegerinck JI, Karlsson J, Maffulli N. Terminology for Achilles tendon related disorders. Knee Surg Sports Traumatol Arthrosc. 2011;19(5):835–41.
5. Attinger CE, Evans KK, Bulan E, Blume P, Cooper P. Angiosomes of the foot and ankle and clinical implications for limb salvage: reconstruction, incisions, and revascularization. Plast Reconstr Surg. 2006;117(7S):261S–93S.
6. Highlander P, Greenhagen RM. Wound complications with posterior midline and posterior medial leg incisions a systematic review. Foot Ankle Spec. 2011;4(6):361–9.
7. Kelikian AS, Sarrafian SK, editors. Sarrafian's anatomy of the foot and ankle: descriptive, topographic, functional. Philadelphia: Lippincott Williams & Wilkins; 2011.
8. DeVries GJ, Summerhays B, Guehlstorf DW. Surgical correction of Haglund's triad using complete detachment and reattachment of the Achilles tendon. J Foot Ankle Surg. 2009;48(4):447–51.
9. Yodlowski ML, Scheller AD, Minos L. Surgical treatment of Achilles tendinitis by decompression of the retrocalcaneal bursa and the superior calcaneal tuberosity. Am J Sports Med. 2002;30(3):318–21.
10. Wagner E, Gould JS, Kneidel M, Fleisig GS, Fowler R. Technique and results of Achilles tendon detachment and reconstruction for insertional Achilles tendinosis. Foot Ankle Int. 2006;27(9):677–84.
11. Paavola M, Orava S, Leppilahti J, Kannus P, Järvinen M. Chronic Achilles tendon overuse injury: complications after surgical treatment an analysis of 432 consecutive patients. Am J Sports Med. 2000;28(1):77–82.

12. Pfeffer G, et al. Operative techniques: foot and ankle surgery. Philadelphia: Saunders; 2010. p. 538–56.
13. Wagner E, Gould JS, Kneidel M, Fleisig GS, Fowler R. Technique and results of Achilles tendon detachment and reconstruction for insertional Achilles tendinosis. Foot Ankle Int. 2006;27(9):677–84.
14. DeOrio MJ, Easley ME. Surgical strategies: insertional Achilles tendinopathy. Foot Ankle Int. 2008;29(5):542–50.
15. Boffeli TJ, Peterson MC. The Keck and Kelly wedge calcaneal osteotomy for Haglund's deformity: a technique for reproducible results. J Foot Ankle Surg. 2012;51(3):398–401.
16. Kolodziej P, Glisson RR, Nunley JA. Risk of avulsion of the Achilles tendon after partial excision for treatment of insertional tendonitis and Haglund's deformity: a biomechanical study. Foot Ankle Int. 1999;20(7):433–7.
17. Beitzel K, Mazzocca AD, Obopilwe E, Boyle JW, McWilliam J, Rincon L, et al. Biomechanical properties of double-and single-row suture anchor repair for surgical treatment of insertional Achilles tendinopathy. Am J Sports Med. 2013;41(7):1642–8.
18. Pilson H, Brown P, Stitzel J, Scott A. Single-row versus double-row repair of the distal Achilles tendon: a biomechanical comparison. J Foot Ankle Surg. 2012;51(6):762–6.
19. Maffulli N, Testa V, Capasso G, Sullo A. Calcific insertional Achilles tendinopathy reattachment with bone anchors. Am J Sports Med. 2004;32(1):174–82.
20. Witt BL, Hyer CF. Achilles tendon reattachment after surgical treatment of insertional tendinosis using the suture bridge technique: a case series. J Foot Ankle Surg. 2012;51(4):487–93.
21. Greenhagen RM, Shinabarger AB, Pearson KT, Burns PR. Intermediate and long-term outcomes of the suture bridge technique for the management of insertional Achilles tendinopathy. Foot Ankle Spec. 2013;6(3):185–90.
22. Roche AJ, Calder JDF. Achilles tendinopathy: a review of the current concepts of treatment. Bone Joint J. 2013;95-B:1299–307.
23. Paavola M, Kannus P, Orava S, Pasanen M, Järvinen M. Surgical treatment for chronic Achilles tendinopathy: a prospective seven month follow up study. Br J Sports Med. 2002;36(3):178–82.
24. Calder JDF, Saxby TS. Surgical treatment of insertional Achilles tendinosis. Foot Ankle Int. 2003;24(2):119–21.
25. McGarvey WC, Palumbo RC, Baxter DE, Leibman BD. Insertional Achilles tendinosis: surgical treatment through a central tendon splitting approach. Foot Ankle Int. 2002;23(1):19–25.
26. Den Hartog BD. Insertional Achilles tendinosis: pathogenesis and treatment. Foot Ankle Clin. 2009;14(4):639–50.
27. Murphy GA. Surgical treatment of non-insertional Achilles tendinitis. Foot Ankle Clin. 2009;14(4):651–61.
28. Falck-Ytter Y, Francis CW, Johanson NA, Curley C, Dahl OE, Schulman S, et al. Prevention of VTE in orthopedic surgery patients: antithrombotic therapy and prevention of thrombosis: American College of Chest Physicians evidence-based clinical practice guidelines. CHEST J. 2012;141(2_suppl):e278S–325S.
29. Lapidus LJ, Ponzer S, Pettersson H, de Bri E. Symptomatic venous thromboembolism and mortality in orthopaedic surgery—an observational study of 45 968 consecutive procedures. BMC Musculoskelet Disord. 2013;14(1):177.

Tarsal Tunnel Surgery

20

Guido LaPorta and Ellianne M. Nasser

Introduction

Tarsal tunnel syndrome is an entrapment neuropathy beneath the flexor retinaculum or distal anatomic tunnels resulting in pressure on the posterior tibial nerve and its branches. Persistent compression of the tibial nerve results in a range of neuritic symptoms that effect the plantar aspect of the foot in a variable distribution. Symptoms often mimic those of other lower extremity pathology thus making diagnosis and treatment difficult.

Etiology of tarsal tunnel syndrome includes space-occupying lesions, hindfoot deformity, varicosities, neurilemoma, hypertrophic flexor retinaculum, post-traumatic fibrosis, and low-lying muscle belly [1–3]. Following successful diagnosis of tarsal tunnel syndrome, conservative treatment is limited and can include anti-inflammatory medications, activity modification, stretching, icing, oral gabapentin or pregabalin, and iontophoresis. Orthotics may be beneficial in a flexible hindfoot deformity [1–4].

Indications of Procedure

Surgical intervention for tarsal tunnel syndrome is warranted following failure of conservative treatment or when there are persistent sensory symptoms, atrophy, or documented Wallerian degeneration. Surgery includes decompression of the posterior tibial nerve and its terminal branches in their anatomic tunnels. Complications with tarsal tunnel decompression include wound dehiscence or infection, recurrent symptoms, seroma, hematoma, subluxation of posterior tibial nerve, calcaneal nerve neuroma, and neuroma of the posterior branch of the saphenous nerve [3–12].

Success rates following surgical intervention for tarsal tunnel syndrome have varied in the literature from 44–96% [1]. Authors have demonstrated that timing of the decompression may influence results as continued compression leads to intraneural fibrosis which can result in muscle atrophy and irreparable nerve damage if not treated [1, 3, 13, 14]. Patients with symptoms greater than a year before surgery have a prolonged time for recovery of sensibility with some having postoperative dysesthesia [14]. Sammarco and Chang found better outcomes in patients with symptoms less than 1 year in a review of 75 tarsal tunnel release procedures [3]. Baba et al. reviewed 34 patients and found that results of tarsal tunnel release were favorable when there was a history of symptoms less than 1 year [13]. Turan et al. reviewed 18 cases of tarsal tunnel decompression in patients with long-standing symptoms (median 60 months). With complete relief of symptoms found in 61% of patients, the authors conclude that surgical decompression is beneficial for long-standing tarsal tunnel syndrome [15].

Contraindications/Limitations

Contraindications to tarsal tunnel release include the presence of another cause of neuritic pain. Electromyogram and nerve conduction studies must be ordered prior to surgical intervention to rule out a more proximal cause of neuritic pain. Patient comorbidities such as diabetes mellitus or alcohol abuse must be evaluated to assess their contribution to patient symptoms. Limitations to tarsal tunnel release include its inability to provide complete relief in patients with intraneural damage.

G. LaPorta (✉)
LaPorta and Associates, PC, 414 East Drinker St. Suite 101, Dunmore, PA 18512, USA
e-mail: glaporta@msn.com

E.M. Nasser
Geisinger Health System, 1800 Mulberry Street, Scranton, PA 18510, USA

M.S. Lee, J.P. Grossman (eds.), *Complications in Foot and Ankle Surgery*, DOI 10.1007/978-3-319-53686-6_20

Technique Pearls and Pitfalls (to Avoid Complications)

Secondary to the risk of wound complications with surgical decompression of the tibial nerve beneath the flexor retinaculum, patients should remain non-weightbearing until the incision site has fully healed and sutures are removed. We routinely utilize an Allgower-Donati suture technique to limit compromise of cutaneous blood flow at the incision site (Fig. 20.1) [16].

Inadequate control of bleeding prior to wound closure places patient at risk for both wound dehiscence as well as postoperative scarring. Prior to closure of the surgical site, the surgeon must drop the tourniquet and control any bleeding. In cases with significant varicosities, a drain may be used to prevent seroma or hematoma. Recognition of seroma or hematoma in a timely fashion is key to prevention of wound complications and/or postoperative scarring. The surgeon must evacuate the hematoma or seroma as well as aim to treat the etiology of its formation.

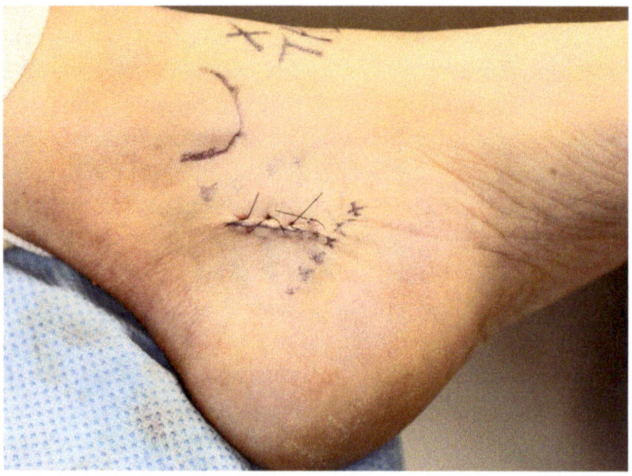

Fig. 20.1 Allgower-Donati suture technique used for closure after tarsal tunnel release

Prior to surgical intervention for tarsal tunnel syndrome, thorough workup must be complete to rule out double crush syndrome and to identify any space-occupying lesions or bony projections contributing to symptoms. Electromyogram and nerve conduction studies must be ordered prior to surgical intervention to rule out a more proximal cause of neuritic pain. Imaging studies should be utilized appropriately to aid the surgeon in the workup and surgical planning (Fig. 20.2). Once workup is complete and the surgeon is prepared to treat any underlying etiology, meticulous surgical technique is paramount in successful tarsal tunnel release. Direct manipulation of the tibial nerve should be minimized [17]. Comprehensive release must be performed with inspection of the nerve in its entirety. Hemostasis must be achieved prior to closure to prevent scarring, hematoma, and infection.

Management of Specific Complications

Recalcitrant Pain

Failure of symptom relief following tarsal tunnel decompression is an unfortunately frequent complication and poses a treatment challenge to the foot and ankle surgeon. Failure of symptom relief can be divided into two categories: (1) patient shows no improvement of symptoms following decompression, and (2) patient shows temporary relief of symptoms followed by recurrence of symptoms. Etiology of

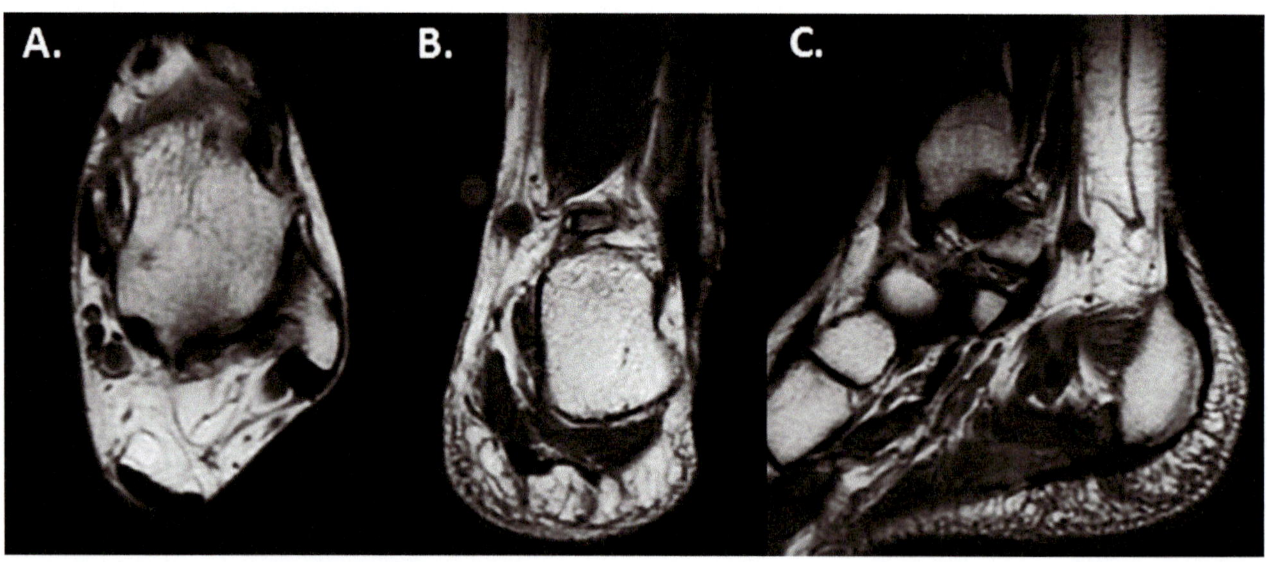

Fig. 20.2 (**a**) Axial, (**b**) coronal, and (**c**) sagittal T1 MRI images depicting schwannoma of the tibial nerve

failure must be established prior to revision surgery or subsequent treatment. Raikin and Minnich presented an algorithm for failed tarsal tunnel syndrome surgery in 2003 [9]. Through experience and current literature, we have adapted this approach as presented in Fig. 20.3. The following paragraphs will outline the algorithm proposed in Fig. 20.3, providing etiologies and treatment plans for each category.

Double Crush Syndrome

Double crush syndrome was first described by Upton and McComas in 1973 to involve both a proximal and distal nerve lesion in the same limb [18]. The authors theorized that a proximal lesion in a nerve would make that nerve more vulnerable to distal lesions. Most literature on double crush syndrome describes the upper extremity; however the theory has been applied to the lower extremity as well [9, 19, 20]. Etiologies of proximal compression of the effected limb include radiculopathy, plexopathy, and proximal tibial nerve compression. Systemic disease such as diabetes or alcohol abuse may cause neurologic symptoms contributing to the double crush syndrome [9, 14].

Proximal tibial nerve compression, or "soleal sling syndrome," is compression of the tibial nerve beneath the fibrous sling between the tibia and fibula at the origin of the soleus muscle [21]. Patients present with numbness, tingling, hypersensitivity, dysesthesia, plantar foot pain, and weakness in the foot or toes. The area of compression occurs approximately 9 cm distal to the medial tibial plateau, making a medial calf approach to the compression site feasible [22]. In a retrospective review of 69 proximal tibial nerve decompressions, Williams et al. stated that all patients had severe pain on physical exam with gentle palpation of the calf 9 cm distal to the popliteal crease [21]. The authors point out that in patients with available electrodiagnostic studies, none of the tests suggested a tibial nerve compression at the level of the soleal sling, thus making it a clinical diagnosis only.

There may be a substantial conduction block between the stimulation sites at the knee and ankle in proximal tibial nerve compression that is not found in tarsal tunnel syndrome. Stimulation of the abductor hallucis muscle at the level of the knee would be markedly reduced in comparison to stimulation at the ankle, with the response of the gastrocnemius muscle at the knee normal, thus indicating a conduction block in the calf [23].

Patients with double crush syndrome who undergo tibial nerve decompression experience either partial relief of symptoms or no relief of symptoms. Following failed tarsal tunnel syndrome in patients with double crush syndrome, repeat tarsal tunnel decompression is not indicated. Treatment is focused on the second "crush": radiculopathy, plexopathy, proximal tibial nerve compression, or systemic disease.

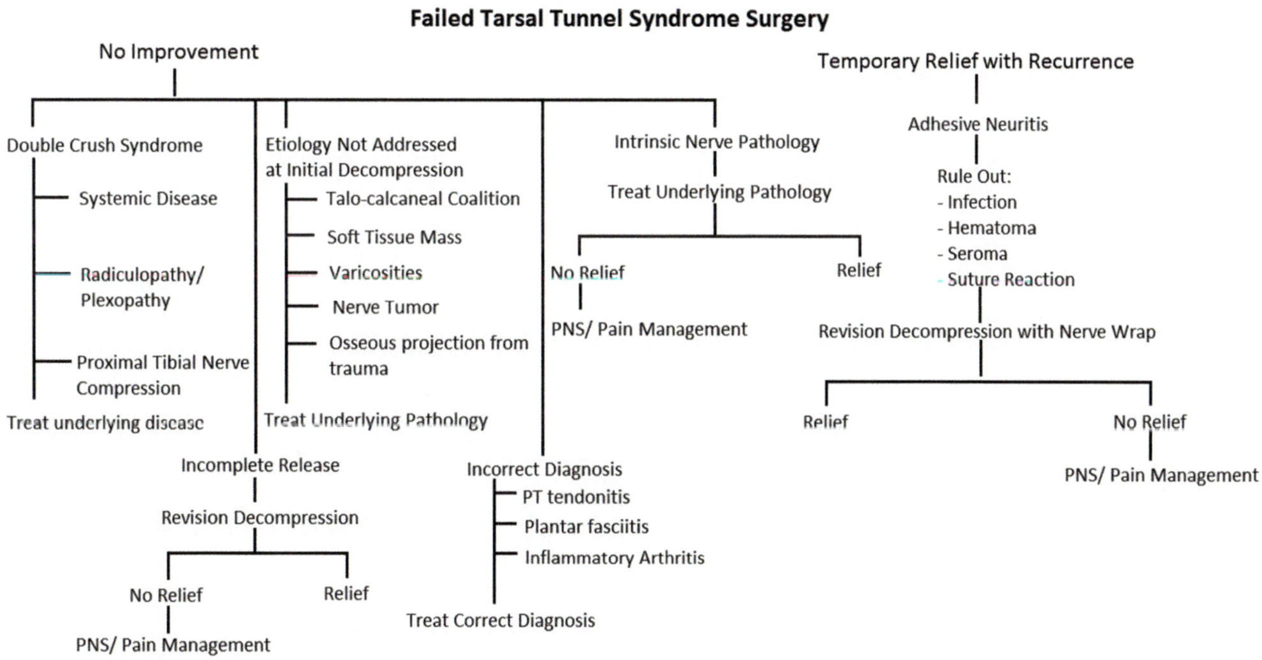

Fig. 20.3 Algorithm for treatment of failed tarsal tunnel syndrome surgery. Failure of symptom relief is divided into two treatment categories: (1) patient shows no improvement of symptoms following decompression, and (2) patient shows temporary relief of symptoms followed by recurrence of symptoms

Incomplete Release

Incomplete initial tarsal tunnel decompression may result in partial improvement or no improvement of symptoms. If the initial procedure was performed by a different physician, review of the operative report as well as inspection of incision size can provide insight as to whether or not a complete release was performed. If initial release was not complete, a second complete tarsal tunnel decompression is indicated. Complete proximal and distal release must be performed including release of the medial and lateral plantar nerve tunnels as well as excision of the septa dividing the nerve tunnels. If relief is not provided following revision decompression, a peripheral nerve stimulator or referral to pain management center is considered.

Etiology not Addressed at Initial Decompression

Space-occupying lesions are often cause for tarsal tunnel syndrome and include soft tissue mass, low-lying muscle belly, talocalcaneal coalition, varicosities, nerve tumor, or post-traumatic osseous projections (Fig. 20.4) [24]. Pfeiffer and Cracchiolo suggest that a space-occupying lesion at the area of the tarsal tunnel producing symptoms is the best indication for operative treatment [8]. If the primary etiology causing nerve compression and pathology is not addressed at time of decompression, patient will complain of only partial improvement of symptoms or no improvement of symptoms. Decompression alone without excising the soft tissue mass, schwannoma, or talocalcaneal coalition, or without ligation of varicosities, will not provide complete relief of symptoms. Revision surgical intervention is warranted to address the etiology of the tarsal tunnel syndrome.

Preoperative imaging studies may provide the surgeon with assessment of soft tissue or bony abnormalities in the tarsal tunnel region for complete preoperative planning. MRI or ultrasound will evaluate the presence of soft tissue mass or nerve tumor in the tarsal tunnel region [25]. Talocalcaneal coalition is best evaluated on CT scan if suspected. We routinely send patients with suspected venous insufficiency and tarsal tunnel symptoms for venous studies. If reflux is present, patients are sent to a vascular surgeon for consult and possible closure of the great saphenous vein prior to surgical decompression of the tarsal tunnel.

Incorrect Diagnosis

Incorrect diagnosis is a common cause for failure of tarsal tunnel syndrome resulting in no improvement of symptoms following tibial nerve decompression. Differential diagnosis includes tibialis posterior tendonitis, plantar fasciitis, calcaneal stress fracture, hindfoot degenerative joint disease, inflammatory arthritis, plantar fibromatosis, gout, sinus tarsi syndrome, and peripheral vascular disease [14]. Repeat tarsal tunnel decompression is not indicated in these patients. Rather, treatment is focused on the correct etiology.

Intrinsic Nerve Pathology

Intraneural damage occurs at the axonal level and may be caused by chronic compression, stretch, traction, crush injury, or systemic disease. As damage is intraneural, extraneural decompression will not alleviate symptoms. Treatment is aimed at addressing the cause of intraneural pathology. Blood sugar control in diabetic patients and treatment of alcohol abuse in patients with alcoholic neuropathy can halt the progression of intraneural damage [9]. Medications used for chronic pain syndromes may influence pain caused by intraneural damage. Through action on both central and peripheral nerve pathways, medications including nonsteroidal anti-inflammatories, steroids, tricyclic antidepressants, serotonin reuptake inhibitors, anti-epileptics, narcotics, calcium channel blockers, antiarrhythmics, sympatholytics, and *N*-methyl-D aspartate antagonists may provide symptomatic relief [20].

Clinical signs of intraneural damage include persistent sensory change, muscle wasting, and abnormal two-point discrimination, indicating actual loss of nerve fibers and Wallerian degeneration [14]. A Tinel sign may be used as an indication of nerve regeneration. Early and late nerve pathology demonstrate distinct muscular and sensory signs and symptoms. Loss of neural input to a muscle (late nerve pathology) secondary to Wallerian degeneration causes actual wasting of the muscle, while early nerve pathology due to compression causes only weakness of the muscle. Late nerve compression with intraneural damage increased the threshold of intensity required to elicit a sensory response, while early nerve pathology causes a hypersensitive response [14].

Easley and Schon reviewed 21 patients with failed tarsal tunnel surgery treated with revision neurolysis using a vein wrap [26]. The authors state that the majority of failures in their series occurred in nerves with intraneural compromise (seven failures out of 17 cases). We do not recommend revision neurolysis in patients with suspected intrinsic nerve pathology. Careful inspection of the tibial nerve during the initial decompression procedure is paramount in the success of the procedure. If scarring is present within the nerve as well as loss of vascular striations, this should be noted in the operative report and used to dictate future treatment if necessary. If treatment of the underlying pathology fails, patients are referred to pain management and/or considered for a peripheral nerve stimulator.

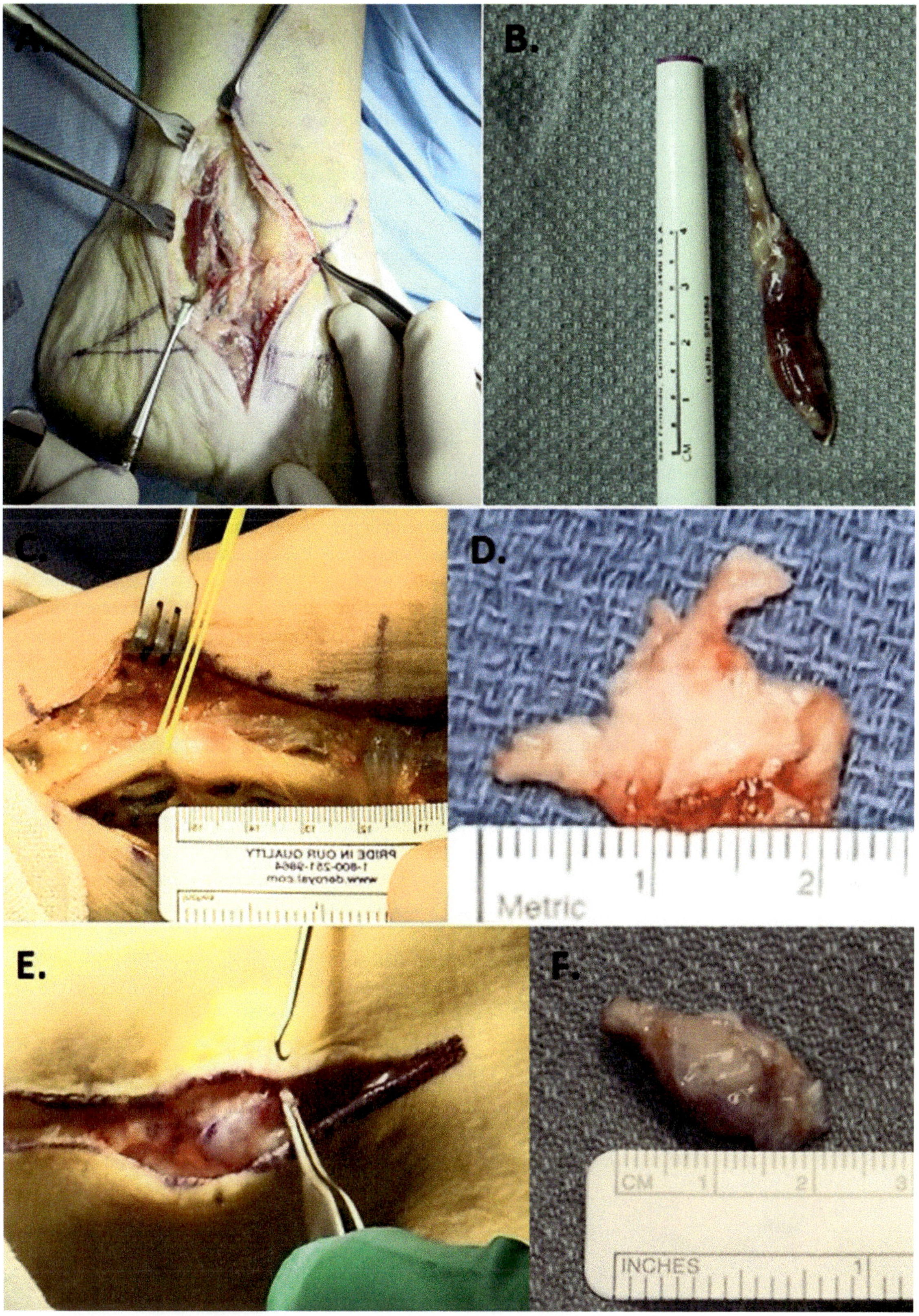

Fig. 20.4 Intraoperative photographs depicting space-occupying lesions of the tarsal tunnel: (**a**, **b**) flexor accessorius, (**c**, **d**) schwannoma of the tibial nerve, and (**e**, **f**) ganglion causing pressure on tarsal tunnel. Decompression of the tarsal tunnel without removal of these space-occupying lesions will fail to relieve patient symptoms

Other Complications

Neuroma of the posterior branch of the saphenous nerve has been reported to cause recurrent pain following tarsal tunnel decompression. Kim and Dellon reviewed 16 patients complaining of pain at the proximal incision site following tarsal tunnel decompression which was relieved by a block of the distal saphenous nerve [6]. All patients underwent resection of the distal saphenous nerve with implantation into the soleus muscle. Excellent relief of pain was achieved in 76% of cases at a mean of 18.5 months [6].

Neuroma of the calcaneal nerve has been reported following tarsal tunnel decompression. Treatment is similar to that of the posterior branch of the saphenous nerve with resection of the neuroma and implantation into the nearest muscle belly, typically the flexor hallucis longus [27].

One report of subluxation of the tibialis posterior following decompression of the posterior tibial tendon is reported in the literature [7]. Langan and Weiss describe a 16-year-old girl who complained of a "slipping sensation" at her medial ankle 2 months following tarsal tunnel decompression. A groove deepening procedure was performed with the periosteum used to reconstruct the flexor retinaculum. Patient was asymptomatic 3 years following the surgical procedure [7].

Rosson et al. report three cases of complicated ganglion excision with tarsal tunnel release resulting in resection of the tibial nerve (three patients), resection of the tibial artery (two patients), and return of the ganglion (three patients) [10]. The authors recommend decompressing intraneural ganglion, stating that recurrent ganglia will arise from the joint rather than the nerve, and therefore the cyst lining may be left intact without risk of recurrence [10]. Meticulous dissection is paramount in all cases of surgical decompression of the tarsal tunnel. Injury to the posterior tibial artery should be repaired by a vascular surgeon.

Entrapments

Patients with adhesive neuritis typically experience symptom relief after initial decompression for a period of 2–4 months after which symptoms return [20]. Compression of the tibial nerve beneath the laciniate ligament occurs near the ankle joint, with postoperative joint motion adding risk for wound complications leading to increased scarring [5]. Many authors have advocated endoscopic, minimally invasive, or modified incisional approaches in an effort to prevent postoperative scarring and adhesive neuritis [5, 28–35]. Despite this, many open approaches may result in recurrent symptoms secondary to external scarring around the previously released nerve. Nerve adhesions prevent gliding of the nerve with ankle and subtalar joint range of motion leading to traction neuritis and pain [36].

Postoperative wound dehiscence with or without infection causes a local inflammatory response increasing risk for adhesive neuritis. Inadequate hemostasis may lead to postoperative bleeding and hematoma which may cause increased scarring surrounding the nerve. If adhesive neuritis is suspected, the surgeon must rule out current infection, hematoma, seroma, or suture reaction. Often patients have a tender, hypertrophic scar at the previous incision site, with decreased mobility of the ankle joint. Pain increases with pressure at the area of scar and with motion of the surrounding joints. Nerve conduction studies in patients with adhesive neuritis typically show slowing of nerve velocities with prolonged latencies. However, studies may be normal if scarring only prevents nerve gliding without compression [9, 37].

Treatment for patients with recurrent symptoms and adhesive neuritis is revision decompression with use of a nerve wrap (Fig. 20.5). Care must be taken to completely release the nerve from the surrounding scar tissue. Incision should start proximal to original incision to begin dissection at healthy nerve. Vein wrapping was initially described in the upper extremity to prevent scarring in peripheral nerves [38]. Collagen grafts were later developed in an effort to decrease surgical time and provide

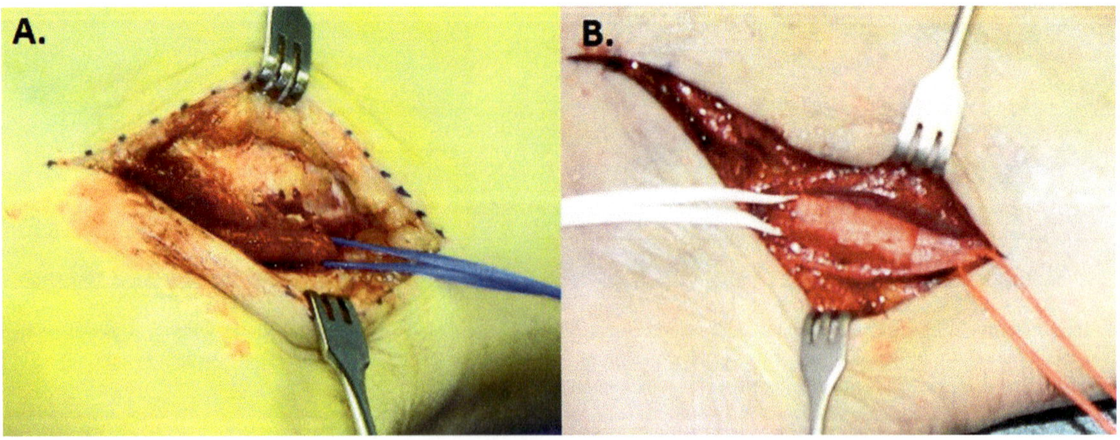

Fig. 20.5 Nerve wrap: Images demonstrate use of a collagen nerve wrap in revision tibial nerve decompression with adhesive neuritis

a more convenient option to treat adhesive neuritis. Both vein and collagen nerve wraps decrease nerve scarring, do not constrict around the nerve, and improve nerve gliding [37].

Easley and Schon reported 25 patients with revision neurolysis for adhesive neuritis confirmed by poor mobility of scar tissue and reproduction of symptoms with ankle range of motion [26]. All patients were treated with a saphenous or umbilical vein wrap. At 1 year, 17 of 25 patients were satisfied, with the eight patients not satisfied showing intraoperative evidence of intrinsic nerve damage.

Collagen nerve wraps are convenient and easy to use. Grafts come split longitudinally in various sizes and are easy to handle. Gould reports no difference or advantage of veins over commercial products; however this data was not analyzed [36]. No clinical data to date has directly compared the use of vein wrapping to collagen grafts for revision neurolysis in adhesive neuritis.

Peripheral Nerve Stimulation

We routinely utilize peripheral nerve stimulation in cases of persistent chronic lower extremity pain after failure of all other treatment including revision neurolysis with or without nerve wrap. Peripheral nerve stimulation is based on the gate mechanism of pain, theorizing that direct stimulation of afferent pain fibers may "interfere" with their transmission and therefore reduce the pain stimulus [20]. Direct stimulation of the nerve is performed placing leads on the tibial nerve just proximal to the flexor retinaculum (Fig. 20.6).

Wound Complications

In symptomatic tarsal tunnel syndrome, the tibial nerve is compressed beneath the laciniate ligament. Surgical exposure for tarsal tunnel release requires an incision crossing both the subtalar and ankle joints. Postoperative motion at these joints increases risk of wound dehiscence. In a review of 32 feet, Pfeiffer and Cracchiolo found a 13% rate of wound complications [8].

Diabetic patients are prone to incision site infection and dehiscence. Wieman and Patel found a 15% incidence in wound complications in a review of 26 diabetic patients who underwent posterior tibial nerve decompression [11]. Wood and Wood found a 12% incidence of wound dehiscence in a review of 33 patients with diabetes who underwent decompression of the tibial, common peroneal, and deep peroneal nerves [12].

Early identification and treatment of wound complications is paramount in the success of tarsal tunnel decompression surgery. Wound infection and dehiscence provide risk for postoperative adhesions causing recurrence of symptoms. Use of drains or disposable wound vacs may improve outcomes and decrease incidence of wound complications.

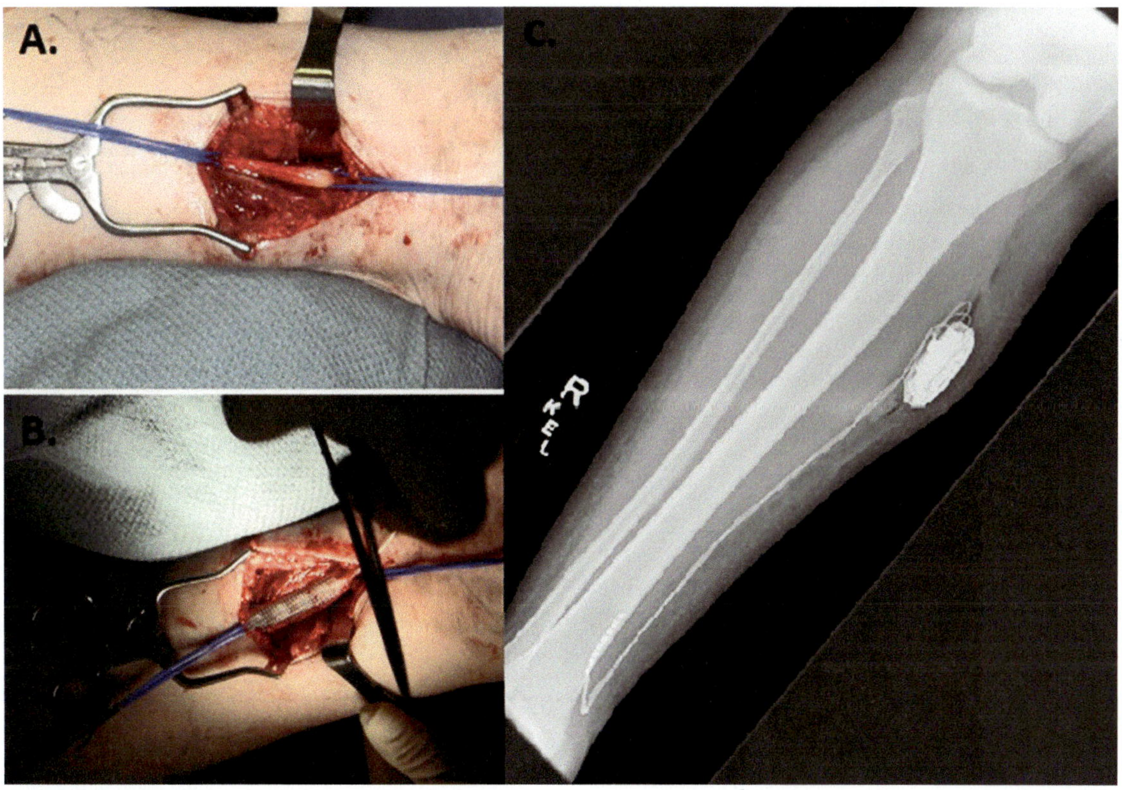

Fig. 20.6 Peripheral nerve stimulator: (**a**) Tibial nerve is isolated proximal to the tarsal tunnel. (**b**) Nerve stimulator lead placed directly on tibial nerve and sutured in place. (**c**) Postoperative radiograph demonstrating lead placement proximal to tarsal tunnel with battery placement in calf

Patients must remain non-weightbearing until the incision site is closed. If wound complications occur, no weightbearing is allowed until full closure of the wound is achieved.

Summary

In the setting of failed tarsal tunnel decompression with persistent symptoms, the surgeon must identify the reason for failure. Outcomes for revision surgical decompression are worse than primary decompression. Patients who fail revision neurolysis will require referral to a pain management center with or without peripheral nerve stimulator insertion.

References

1. Ahmad M, Tsang K, Makenny PJ, Adedapo AO. Tarsal tunnel syndrome: a literature review. J Foot Ankle Surg. 2012;18:149–52.
2. Franson J, Baravarian B. Tarsal tunnel syndrome: a compression neuropathy involving four distinct tunnels. Clin Podiatr Med Surg. 2006;23:597–609.
3. Sammarco GJ, Chang L. Outcome of surgical treatment of tarsal tunnel syndrome. Foot Ankle Int. 2003;24:125–31.
4. Gould JS. Tarsal tunnel syndrome. Foot Ankle Clin N Am. 2011;16:275–86.
5. Ducic I, Felder J. Tibial nerve decompression: reliable exposure using shorter incisions. Microsurgery. 2012;32:533–8.
6. Kim J, Dellon AL. Pain at the site of tarsal tunnel incision due to neuroma of the posterior branch of the saphenous nerve. J Am Podiatr Med Assoc. 2001;91:109–13.
7. Langan P, Weiss CA. Subluxation of the tibialis posterior, a complication of tarsal tunnel decompression. Clin Orthop Relat Res. 1980;146:226–7.
8. Pfeiffer WH, Cracchiolo A. Clinical results after tarsal tunnel decompression. J Bone Joint Surg. 1994;76-A:1222–30.
9. Raikin SM, Minnich JM. Failed tarsal tunnel syndrome surgery. Foot Ankle Clin N Am. 2003;8:159–74.
10. Rosson GD, Spinner RJ, Dellon AL. Tarsal tunnel surgery for treatment of tarsal ganglion: a rewarding operation with devastating potential complications. J Am Podiatr Med Assoc. 2005;95:459–63.
11. Wieman TJ, Patel VG. Treatment of hyperesthetic neuropathic pain in diabetics: decompression of the tarsal tunnel. Ann Surg. 1995;221:660–5.
12. Wood WA, Wood MA. Decompression of peripheral nerves for diabetic neuropathy in the lower extremity. J Foot Ankle Surg. 2003;42:268–75.
13. Baba H, Wada M, Annen S, Azuchi M, Imura S, Tomita K. The tarsal tunnel syndrome: evaluation of surgical results using multivariate analysis. Int Orthop. 1997;21:67–71.
14. Mackinnon SE, Dellon AL. Surgery of the peripheral nerve. New York: Theime; 1988.
15. Turan I, Rivero-Melian C, Guntner P, Rolf C. Tarsal tunnel syndrome: outcome of surgery in longstanding cases. Clin Orthop Relat Res. 1997;343:151–6.
16. Sagi HC, Papp S, Dipasquale T. The effect of suture pattern and tension on cutaneous blood flow as assessed by laser Doppler flowmetry in a pig model. J Orthop Trauma. 2008;22:171–5.
17. Mahan KT, Rock JR, Hillstrom HJ. Tarsal tunnel syndrome: a retrospective study. J Am Podiatr Med Assoc. 1996;88:81–91.
18. Upton AR, McComas AJ. The double crush in nerve entrapment syndromes. Lancet. 1973;2:359–62.
19. Borgia AV, Hruska JK, Braun K. Double crush syndrome in the lower extremity: a case report. J Am Podiatr Med Assoc. 2012;102:330–3.
20. Schon LC, Easley ME. Chronic Pain. In: Myerson MS, editor. Foot and ankle disorders. Philadelphia: WB Saunders; 2000. p. 851–81.
21. Williams EH, Rosson GD, Hagan RR, Hashemi SS, Dellon AL. Soleal sling syndrome (proximal tibial nerve compression): results of surgical decompression. Plast Reconstr Surg. 2012;129:454–62.
22. Williams EH, Williams CG, Rosson GD, Dellon LA. Anatomic site for proximal tibial nerve compression: a cadaver study. Ann Plast Surg. 2009;62:322–5.
23. Glennon TP. Electrodiagnosis of nerve entrapment syndromes that produce symptoms in the foot and ankle. In: Myerson MS, editor. Foot and ankle disorders. Philadelphia: WB Saunders; 2000. p. 800–7.
24. Yoo JH, Kim EH, Kim BS, Cha JG. Tarsal coalition as a cause of failed tarsal tunnel release for tarsal tunnel syndrome. Orthopedics. 2009;32:285–6.
25. Sung K, Park S. Short term operative outcome of tarsal tunnel syndrome due to benign space-occupying lesions. Foot Ankle Int. 2009;30:741–5.
26. Easley ME, Schon LC. Peripheral nerve vein wrapping for intractable lower extremity pain. Foot Ankle Int. 2000;21:492–500.
27. Wagner E, Ortiz C. The painful neuroma and the use of conduits. Foot Ankle Clin N Am. 2011;16:295–304.
28. Bezerra MJC, Leite JAD, Neto JE, Romero S. Endoscopic release of the tarsal tunnel: a suggested surgical approach. Acta Ortop Bras. 2005;13(1):46–8.
29. Day III FN, Naples JJ. Endoscopic tarsal tunnel release: update 96. J Foot Ankle Surg. 1996;35(3):225–9.
30. Day III FN, Naples JJ. Tarsal tunnel syndrome: an endoscopic approach with 4- to 28-month follow-up. J Foot Ankle Surg. 1994;33(3):244–8.
31. El Shazly O, El Shazly A, Desouky A, El Zohiery AK, Sakr HM. Anatomical bases of endoscopic tarsal tunnel release: anatomical and ultra-sonographic study with a preliminary case report. Surg Radiol Anat. 2011;33:929–36.
32. Gkotsoulis EN, Simonson DC, Roukis TS. Outcomes and safety of endoscopic tarsal tunnel decompression: a systematic review. Foot Ankle Spec. 2013;7(1):57–60.
33. Jolly GP. Tarsal tunnel syndrome: can a minimally invasive release be advantageous? Podiatry Today. 2009;3(22):30–34
34. Krishnan KG. Endoscopic decompression of the tarsal tunnel. Tech Foot Ankle Surg. 2010;9(2):52–7.
35. Krishnan KG, Pinzer T, Schackert G. A novel endoscopic technique in treating single nerve entrapment syndromes with special attention to ulnar nerve transposition and tarsal tunnel release: clinical application. Neurosurgery. 2006;59(1):89–100.
36. Gould JS. The failed tarsal tunnel release. Foot Ankle Clin N Am. 2011;16:287–93.
37. Masear VR. Nerve wrapping. Foot Ankle Clin N Am. 2011;16: 327–37.
38. Masear VR, Tulloss JR, St. Mary E, Meyer RD. Venous wrapping of nerves to prevent scarring. J Hand Surg. 1990;15A:817–8.

Complications of Stage II Flatfoot Surgery

21

Alan Catanzariti and Collin M. Zdenek

This chapter will focus on complications following surgery to address stage II adult acquired flatfoot. These procedures include the joint-sparring procedures of the hindfoot and medial column. Specifically, the chapter will discuss complications that include:

- Failed repair of posterior tibial tendon and flexor digitorum longus tendon transfer
- Undercorrection with periarticular osteotomies
- Overcorrection with medial displacement osteotomy of the calcaneus
- Overcorrection and lateral column overload following lateral column lengthening
- Nonunion and malunion following lateral column lengthening
- Nonunion following medial column arthrodesis of the naviculocuneiform and first tarsometatarsal joints
- Failure to address equinus
- Residual forefoot varus
- Progressive deformity following Kidner procedures
- Failed arthroereisis

Failed Repair of the Posterior Tibial Tendon and Flexor Digitorum Longus Transfer

Failure to address underlying osseous deformities can result in failed repair of the posterior tibial tendon (PTT) and/or transfer of the flexor digitorum longus (FDL) tendon. Regardless of the type of repair that is employed to address a diseased PTT, residual symptoms or recurrence is likely when flatfoot deformity persists. Failure of isolated tendon transfer or tenodesis can result from persistent muscle imbalance when the pull of the Achilles tendon remains lateral to the axis of the subtalar joint and continues to be a valgus deforming force on the hindfoot [1]. FDL tendon transfer may eventually be unsuccessful without osseous procedures that provide long-term biomechanical protection [2]. One study demonstrated that FDL tendon transfer combined with medial displacement calcaneal osteotomy resulted in significant reduction in load on the medial column relative to FDL transfer alone [3]. The PTT may undergo the same degenerative process as prior to surgery when osseous deformity persists. Tendinosis with corresponding symptoms will result over time, depending on the patient's activity level, BMI, severity of deformity, etc. Therefore, it is important to recognize and address osseous deformity when repairing the PTT. This is important not only for stage II deformities, but stage I deformities as well. Even a subtle flatfoot deformity can strain the PTT with subsequent tendinosis and dysfunction. Although some studies have reported improved functional outcomes and pain relief for stage II AAFF deformities with tendon transfers alone, recurrence occurs when residual deformity persists [1]. DiDomenico et al. performed double calcaneal osteotomy and posterior muscle group lengthening in nine flat feet on eight patients with postoperative follow-up of 12 months and found a statistically significant change in radiographic angles including: talar-first metatarsal, talocalcaneal, calcaneal inclination, and talar declination angles. This demonstrates the importance of recognizing the need for osseous realignment as opposed to soft tissue procedures alone [4].

Repair of PTT will fail if the muscle-tendon unit is no longer functional. The muscle-tendon unit can become dysfunctional in long-standing cases of AAFF. The PTT is usually beyond salvage in these situations. Preserving the tendon can result in persistent symptoms following surgery as well as residual dysfunction. Even if osseous realignment has been achieved, PTT dysfunction will persist. Viability of

A. Catanzariti (✉)
West Penn Hospital, The Foot and Ankle Institute, 4800 Friendship Avenue, North Tower, 1st Floor, Pittsburgh, PA 15524, USA
e-mail: alan.catanzariti@ahn.org

C.M. Zdenek
Mountain View Center, Palo Alto Medcal Foundation, 701E El Camino Real, Mountain View, CA 94040, USA
e-mail: colinzdenek@gmail.com

M.S. Lee, J.P. Grossman (eds.), *Complications in Foot and Ankle Surgery*, DOI 10.1007/978-3-319-53686-6_21

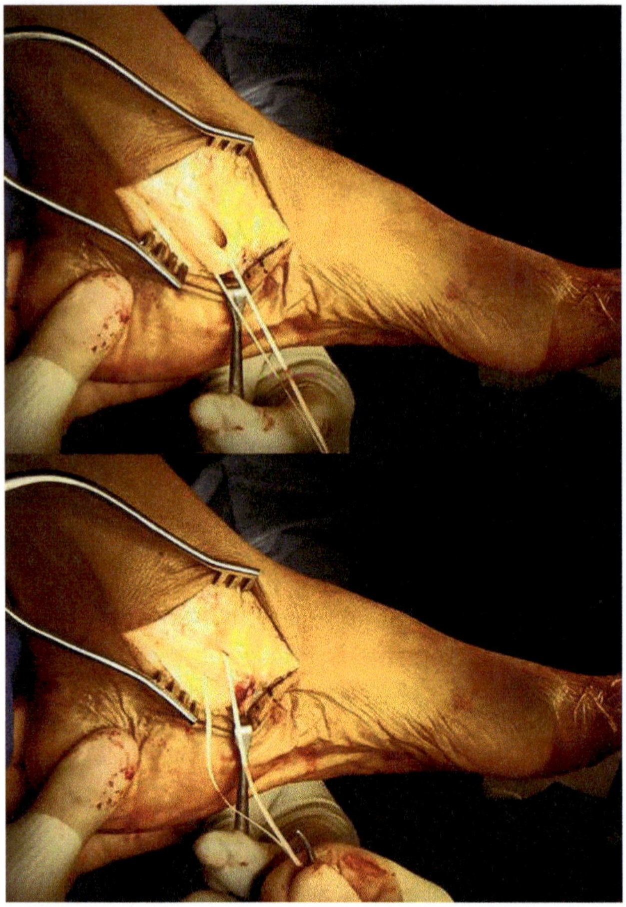

Fig. 21.1 A-B Intraoperative assessment of the posterior tibial tendon. Elasticity of the muscle-tendon unit can be determined by pulling on the tendon

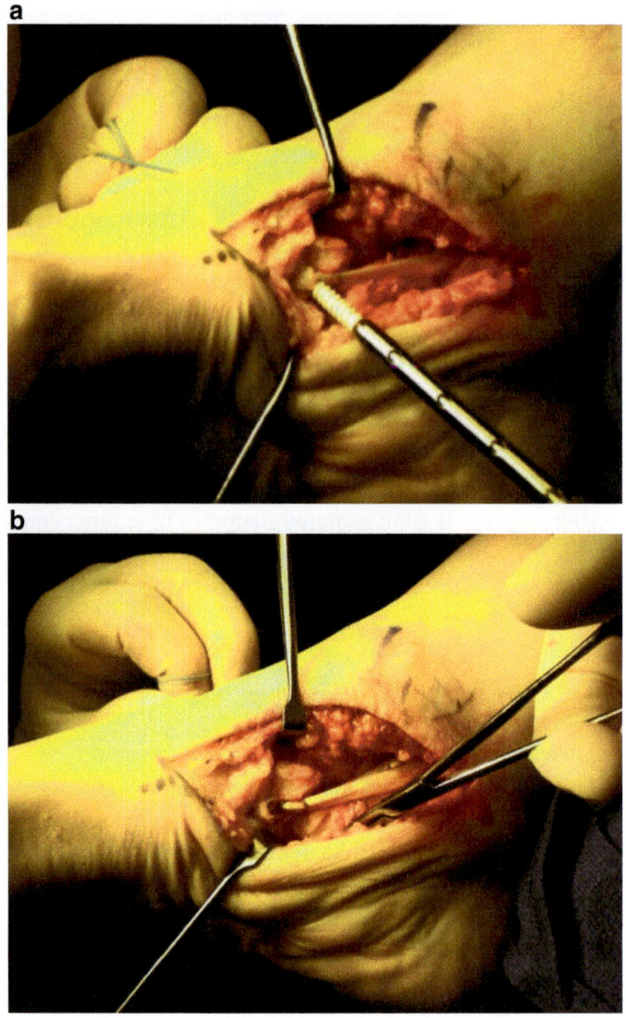

Fig. 21.2 A-B Tenodesis of the Flexor digitorum longus tendon into the navicular with an absorbable interference screw

the muscle-tendon unit can be determined by pulling on the tendon (Fig. 21.1). A viable tendon will demonstrate elasticity, springing back into its original position, whereas a nonviable muscle-tendon unit will have virtually no elasticity.

Leaving behind the pathologic tendon at the time of surgery can result in persistent symptoms, as diseased tendon is often a pain generator and contributes to the symptom complex. Simple debridement with repair of the PTT may be inadequate when tendinosis is pronounced. These situations often warrant complete evacuation of the diseased PTT, and tendon transfer should be considered as an adjunct procedure.

Insufficient tendon length and technically inadequate anchoring techniques can also result in an increased likelihood of failed correction. However, with the recent advances in tenodesis techniques, this is not a common complication (Fig. 21.2).

Undercorrection with Periarticular Osteotomies

Undercorrection of stage II AAFF will result in a foot that remains unbalanced and predisposed to recurrence. Although symptoms will initially improve, long-term prognosis is guarded and recurrent deformity is possible. This is not uncommon when PTT repair is combined with an isolated medial calcaneal displacement osteotomy (MCO) and no other osseous procedures for late stage II AAFF. Although FDL tendon transfer with an isolated MCO has been described as an effective surgical approach to address less severe cases of stage II AAFF, it may not be adequate to correct more severe cases of stage II AAFF [1]. Myerson et al. found 97% of participants experienced pain relief and 94%

showed improvement of function in 129 patients with stage II AAFF who underwent an FDL tendon transfer and a MCO. They recommend this combination of procedures if the patient has a flexible flatfoot, insignificant fixed forefoot supination, and less than 30% uncovering of the talonavicular joint on a weight-bearing AP X-ray [1]. FDL transfer and MCO in patients with deformities that go beyond these parameters may result in unacceptable outcomes. Additional procedures are needed for late stage II deformity [1, 2, 5]. In one study, patients who demonstrated undercorrection with a MCO, based on preoperative and postoperative hindfoot alignment radiographs, experienced less subjective improvement as opposed to a mild varus cohort [6]. The researchers concluded that patients who have residual postoperative valgus hindfoot moment arms continue to experience the everting pull of the Achilles tendon resulting in high loads along the medial longitudinal arch [6]. A radiographic study of 40 patients treated with either lateral column lengthening (LCL) or MCO demonstrated that LCL provided greater correction of the longitudinal arch and realignment of the medial column in comparison with the MCO [7].

Nonetheless, medial displacement osteotomy of the calcaneus is an effective procedure. A prospective study evaluated 30 patients with stage II AAFD undergoing flatfoot reconstruction. Preoperative and postoperative radiographs were reviewed to assess for correction in hindfoot alignment, which was measured by the change in hindfoot moment arm [8]. Correction in hindfoot alignment was primarily determined by the MCO, and concomitant procedures, including LCL, had a much lesser effect on hindfoot alignment during reconstruction [8]. More importantly, although the amount of LCL performed was positively correlated with the change in moment arm as an individual variable, the strength of the correlation was much lower than that of the MCO [8]. The authors concluded that the hindfoot alignment view can serve as a valuable preoperative measurement to help surgeons determine the proper amount of correction that is required (Fig. 21.3) [8]. Conti et al. assessed the relationship between postoperative hindfoot alignment following an MCO for stage II AAFD and patient outcomes. Evaluation was performed on 55 patients who underwent reconstruction for a stage II AAFF. Hindfoot alignment radiographs were taken before and after surgery. Average follow-up was 3.1 years. They concluded that hindfoot alignment between 0 and 5 mm of varus following stage II AAFF reconstruction was associated with the greatest improvement in clinical outcomes [6].

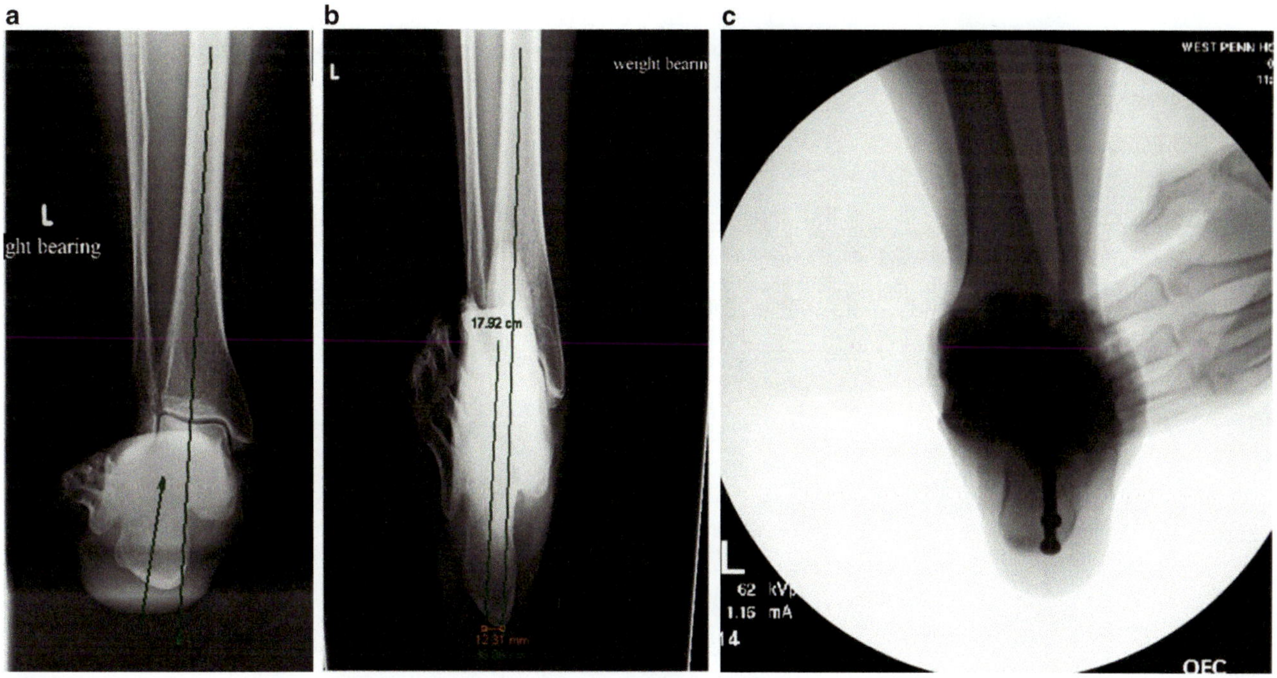

Fig. 21.3 A-B Long-leg axial and hindfoot alignment x-rays. C Intraoperative axial radiograph demonstrating realignment following medial displacement osteotomy of the calcaneus

Undercorrection of medial displacement osteotomies can result from technical errors, especially when the osteotomy is performed too proximal. The intrinsic muscles, plantar fascia, etc. originate from the plantar aspect of the tuber segment. Displacement in this area can be hindered by these soft tissue attachments and result in insufficient translation and undercorrection. Medial displacement can often be facilitated by releasing the plantar structures. Osteotomy placement distal to the plantar intrinsic muscles allows easier medial translation of the tuber segment (Fig. 21.4).

Undercorrection can also result from inadequate lengthening of the lateral column at the time of surgery or loss of correction afterward due to bone graft resorption. Bone graft resorption can occur with premature weight-bearing, inadequate fixation, or inappropriate graft composition. According to Dayton et al., lateral column length must be maintained postoperatively to obtain an effective long-term correction. In their study, 22 patients underwent bone grafting for lateral column lengthening (LCL) using the traditional non-fixated technique. Conversely, 13 patients had the graft fixated with a locking plate to prevent compressive forces on the graft. Calcaneal length was measured 10 days and 12 weeks postoperatively to ascertain the mean amount of calcaneal shortening. Their results demonstrated that the mean amount of calcaneal shortening in the non-fixated group was 2.5 mm (range 0–6 mm). The mean amount of calcaneal shortening in the fixated group was 1.0 mm (range 0–3) [9]. These results might explain postoperative undercorrection following LCL without fixation. Locking plate fixation also reduced anterior displacement of calcaneal fragments [9]. In a recent study of 24 LCL patients, a wedge locking plate was found to be more effective in maintaining the mid-calcaneal length time when compared with a tricortical allograft wedge [10]. The mean decrease in mid-calcaneal length was greater for the tricortical allograft wedge group (2.8 ± 0.7 mm) than for the wedge locking plate group (0.6 ± 0.7 mm) at 6 months following surgery. Titanium trusses might also be effective in maintaining length following LCL (Fig. 21.5).

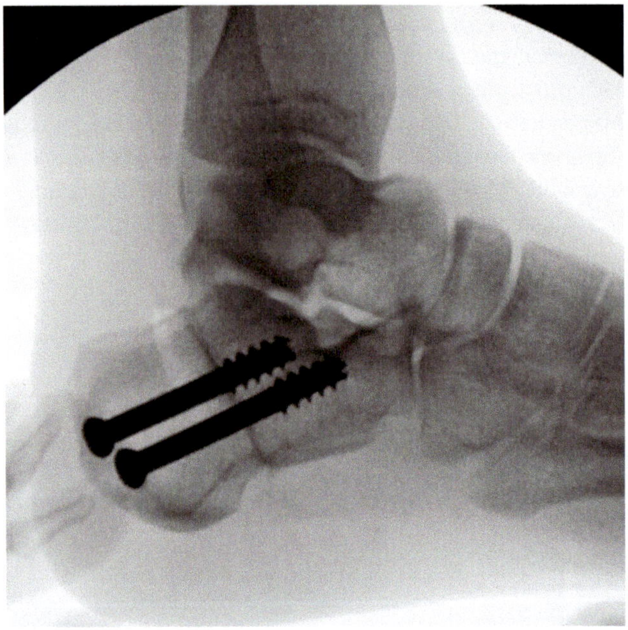

Fig. 21.4 Lateral radiograph demonstrating placement of a medial displacement calcaneal osteotomy in the mid-substance of the calcaneus. The mid substance of the calcaneus is in ideal location for the medial displacement osteotomy

To avoid undercorrection/overcorrection with LCL procedures, one can implement digital planning for LCL as proposed by Siddiqui and Lamm. Preoperative digital planning accurately predicted the calcaneal graft size used during LCL when compared with the actual graft size utilized by the surgeon who was unaware of the predicted graft size. The preoperative graft measurement compared with the actual graft placed was within 0.4 mm (±1.8 mm) [11].

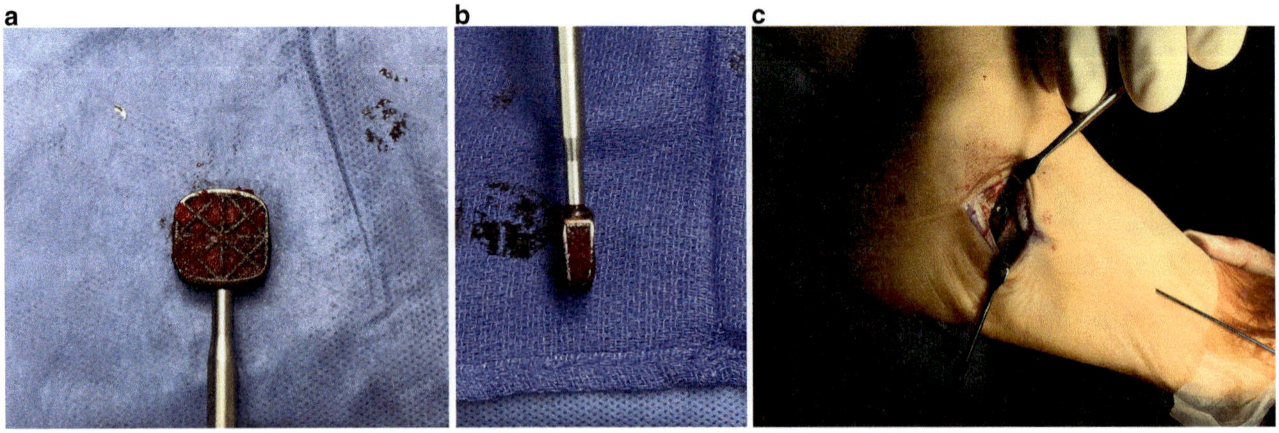

Fig. 21.5 Trial wedges used to ascertain the appropriate amount of lateral column lengthening

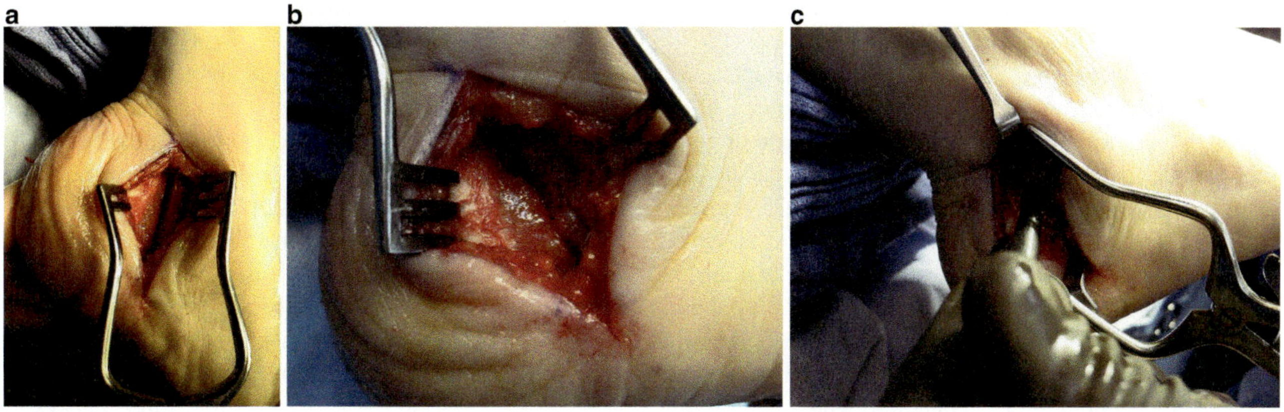

Fig. 21.6 A-C. Osteoplasty of the lateral overhang of bone following medial displacement. This procedure helps to decompress the lateral wound

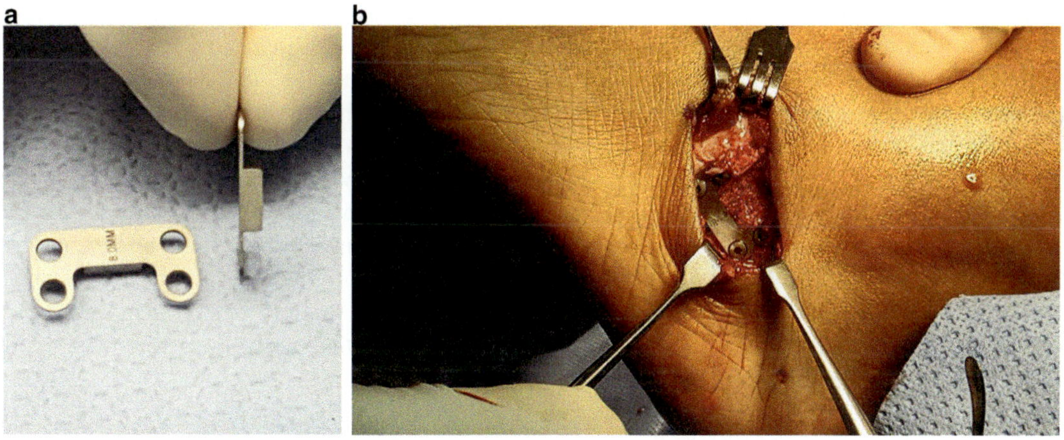

Fig. 21.7 A-B Lateral column lengthening with a wedge plate and BMA –soaked cancellous allograft bone

The authors prefer utilizing both MCO and LCL for most cases of stage II AAFF. [12] This provides the latitude to modify both osteotomies as needed and requires less displacement at both sites. This preserves a greater degree of hindfoot motion and results in less traction on neural structures. One can "dial in" the necessary correction at both sites with finer control. Overzealous displacement of the tuber segment can place excess tension on the lateral skin, resulting in wound dehiscence. We recommend osteoplasty of the overhanging portion of the calcaneus following displacement to help decompress the lateral skin (Fig. 21.6). Nonetheless, the risk of wound problems remains a potential problem with a large displacement.

Large amounts of distraction along the lateral column can result in lateral column overload, traction neuritis, and disruption of the planter soft tissues that stabilize the distal segment of the calcaneus with subsequent sagittal plane displacement and extended convalescence to allow adequate incorporation of the bone graft. The authors rarely use a graft size greater than 8.0 mm when combining LCL with a medial displacement osteotomy. Additionally, we no longer use structural grafts. Rather, we prefer lateral plates that maintain distraction and then "backfill" with bone graft (Fig. 21.7). The process of backfilling is carried out with a combination of frozen cancellous chips, bone marrow aspirate, and demineralized bone matrix putty. The plates allow for precise correction that can easily be changed during the procedure. Titanium trusses afford the same benefits.

Overcorrection with Medial Displacement Osteotomy of the Calcaneus

Overcorrection of hindfoot alignment may shift plantar pressures laterally and has the potential to cause symptoms in the lateral foot. Hadfield et al. demonstrated that medial translation of the calcaneus resulted in increased peak pressures in the lateral forefoot as well as the lateral aspect of the heel [13]. The average pressure over the 1st and 2nd metatarsal regions of the forefoot decreased significantly after a MCO. However there was a significant increase in maximum forefoot pressure over the area of the 3rd–5th metatarsals [13]. Overcorrection of hindfoot alignment may shift plantar pressures laterally which can lead to discomfort along the lateral column [13]. The Achilles tendon is able to assist the PTT with inversion of the heel when the insertion point on the calcaneus is medial to the mid-tibial axis; however, overcorrection secondary to medial translation of the heel may result in symptoms due to lateral weight-bearing and/or excessive stiffness.

It is important to assess the magnitude of deformity and suppleness of soft tissues preoperatively as well as intraoperatively so that the appropriate amount of correction is obtained at the time of surgery. Furthermore, the amount of correction obtained with other procedures, such as lateral column lengthening, must also be taken into account. One should not translate the tuber segment the same amount for every case. Rather, the amount of displacement should be based on these factors.

Overcorrection and Lateral Column Overload Following Lateral Column Lengthening

Lateral column overload can result from overcorrection, failure to recognize/address forefoot varus, and failure to recognize/address medial column instability. LCL causes a significant shift of plantar load to lateral column, decreased contact in the medial midfoot through increased TN coverage, and higher maximum mean plantar pressures along the lateral midfoot [14]. A cadaveric study found significantly decreased talonavicular abduction and increased lateral column plantar pressures as they increased the amount of LCL performed from 6 to 10 mm. These findings suggest that overcorrection of the abduction deformity in patients with stage II AAFD may lead to less than ideal outcomes [15].

Ellis et al. performed a comparative cohort study with 20 patients, ten of which developed lateral column pain after undergoing a LCL procedure with additional adjunctive procedures [16]. The authors hypothesized that the patients with postoperative pain would have an increase in lateral column pressure measured by an EMED-ST plantar pressure platform. Results demonstrated a positive correlation with patients experiencing postoperative pain and an increased maximum force to the lateral aspect of the midfoot. Interestingly, the increased lateral plantar pressures did not correlate with excessive lengthening according to their radiographic measurements [17].

One of the technical challenges with LCL is determining the appropriate graft size or amount of lengthening. Unfortunately, there are no guidelines for estimating the necessary amount of LCL. Determination of graft size should be based on the degree of deformity and the suppleness of the soft tissues. In most cases, this is an intraoperative decision. Although intraoperative fluoroscopy (AP and lateral views) can help, simulated weight-bearing fluoroscopy is of limited value. It is difficult to simulate a patient's body weight while trying to obtain appropriate radiographic views during surgery. Manual eversion testing is important following graft placement to ascertain range of motion. Our preference is to maintain at least 1/3–1/2 of eversion following LCL. Otherwise, patients may experience difficulty off-loading the lateral column during the mid-stance phase of gait. Some authors have reported the use of trial wedges as an effective way to determine appropriate graft size (Fig. 21.8). However, other reports suggest that trial wedges have limited accuracy and predictability [17].

Preoperative evaluation should always include a thorough assessment of the forefoot to hindfoot position, especially with the foot in a corrected position. This should unmask forefoot varus, which can be addressed during surgery with a medial column procedure (NC arthrodesis, 1st TMT arthrodesis, or cuneiform osteotomy). It is also important to evaluate the medial column for instability. Although the forefoot might be parallel to the hindfoot when the foot is placed into a corrected position during the preoperative assessment, one

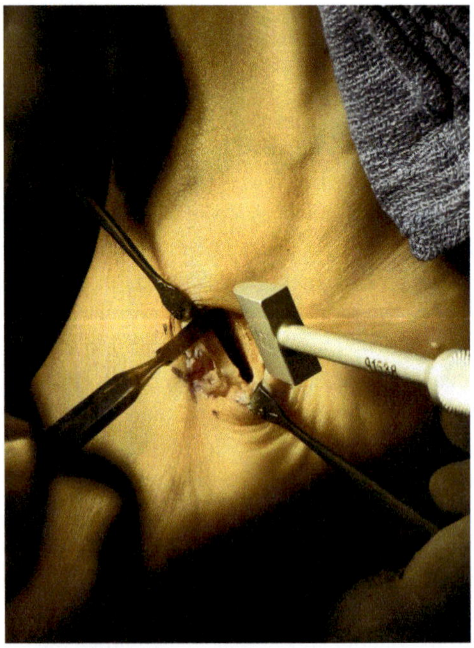

Fig. 21.8 Trial wedges used to ascertain the appropriate amount of lateral column lengthening

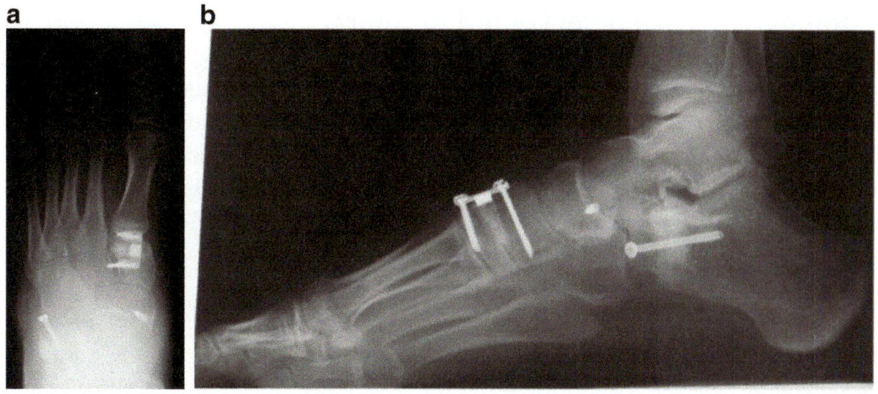

Fig. 21.9 Dorsal opening wedge osteotomy of the medial cuneiform to address forefoot varus and lateral column overload

must also evaluate medial column stability. Failure to recognize instability can result in overload to the lateral column with corresponding symptoms. Instability can be treated surgically with medial column stabilization procedures.

A study of 55 patients by Deland et al. reviewed postoperative talonavicular joint radiographic measurements of patients following reconstruction of stage II adult acquired flatfoot deformity. A postoperative talonavicular joint position of adduction was associated with decreased patient outcomes in daily activities and quality of life compared with an abducted position [18]. The authors were able to correlate postoperative midfoot radiographic alignment with clinical outcomes. There was no statistically significant difference between BMI, sex, and age between the midfoot groups. All patients underwent MCO, 39 LCL, 28 1st TMT arthrodesis, 24 medial cuneiform osteotomies, and five spring ligament repairs. The amount of LCL performed in the abducted and adducted groups was not significantly different, which indicates that the results of this study do not depend on how much the midfoot position was changed but rather on the final postoperative radiographic alignment [18].

Lateral column overload can result in significant pain and discomfort [17]. Although this is often a transient problem, and most cases improve within the first postoperative year, some patients experience recalcitrant symptoms. This is a rather challenging problem to manage. Orthotics, nonsteroidal anti-inflammatory medications, topical analgesics, and physical therapy can provide some benefit.

Ultimately, patient's failing non-operative therapy will require revision surgery. In most cases, the authors prefer NC arthrodesis or first cuneiform osteotomy. Although both procedures will impart stability to the medial column, NC arthrodesis is ideal to stabilize the medial column. However, if lateral column overload is primarily a result of forefoot varus, then a plantar-flexion cuneiform osteotomy is acceptable. A biomechanical study evaluated LCL procedures and a simulated FDL tendon transfer on eight cadaveric limbs. Results demonstrated a statistically significant decrease in lateral forefoot pressure after adding a medial cuneiform osteotomy. Additionally, there was a corresponding increase in medial column pressures. These findings suggested that adjuvant medial cuneiform osteotomies are successful in redistributing load to the medial column in patients undergoing a LCL (Fig. 21.9) [19].

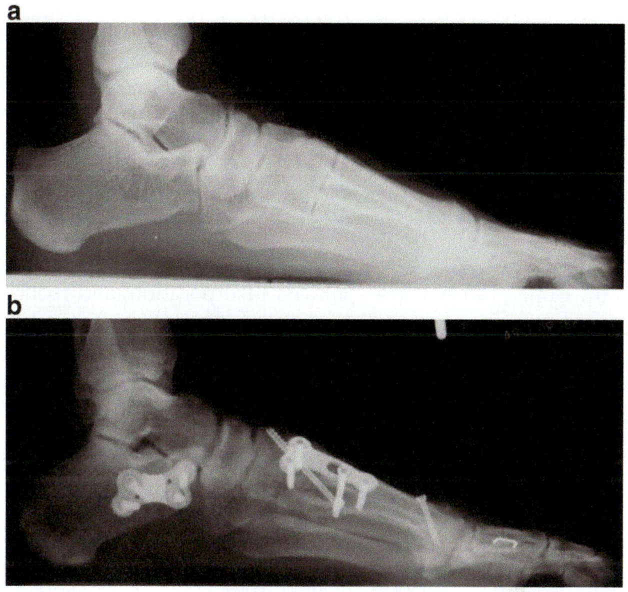

Fig. 21.10 Low-profile plate being utilized to secure the bone graft following lateral column lengthening

The sural nerve is always at risk for injury with virtually any approach to the lateral calcaneus. Traction neuritis is not uncommon, especially with a substantial amount of lengthening. Although this is often transient, patients can experience some degree of permanent numbness. We often combine LCL with MCO so that a smaller degree of correction is necessary at the LCL site. This will limit traction on the neural structures. Additionally, various fixation devices can be potential sources of direct irritation to the nerve. Low profile devices are ideal in this area (Fig. 21.10). This should be explained in the preoperative consultation, especially with larger deformities.

Nonunion and Malunion Following Lateral Column Lengthening

LCL is a commonly used procedure to address stage II AAFF. Good outcomes have been well documented. The lateral column can be lengthened through either distraction arthrodesis of the calcaneocuboid joint (CCJ) or mid-substance osteotomy of the calcaneus.

Distraction arthrodesis of the CCJ has been utilized as a method of LCL [20]. This procedure requires resection of the articular surfaces and insertion of a structural bone graft. Nonunion is a known complication following CCJ distraction arthrodesis. Although CCJ distraction arthrodesis has been an effective procedure in restoring alignment in stage II AAFF, the incidence of nonunion has been relatively high. Toolan et al. evaluated a total of 36 patients that underwent a distraction arthrodesis of the CCJ with additional adjunctive procedures including an FDL tendon transfer. Their results demonstrated a 20% nonunion rate. In addition 71% of the patients required an additional operative procedure such as removal of hardware, bone grafting of nonunion site, or additional corrective osteotomies for residual deformities [20]. Bone graft collapse, delayed incorporation, and recurrent deformity have been reported with CCJ bone block arthrodesis (Fig. 21.11). Furthermore, the convalescence associated with this procedure is extended compared to LCL through the mid-substance of the calcaneus.

Haeseker et al. performed a retrospective comparison of two groups with stage II AAFF deformity. A total of 35 patients were involved in the study in which 16 feet (group 1) underwent a CCJ distraction arthrodesis and 21 feet (group 2) underwent a calcaneal lengthening osteotomy. AOFAS ankle-hindfoot scores demonstrated a statistically significant difference in their results. At a mean follow-up of 42.4 months, group I AOFAS score was 71.9 and group 2 was 84.9. The nonunion and hardware removal rate was 6.25% and 31.25% for group 1, compared to 5.26% and 10.53% for group 2. Two patients were dissatisfied with the CCJ distraction and three patients (21.43%) would not repeat the same procedure again. No patients were dissatisfied and only one (5.26%) patient stated they would not repeat the same procedure in the calcaneal osteotomy group. Due to the higher AOFAS score, the authors believe patients with stage II AAFF would better benefit from a LCL through a mid-substance calcaneus osteotomy as opposed to a distraction arthrodesis of the CCJ [21].

Although degenerative changes of the CCJ have been described following LCL through a calcaneal osteotomy, these changes may not be clinically significant. Radiographic signs of CCJ arthritis can be seen following periarticular osteotomies for stage II AAFF; however radiographic signs of DJD do not correlate with clinic findings. These patients are most often asymptomatic [22].

a

b

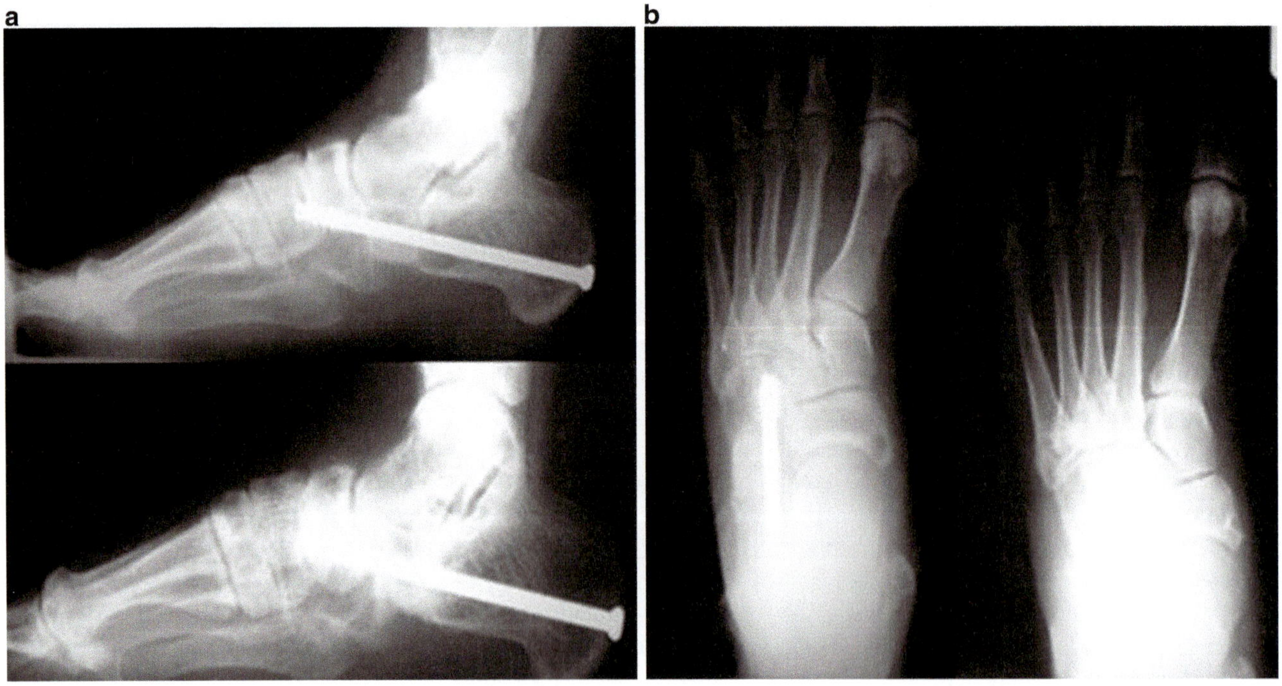

Fig. 21.11 A-B. Radiographs demonstrating calcaneocuboid bone block arthrodesis to accomplished lateral column lengthening. Subsequent graft collapse and loss of correction. This was revised into a triple arthrodesis

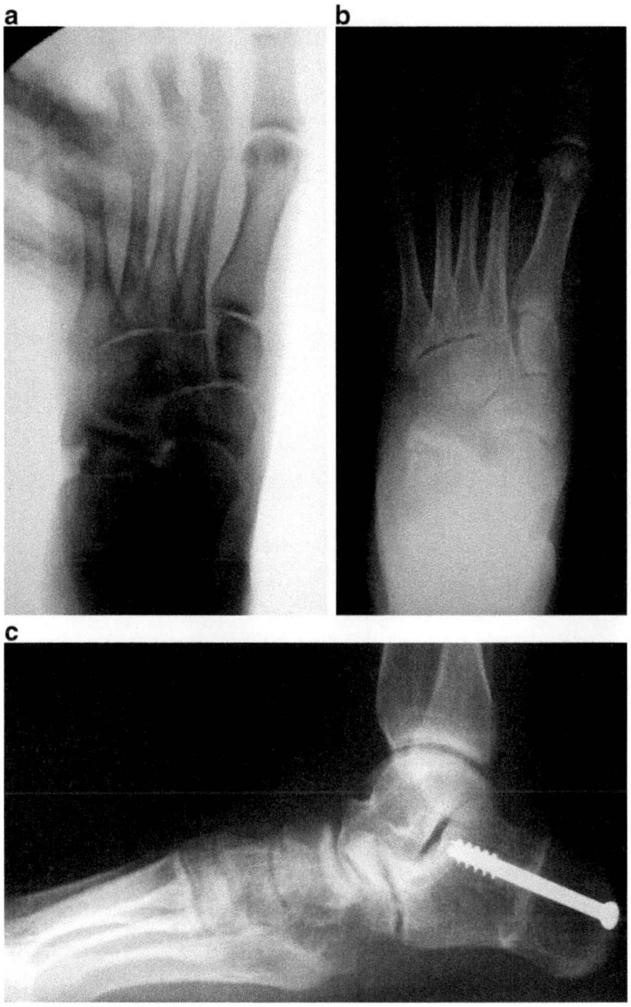

Fig. 21.12 A-C. Radiographs demonstrating graft collapse and subsequent loss of correction following lateral column lengthening with allograft bone through the mid substance of the calcaneus

Although LCL within the mid-substance of the calcaneus has a much lower incidence of nonunion relative to CCJ bone block arthrodesis, nonunion can still occur. Nonunion can result in loss of correction, sagittal plane malalignment, and recurrent flatfoot deformity (Fig. 21.12).

Nonunion can develop secondary to premature weight-bearing, lack of or inappropriate fixation, poor host factors, etc. Controversy exists regarding the need for fixation of mid-substance LCL within the calcaneus. Although good outcomes have been reported without fixation, complications have been reported as well.

Loss of correction secondary to bone graft resorption has been reported following LCL. This can obviously result in a loss of correction and residual flatfoot deformity (Fig. 21.11). In addition to securing or stabilizing osseous segments to promote healing, certain fixation devices will maintain long-term correction. The use of fixation can minimize graft resorption as well as prevent sagittal plane displacement of the distal calcaneal segment [9].

The revision of nonunion or graft collapse often requires debridement, bone grafting, and fixation. Our preference has been frozen femoral head allograft combined with bone marrow aspirate. These grafts must be large enough to restore alignment and make up for any bone loss. Fixation is accomplished with a locking plate.

Nonunion Following Medial Column Stabilization Through Naviculocuneiform or First Tarsometatarsal Arthrodesis

Nonunion is possible following any arthrodesis procedure. Both TMT and NC arthrodesis are procedures utilized in stage II AAFF to address medial column instability. Nonunion can be managed with non-operative therapy such as immobilization, non-weight-bearing, bone growth stimulation, etc. if alignment is maintained. However, if there is sagittal plane malalignment, then revision surgery is required (Fig. 21.13). In these cases, both union and realignment are necessary. Revision surgery should include some type of bone grafting and/or orthobiologic, adequate fixation, immobilization, and non-weight-bearing (Fig. 21.14). Obviously, any poor host factors such as vitamin D deficiency, uncontrolled diabetes mellitus, etc. should also be addressed to enhance union.

Failure to Address Equinus

Equinus deformity must be thoroughly evaluated and appropriately addressed as part of stage II AAFF reconstruction. Virtually all patients with stage II AAFF have some degree of equinus. Patients can lose up to 15° of dorsiflexion after LCL [9, 23]. Residual equinus can result in significant forces through the midfoot during axial loading with subsequent breakdown of the flatfoot reconstruction.

Residual Forefoot Varus

Forefoot varus, if not addressed or unrecognized, can potentiate lateral column discomfort following hindfoot reconstruction due to lateral forefoot overload [18, 24].

The Cotton osteotomy, a plantar-flexion osteotomy of the medial cuneiform, is an adjunctive procedure that has been recommended following realignment of the hindfoot. When the hindfoot is surgically corrected during AAFF reconstruction, forefoot varus may become unmasked. This deformity should be addressed [24, 25] during reconstruction.

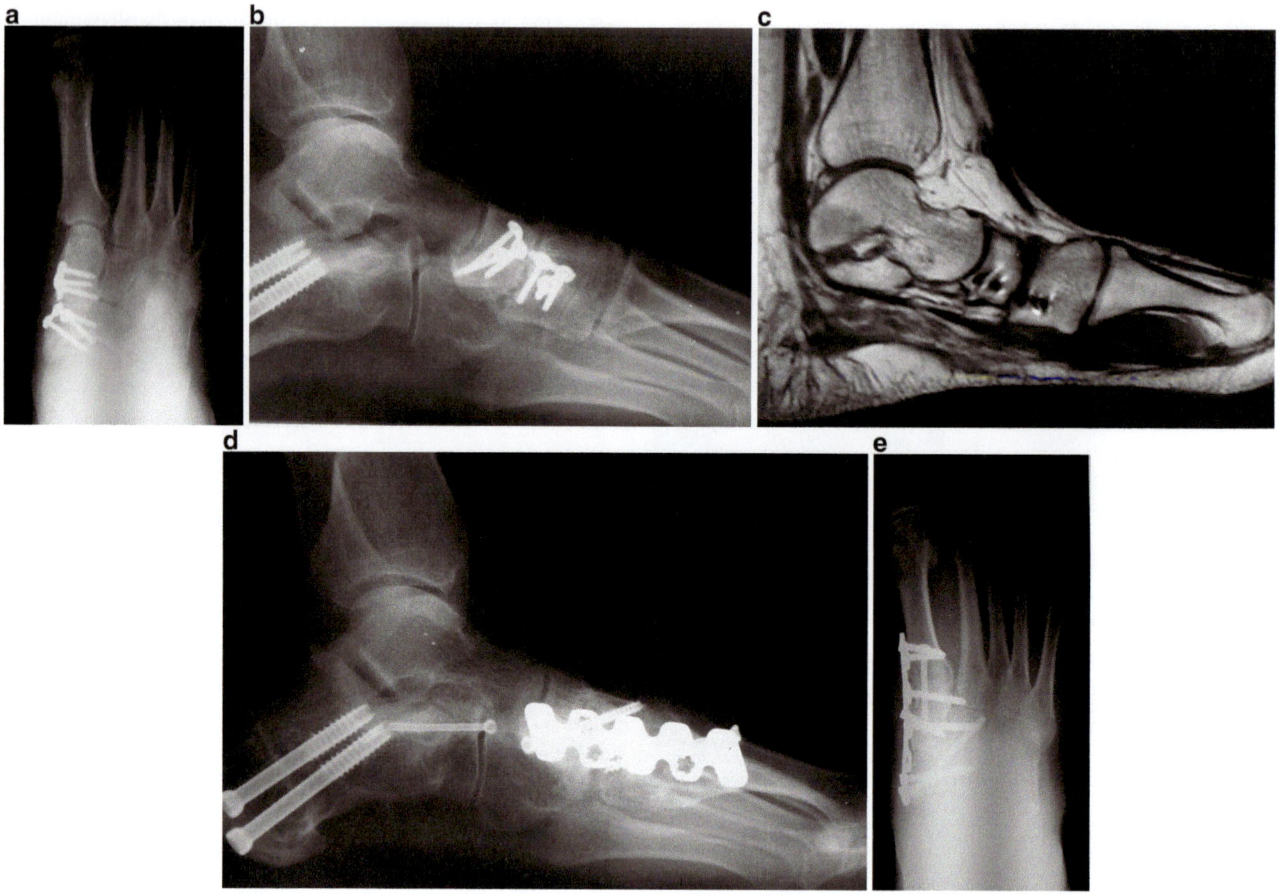

Fig. 21.13 A-C. Nonunion of the naviculocuneiform joint following flatfoot reconstruction. D&E. Revision is performed with autogenous bone graft and plate fixation that extend the fusion mass to incorporate the 1st tarsometatarsal joint

Failure to recognize and correct residual forefoot varus deformity following hindfoot realignment may lead to failure and recurrence of the flatfoot deformity [24, 26]. The medial Cotton osteotomy has been shown to correct the forefoot varus component of AAFF with evidence of improvement in radiographic parameters including lateral talus-first metatarsal angle, calcaneal pitch, and medial cuneiform-to-floor distance [25].

Progressive Deformity Following Kidner Procedures

Resection of a symptomatic os tibiale externum with advancement of the posterior tibial tendon (Kidner procedure) is an effective procedure. However, a symptomatic os tibiale externum is often associated with a flexible flatfoot deformity. In those cases where the flatfoot deformity is significant, i.e., stage II AAFF, performing an isolated Kidner procedure without addressing the underlying skeletal deformity can result in progression of the deformity. Unfortunately, disruption of the medial soft tissue structures associated with resection of the os tibiale externum will often result in progression of the flatfoot deformity. Progression is not uncommon when these soft tissue constraints are absent. These patients may require revision surgery to address the flatfoot deformity and associated symptoms. Procedures should be chosen based on the type and degree of deformity.

Arthroereisis

Subtalar joint arthroereisis has been recommended as an adjunct procedure for stage II AAFF. A cadaveric study demonstrated that the addition of arthroereisis to a MCO and FDL transfer in severe AAFF resulted in increased correction of the deformity and did not cause adverse biomechanical consequences as opposed to simply performing a FDL transfer and medializing calcaneal osteotomy [5]. Various

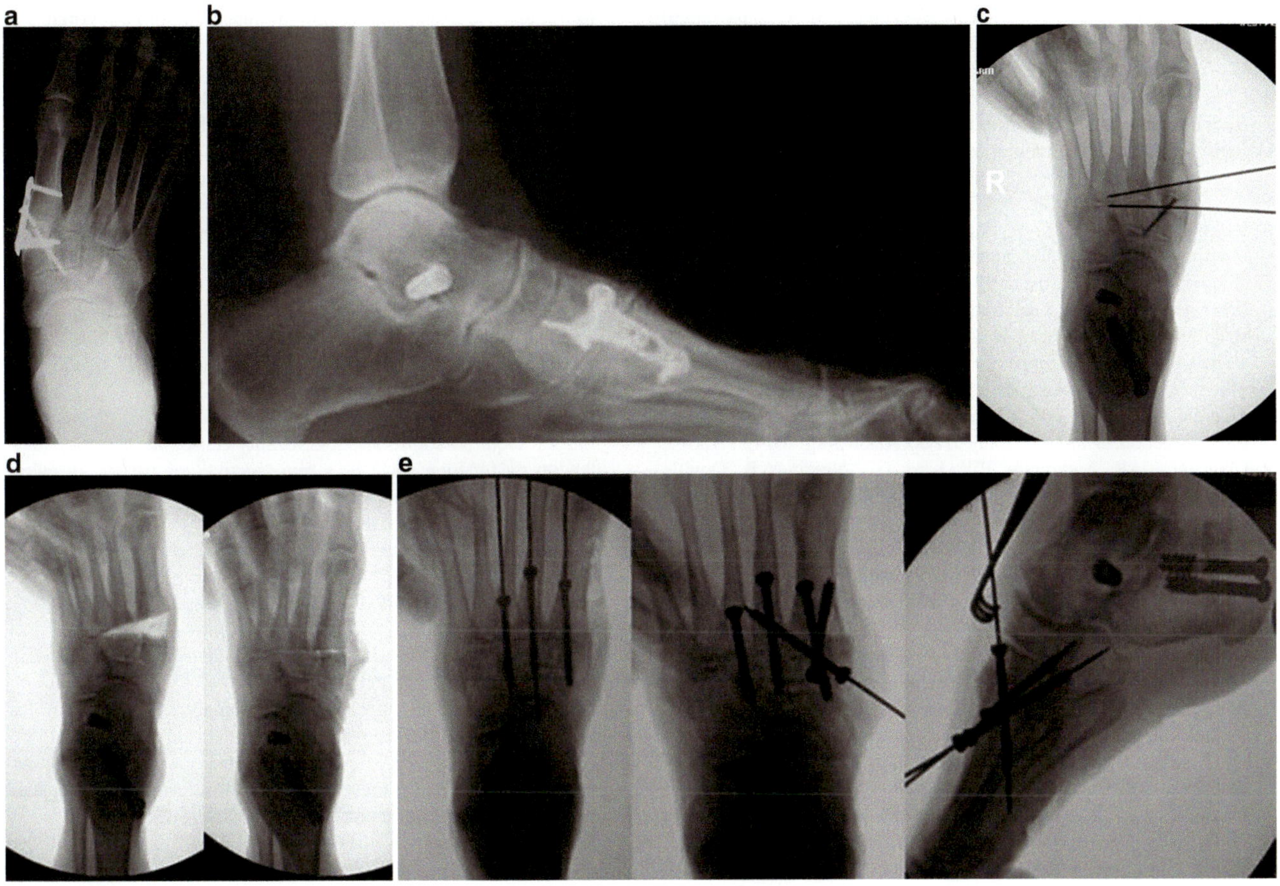

Fig. 21.14 A-B. Nonunion of the 1st tarsometatarsal joint following flatfoot reconstruction. C-E. Revision is performed with a midfoot osteotomy and medial displacement osteotomy of the calcaneus

complications have been noted, including overcorrection with persistent sinus tarsi pain and implant displacement. This can be addressed by removing the implant. However, controversy exists regarding the use of this procedure in adults.

Summary

Stage II AAFF reconstruction with double is a sound operation to relieve symptoms, improve function, and improve quality of life. Furthermore, this is a joint-sparing operation that is durable and predictable. One of the surgical goals is to prevent progression and the need for future arthrodesis. Nonetheless, complications do occur. Fortunately, many of these complications are avoidable with appropriate planning. Additionally, addressing these complications is straightforward. Management should be based on reasons for failure of the index operation.

References

1. Myerson MS, Badekas A, Schon LC. Treatment of stage II posterior tibial tendon rupture with flexor digitorum longus tendon transfer and calcaneal osteotomy. Foot Ankle Int. 2004;25(7):445–50.
2. Guyton GP, Jeng C, Krieger LE, Mann RA. Flexor digitorum longus transfer and medial displacement calcaneal osteotomy for posterior tibial tendon dysfunction: a middle-term clinical follow-up. Foot Ankle Int. 2004;22(8):627–32.
3. Arangio GA, Salathe EP. A biomechanical analysis of posterior tibial tendon dysfunction, medial displacement calcaneal osteotomy and flexor digitorum longus transfer in adult acquired flatfoot. Clin Biomech. 2009;24(6):530.
4. DiDomenico L, Stein DY, Wargo-Dorsey M. Treatment of posterior tibial tendon dysfunction without flexor digitorum tendon transfer: A retrospective study of 34 patients. J. Foot Ankle Surg. 2011;50(3):293–8.
5. Vora AM, Tien TR, Parks BG, Schon LC. Correction of moderate and severe acquired flexible flatfoot with medializing calcaneal osteotomy and flexor digitorum longus transfer. J Bone Joint Surg Am. 2006;88(8):1726–34.
6. Conti MS, Ellis SJ, Chan JY, Do HT, Deland JT. Optimal position of the heel following reconstruction of the stage II adult-acquired flatfoot deformity. Foot Ankle Int. 2015;36(8):919–27.

7. Chi TD, Toolan BC, Sangeorzan BJ, Hansen Jr ST. The lateral column lengthening and medial column stabilization procedures. Clin Orthop Relat Res. 1999;365:81–90.
8. Chan JT, Williams BR, Nair P, Yound E, Sofka C, Deland JT, Ellis SJ. The contribution of medializing calcaneal osteotomy on hindfoot alignment in the reconstruction of the stage II adult acquired flatfoot deformity. Foot Ankle Int. 2013;34(2):159–66.
9. Dayton P, Prins DB, Smith DE, Feilmeier MJ. Effectiveness of a locking plate in preserving midcalcaneal length and positional outcome after Evans calcaneal osteotomy: a retrospective pilot study. J. Foot Ankle Surg. 2013;52:710–3.
10. Protzman NM, Wobst GM, Storts EC, Mulhern JL, McCarroll RE, Brigido SA. Mid-calcaneal length after Evans calcaneal osteotomy: a retrospective comparison of wedge locking plates and tricortical allograft wedges. J. Foot Ankle Surg. 2015;54(5):900–4.
11. Siddiqui NA, Lamm BM. Digital planning for foot and ankle deformity correction: Evans osteotomy. J. Foot Ankle Surg. 2014;53:700–5.
12. Catanzariti AR, Mendicino RW, King GL, Neerings B. Double calcaneal osteotomy realignment considerations in eight patients. J Am Podiatr Med Assoc. 2005;95(1):53–9.
13. Hadfield MH, Snyder JW, Liacouras PC, Owen JR, Wayne JS, Adelaar RS. Effects of medializing calcaneal osteotomy on Achilles tendon lengthening and plantar foot pressures. Foot Ankle Int. 2003;24(7):523–9.
14. Conti MS, Chan JT, Do HT, Ellis SJ, Deland JT. Correlation of postoperative midfoot position with outcome following reconstruction of the stage II adult acquired flatfoot deformity. Foot Ankle Int. 2015;36(3):239–47.
15. Oh I, Imhauser C, Choi D, Willims B, Ellis S, Deland J. Sensitivity of plantar pressure and talonavicular alignment on lateral column lengthening in flatfoot reconstruction. J Bone Joint Surg Am. 2013;95(12):1094–100.
16. Ellis SJ, Williams BR, Garg R, Campbell G, Pavlov H, Deland JT. Incidence of plantar lateral foot pain before and after the use of trial metal wedges in lateral column lengthening. Foot Ankle Int. 2011;32(7):665–73.
17. Ellis SJ, Yu JC, Johnson AH, Elliot A, O'Malley M, Deland J. Plantar pressures in patients with and without lateral foot pain after lateral column lengthening. J Bone Joint Surg Am. 2010;92(1):81–91.
18. Deland JT. Adult acquired flatfoot deformity. J Am Acad Orthop Surg. 2008;16:399–406.
19. Benthien RA, Parks BG, Guyton GP, Schon LC. Lateral column calcaneal lengthening, flexor digitorum longus transfer and opening wedge medial cuneiform osteotomy for flexible flatfoot: a biomechanical study. Foot Ankle Int. 2007;28(1):70–7.
20. Toolan BC, Sangeorzan BJ, Hansen Jr ST. Complex reconstruction for the treatment of dorsolateral peritalar subluxation of the foot. J Bone Joint Surg Am. 1999;81(11):1545–60.
21. Haeseker GA, Mureau MA, Faber FWM. Lateral column lengthening for acquired adult flatfoot deformity caused by posterior tibial tendon dysfunction stage II: a retrospective comparison of calcaneus osteotomy with calcaneocuboid distraction arthrodesis. J Foot Ankle Surg. 2010;49(4):380–4.
22. Moseir-LaClair S, Pomeroy G, Manoli A. Intermediate follow-up on the double osteotomy and tendon transfer procedure for stage II posterior tibial tendon insufficiency. Foot Ankle Int. 2001; 22(4):283–91.
23. DeYoe BE, Wood J. The Evans calcaneal osteotomy. Clin Podiatr Med Surg. 2005;22(2):265–76.
24. Evans EL, Catanzariti AR. Forefoot supinatus. Clin Podiatr Med Surg. 2014;31(3):405–13.
25. Hirose CB, Johnson JE. Plantarflexion opening wedge medial cuneiform osteotomy for correction of fixed forefoot varus associated with flatfoot deformity. Foot Ankle Int. 2004;25(8):568–74.
26. Lutz M, Myerson M. Radiographic analysis of an opening wedge osteotomy of the medial cuneiform. Foot Ankle Int. 2011;32(3): 278–87.

22 Flatfoot Surgery

Glenn Weinraub

Posterior tibial tendon dysfunction (PTTD) is a complex multiplanar deformity that represents a technically challenging treatment plan for the foot and ankle surgeon. While there have been numerous procedures described for the treatment of PTTD, an algorithmic classification system has been designed to help aid the foot and ankle surgeon in selective procedures. While this classification system aids in the selection of procedures there is no algorithmic approach for the management of complications associated with surgical correction of the symptomatic flatfoot. This chapter, while not all inclusive for all flatfoot surgical procedures, will outline the biomechanics of a symptomatic flatfoot, highlight an algorithmic approach to procedure selection, and focus on management strategies for complications associated with the most common procedures performed for the treatment of Adult flatfoot/PTTD.

Biomechanics

Understanding the biomechanics of the hindfoot complex and the role of the posterior tibial tendon is paramount in surgical reconstruction of a symptomatic flatfoot. The development of PTTD is considered multifactorial with failure of both static and dynamic stabilizers. Static stabilizers of the hindfoot are the interosseous ligaments, joint capsular complexes, and structural bony architecture. Dynamic stabilizers are the intrinsic and extrinsic myotendinous units of the foot and the leg. While it is a combination of these factors that lead to the development of a symptomatic flatfoot, the posterior tibial tendon still plays a crucial role in the development of the pathologic flatfoot [1]. The posterior tibial tendon (PTT) acts upon three functional joints: the tibiotalar, subtalar, and midtarsal joints. It acts as primary stabilizer of the foot from heel contact to late midstance [2]. During gait, normal biomechanics have shown that the PTT acts to decelerate subtalar joint (STJ) pronation from heel strike through midstance. The PTT then accelerates STJ supination by imparting stability at late midstance, through the midtarsal joint, and helps aid in heel lift and propulsion by providing proximal stability of the foot [3]. Abnormal mechanics of the PTT have shown that it places undo stress on the soft tissue structures that causes stretching and a predictable sequelae of deformity. The flatfoot develops through increased forefoot abduction on the rearfoot, increased hindfoot valgus, progression of an apropulsive gait, and a pain complex that begins medially and then progresses laterally with increasing deformity [4].

G. Weinraub (✉)
Department of Orthopedic Surgery, Kaiser Permanente, 2500 Merced St, San Leandro, CA 94577, USA
e-mail: Gmweinraub@gmail.com

Indications

Understanding the pathomechanics and development of a symptomatic flatfoot is paramount in procedure selection after failure of conservative care. Conservative care often includes immobilization and rehabilitation with supportive inserts and bracing as the mainstays. When conservative care has failed, proper clinical examination of the flatfoot is needed to determine the correct collection of surgical procedures to perform. Again this process is typically due to multiplanar deformities with often one plane of deformity predominating. Clinical examination typically reveals pain initially along the course of the posterior tibial tendon and spring ligament complex and through time can progress to lateral subtalar pain through impingement. Patients will often present with weakness and pain with strength testing of the posterior tibial tendon and eventually through prolonged progressions of the pathology may show an inability to perform single leg heel raises with loss of calcaneal inversion. Based on planal dominance those with predominant transverse plane deformity will show increased forefoot abduction on the rearfoot which clinically will manifest as the "too many toes sign" when viewed from behind. If there is a

M.S. Lee, J.P. Grossman (eds.), *Complications in Foot and Ankle Surgery*, DOI 10.1007/978-3-319-53686-6_22

predominance of frontal plane deformity you will often see increased calcaneal eversion when the patient is standing in their angle and base of gait [1]. With frontal plane dominance it is important to establish if the deformity is reducible, by utilizing the Hubscher maneuver (establishment of an arch via the windlass mechanism as one dorsiflexes the hallux) and also by ipsilateral external rotation of the leg. If the deformity is reducible one should see a resolution of the deformity through external rotation of the leg. One of the biggest drivers in the development of a symptomatic flatfoot is the role of equinus. Determining if the patient has a gastrosoleal versus gastrocnemius equinus can be achieved with the Silverskiold test. These are some tests that can be performed for the evaluation of PTTD.

Classification

There have been many attempts in classification of PTTD. Most of these classifications are purely descriptive along the course of progression of the disease. While helpful in describing the progression of the disease process they are typically not helpful in aiding in decision making with surgical reconstruction. Several classifications include Conti which is based on magnetic resonance imaging (MRI) but this staging system does not often correlate to intra-operative findings [5]. Johnson and Strom classified PTTD based on clinical signs in combination with the pathological condition of the posterior tibial tendon [6]. We prefer the more comprehensive classification of Weinraub and Heilala as it aids in the development of a surgical treatment plan for PTTD (Table 22.1).

Management of Complications

Surgical intervention for the acquired flatfoot may fail for any number of reasons. Below we will outline the most common reasons for failure and provide management strategies for the most common complications.

Equinus

Equinus has been shown to be present in up to 96% of biomechanically induced foot pain [6]. Equinus has shown to be pathologic and present in the development of the pathologic flatfoot. Compensation for ankle equinus often results in midtarsal and subtalar pronation with a demonstrated three fold arch deforming force of the Achilles tendon over the posterior tibial tendon by Thordarson and colleagues [7]. Hibbs was the first to advocate a tendo-Achilles lengthening procedure as part of the treatment for pes planus deformity. An unaddressed equinus forces the calcaneus into a valgus position and limits subtalar joint inversion. Therefore, in order to get the calcaneus into a rectus position a posterior muscle group lengthening procedure should be considered. Failure to identify the equinus component when surgically reconstructing the symptomatic flatfoot predisposes the surgeon to less than desirable results.

Undercorrection

While there are many options for surgical reconstruction of PTTD refractory to conservative care one of the most common complications encountered is undercorrection of the

Table 22.1 Algorithmic approach to posterior tibial tendon dysfunction

	Grade (dictates osseous procedures)		
	Grade A, no deformity	Grade B, reducible deformity (pre-existing or acquired)	Grade C, rigid deformity
Stage (Dictates soft tissue procedures)	No osseous procedures	Joint sparing osseous	Selected arthrodesis
Stage 1 Acute inflammation, tendinitis with minimal tendinosis	Tenosynovectomy Possible augmentation of static soft tissue support	Tenosynovectomy Augmentation of static soft tissue support Evans versus medial displacement osteotomy	
Stage 2 Tendinosis with medial attenuation and insufficiency of soft tissue static and dynamic stabilizers	Medial debridement Augmentation of static stabilizers FDL transfer versus Kidner	Medial debridement Augmentation FDL versus Kidner Evans versus medial displacement calcaneal osteotomy	Selective arthrodesis Selective augmentation
Stage 3 Advanced attenuation or rupture of tendon or medial supportive structures	Medial debridement Augmentation of static stabilizers Tendon replacement via transfer, interposition, or grafting	Medial debridement Tendon replacement via transfer, interposition, or graft Evans versus medial displacement osteotomy	Selective arthrodesis Selective augmentation Selective replacement

Deformities are graded as: no planar deformity (A), reducible planar deformity (B), or rigid, non-reducible deformity (C). Grading dictates which type of osseous procedure, if any, to perform. The continuum of soft tissue pathology from acute tenosynovitis, to frank rupture, is stage. Staging dictates which soft tissue procedures are to be performed. The combining of the Grade and Stage leads to a comprehensive treatment algorithm. All require evaluation for, and correction of, any equinus deformity

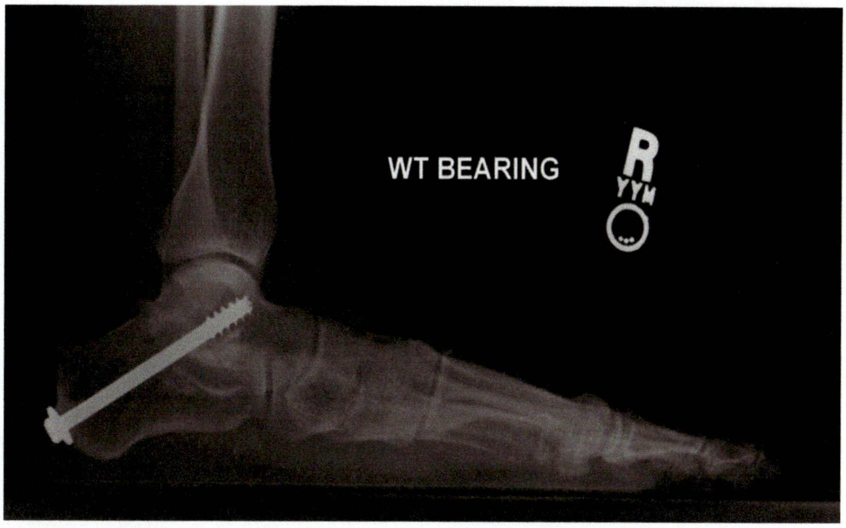

Fig. 22.1 A 48-year-old female with isolated subtalar fusion with continued pain and under correction with anterior break in cyma line and negative Mearys angle

deformity. Undercorrection can occur with joint sparing as well as joint destructive procedures. Failure to correct the deformity leads to continued pain and disability and further progression of PTTD. Identifying all planes of deformity is important in the reconstruction of PTTD.

Undercorrection in the transverse plane can lead to continued pain along the posterior tibial tendon and lateral impingement of the subtalar joint (Fig. 22.1). Procedures commonly used for the correction of transverse plane deformity focus on lengthening of the lateral column. This is commonly approached through either an Evans osteotomy or calcaneocuboid distraction arthrodesis (CCJ) (Fig. 22.2).

In situ/undercorrected triple arthrodesis of a stage IIIC PTTD does not correct for any deformity and often leads to continued pain and disability. In situ fusion is often multiplanar and results in a post-operative foot that is malaligned and stiff. Revision of an in situ arthrodesis often requires takedown of the existing fusion and techniques to realign the hindfoot in a rectus position. Multiple examples can be seen below on management strategies for malaligned double or triple arthrodesis.

When confronted with a "mal-aligned in-situ" arthrodesis requiring revision, the authors have had good success with an intra-operative protocol that entails initial takedown of the previous fusion sites, followed by a realignment lateral column lengthening (either Evans or CCJ distraction) that essentially "dials in" the correction in all three planes in the same manner a virgin lateral column lengthening procedure does. The talonavicular and subtalar joints are then fixated in this new revised alignment (Fig. 22.3).

Surgical approach for an end stage PTTD typically involves doing a triple or double arthrodesis. Traditionally a triple arthrodesis is approached through a lateral primary incision. Joint resection occurs laterally as well as positioning the foot for final alignment and fixation. The end stage PTTD that requires triple or double arthrodesis will have a hindfoot valgus and surgical resection laterally can make it hard to place the foot into correct alignment and avoid a valgus malalignment. The author routinely performs a medial approach—double arthrodesis for end stage PTTD (Fig. 22.4). This allows adequate correction of the valgus component of the hindfoot through medial joint resection. Astion and colleagues have shown that after isolated arthrodesis of the talonavicular and subtalar joints there is no motion left in the calcaneocuboid joint [8, 9].

Lateral Column Lengthening Complications

When addressing transverse plane deformities through lateral column lengthening procedures there are a number of complications that can occur. Evans osteotomy is a calcaneal osteotomy performed through the anterior aspect of the calcaneus utilizing either an allograft of autograft as a wedge to elongate the calcaneus. The same principle is applied with a CCJ arthrodesis with the exception that this is a joint destructive procedure. Both procedures involve lengthening the lateral column to correct for transverse plane deformity associated with PTTD.

Graft subsidence is a cause of undercorrection when performing an Evans osteotomy or CCJ arthrodesis (Fig. 22.5a, b). If subsidence does occur, performing revision lateral column procedures is acceptable but utilizing adequate fixation is preferred to avoid the complication again. Locked plating techniques to bridge the osteotomy can be performed for stabilization and successful union (Fig. 22.5c, d).

Complications with the Evans osteotomy occur with capital fragment displacement/rotation, non-union as the graft doesn't incorporate into the calcaneus, and graft subsidence. The author frequently utilizes provisional fixation when performing the osteotomy through the capital fragment to avoid displacement. As the graft is typically press fit, fixation is often not required but often utilized to avoid this complication. Multiple fixation

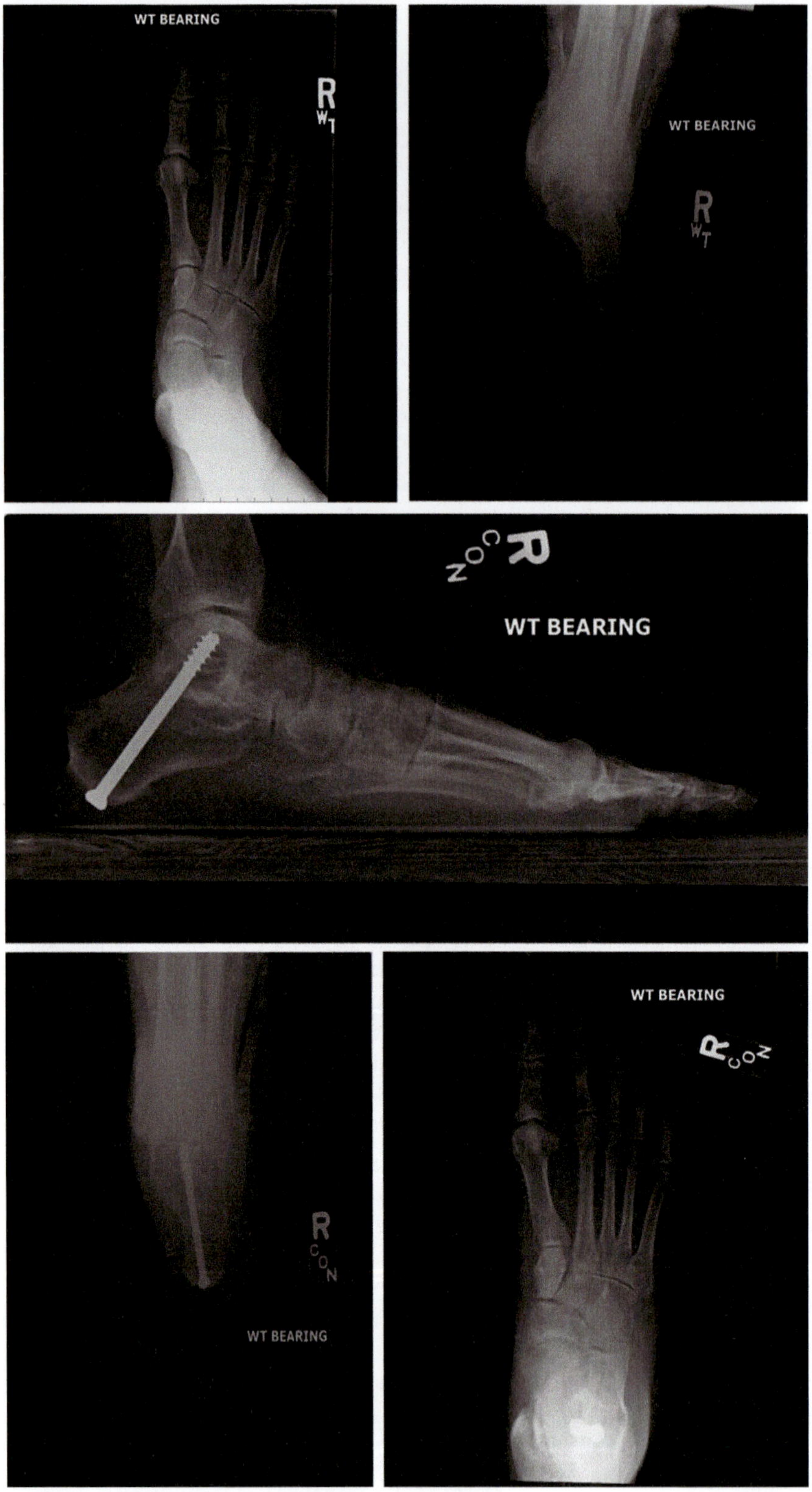

Fig. 22.2 Revision subtalar fusion with Evans osteotomy to correct for transverse plane deformity. Note straight lateral column, rectus heel calcaneal alignment, and normal Mearys angle. (Photos courtesy of G. Weinraub)

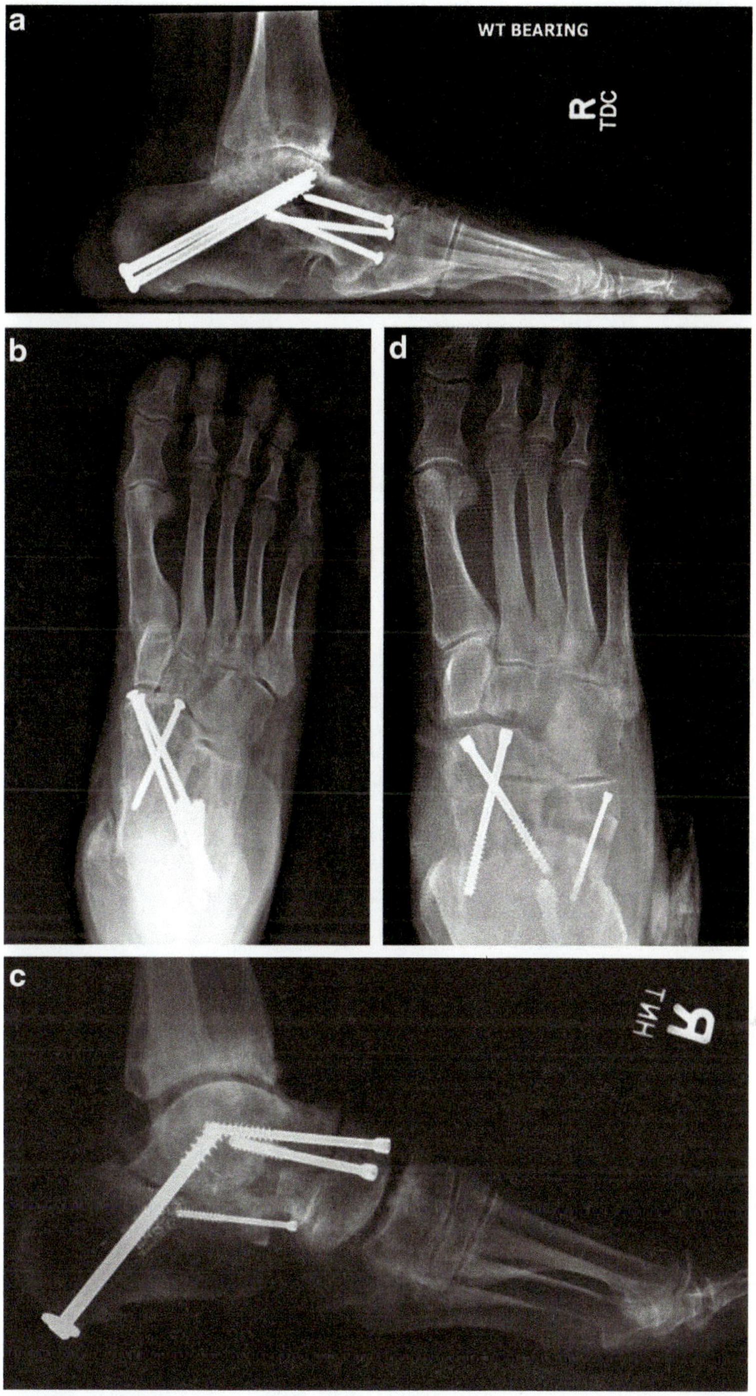

Fig. 22.3 (**a**, **b**) Preoperative mal-aligned in situ fusion. (**c, d**). Correction via "take down" of previous fusion sites to mobilize entire hindfoot complex. An Evans osteotomy with allograft was used to lengthen the lateral column to affect "triplane" correction with subsequent fusion of the STJ and TNJ. These are immediate post-op radiographs to illustrate the powerful restorative potential of the Evans osteotomy. (Photos courtesy of G. Weinraub)

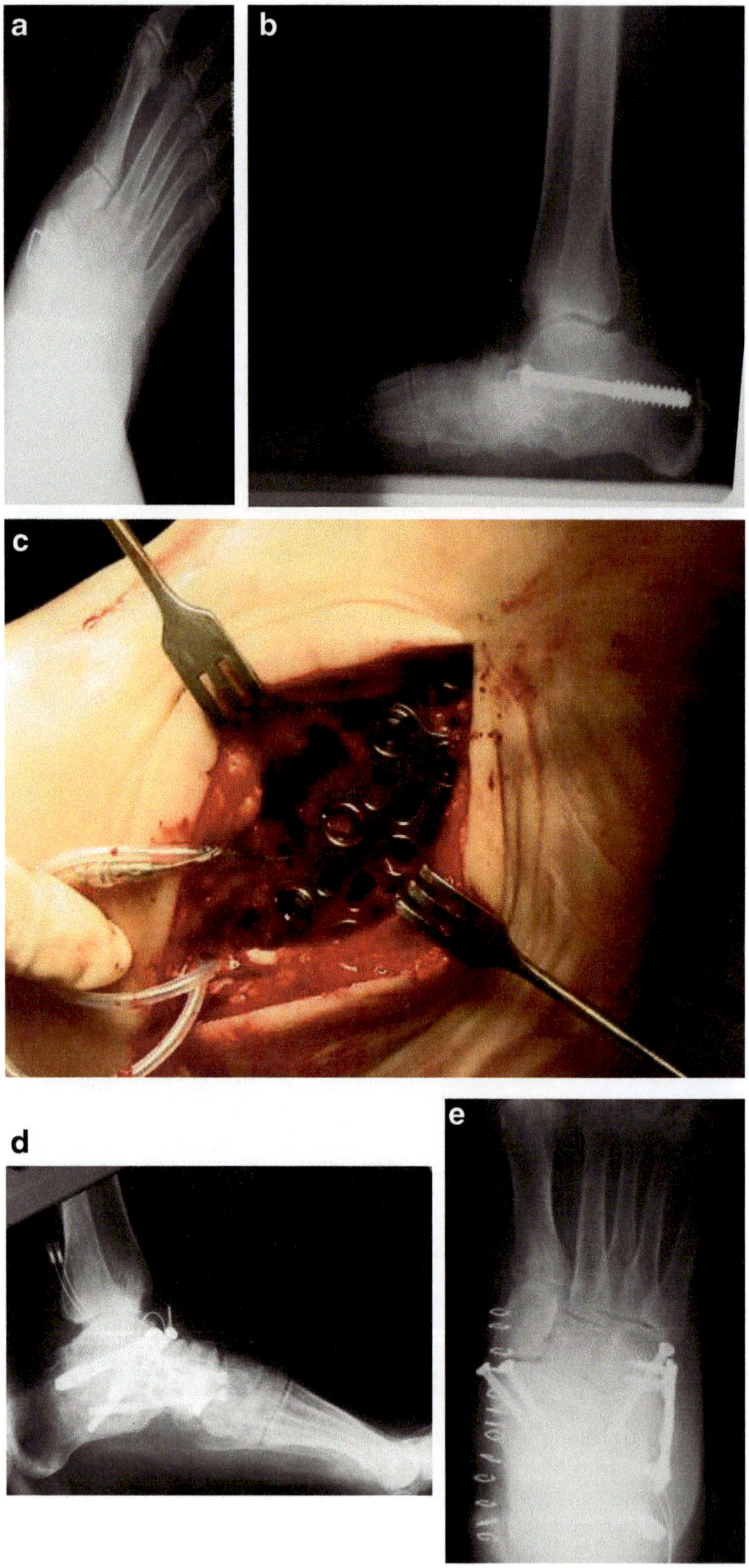

Fig. 22.4 (**a**, **b**) In situ triple arthrodesis for PTTD (Pre op) (Photos courtesy of G. Weinraub). (**c**) This patient underwent revision triple arthrodesis with CCJ distraction arthrodesis using cervical locking plate. (**d**, **e**) Post-operative radiographs showing revision triple arthrodesis with CCJ distraction arthrodesis (Photos courtesy of G. Weinraub)

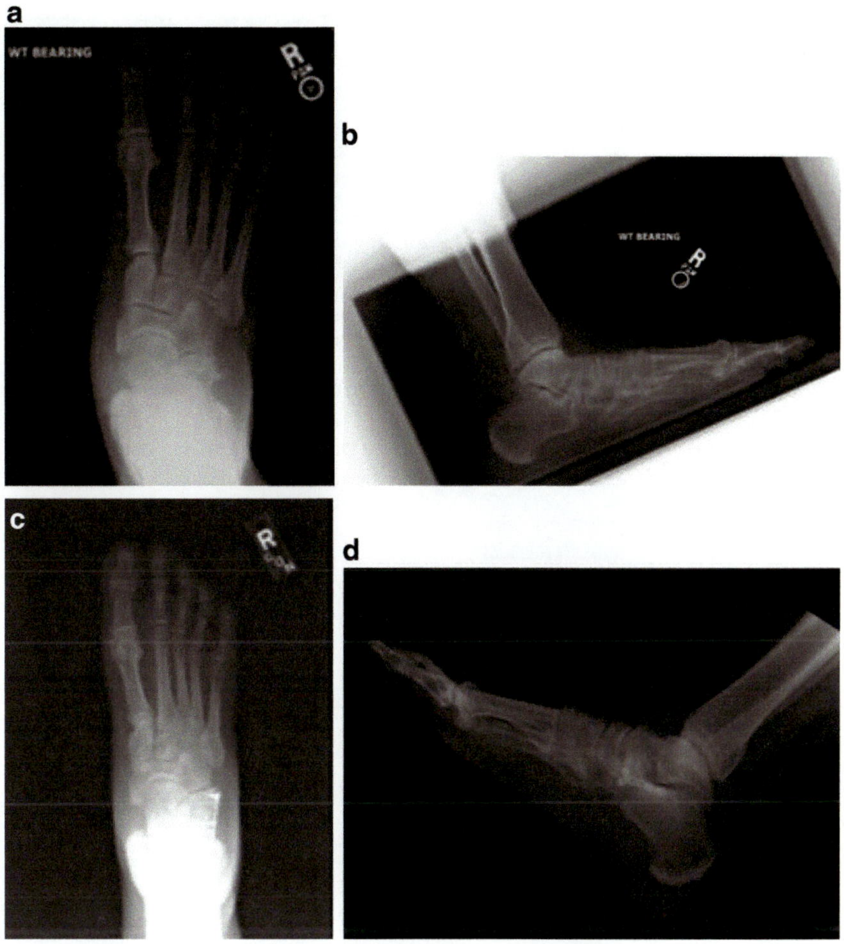

Fig. 22.5 (**a**, **b**) Graft subsidence due to non-compliance. (**c**, **d**) Graft revision with new allograft and plate fixation

options are available for fixation of the Evans osteotomy including K wire fixation, single screw options, and plate fixation. Failure to avoid capital fragment displacement or rotation can result in incongruency of the calcaneocuboid joint and lead to painful degenerative arthrosis [10] (Fig. 22.6).

A common complication shared between these two procedures involves non-union of the graft at either the osteotomy site for the Evans or non-union at the fusion site when performing a CCJ arthrodesis (Fig. 22.6). Both allograft and autograft have been utilized to accomplish this procedure. Non-union rates have been studied between the two procedures and historically the CCJ arthrodesis has had higher non-union rates up to 20% when compared to the Evans osteotomy with non-union rates around 5% [11–14]. Studies have also shown comparable rates of fusion when using tri-cortical allograft versus autograft. According to Grier et al., they showed a union rate of 70% when using autograft from the iliac crest versus 94% union rate when using allograft and protein rich plasma associated with the graft for lateral column lengthening procedures of either Evans osteotomy or CCJ arthrodesis [15].

Medial Column Complications

When surgically reconstructing a symptomatic flatfoot often a medial column deformity can exist or progress with a long standing flatfoot. With surgical realignment of the flatfoot one needs to address the medial column after positioning of the hindfoot and correction of the lateral column. Compensation of hindfoot valgus through the medial column often happens through the 1st Metatarsal cuneiform joint (MCJ) or Naviculocuneiform joint. This can typically be indentified on a lateral radiograph. Prior to performing a surgical reconstruction, identifying if the medial column deformity is reducible can be achieved through recreation of the Windlass mechanism and a lateral radiograph can be taken to see if the sagittal plane faulting resolves (Jacks test) [16]. By defining the level of the medial column faulting then one can decide which procedure to employ for correction of forefoot varus. Naviculocuneiform arthrodesis, 1st MCJ, or cotton osteotomies have been described for the correction for residual forefoot varus.

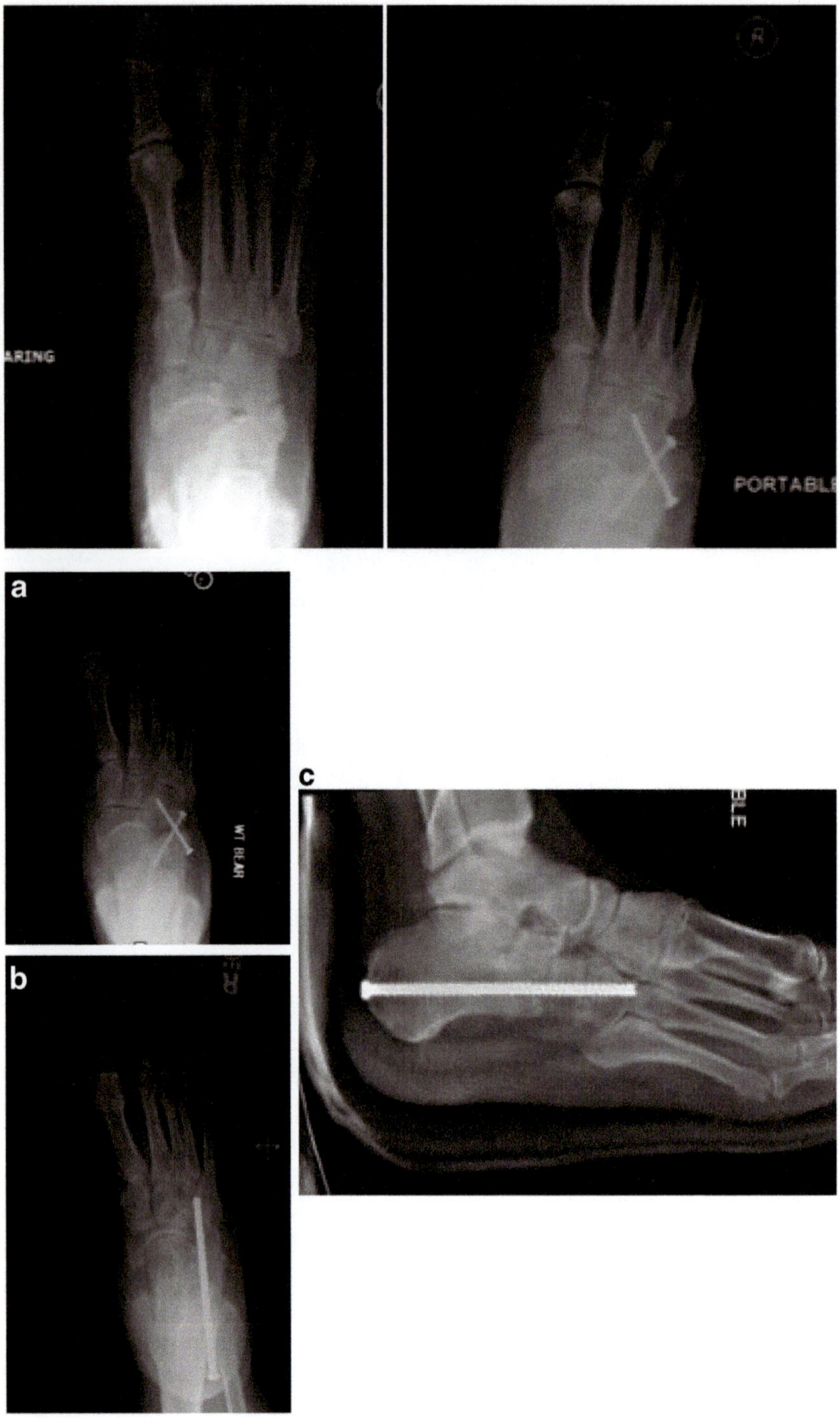

Fig. 22.6 Evans revision resulted in CCJ arthrosis which was converted to a CCJ arthrodesis. (**a**) CCJ arthrodesis non-union. (**b**, **c**) Revision CCJ arthrodesis after above non-union. (Photos courtesy of G. Weinraub)

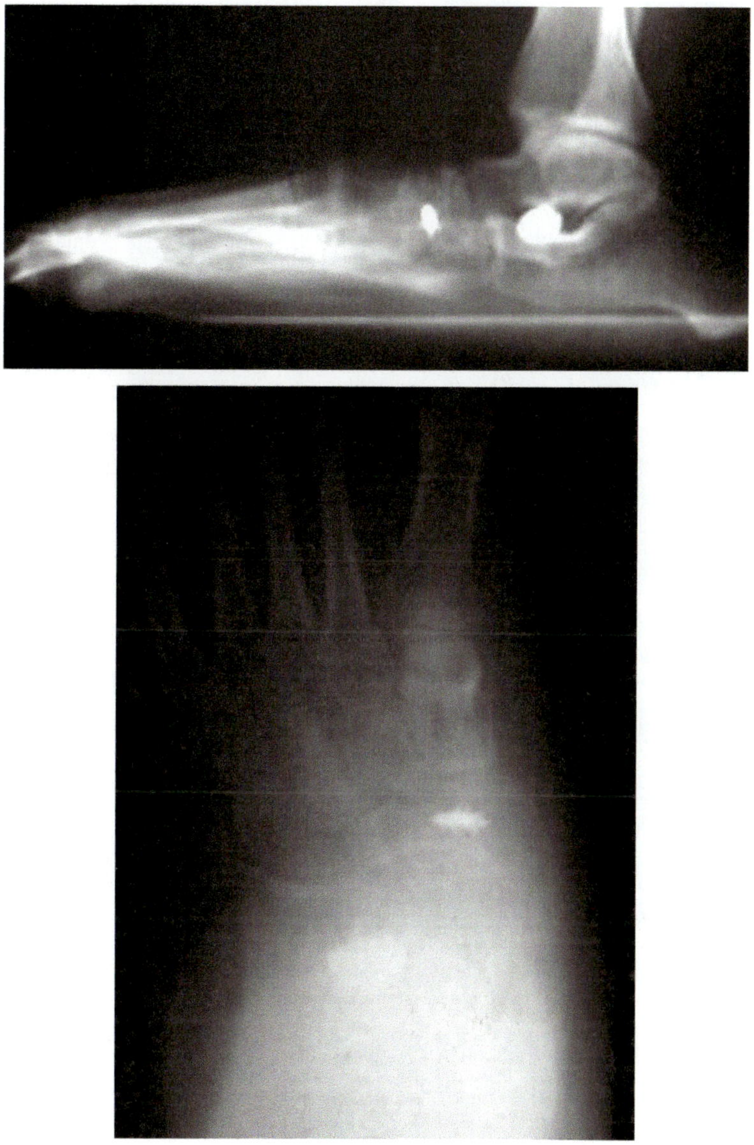

Fig. 22.7 Teenager that underwent Kidner with arthroeresis with continued spastic pes planovalgus (Photos courtesy of G. Weinraub)

Failed Arthroeresis

Subtalar arthroeresis has been used for the correction of hindfoot valgus by blocking subtalar pronation. There have been an increasing number of surgical failures due to arthroeresis used as single procedures for the correction of symptomatic flatfoot deformity. The ease of the procedure has lulled many surgeons into using this device for all deformities without any regard for ancillary flatfoot procedures (Fig. 22.7). Pain and cystic formation have been implicated as complications associated with subtalar arthroeresis. In failed cases with associated sinus tarsi pain, subtalar joint arthrosis, or peri-implant cyst formation a subtalar arthrodesis may be the revision procedure of choice [17] (Fig. 22.8).

Deltoid Insufficiencies, Missed Stage 4

As PTTD progresses the static soft tissue structures continue to be affected and ultimately will progress to yield talar tilt with subsequent valgus ankle joint deformity. The deltoid becomes incompetent and can no longer resist tibiotalar tilting. Harper demonstrated that sectioning of the deep and superficial deep components of the deltoid ligament produces an average of 14 degrees of valgus talar tilting [18]. Early in the development of the Stage IV PTTD the valgus ankle is reducible with minimal tibiotalar arthritis and surgical reconstruction of the medial soft tissue structures is possible. As it further progress the ankle becomes rigid more arthritis develops and reconstruction for ankle preservation is often not

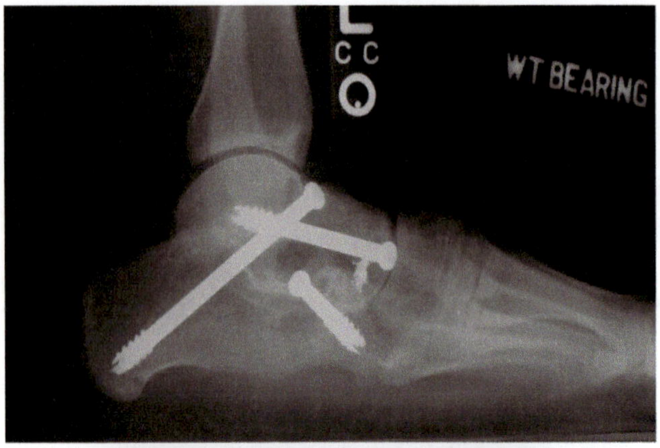

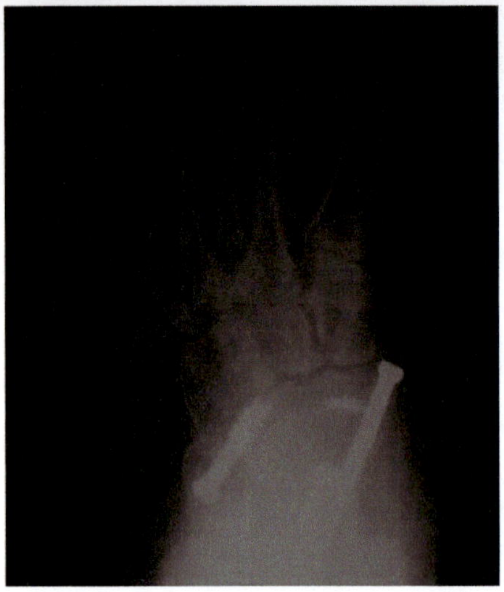

Fig. 22.8 Intra-operatively patient was noted to have large extensive STJ posterior facet arthritis, as such the patient converted to a triple arthrodesis

possible. Determining if an ankle valgus is reducible or not can be demonstrated under fluoroscopy with a varus thrust and realignment of the talus within the mortise.

Recognizing the valgus ankle component when evaluating patients is important. PTTD Stage IV A (reducible ankle valgus) can be managed with selective hindfoot fusions based on pathology but the primary operation for realignment of the ankle joint is reconstruction of the deltoid ligament complex. Numerous reports of deltoid ligament reconstruction have been reported. Autograft or allograft reconstruction is favored over direct repair of the tissues, as direct repair has been shown to ultimately fail due to the poor quality of tissue during the Stage IV disease. When Stage IV PTTD is unrecognized, patients have poorer outcomes and continued disability with pain. Management of complications tends to be difficult and revision surgery is often necessary with missed Stage IV PTTD.

Position of a triple arthrodesis or double arthrodesis needs to be carefully evaluated as the cause of failure of the deltoid ligament and talar tilt. Malunion of a valgus hindfoot is one of the largest contributing factors following a triple arthrodesis [19]. It has been shown that a triple arthrodesis fused in valgus or in situ position will lead to a 76% increase strain on the deltoid ligament complex [20].

An example of a revision Stage IV PTTD is outlined below (Fig. 22.9). The patient underwent ankle fusion for ankle arthritis but the acquired flatfoot was unrecognized as the driving force for the development of the ankle arthritis. They had successful fusion of the ankle joint but the foot continued to swing into valgus as the flatfoot was not addressed the fibula was taken down and no longer able to act as a strut. Clinical and radiographs can be followed for the management of this patient and reconstruction of their deformity.

More commonly is the unrecognized Stage IV A PTTD where the patient undergoes triple arthrodesis for end stage PTTD. The foot will be well aligned underneath the long axis of the leg but do to the laxity in the medial structures the foot can continue to drift into valgus through the ankle joint. If the ankle valgus is identified and there is significant arthritis within the ankle joint, ankle replacement surgery versus pantalar arthrodesis/Tibiotalar arthrodesis (TTC) may be considered. While pantalar arthrodesis/TTC is successful in realigning Stage IV PTTD, there have been many studies identifying the higher risk of non-union, residual pain, increased energy expenditure and decreased function with TTC and pantalar arthrodesis [21, 22]. More recently many authors have proposed double or triple arthrodesis combined with total ankle arthroplasty. Lewis and colleagues recently have shown improvement in pain and functional outcome with ipsilateral hindfoot fusions combined with TAR. Long-term follow-up for these patients is needed as the average follow-up was an average of 3.2 years but shows promising results for Stage IV B PTTD [23]. Survivorship of the implant depends on the realignment of the hindfoot complex with or without deltoid reconstruction [24–26].

Summary PTTD is a complex multiplanar pathology with multiple options for surgical reconstruction. Due to the varying number of surgical procedures and approaches for addressing the deformities associated with PTTD the surgeon must be prepared to encounter complications associated with surgical reconstruction.

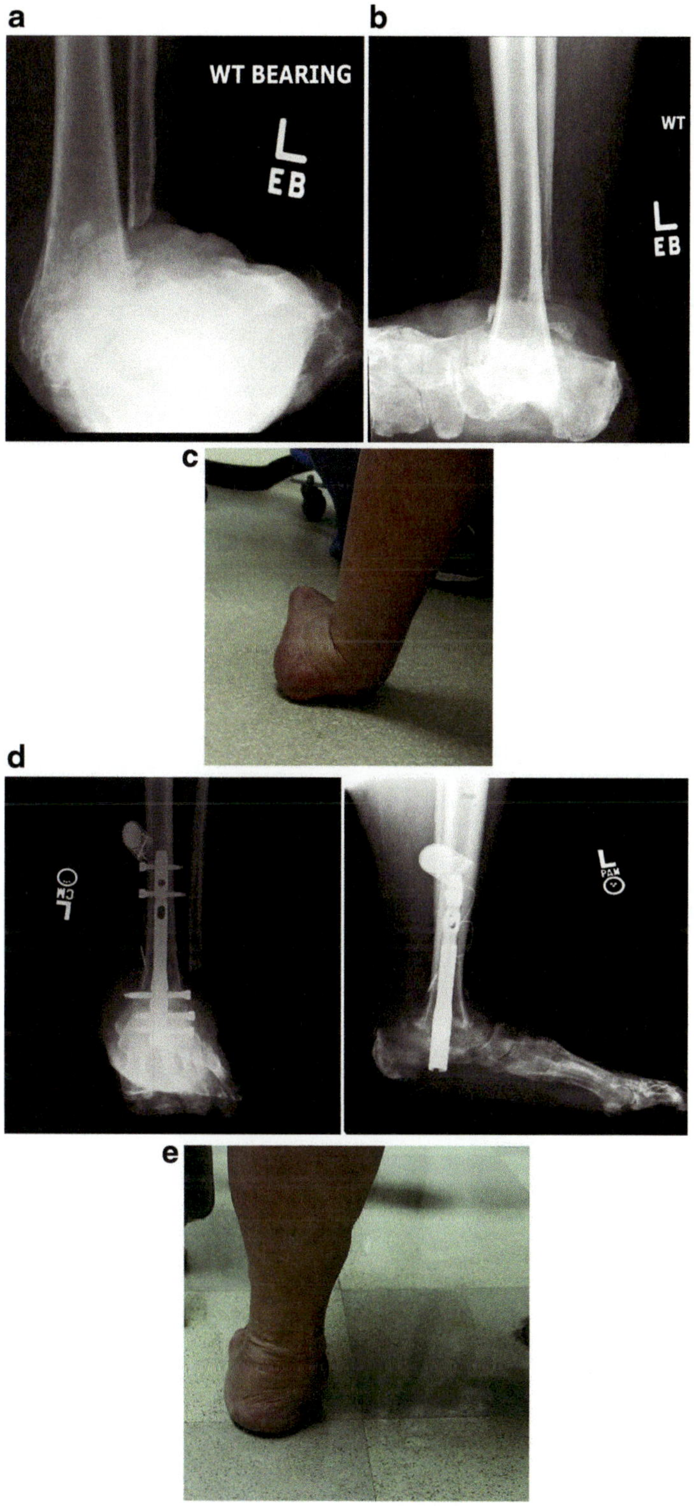

Fig. 22.9 (**a**, **b**) Example of Missed Stage IV PTTD. Patient underwent successful ankle fusion but PTTD was unrecognized. (Photos courtesy of G. Weinraub). (**c**) Clinical photo of Missed Stage IV PTTD with ankle fusion. (Photos courtesy of G. Weinraub). (**d**, **c**) Post-operative radiographs with salvage tibiotalocalcaneal arthrodesis using intramedullary nailing technique. (Photos courtesy of G. Weinraub). (**e**) Clinical photo demonstrating rectus foot and ankle alignment following salvage procedure (Photos courtesy of G. Weinraub)

References

1. Weinraub GM, Saraiya MJ. Adult flatfoot/posterior tibial tendon dysfunction: classification and treatment. Clin Podiatr Med Surg. 2002;19(3):345–70.
2. Weinraub GM, Heilala MA. Adult flatfoot/posterior tibial tendon dysfunction: outcomes analysis of surgical treatment utilizing an algorithmic approach. J Foot Ankle Surg. 2000;39(6):359–64.
3. Root ML, Orien WP, Weed JH. Normal and abnormal function of the foot: Clinical Biomechanics.
4. Myerson MS. Adult acquired flatfoot deformity: treatment of dysfunction of the posterior tibial tendon. J Bone Joint Surg. 1996;78-A(5):780–92.
5. Conti S, Michelson J, Jahss MD. Rupture of the posterior tibial tendon. J Bone Joint Surg. 1990;72A:884–8.
6. Hill RS. Ankle Equinus: prevalence and linkage to common foot pathology. J Am Podiatr Med Assoc. 1995;85:295–300.
7. Thordarson DB, Schmotzer H, Chon J, et al. Dynamic support of the human longitudinal arch. A biomechanical evaluation. Clin Orthop Relat Res. 1995;316:165–72.
8. Astion DJ, Deland JT, Otis JC, et al. Motion of the hindfoot after simulated arthrodesis. J Bone Joint Surg. 1997;79-A(2):241–6.
9. Weinraub GM, Schuberth JM, Lee M, Rush S, Ford L, Neufeld J. Isolated medial incisional approach to subtalar and talonavicular arthrodesis. J Foot Ankle Surg. 2010;49:326–30.
10. Mosier-LaClair S, Pomeroy G, Manoli A. Operative treatment of the difficult stage 2 adult acquired flatfoot deformity. Foot Ankle Clin. 2001;6:95–119.
11. Toolan BC, Sangeorzan BJ, Hansen ST. Complex reconstruction for the treatment of dorsolateral peritalar subluxation of the foot. JBJS. 1999;81-A:1545–60.
12. Chi TD, Toolan BC, Sangeorzan BJ, Hansen ST. The lateral column lengthening and medial column stabiliztion procedures. CORR. 1999;365:81–90.
13. Conti SF, Wong TS. Osteolysis of structural autograft after calcaneocuboid distraction arthrodesis for stage II posterior tibial tendon dysfunction. Foot Ankle Int. 2002;23:521–9.
14. Hinterman B, Valderrabano V, Kundert HP. Lengthening of the lateral column and reconstruction of the medial soft tissue for treatment of acquired flatfoot deformity associated with insufficiency of the posterior tibial tendon. Foot Ankle Int. 1999;20:622–9.
15. Grier GM, Waling AK. The use of tricortical autograft vs allograft in lateral column lengthening for adult acquired flatfoot deformity: an analysis of union rates and complications. Foot Ankle Int. 2010;31:760–9.
16. Budny AM, Grossman JP. Naviculocuneiform arthrodesis. Clin Podiatr Med Surg. 2007;24:753–63.
17. Rockett AK, Magnum G, Mendicino SS. Bilateral intraosseous cystic formation in the talus: a complication of subtalar arthroereisis. J Foot Ankle Surg. 1998;37(5):421–5.
18. Harper MC. Deltoid ligament: an antatomical evaluation of function. Foot Ankle. 1987;8:19–22.
19. Bohay DR, Anderson JG. Stage IV posterior tibial tendon insufficiency: the tilted ankle. Foot Ankle Clin. 2003;8:619–36.
20. Resnick RB, Jahss MH, Choueka J, et al. Deltoid ligament forces after tibialis posterior tendon rupture: effects of triple arthrodesis an calcaneal displacement osteotomies. Foot Ankle Int. 1995;16:14–20.
21. Barrett GR, Meyer LC, Bray III EW, et al. Pantalar arthrodesis: a long-term follow-up. Foot Ankle. 1981;1:279–83.
22. Chou LB, Mann RA, Yaszay B, et al. Tibiotalocalcaneal arthrodesis. Foot Ankle Int. 2000;21:804–8.
23. Lewis J, Adams S, Queen R, et al. Outcomes after total ankle replacement in association with ipsilateral hindfoot arthrodesis. Foot Ankle Int. 2014;35(6):535–42.
24. Johnson KA, Strom DE. Tibialis posterior tendon insufficiency: diagnosis and treatment. Clin Orthop. 1989;239:197–206.
25. Frey C, Shereff M, Greenidge N. Vascularity of the posterior tibial tendon. J Bone Joint Surg Am. 1990;72:884–8.
26. Rush SM. Reconstructive options for failed flatfoot surgery. Clin Podiatr Med Surg. 2007;24:779–88.

Pes Cavovarus Surgery

23

Richard Derner

Overview

Surgical correction of the cavovarus foot deformity can be extremely challenging. Not only are you dealing with a very complex foot structure but also understanding the neurological etiology is critical to a successful outcome. Cavovarus deformity can be caused from either static contracture or dynamic contracture. When treating patients with dynamic contractures, where there is a progressive nature to the deformity, long-term outcomes are especially difficult to predict [1]. Static contractures, on the other hand, are easier to predict, and treatment is more straightforward. This chapter is intended to identify the crucial elements of procedure selection, discuss technical pearls for the commonly performed reconstructive procedures to prevent complications, and review specific complications and ways to manage them effectively.

Before delving into technical pearls and management of complications, it is important to attempt to define the deformity being discussed in this chapter. Although there is no universally accepted definition, the cavovarus foot can be described as a spectrum of foot shapes that all have a high arch in common. The more severe deformity is commonly fixed in position as opposed to the less affected non-fixed foot structure. The high arch may present with a variety of findings, such as a high calcaneal inclination angle in the hindfoot, plantarflexion of the forefoot, metatarsus adductus, or the apex of deformity within the midfoot [2].

The major components of a cavovarus foot structure are increased inclination, varus of the hindfoot, plantarflexion of the midfoot, and adduction and varus within the forefoot as noted on X-rays [2, 3] (Figs. 23.1, 23.2, 23.3, 23.4, and 23.5).

R. Derner (✉)
Past President, American College of Foot and Ankle Surgeons, Department of Orthopedics INOVA Fairfax Medical Campus, 3300 Gallows Road, Falls Church, VA 22042, USA
e-mail: Richd87@mac.com

Numerous means of classifying the cavovarus deformity have been devised throughout the years. These classification schemes have been based on the apex of the deformity, the reducibility of the deformity, the associated conditions with the deformity, and the etiology of the deformity [4–6]. All of these considerations have their merit in the optimal surgical management of the cavovarus foot.

A critical component to the management of the cavovarus foot deformity is understanding the neuromuscular imbalances that are present. This deformity has long been thought to stem from underlying neurological disorder and be a primary cause in the development of the cavus foot. Identifying the specific pattern of muscular imbalance is essential in the surgical management of patients with a cavovarus foot as osseous correction alone is often insufficient in preventing recurrence of the deformity. In some neuromuscular diseases, muscle strength progressively worsens, and not realizing the etiological factor at the time of surgery dooms the patient to ultimate failure and recurrence of the cavovarus foot deformity.

Surgical Decision Making

The determination of the ideal approach for surgical intervention is dependent upon several important considerations that should be identified during the preoperative evaluation: Where is the apex of the deformity? What type of cavovarus deformity is identified (i.e., forefoot cavus, midfoot cavus, global cavus)? What is the first ray position? Is this deformity fixed or non-fixed? Finally, and most importantly, it is imperative to identify all forces causing imbalance in the foot. A careful examination of all muscles acting on the foot will provide invaluable information on how to dynamically balance the cavovarus foot. Commonly, muscle testing will demonstrate overpowering of the tibialis anterior muscle by the peroneus longus muscle with a plantarflexed first ray and overpowering of the peroneus brevis muscle by the posterior tibial muscle in the varus foot deformity [4, 7, 8].

M.S. Lee, J.P. Grossman (eds.), *Complications in Foot and Ankle Surgery*, DOI 10.1007/978-3-319-53686-6_23

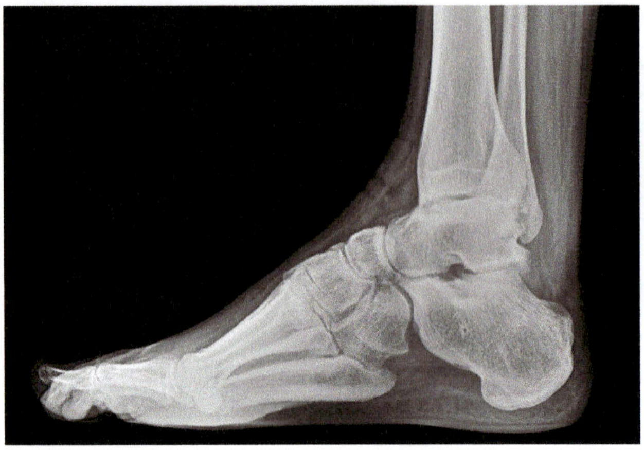

Fig. 23.1 Increase in calcaneal inclination (X-ray) angle

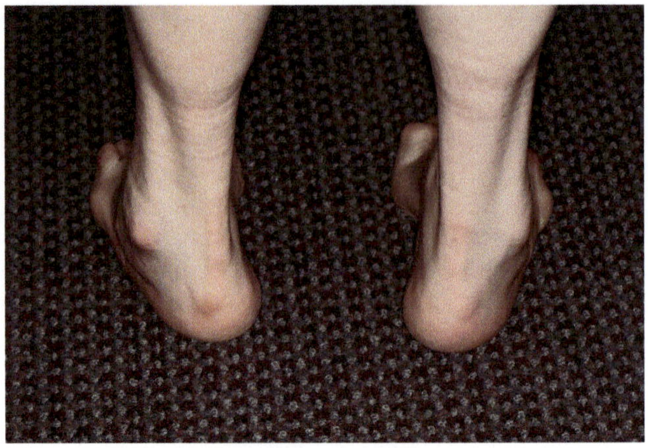

Fig. 23.4 Bilateral calcaneal varus (clinical)

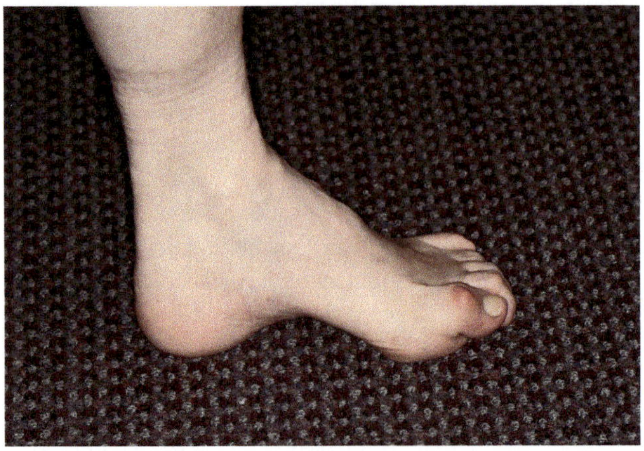

Fig. 23.2 Increase in calcaneal inclination angle (clinical)

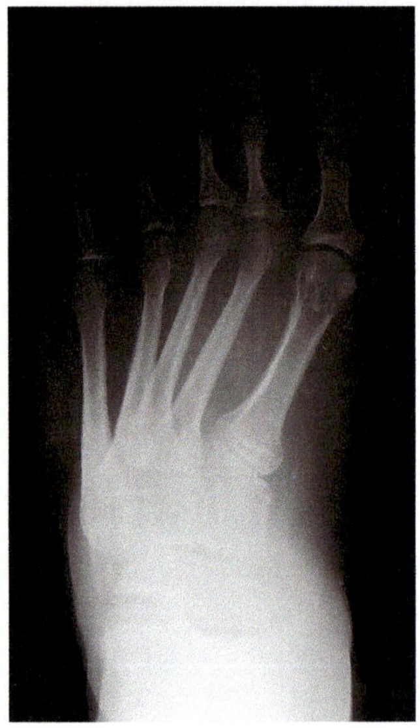

Fig. 23.5 Metatarsus adductus

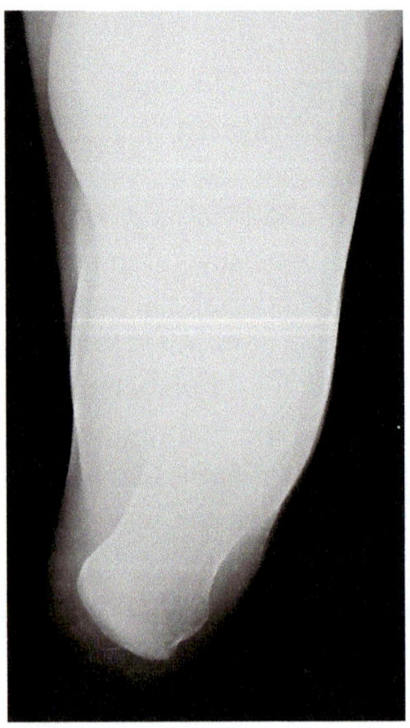

Fig. 23.3 Calcaneal varus (X-ray)

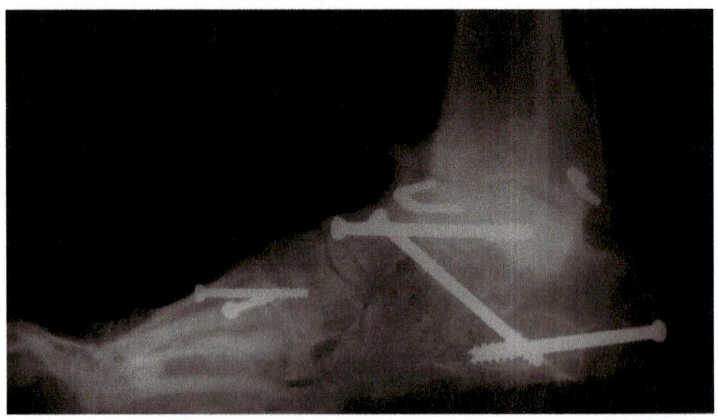

Fig. 23.6 Long-term follow-up: triple arthrodesis with severe adjacent-joint arthritis

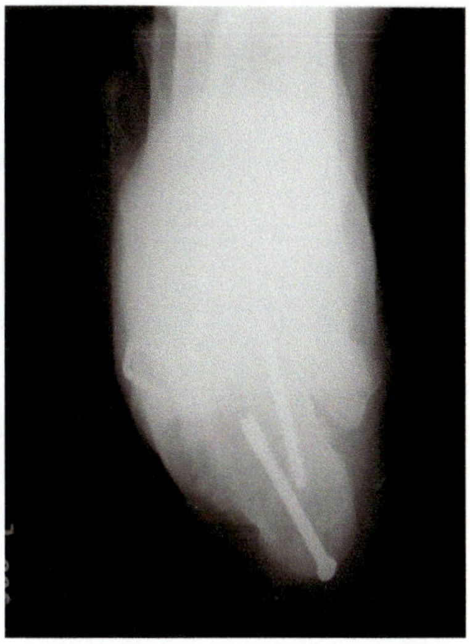

Fig. 23.7 Long-term follow-up: triple arthrodesis with ankle varus and recurrence of the varus deformity

Once this information has been ascertained, surgical correction is largely based on the utilization of both osseous and soft tissue procedures. The ideal combination of osseous and soft tissue procedures has not been identified for each pathological condition. It would be impossible to formulate such an algorithm due to the variation in severity of deformity, difference in patient anatomy, etiology of the deformity, and other varying factors. There is no single procedure or combination of procedures that has been found to offer reliably good long-term results across the cavovarus landscape. However, there are some basic concepts which much be considered.

Generally, in the milder or non-fixed cavovarus deformity, lesser metatarsophalangeal joint releases with digital arthrodesis are indicated along with soft tissue procedures such as the Jones tenosuspension and Hibbs tendon transfer. Osteotomies such as a dorsiflexory wedge osteotomy of the first metatarsal are indicated to reduce the plantarflexion deformity of the first ray [9–12].

In the more severe, fixed deformities demonstrating hindfoot involvement, calcaneal and midfoot osteotomies in conjunction with soft tissue procedures such as tendon transfers are often utilized. Commonly performed osseous surgical procedures within the rearfoot and midfoot include the Dwyer calcaneal osteotomy and Cole midfoot osteotomy. In the severe, fixed cavovarus deformity, calcaneal and midfoot osteotomies as well as midfoot and hindfoot arthrodesis are indicated [4, 13–16].

The question of when arthrodesis is indicated is a difficult one to answer. Preserving the viability of hindfoot and midfoot joints is important for sustained symptomatic relief and avoidance of additional surgical procedures (Figs. 23.6 and 23.7). It is accepted that triple arthrodesis ought to be avoided as long-term follow-up on the triple arthrodesis in several studies has demonstrated ankle pain and the development of premature arthritis in more than half of operated feet [17]. Therefore, triple arthrodesis is felt to serve better as a salvage procedure for cases with severe arthritis or in cases of recurrence following failed corrective osteotomies [18–21]. The pantalar arthrodesis is also reserved as a salvage procedure when no other options exist for these patients.

Steindler Stripping

Indications and Planning

Contracture of the plantar fascia and plantar intrinsic muscular is invariably present in the moderate to severe cavovarus foot. First described in 1920, Steindler stripping is complete release of the plantar fascia, flexor digitorum brevis muscle, and abductor halluces [22, 23]. This procedure is unlikely to be performed as an isolated procedure, as it is usually followed by bony correction of structural deformity. Release of the plantar fascia is a pivotal part of the correction of the cavus foot. It is this reason that a Steindler stripping is the first procedure performed on a cavus reconstruction. Mobilization of the rearfoot and reduction of the deformity after osteotomy are much easier if this release is performed.

Contraindications/Limitations

A Steindler stripping is almost always never performed alone, but in combination of one or more osseous procedures. It should be performed only on the severe cavovarus deformity, but not on the mild one. In less severe cases, release of the plantar soft tissue structures would not be necessary to allow for lowering of the longitudinal arch.

Technique, Pearls and Pitfalls

Incision placement for the Steindler stripping should be based on the other procedures required to correct the cavus deformity. When performed in combination with the Dwyer calcaneal osteotomy, the procedure can be performed by minimally elongating the lateral incision to meet the inferior border of the calcaneus. A curved mayo scissor is preferred with the curvature faced proximally to avoid the neurovascular structures as the muscle and ligament are transected (Fig. 23.8). Care must be taken to avoid cutting the skin on the medial side of the foot. Otherwise a painful scar may result. This modification of the original Steindler procedure is technically easy to perform as well as reproducible results.

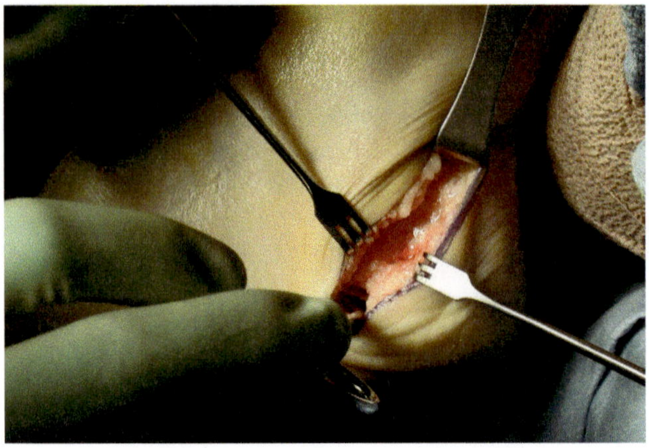

Fig. 23.8 Plantar fascia visualized through extended Dwyer incision

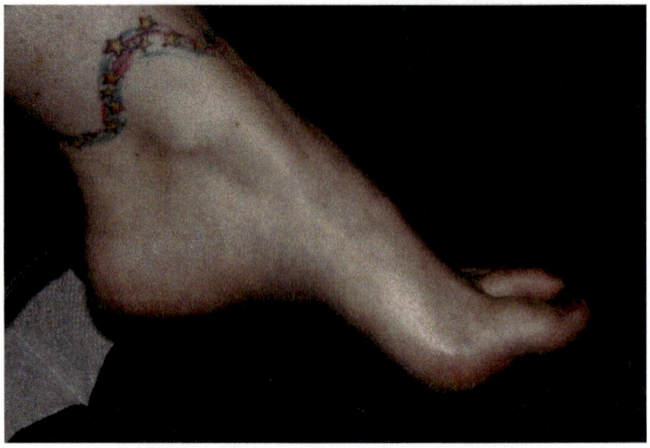

Fig. 23.9 Fixed forefoot deformity causing pseudoequinus with weight bearing

If a calcaneal osteotomy is not indicated, the procedure is performed through a medial longitudinal incision adjacent to the calcaneus and along the glabrous junction.

One of the most common pitfalls of the procedure is incomplete release of the fascia. If performed through the lateral approach, it is imperative that the medial band and the abductor hallucis be completely transected. Injury to any neurovascular structure is unlikely with this procedure, but care must be taken. Modifications have been reported to help avoid damaging the plantar neurovascular [24, 25]. Regardless of the technique performed, a complete release must be performed to help mobilize the rearfoot in severe cavovarus feet.

Achilles Tendon Lengthening

Indications

Lengthening of the Achilles tendon is performed when there is a gastroc-soleus equinus diagnosed on examination. The Achilles tendon is not necessarily strong but contracted in patients with cavovarus deformity. Muscle testing and charger lateral ankle (forced maximum dorsiflexion view) radiographs should be obtained to confirm a contracted Achilles tendon and adequate talar excursion if the tendon is to be lengthened. If the talus is already maximally dorsiflexed within the ankle joint, no type of posterior soft tissue release or lengthening will allow additional dorsiflexion of the talus in the ankle.

A cavovarus deformity normally does not benefit from an Achilles tendon lengthening. Performing an Achilles tendon lengthening, thus resulting in its weakening, can in fact make the cavus foot more severe. The heel cord is resisting further contracture to the high-arched foot. Patient presenting with a presumed tight heel cord most often has a pseudoequinus deformity, which makes your physical exam that more important [26]. The fixed plantarflexed position of the forefoot upon the rearfoot causes the talus to dorsiflex within the ankle joint in order to get the forefoot on the same plane as the rearfoot (Fig. 23.9). Azmaipairashvili et al. noted the heel cord may appear tight but the os calcis is in calcaneus and should never be part of the corrective procedure [27] (Fig. 23.10).

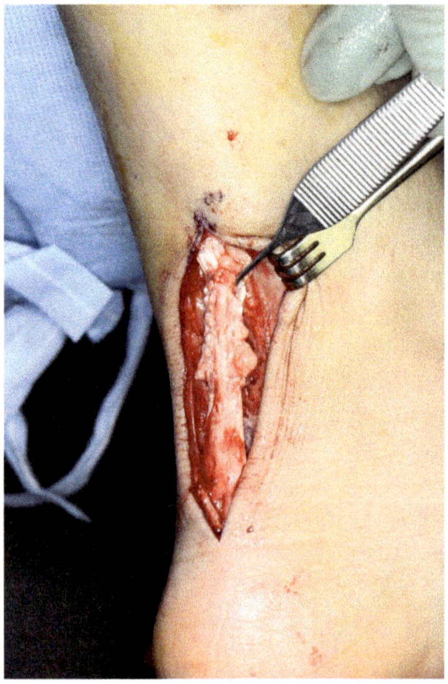

Fig. 23.10 TAL open technique

Contraindications/Limitations

As mentioned, adequate motion about the ankle joint must be present when lengthening the Achilles tendon. Pseudoequinus should be corrected prior to attempting the Achilles lengthening or overlengthening can result. Specifically, dorsiflexion of the forefoot/midfoot will functionally plantarflex the talus within the ankle joint and thus improve ankle joint range of motion. This may prevent the need to lengthen the heel cord. It is also important to evaluate for a bony block equinus. Talar neck abutment dorsally against the tibia will prevent any improvement to the dorsiflexion range of motion about the ankle with lengthening of the Achilles tendon. This would potentially create a calcaneus gait and worsen the already cavus foot [28, 29].

Technique, Pearls and Pitfalls

The Achilles tendon lengthening can be performed either open or percutaneous. The advantage to the open "Z" technique allows for a more precise degree of lengthening. The lengthening is obtained by bisecting the tendon anterior to posterior and exiting proximally posteriorly and anteriorly distally. The bisection must be long enough to allow for overlap of the tendon after released and held to the correct length. The Achilles is repaired with a lateral trap suture technique with nonabsorbable 2-0 suture. This open technique can result in overlengthening and rupture, but both are rare complications. Care must be taken to not perform this procedure until after the osseous work has been completed within the foot to prevent excessive lengthening or undercorrection.

Percutaneous TAL or triple hemisection is another option with the tendon being cut three times, two finger breaths apart with the tendon being cut from the center medialward then lateralward, and finally a medial hemisection through the tendon. Care must be made to cut this correctly or an overlengthening/calcaneal gait is a distinct possibility. If too little is cut, then undercorrection is very probable.

Management of Complication

The most common complication of an open TAL is wound complications. Care must be taken to perform this procedure in an atraumatic technique. Wound care and other conservative measure are often times enough to solve this problem.

Overcorrection of the Achilles tendon lengthening is a potentially devastating problem for the patient with cavovarus or most any foot structure. Once conservative care including extensive physical therapy fails to resolve or strengthen this tendon adequately, surgical intervention is required. An open technique to structurally shorten this tendon alone or in combination with an FHL tendon or peroneal tendon transfer should be considered [28, 29]. Unfortunately, a heel ulcer (Figs. 23.11 and 23.12) may result from overlengthening, ultimately requiring an ankle joint arthrodesis to resolve this problem.

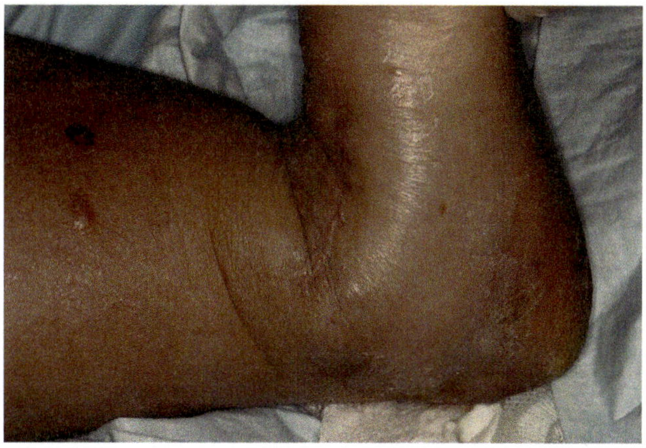

Fig. 23.11 Calcaneal gait following Achilles tendon lengthening

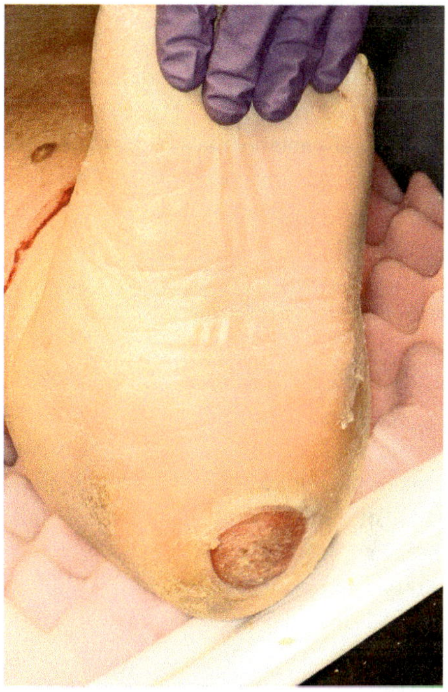

Fig. 23.12 Calcaneal gait with plantar heel ulcer

Tibialis Anterior Tendon Transfer

Indications

The tibialis anterior tendon creates a dynamic supination force to the forefoot with an unopposed pull from the weakened evertors. The indication of the tibialis anterior transfer is to balance the inversion/eversion pull of the forefoot and/or remove the deforming force of the inverted foot.

Transfer of the tibialis anterior in whole or part (split tibialis anterior tendon transfer or STATT) can be part of the treatment for the varus component in the cavovarus foot deformity. It is imperative to determine the underlying etiology of the cavovarus foot structure since specific conditions result in ultimate weakness of the tibialis anterior muscle [30, 31]. Relying on this tendon in the long term may result in minimal improvement or recurrence of the varus deformity. Shapiro and Bresnan noted that weakness over time makes transfer of this tendon inadvisable [32].

It is rare that the tibialis anterior tendon transfer is performed as an isolated procedure. Bony and soft tissue procedures are often necessary for successful correction due to the complicated nature of the deformity [4, 6, 30, 33].

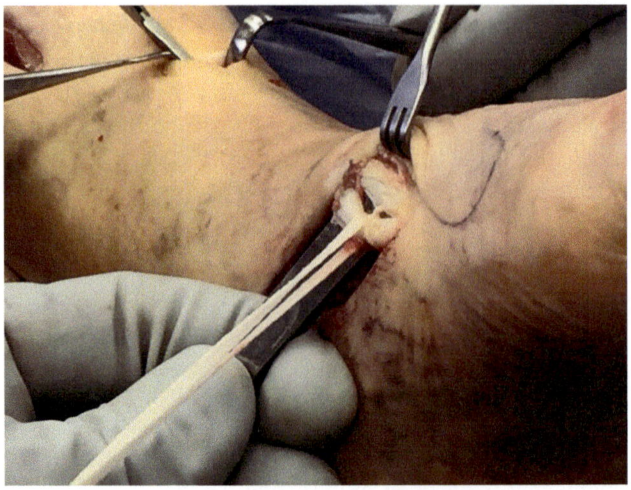

Fig. 23.13 Medial incision for tibialis anterior transfer; umbilical tape used to split the tendon

Contraindications/Limitations

The tibialis anterior tendon transfer has few contraindications. This procedure, as discussed earlier, should be rarely performed in isolation or with disease processes that result in weakening of the tendon. An in-depth physical examination of the tendon should be performed before any procedure takes place. The strength of the tibialis anterior must be accurately quantified to retain functionality. It is important to remember that one grade of muscle strength is typically lost during a tendon transfer [34].

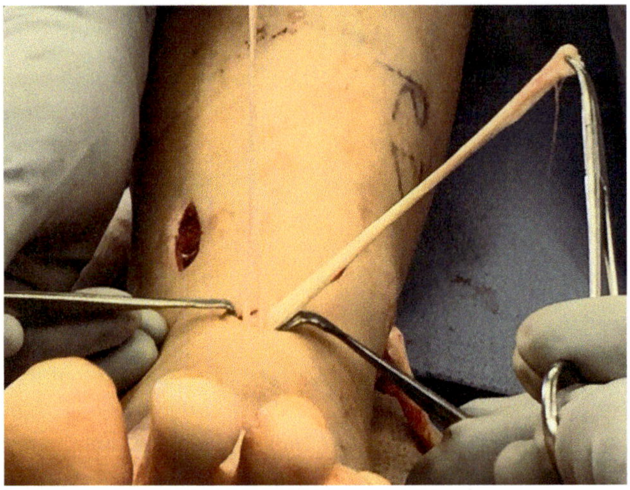

Fig. 23.14 Anterior central incision (second incision) for TA transfer

Technique, Pearls and Pitfalls

The tibialis anterior tendon transfer is performed through a three-incision approach. The first incision is made over the insertion of the tibialis anterior (Fig. 23.13). A dorsal medial incision is made at the navicular-cuneiform joint and extending to the base of the metatarsal. The tendon is fully released from its insertion.

A second incision is made to the anterior-medial aspect of the leg directly over the palpated tibialis anterior tendon (Fig. 23.14). It is important that the incision is made proximal to the extensor retinaculum to prevent bowstringing of the tendon. Other techniques have been described where the tendon is passed superficial to the retinaculum [35]. If strength is to be optimized, the tendon is placed above the retinaculum. If the tendon excursion is more important, then the tendon is passed under the retinaculum within the sheath of the common extensor. Once the tendon is visualized, it is pulled proximal through the anterior-medial leg incision.

The third incision is made on the anterior-lateral of the foot. The incision can be made overlying the lateral cuneiform or the cuboid depending on the surgeon preference and correction desired. The more eversion required, then placement of the tendon should be within the cuboid; this provides a better mechanical advantage for the tendon. In our institution, the tendon is routed to the lateral cuneiform if mild to moderate correction is needed (Fig. 23.15). A more lateral incision over the cuboid is performed if a greater correction is needed. When performing a STATT, the split tendon is transferred to the lateral cuneiform or cuboid; thus, a lateral incision is needed.

An interference screw or anchor is then placed into the lateral cuneiform or cuboid with the tendon properly tensioned. The foot should be in a neutral position. Before the interference screw is inserted, it is important you check the positioning to make sure you have the correction needed. Once the interference screw is inserted, the author uses a suture button to augment the transferred tendon.

Management of Complications

Complications are rare when performing the tibialis anterior tendon transfer. Transient tendonitis as well as the prominence of the tendon along the anterior leg is the most common complication if one fails to transfer the tendon

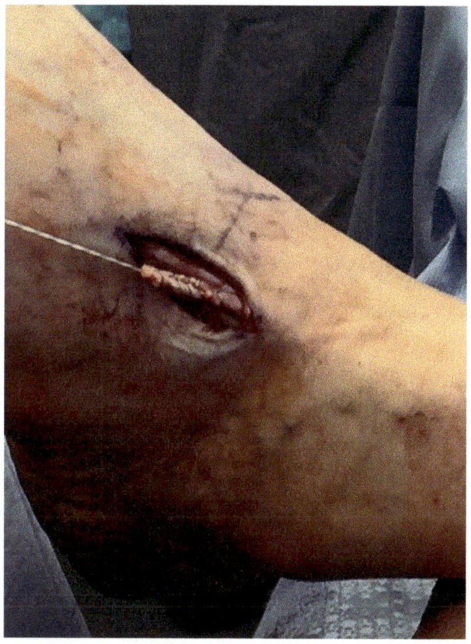

Fig. 23.15 Incision site for placement of TA tendon into the third cuneiform or cuboid

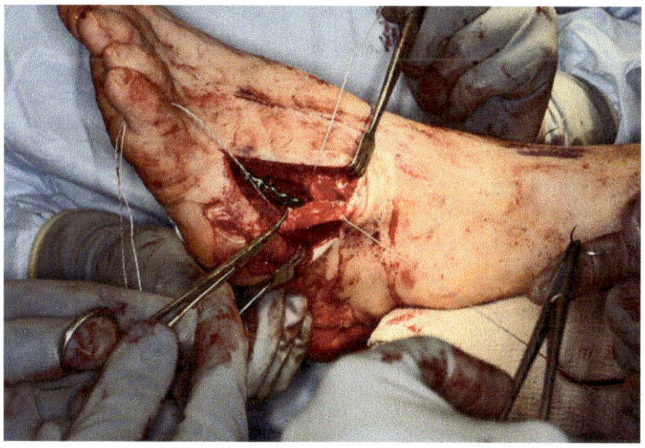

Fig. 23.16 Insertion of TA into lateral cuneiform

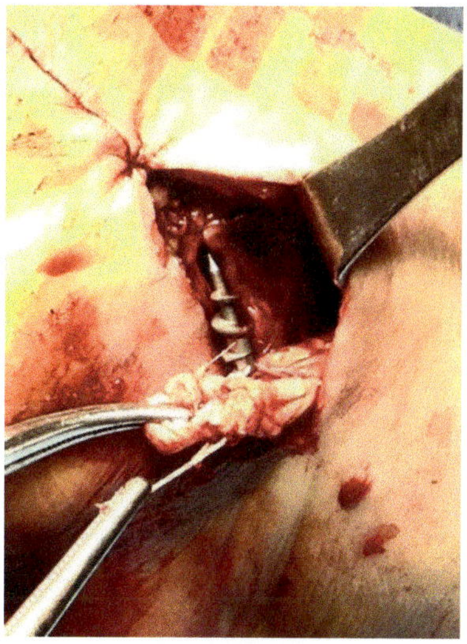

Fig. 23.17 Failure of TA tendon transfer at insertion site

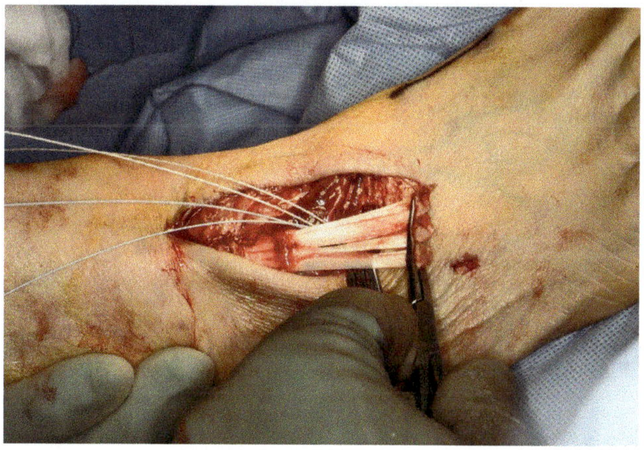

Fig. 23.18 Tendon preparation for Hibbs

under the extensor retinaculum. The patient most often will do well with physical therapy and conservative treatment [36]. This is considered an in-phase transfer, and education is not usually necessary for muscle function.

Failure of the tendon attachment is the most common significant complication requiring surgical repair [34]. Failure of the fixation technique used is often to blame, which would include poor bone stock quality (Figs. 23.16 and 23.17). A suture button is often added to secure the interference screw used due to this complication. A corkscrew-type anchor is another viable option for repair of tendon insertional rupture. It is imperative that the patient is immobilized a minimum of 4–6 weeks postoperatively to prevent recurrent failure at the attachment site (Figs. 23.18 and 23.19).

Overcorrection, although rare, is also a complication that can be very detrimental if not addressed. This results from tightening the tendon too much as the tendon is fixed to the bone. Excessive tightening creates a significant spasm to the tendon resulting in minimal eversion/inversion motion. If this is encountered, correction is required with lengthening of the tendon or removing the interference screw to decrease the tension on the tendon. Another option is for the tendon to be transferred medially to restore the inversion-to-eversion balance relationship [36].

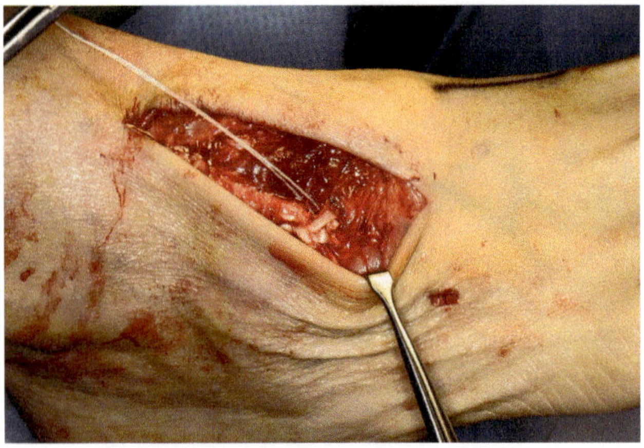

Fig. 23.19 Anchor attachment and suturing for Hibbs

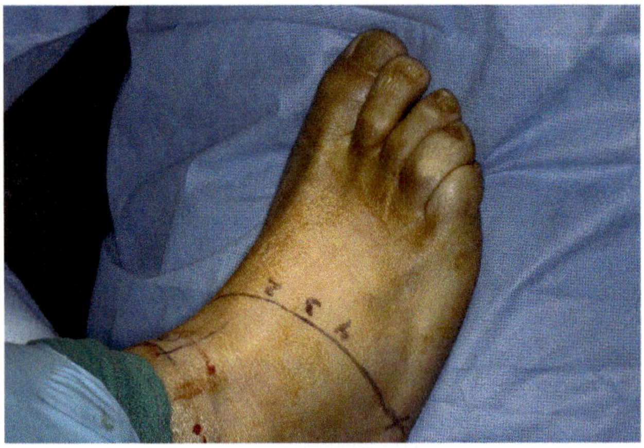

Fig. 23.20 Smith's lines to aid in incision placement

Undercorrection can occur if the tendon is not placed under proper tension when attached to the bone. Everting the foot past neutral with attachment should permit some inversion. Inadequate tension will lose the function of this tendon transfer and further loss of dorsiflexion of the foot.

Hibbs Tenosuspension

Indications

In the flexible cavus foot with the presence of claw toes, the Hibbs tenosuspension can be employed to reduce the deforming force or dorsal contracture of the lesser digits at the MTPJs. This transfer of the four slips of the extensor digitorum longus into the middle or lateral cuneiform allows continued dorsiflexion strength at the ankle without the contracture to the lesser toes. The advantages of this procedure like the tibialis anterior, STATT, and Jones tendon transfer are that they are all in-phase tendon transfers and relatively easy to perform.

Contraindications/Limitations

Transfer of any tendon that is already weak will only weaken and not perform as intended [34, 36]. Therefore, the long common extensor must be strong enough to allow for an effective transfer. The goal of this procedure is not to dorsiflex the metatarsals if transferred into each individual metatarsal but only aid in dorsiflexion at the ankle joint. The goal is to remove the deforming force of dorsiflexion at the metatarsophalangeal joints and aid in dorsiflexion at the ankle joint.

Technique, Pearls and Pitfalls

The Hibbs tenosuspension is often not performed alone but in combination with other procedures including hammertoe repair, lesser metatarsal osteotomies, Lisfranc, or midfoot fusions/osteotomies. Either using Smith's lines or fluoroscopy as an aid, the incision is centered over the lateral cuneiform (Fig. 23.20). The key is to be on the lateral aspect of the longitudinal midtarsal joint axis. This will allow the transfer to aid pronation of the forefoot with active dorsiflexion postoperatively. Care must be given as to the location if a posterior tibial tendon is being transferred as well. There is only so much anatomic area to attach tendons into the bone.

The four slips of the common extensor tendon are then sutured together for the transfer. A drill hole will then be made either into the lateral cuneiform or the cuboid. The same technique as the tibialis anterior tendon transfer is then performed. The foot is placed in a neutral position, then the tendon is tensioned and passed through the drill hole, and an interference screw is then placed. A suture button is attached to the plantar foot again to aid and augment the transfer.

Poor tensioning of the tendon at the attachment to the bone will significantly weaken the tendon and result in an ineffective dorsiflexion. Tendinitis or spasm may result if the attachment is overtightened to the bone. It is critical not to use a cutting needle when suturing the tendon ends together for transfer and attachment. This may result in rupture of the long extensor tendon due to weakening by the needle weaving through the tendon repeatedly.

Consideration must also be given to reattachment of the distal ends of the tendon slips into the short extensor tendons. If the transfer is being made to increase dorsiflexion at the ankle and not for the severe contracture of the lesser toes, it is possible for the flexor tendons to overpower the short extensors resulting in significant plantarflexion of the toes. This has resulted in a dragging and/or tripping on these toes.

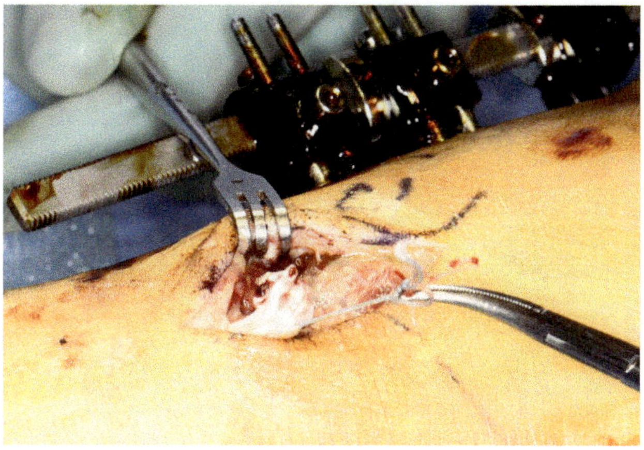

Fig. 23.21 Rupture of EDL after Hibbs tenosuspension

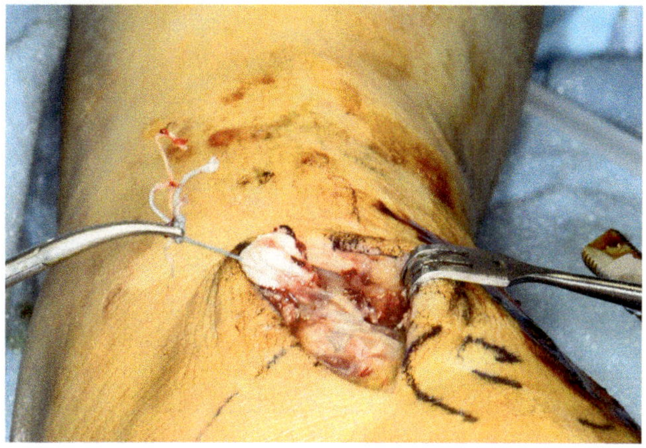

Fig. 23.22 Failure of tendon-to-bone attachment

Management of Complications

Complications are fortunately rare but can occur when performing the Hibbs tenosuspension. Failure of tendon-to-bone attachment is the most common obstacle (Figs. 23.21 and 23.22). Failure of either an interference screw or screw anchor can occur. The patient must be cast immobilized for 4 weeks postoperatively and careful weight bearing afterward to prevent rupture of the attachment.

If rupture occurs, then early diagnosis and treatment are required. Based on the location of the initial attachment, either the reattachment with a larger interference screw with augmentation of a surgical button through the plantar aspect of the foot or use of a corkscrew-type anchor can be utilized.

Bone quality should be assessed when using any bone-type anchor, and augmentation should be done on initial attachment. Augmenting the attachment with suture to periosteum is also beneficial in securing the tendon and treating or preventing rupture.

If flexor digital contracture results from failure to reattach the distal slips to the long extensor tendon to the brevis tendons, then surgery is required. Digital flexor tendon release may be necessary if attachment of the distal extensor slips is not enough to stabilize the toes.

Insufficient length of the tendon for transfer and lack of physiologic tension on the tendon after transfer are two other complications. Typically the tendons are transected at the midshaft region of the lesser metatarsals to allow for more than enough length for transfer. If there is too little tendon available to attach into the lateral cuneiform, then attachment into the talar neck may be required. The foot should be held at 90° to the leg during transfer to ensure proper tension of the tendon complex. If performed correctly in the appropriate patient, this procedure will both correct claw toe deformity and aid in correction of flexible forefoot cavus deformity.

Posterior Tibial Tendon Transfer

Introduction

When correcting the cavovarus foot, proper balancing of muscles is just as important as correction of structural bony deformity. In the cavovarus, the foot posterior tibial tendon (PTT) is commonly a main source for the varus component of the deformity as a result of overpowering the weak peroneus brevis tendon.

Transferring the tendon accomplishes two important goals. First, the removal of the deforming inverted or varus force on the foot structure [2, 4, 7, 27]. There is some question as to the potential complications to the foot structure on PTT transfer; however, the release of the tendon does not cause a subsequent planovalgus deformity [37]. The potential to augment dorsiflexion at the ankle joint is also a major benefit. In severe cases of cavovarus deformity, there is weakness of the extensor tendons and drop foot results. Transfer of the PTT to the dorsum of the foot neutralizes the weakness of the extensor tendons [36, 38, 39].

Indications

When transferring the PTT from the medial foot to the dorsal midfoot, one must remember that this tendon will be out of phase with the rest of the anterior extrinsic muscles. Therefore, extensive neuromuscular re-education must be performed if possible prior to surgery as well as postoperatively, or the tendon must be used for static correction of the varus deformity [39–41]. Transfer of the PTT is performed on patients with significant varus deformity of the foot as well as weakness of dorsiflexors of the foot causing drop foot. The goal is to restore a more normal heel-to-toe gait.

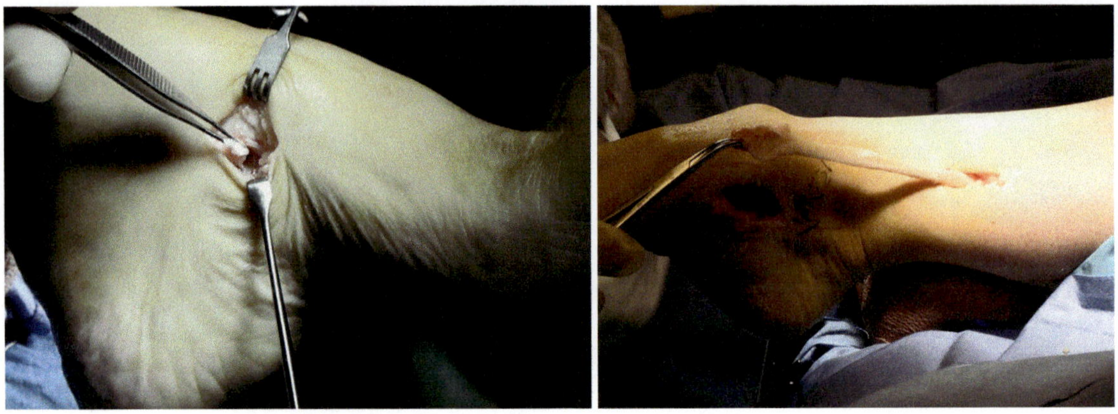

Fig. 23.23 Detachment of the PT tendon from the navicular tuberosity

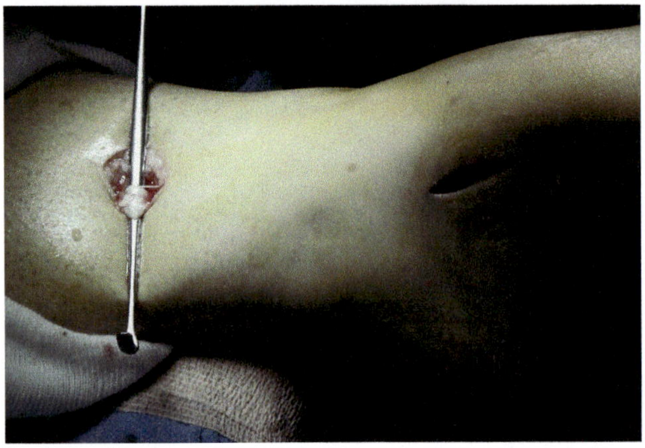

Fig. 23.24 Identification of PT tendon proximal-medial, lower leg

Contraindications/Limitations

The transfer of the PTT to the dorsum of the foot is only performed when there is a significant varus/adducted deformity of the foot, typically with weakness or absent function of the peroneus brevis tendon. The tendon must be strong enough to give enough function once transferred knowing one grade of muscle strength will be lost after transfer [35, 41, 42].

Fixed deformity must be corrected prior to transfer of the PTT. If ignored, tendon transfer will be for naught since no increased motion will result. This correction would either be done by osteotomy or in severe cases, triple arthrodesis. Adequate motion at the ankle is required, and pseudoequinus must also be addressed with either midfoot fusion or osteotomy to lower the arch and place the talus into a functional position within the ankle joint. If equinus is still present, then an Achilles lengthening or gastrocnemius recession is required to allow the PTT transfer to function properly.

Technique

The technique most often performed is through a four-incision technique popularized by Hsu and Hoffer [42]. A medial incision is placed over the PTT insertion onto the navicular. Dissection to the distal tendon and navicular is followed by release of the tendon distal to the navicular tuberosity over the medial cuneiform to ensure maximum length of the harvested tendon (Fig. 23.23).

A second incision is then placed along the posterior/medial border of the tibia at the myotendinous junction of the tibialis posterior approximately 15–20 cm proximal to the ankle joint. Dissection to the posterior tendons is performed, and the PTT is usually located deep to the flexor digitorum longus tendon directly on the posterior/medial tibia. It is beneficial if you pull on the distal end of the tendon to help find the tendon in this medial incision (Fig. 23.24).

The third incision is placed slightly distal to the second incision just anterior/medial to the fibula. Dissection is performed through the subcutaneous tissue, lateral to the extensor digitorum longus and interosseous membrane. The anterior muscles are retracted and pushed aside to visualize the interosseous membrane. A 4 cm opening is made through the interosseous membrane carefully. The neurovascular structures are just deep to the membrane at this point. A portion of at least 2 cm of the membrane should be removed to allow for adequate movement of the transferred tendon through this hole as the tendon is transferred (Fig. 23.25).

The fourth incision is made directly over the lateral cuneiform. With the foot held at 90° to the leg, the PTT is then inserted into the lateral cuneiform through a trephine hole with a suture button, utilizing an interference screw, or with the surgeons' anchoring system of choice (Fig. 23.26).

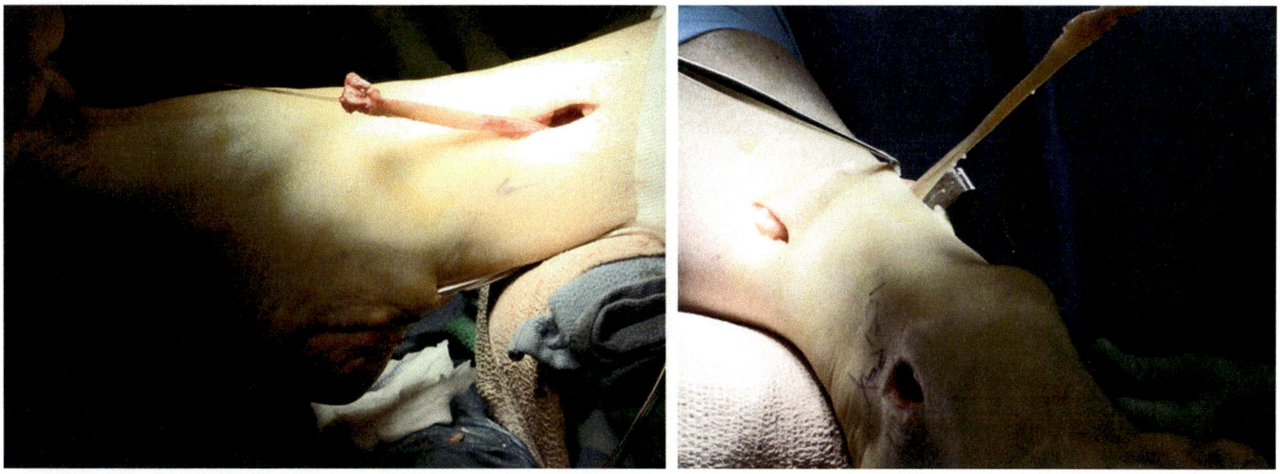

Fig. 23.25 Lateral incision for PT tendon transfer

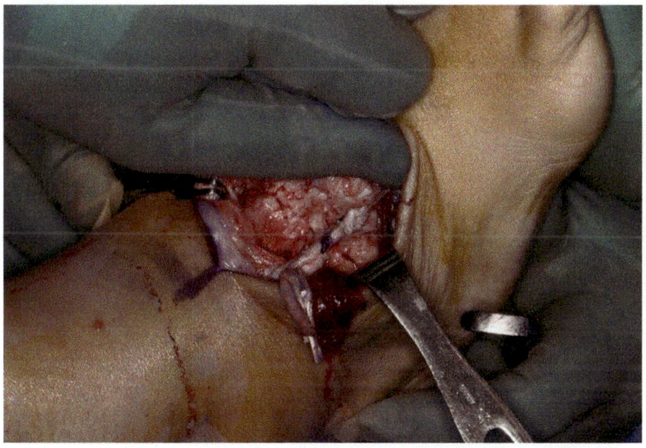

Fig. 23.26 PT tendon ready for insertion to cuneiform or cuboid

Pearls and Pitfalls

Maximal length must be obtained of the tendon at the medial navicular harvest site. Without proper length, the tendon may not reach the lateral cuneiform or cuboid for insertion. Harvesting a small section of the navicular tuberosity and then careful dissection of the tendon off of that bone can ensure maximal length. Proper mobilization of the tendon as it passes through the interosseous membrane can be another source of difficulty during the procedure. If the window in the membrane is not large enough, there can be stenosis of the tendon causing inability to gain proper length as well as lack of excursion when contracted.

There are two options for routing of the tendon once passed through the interosseous membrane. Transfer of the PTT deep to the extensor retinaculum allows for enhanced tendon excursion but gives up strength of the tendon since it is closer to the axis of motion (the ankle joint). If the tendon is not passed deep to the extensor retinaculum, but within the subcutaneous tissue, then the tendon will lose the pulley mechanism and gain strength in transfer. Unfortunately, there will be an obvious bowstring effect to the tendon when it is above the extensor retinaculum [43, 44]. This phenomenon is represented by the Blix curve, which describes the relationship of muscle length and contractile force [8].

Finally, the foot must be held in the correct position to allow for proper tensioning of the tendon during tendon attachment. The tendon should be secured with the foot in the resting neutral position with adequate tension to place the muscle at its resting length [42]. Excessive tension on the transferred tendon will cause the tendon not to function properly and result in more of a tenodesis [8, 36, 42–45].

We have found that the best method of securing the tendon at its appropriate length is by interference screw augmented with a surgical button plantarly on the foot. Once the hole within the lateral cuneiform is made to secure the tendon, the tendon is passed via a Keith needle through this hole and out the bottom of the foot. The foot is then dorsiflexed as the tendon is pulled through the hole. Once the proper position has been established, the tendon is secured with the interference screw.

This technique allows for independent determination of the proper amount of tension by pulling the tendon distally as the foot is dorsiflexed. The PTT is being transferred out of phase, and while neuromuscular re-education can be performed, initially the tension on the tendon will provide for the deformity correction.

Management of Complications

The transfer of the PTT to the dorsum of the foot through the interosseous membrane has the potential for a great deal of complications. Knowledge of the anatomy is a requirement, and this procedure should not be considered unless the surgeon has an understanding of the potential untoward effects. Failure to obtain adequate length is one of the most common shortcomings of this procedure. Attachments will either be by corkscrew-type anchor or tendon weave, the latter being the less efficient method of attachment and can potentially weaken the tendon transfer further. The better option, if the tendon is too short to attach to either cuneiforms or cuboid, would be to attach the tendon to the talar neck. This is a better method to secure the tendon to the bone directly. Due to the close proximity of the tendon insertion to the ankle joint axis, effective dorsiflexion is greatly reduced [36, 45].

Rupture of the attachment is always a possibility as mentioned earlier with the other tendon transfers. Repair is similar with augmenting the anchor method and the use of a surgical button. It is critical that the diagnosis is made early so there is no significant degree of retraction of the tendon proximally. If there is retraction of the tendon, then a graft may be necessary to aid in reattachment. Otherwise, a more proximal attachment may be required. Bone quality plays a significant role as to how well a tendon will attach to and maintain its attachment. Interference screws or anchors will only work as well as the quality or density of the bone where it is being applied. Therefore, augmentation of the tendon attachment should be considered if there is questionable bone quality.

Due to the proximity of the neurovascular bundle during the transfer of the tendon through the interosseous membrane, potential for injury can result. A vascular surgeon may be required if injury is extensive to the posterior tibial artery in this location. Care must be given when windowing the interosseous membrane and transfer of the PTT through this opening.

An adhesion of the posterior tibial muscle and tendon as it passes through the interosseous membrane is also a complication that results in poor excursion of this muscle and poor functional outcome. Too small of a window in the interosseous membrane or too acute of an angle the muscle and tendon travel from the posterior muscle compartment to the anterior compartment can limit the excursion of this tendon transfer. To avoid this complication, a larger window should be employed within the interosseous membrane. In addition, a more proximal skin incision must be made medially than anterolateral to create an appropriate transfer of the tendon. If either of these important points is not carried out, then a poor result is inevitable [36, 43, 44].

Peroneus Longus to Peroneus Brevis Tendon Transfer

Indications

In the cavovarus foot, especially with Charcot-Marie-Tooth, it is common to have normal function and strength of the peroneus longus (PL) muscle. Due to the progressive nature of the disease, classically there are decreased function and strength of the tibialis anterior (TA) as well as, and more importantly, the peroneus brevis (PB) tendon. With weakening of the TA tendon, the PL will overpower the TA muscle, thus creating a plantarflexion of the first ray and specifically the first metatarsal [1, 7, 38, 46, 47]. Tenodesis of the PL to the PB decreases the plantarflexion pull of the first ray, as well as increases the eversion force that the PB applies to the fifth metatarsal base. This transfer will increase eversion strength by its new attachment to the base of the fifth metatarsal. Removing the plantarflexion ability of the PL tendon

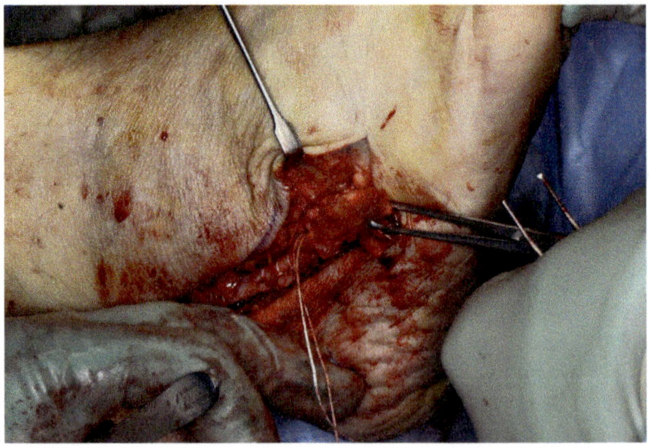

Fig. 23.27 Peroneus longus and brevis

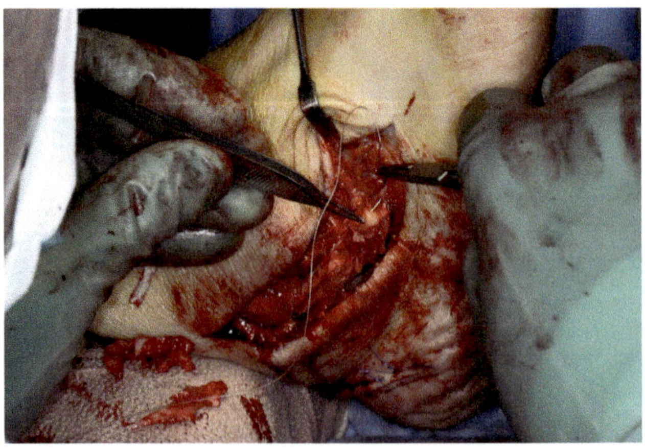

Fig. 23.28 Peroneus longus to brevis transfer

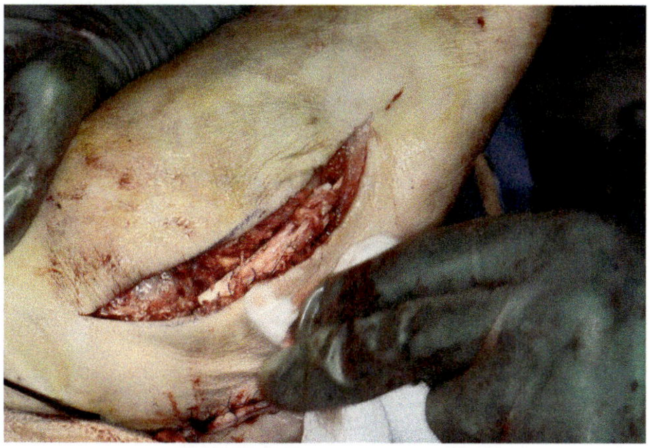

Fig. 23.29 Note the distal tenodesis with slight overlap

on the first ray also prevents continued supination of the foot, exacerbating the cavovarus deformity. Although the PL tendon everts the foot in open kinetic chain, it is a supinator of the foot in closed kinetic chain. Transfer of the PL to PB negates this effect [38, 48].

Technique, Pearls and Pitfalls

The peroneal tendons can be accessed by an incision from the base of the fifth metatarsal to the lateral malleolus. After isolating the peroneal tendons, the PL tendon is released as it courses plantar to the cuboid. Tenodesis of the tendons is then performed with a nonabsorbable suture as the foot is held in maximum eversion.

If a calcaneal osteotomy or midfoot osteotomy is performed, those procedures should be completed prior to transfer, as the tension of the tenodesis and positioning of the foot will change. If an os peroneum is present, it should be removed prior to tenodesis. Along with standard tenodesis, the PL tendon can also be woven in a pulvertaft fashion through the PB tendon. The tenodesis must be performed 5 cm distal to the retinaculum to permit adequate excursion of the tendon. This is similar to repair for a ruptured PB tendon with PL tenodesis. One can also tenodese these two tendons proximally above the peroneal retinaculum [49].

The result of this proximal tenodesis would be continued pull on the first ray by the PL tendon but has less effect as an evertor of the foot. This would have to be high enough above the retinaculum at least 3 cm to allow for proper excursion of the tendon as well [49, 50]. A distal transfer is preferred, almost an end-to-end attachment with a small degree of tendon overlap. Less overlap results in a less bulky tenodesis which is tolerated better by patients as well as less irritation to the lateral dorsal cutaneous nerve (Figs. 23.27, 23.28, and 23.29).

Management of Complications

Similar to all tendon transfers, rupture of the tenodesis can occur. Treatment is performed with either approximation of the edges or augmentation with either auto- or allograft. Semitendinosus allograft is often times used as an allograft and performed shortly after the rupture is diagnosed. Immediate repair with intercalary allograft has been shown to be successful in failed peroneal tendon patients [51].

Proper tension, as with all tendon transfers, is critical for success and effectiveness of the tendon transfer. An appropriate amount of tension on the tendon repair is necessary to allow for proper contracture of the tendon. Laxity in the approximation of the tendon ends minimizes the effectiveness of the transfer. Excessive tightening of the tendon edges can lead to rupture of the approximation or symptoms of tendinitis. Suture reaction is also a concern, and nonabsorbable suture is typically the choice of suture in this transfer. Care must be taken not to use excessive amounts of nonabsorbable suture for the potential of suture reaction and soft tissue irritation.

If a tendon transfer causes pain due to the thickness at the suture site, debulking will need to be performed. Care must be taken to maintain the integrity of the transfer, and one cannot sacrifice the strength necessary for tendon function.

The question of inadvertent consequences of any procedure must be looked at prior to performing such procedure. For example, since the function of the PL tendon is to plantarflex the first ray, will removing the tendon cause elevation of the first ray? The answer is no; there are no reports of metatarsus primus elevatus after transfer of the PL. If one is concerned, then a first metatarsal cuneiform arthrodesis can be performed to stabilize the first ray and elevate into a more functional position if necessary.

Jones Tenosuspension

Indications

It is not unusual for the cavus foot deformity to present with a hallux malleus deformity, along with an overactive extensor hallucis longus (EHL) tendon. However, the extensor tendon is not necessarily overpowering the long flexor tendon but causes a contracture of the metatarsophalangeal joint (MTPJ) and interphalangeal joint (IPJ) as a result of the loss of intrinsic muscles to the great toe [52].

Combined with the presence of a plantarflexed first ray, there is a mechanical advantage for the great toe to dorsiflex at the MTPJ. The Jones tenosuspension most importantly removes the deforming force from the hallux. Moving the insertion of the EHL tendon to the neck of the metatarsal, or

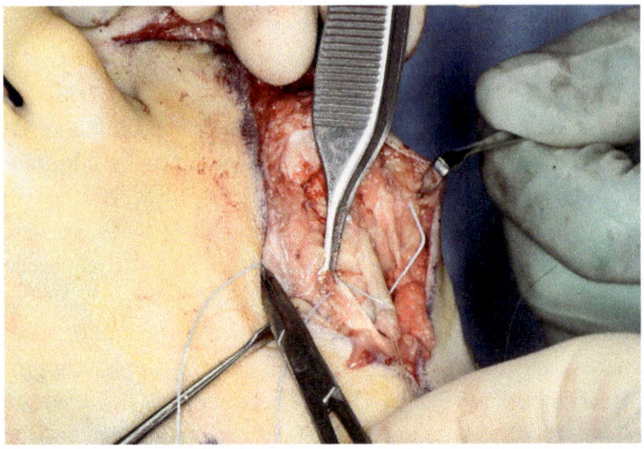

Fig. 23.30 EHL tendon being transferred for Jones procedure

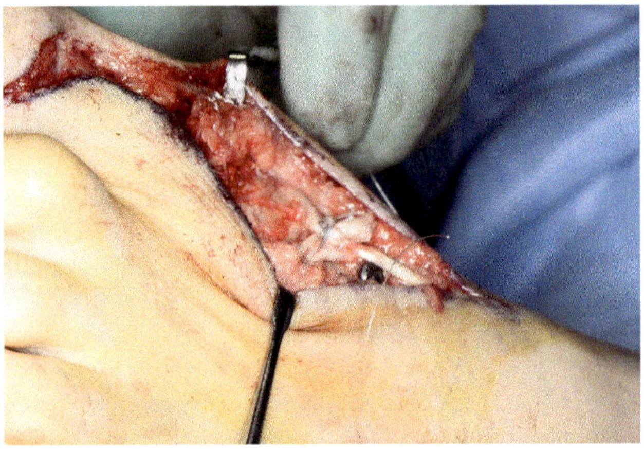

Fig. 23.31 EHL being wrapped upon itself and sutured. Note the screw for DFWO

even more proximally, also reduces the retrograde pressure to the first metatarsal. Dorsiflexion is maintained at the ankle after the tendon transfer is completed. It is important to realize that the goal to transfer of the EHL tendon to the first metatarsal is not to elevate the first metatarsal but only to remove the deforming force to the hallux [53, 54].

With a fixed plantarflexed first ray deformity, a dorsiflexory wedge osteotomy must be performed to elevate the first metatarsal. The osteotomy needs to be performed first, followed by the tendon transfer. The fixation and technique used is a single 4.0 mm screw, but many other fixation techniques are described.

Technique, Pearls and Pitfalls

Linear incision is made over the distal one-third of the first metatarsal to the dorsal aspect of the interphalangeal (IP) joint. Dissection is first performed to the IP joint, and the EHL tendon is released with a 5–10 mm distal stump left

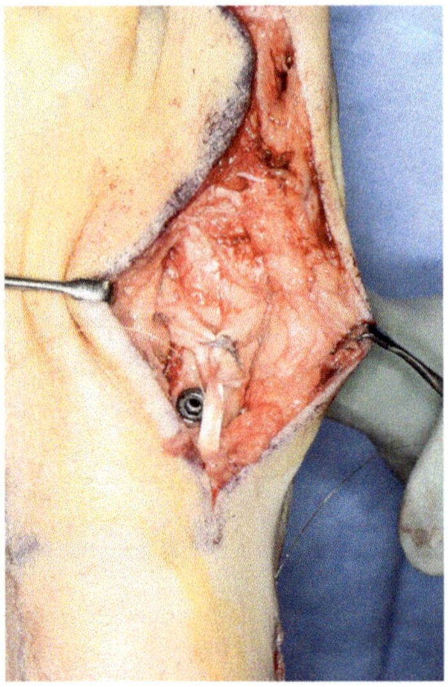

Fig. 23.32 Jones tenosuspension with DFWO

attached to the distal phalanx. After release of the tendon, the IP joint is prepared for arthrodesis with joint resection, and then the arthrodesis is performed with screws or K-wires at the surgeon's discretion. The EHL is then released from the first MTP joint, and dissection is progressed to the metatarsal neck. A trephine hole is then placed from medial to lateral, and the proximal stump of the tendon is routed through the trephine hole and sutured onto itself with the foot held at 90° and proper tension applied to the tendon.

The Jones tenosuspension is one of the most common tendon transfers for hallux malleus and cavus forefoot deformities. There are a few pearls that can help make the transfer easier for the practitioner. As mentioned earlier, the first metatarsal osteotomy should be performed first if one is planning on elevating the first ray during the time of surgery. Once this is completed, then the drill hole is made from medial to lateral. A bone clamp to augment fixation during the drilling will decrease the forces on the osteotomy. The drill size should be carefully selected, as too big of a drill hole will create a larger stress riser than a smaller drill hole. Too small of a hole will make the transfer tedious and very time-consuming.

The tendon is typically routed from lateral to medial if at all possible (Fig. 23.30). The tendon end is typically sutured to approximate the tendon end to allow for easier transfer (Figs. 23.31, 23.32, and 23.33). Once done, this suture can be brought through the bone with a small tendon passer. An older technique is to pass an independent suture from medial to lateral through the hole in the first metatarsal then back again from lateral to medial creating a loop of suture on the lateral side of the bone. The suture from the tendon is placed within the loop, and the suture pulled medially to pass the suture. The tendon then follows as the suture is pulled. An old-school technique to pass this suture is to use a Frazier tip. The tip is placed

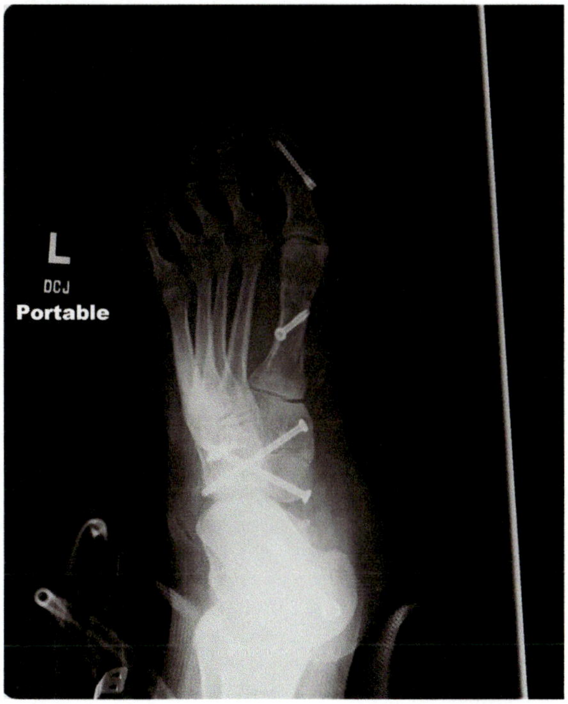

Fig. 23.33 DFWO and IPJ fusion with Jones tenosuspension

in the drill hole, and the suction pulls the suture from the end of the tendon as the suction is pulled from the bone slowly.

The Jones tenosuspension is often performed in conjunction with a hallux IPJ arthrodesis, which today is called a "modified Jones procedure." It is the author's opinion that the IPJ fusion should always be performed in conjunction with the transfer to stabilize the digit and prevent further contracture after removing the EHL tendon.

The main pitfall with any tendon transfer, including the Jones, is the lack of adequate length to properly transfer and attach the tendon. In the Jones, it is important to harvest the tendon no more than 1 cm from the insertion on to the distal phalanx. In the Jones, if proper length is not obtained, one will not be able to route the tendon through the metatarsal neck and have enough length to suture it onto itself. Location of the hole within the metatarsal can be another pitfall, if not placed correctly. If the hole is placed too distal, there may not be enough tendon to route through and reattach to itself, and if it is placed too proximal, the lever arm of the EHL will be decreased, decreasing the mechanical force of the EHL tendon.

Fracture of the metatarsal is also a known complication. A hole within the first metatarsal creates a stress riser within the bone. Therefore, one must be careful about how large a hole is made within the first metatarsal. If enough force is applied to the bone, a fracture and subsequent elevation will occur to the first metatarsal. If a fracture occurs, then repair may be required depending on the sagittal plane displacement of the distal fragment.

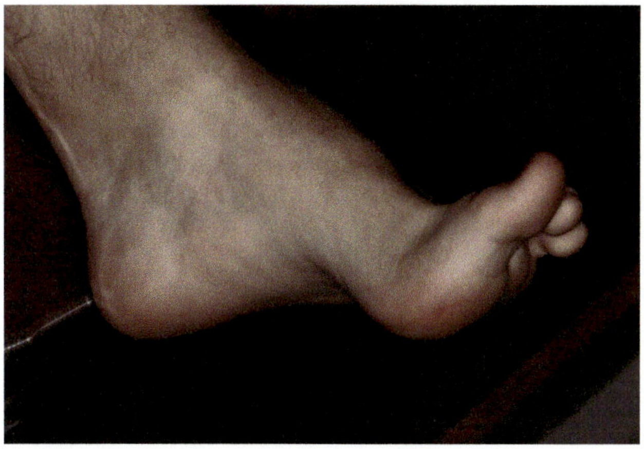

Fig. 23.34 Fixed severe plantarflexed position of the first ray

Management of Complications

Complications of the Jones tenosuspension are rare. Tendon insertion rupture is always a possibility, and early recognition and reattachment are critical. A more proximal attachment may be required if tendon length is an issue. Attachment to the tibialis anterior tendon, or to the proximal portion of the first metatarsal, is two options for reattachment.

As mentioned earlier, fracture of the first metatarsal through the drill hole can occur. The more proximal the hole within the first metatarsal, the higher the possibility for fracture. A lever arm is created from the ground to the hole within the first metatarsal. Therefore, a hole within the metatarsal head region is best to avoid this potential complication.

Dorsiflexory Wedge Osteotomy (DFWO) of the First Metatarsal

Indications

In the cavus foot, fixed plantarflexion of the first metatarsal is a usual finding. Pain due to overloading of this first metatarsal is a common indication to elevate this first metatarsal [26, 37]. The moderate or severe cavus foot structure will often require an elevation osteotomy to the first metatarsal. A strong PL tendon overpowers the TA tendon in patients with CMT resulting in plantarflexion of the first metatarsal. The Coleman block test is performed to evaluate whether the heel varus is due to a structural deformity within the calcaneus or a result of the first ray being plantarflexed [37]. This plantarflexed-fixed position of the first metatarsal subsequently inverts the heel in closed kinetic chain. Therefore, lateral ankle instability, varus heel deformity, lateral foot pain, and residual heel varus may all be a result of a significantly fixed position plantarflexed first ray (Fig. 23.34).

Technique, Pearls and Pitfalls

A 5 cm incision is made along the dorsal aspect of the first metatarsal at the proximal metaphyseal-diaphyseal level. After exposure of the bone, 2 cm distal to the first tarsometatarsal joint, a dorsal-distal to proximal-plantar wedge is removed from metatarsal with the osteotomy directed in a 45° angle to the first tarsometatarsal joint. The size of the wedge removed is based on the severity of plantarflexion. Following removal of the wedge, the osteotomy can be fixated with a dorsal-proximal to distal-plantar interfragmentary compression screw.

While other techniques will call for a more vertical wedge removed from the base of the metatarsal, the technique described above allows for interfragmentary screw fixation, rather than relying on a plate or tension band technique. When making the osteotomy, the proximal cut is made first; however, care is taken to not violate the plantar cortex. After the distal cut is performed and the wedge is removed, the plantar hinge should remain intact, which will prevent any rotation deformity. Manual reduction of the osteotomy with bone reduction forceps is performed, or dorsal pressure to the first metatarsal head plantarly can be made. However, if gaping is noted, then the osteotomy is feathered to closure to allow for reduction with a sagittal saw.

If the plantar hinge is violated, the surgeon should add another point of fixation to prevent transverse plane instability. The more proximal the osteotomy is performed, the more correction will be obtained, with less bone removed, so placement of the osteotomy is of great importance. The DFWO of the first metatarsal should be performed after any rearfoot correction, as this will prevent over- or undercorrection of the first metatarsal alignment [53].

The medial dorsal cutaneous nerve is located near the base of the first metatarsal and traverses in an oblique manner from proximal lateral to distal medial. Care must be taken to identify and retract this nerve in order to prevent inadvertent transection or entrapment.

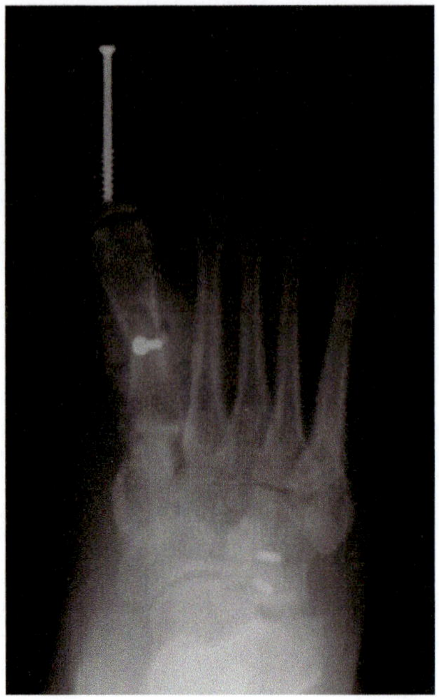

Fig. 23.35 First metatarsal fracture following DFWO

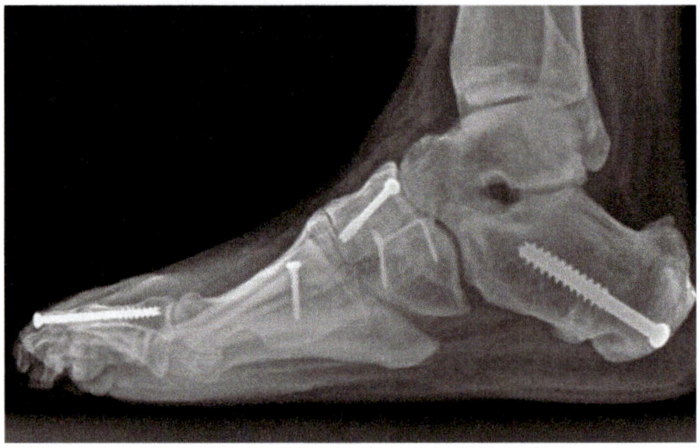

Fig. 23.36 First metatarsal fracture with bone remodeling

Management of Complications

Complications of the DFWO are most often avoidable. Leeuwesteijn et al. demonstrated minimal complications in short-term to midterm outcomes employing a proximal dorsiflexion osteotomy with combined soft tissue procedures. They showed 90% satisfactory results in 33 patients or 52 feet [12]. However, undercorrection and overcorrection are most common. Failure to remove adequate amount of the bone from the first metatarsal bone may result in persistent varus foot deformity or continued pain subfirst metatarsal or fracture of the osteotomy. Further elevation may be required to correct this problem if conservative care fails to relieve symptoms and alignment issues.

Fracture of the first metatarsal can also result if there is inadequate amount of elevation. This may also be due to premature weight bearing postoperatively. Treatment is based on the amount of elevation post fracture and clinical evaluation subsequently. Most often, the patient is casted non-weight bearing to allow for consolidation (Figs. 23.35 and 23.36).

If severe, repair of the displaced fracture is required. Additional bone should be removed to elevate the distal portion of the first metatarsal if possible, and then appropriate fixation is performed. Screw fixation is not enough, and a plate should be employed for fixation of the metatarsal.

Overcorrection resulting in hallux rigidus and transfer lesser metatarsalgia may also occur [53]. If this is the case, an opening wedge osteotomy is performed to place the first metatarsal into a better functional position.

Multiple Lesser Metatarsal Osteotomies

Cavus foot deformity with plantarflexion of all the metatarsals usually presents with clinical symptoms of diffuse lesser metatarsalgia, painful lesions to the forefoot, and claw toe deformity. There is often a fixed plantarflexed position of all the metatarsals with distal migration of the fat pad noted. Lesser metatarsal osteotomies are usually performed with an anterior cavus. The apex of the deformity is located closer to the forefoot [11, 16].

Most importantly, lesser metatarsal osteotomies are employed in lieu of fusion procedures in order to maintain motion within the foot and prevent adjacent joint arthrosis in the long term. A few additional benefits to lesser metatarsal osteotomies are that arthrodesis is avoided, maintaining flexibility of the foot, and they are also considered to be technically easier to perform [14, 16].

Technique, Pearls and Pitfalls

The lesser metatarsal osteotomies are usually performed through three separate incisions on the dorsum of the foot. The medial incision is located over the first metatarsal, the second incision placed between the second and third metatarsal shafts, and the lateral incision created between the fourth and fifth metatarsal shafts. It is easier to perform all of the dissection prior to performing the metatarsal osteotomies.

The second metatarsal is cut first and then temporarily fixated with a bone clamp. The oblique osteotomy is made at the proximal metaphyseal-diaphyseal junction with the wedge being dorsal-distal and then feathered to closure. Once the position is considered acceptable, screw fixation is employed in a standard AO technique with either a 2.0 or 2.7 mm screw. The third metatarsal followed by the fourth and then fifth metatarsals is cut and fixated. This technique of sagittal plane alignment is done only by feel. There is no scientific or radiographic assessment to determine the "correct" position of the metatarsal. Finally, the first metatarsal osteotomy is made and fixated. The amount of elevation of this bone is directly related to the position of the second metatarsal.

Meary's angle is evaluated with the foot loaded as best as possible intraoperatively to help confirm reduction of the anterior cavus foot structure. Postoperatively the patient is non-weight bearing for approximately 4–6 weeks.

There are many pearls to help minimize complications for this not-so-benign procedure. Intraoperative X-ray prior to incision helps confirm proper skin incision placement between the metatarsals. Too medial or lateral of a skin incision will challenge healing of the skin islands as well as make exposure to the bone cuts more challenging. Dissection is carried out on all of the metatarsals prior to making bone cuts. This allows for continued progressive osteotomies, once they have been prepared. As with any oblique osteotomy, care should be taken to make the dorsal wing big enough to allow for screw fixation. Too short of a wing will make fixation difficult and lead to fracture.

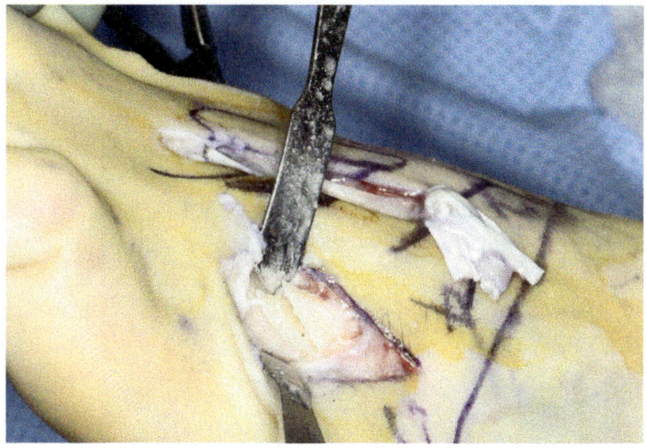

Fig. 23.37 Wafer of wedge resected to decrease risk of overcorrection

The second metatarsal being the keystone is cut first. The position of the second metatarsal will determine how much to elevate the other metatarsals. This metatarsal is the most stable, meaning less range of motion in the sagittal plane. Therefore, this allows for good judgment for the other metatarsals, as they are elevated into proper position with the hope to minimize transfer lesions.

The goal here is to minimize too little or too much elevation of the metatarsals. Failure to place the metatarsals on the same plane will result in either continued metatarsalgia or transfer type lesions.

The basal osteotomy employed to elevate the metatarsal is a powerful osteotomy. A small wedge of the bone resected from the proximal portion of the metatarsal can elevate the metatarsal significantly more than the same amount of the bone resected from the distal portion of the metatarsal. A smaller wedge of the bone resected to elevate the metatarsal is better than too much (Fig. 23.37). Too much elevation of the fifth metatarsal can cause prominence of its base and subsequently a painful lesion. For this reason, there is only so much elevation that can be done to the fifth metatarsal and the others as well.

Care must be taken to feather the osteotomy rather than creating a complete through and through cut. Cutting completely through the bone will create an unstable distal fragment and a very challenging problem to fixate. Testing the ability to close the osteotomy often as the cut is made helps

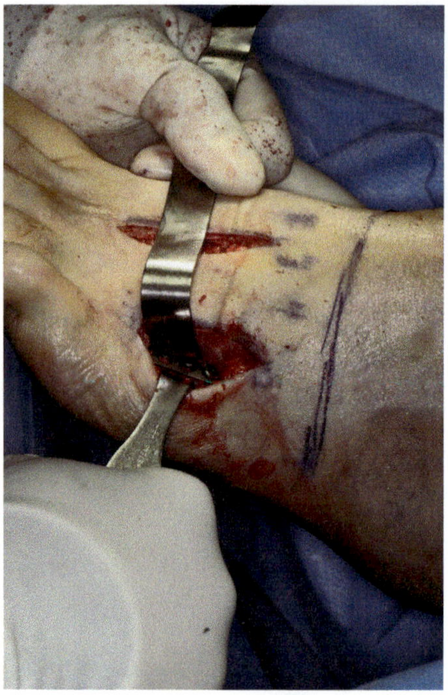

Fig. 23.38 Plate fixation of fifth metatarsal for accidental complete osteotomy

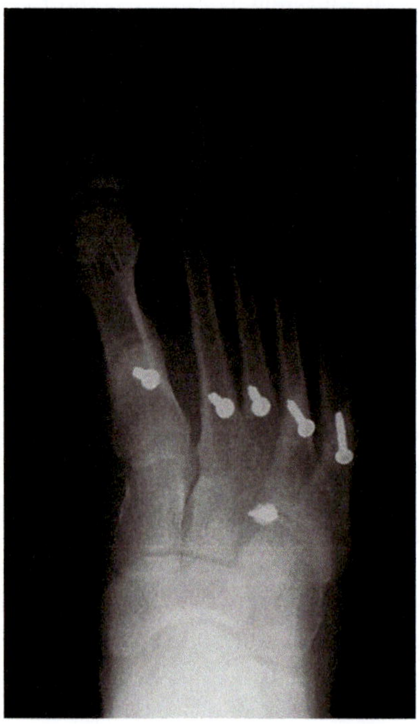

Fig. 23.39 Screw fixation of lesser metatarsal osteotomies

prevent a very challenging complication. Once the proper depth of the osteotomy is confirmed, then continued cutting in a reciprocal fashion to elevate the bone to its final position takes place. Fixation is either performed by screw fixation alone or by plate fixation if added stability is required (Figs. 23.38 and 23.39).

Management of Complications

According to the literature, complications are not very common for multiple lesser metatarsal osteotomies [11, 14, 48, 55]. However, there are several known complications which can occur and must be treated. Not knowing the indications and contraindications for multiple elevational osteotomies usually leads to failure and poor outcome. A non-fixed cavus deformity and supple cavus with global forefoot pain without arthritic rearfoot joints are the indications for this procedure. If arthrosis is noted to Lisfranc joint, then global fusion of these joints is required and not lesser metatarsal osteotomies. The apex of the cavus deformity must be ascertained preoperatively. A forefoot cavus is the only indication for this technique.

There are several intraoperative complications associated with this surgical procedure. Location of the osteotomy and technique are very important in a successful outcome of this procedure. Due to the increased declination of the metatarsal, the cut must be long enough if screw fixation is to be performed. Otherwise, the osteotomy will be too short and be unable to accommodate a screw. If the screw is placed too close to the osteotomy, this will most likely lead to fracture of the "beak," ultimately leading to instability of the osteotomy. Proper countersinking is critical to allow for the screw head to seat properly to compress this osteotomy and prevent fracture. A cannulated screw may be utilized as well to help confirm placement prior to placing the screw across the osteotomy.

A strategy for failure of screw fixation is necessary in any surgery and especially here. If this screw does not hold, then a larger diameter screw may work. If there is fracture of the dorsal fragment, and the single screw fails, then plate fixation of the metatarsal is required. There is really no need for a locked plate in this situation, as the bone quality is quite excellent in this high cortical region.

Over- and undercorrection are the most common postoperative complications associated with multiple lesser metatarsal osteotomies [11, 55]. Determining the correct sagittal plane alignment of all the metatarsals is perhaps the most challenging part about multiple osteotomies. Managing postoperatively is usually conservative with orthotic offloading techniques. However, failure to respond conservatively will necessitate an additional osteotomy. This can be performed either proximally or distally, but may be easier to align if performed more distally. An offset V-osteotomy is a great choice to elevate the metatarsal bone, but other options are available at the surgeon's preference. Plantarflexion of a metatarsal for an overcorrected metatarsal is done in a simi-

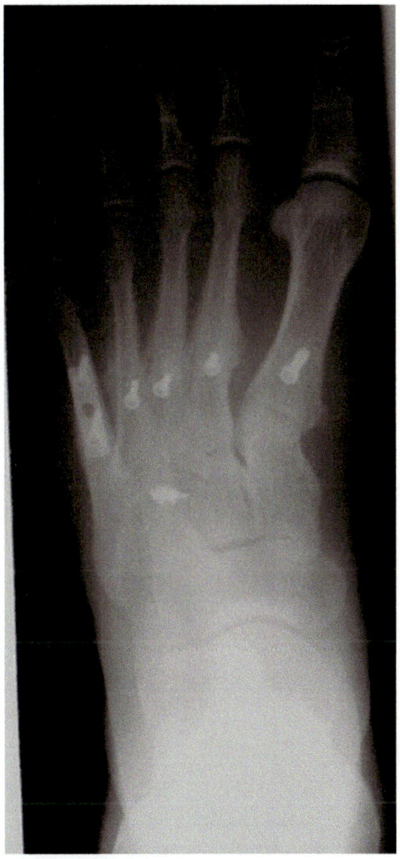

Fig. 23.40 Stress fracture of lesser metatarsals with plate fixation of the fifth metatarsal

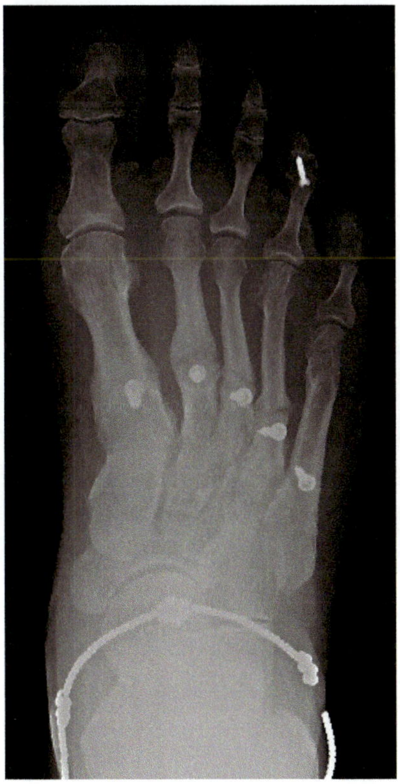

Fig. 23.41 Nonunion of second, third, and fourth metatarsals

lar manner with the offset V-osteotomy. An opening osteotomy with bone graft is another alternative to plantarflex the metatarsal as well, but this is a more complex procedure and comes with its own set of complications.

Stress fractures can occur after lesser metatarsal osteotomies due to the difficulty of alignment and excessive force resulting in fracture at the screw site (Fig. 23.40). This issue is often treated with immobilization and time. This often resolves with conservative measures.

Nonunions of lesser metatarsal osteotomies have been documented to be very low and often resolve with conservative treatment (Fig. 23.41) [11, 14]. Treatment of nonunions for lesser metatarsals is similar as to any nonunion. Initial conservative care of non-weight bearing and cast immobilization with bone stimulator are performed. If conservative management fails, then surgical intervention including resection of the nonunion, bone graft, and fixation is advocated.

The bone graft can either be intercalary or inlay depending on the goal and problem being treated. Plate fixation is often required for adequate fixation. Care must be taken as to carefully establish the final position of the metatarsal to avoid transfer lesions and metatarsalgia.

Cole Midfoot Osteotomy

Indications

There are a number of midfoot osteotomies that have been proposed to correct pes cavus deformity. All are based on apex of deformity and overall reduction in the sagittal plane for anterior cavus. The most common is the Cole procedure, first described by Saunders in 1935 and then published and popularized by Cole in 1940 [56, 57]. It is the most common osteotomy/arthrodesis performed today for moderate cavus deformity.

The Cole osteotomy is performed for a midfoot and combined rearfoot cavus deformity. The osteotomy is achieved by removing a dorsally based wedge combining an osteotomy through the cuboid and fusion of the navicular with the cuneiform bones [57]. This osteotomy/arthrodesis corrects for sagittal plane cavus deformities specifically by improving Meary's angle [58–60]. This alone or in combination with a dorsiflexory wedge osteotomy of the first metatarsal lowers the arch into more anatomic position.

Contraindications/Limitations

One of the advantages to the Cole osteotomy is the preservation of the essential joints of the foot. It is important that the rearfoot joints are assessed, and there is no evidence of arthrosis to the subtalar, midtarsal, and ankle joints. A fusion of the naviculocuneiform joints will cause additional stress on the adjacent joints, especially the talonavicular joint.

Motion at these rearfoot joints will continue to allow for adaptation with ambulation. If arthrosis is noted, then a triple or midtarsal arthrodesis with sagittal plane correction would be necessary.

The Cole osteotomy allows for purely sagittal plane correction. Removal of more bone dorsally from the medial cuneiform may improve the varus deformity, but not to the degree one would think. Therefore, a first metatarsal dorsiflexory osteotomy would be necessary in addition to the Cole to resolve the forefoot varus deformity [58–60].

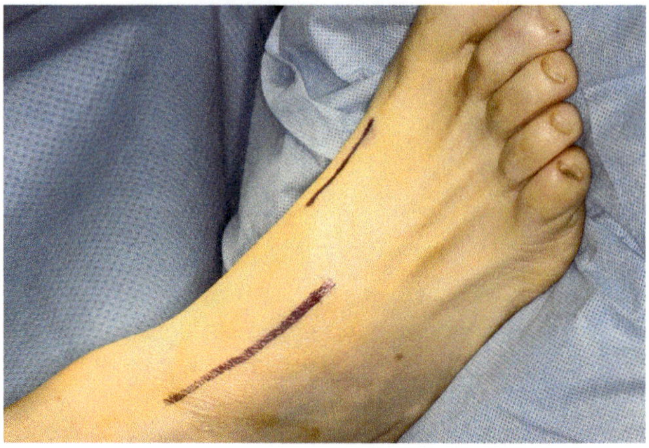

Fig. 23.42 The single dorsal incision placement for Cole osteotomy and DFWO

Technique, Pearls and Pitfalls

There are two different incisional approaches to the Cole osteotomy: the dual-incision approach and the single dorsal central one (Fig. 23.42). In the two-incision approach, if a PT tendon transfer is to be performed in combination with the Cole, then that medial incision is used. A second lateral incision is made overlying cuboid. Subperiosteal dissection is performed with care taken to avoid the neurovascular structures. Once the two incisions are connected, the osteotomy is performed. The proximal osteotomy is the first to be performed and is oriented nearly vertical to the foot. This bone cut is started just proximal to the naviculocuneiform joint and extended laterally to the midpoint of the cuboid.

The second osteotomy is performed next in which it is oriented to converge plantarly. The osteotomy begins on the distal aspect of the naviculocuneiform joint and exits laterally on the cuboid. Usually a 1–1.5 cm wedge is made during this osteotomy. The amount can vary pending the deformity present and can be assessed on a lateral X-ray intraoperatively to ensure adequate resection.

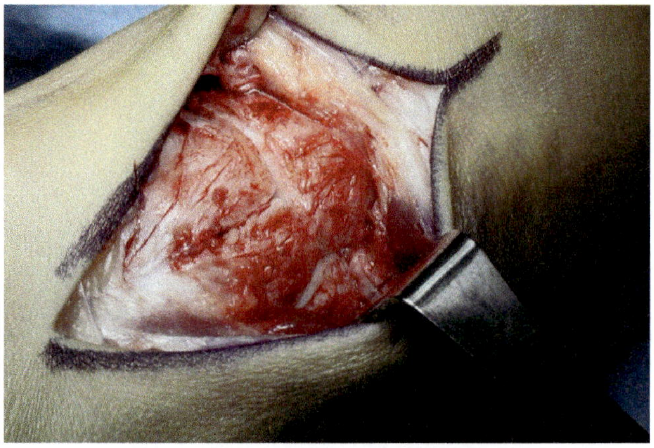

Fig. 23.43 Cole osteotomy through single-incision approach

The forefoot is then dorsiflexed upon the rearfoot to compress the osteotomy. Feathering may be needed to achieve a well-opposed osteotomy. Temporary fixation is then used once the desired position is confirmed under fluoroscopy. Final fixation is then performed using two or three 4.0 mm cannulated screws. The first screw is started at the medial cuneiform and oriented into the lateral navicular. The second screw is started at the lateral cuneiform and oriented into the medial navicular. It is important that fluoroscopy be used throughout this process to avoid screw placement into the talonavicular joint. A third screw is then placed orienting from the navicular tuberosity into the medial cuneiform.

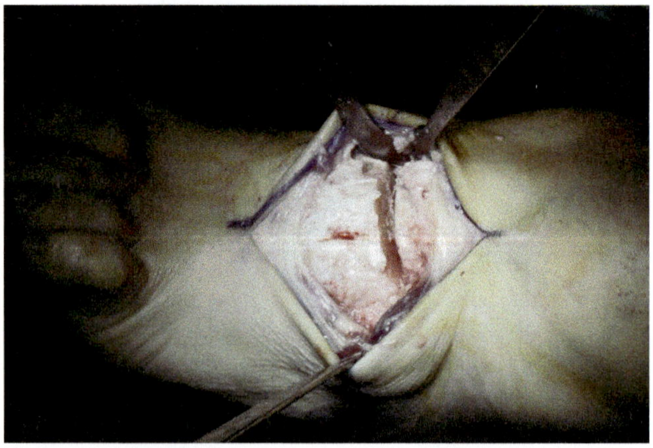

Fig. 23.44 Another view of the Cole osteotomy through single-incision approach

Incision placement is critical in obtaining proper exposure for this osteotomy. A single dorsal linear incision is preferred, which allows for direct visualization to the dorsum of the entire midfoot (Figs. 23.43 and 23.44). The limitation of this incision is the need to directly mobilize the neurovascular bundle medially. If the dissection is started lateral to the neurovascular bundle, subperiosteal dissection will avoid injury to these vital structures. The two-incision approach, medial and lateral, better protects for injury to the neurovascular structures, but visualization is limited in comparison.

Once the dissection has been carried out, it is critical to make a precise cut within the navicular, cuneiforms, and

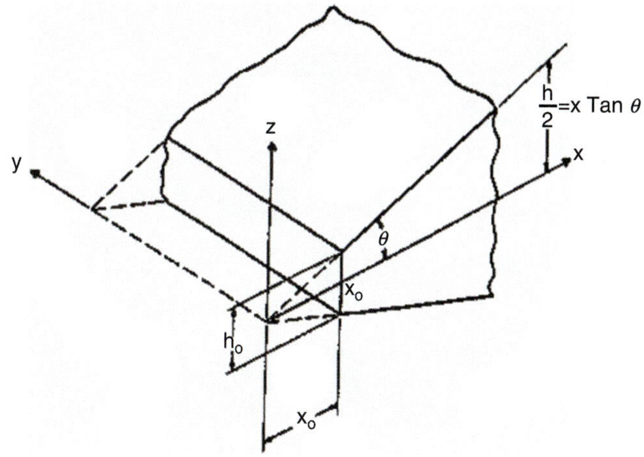

Fig. 23.45 Truncated wedge (*solid line*) vs. traditional wedge (*dotted line*)

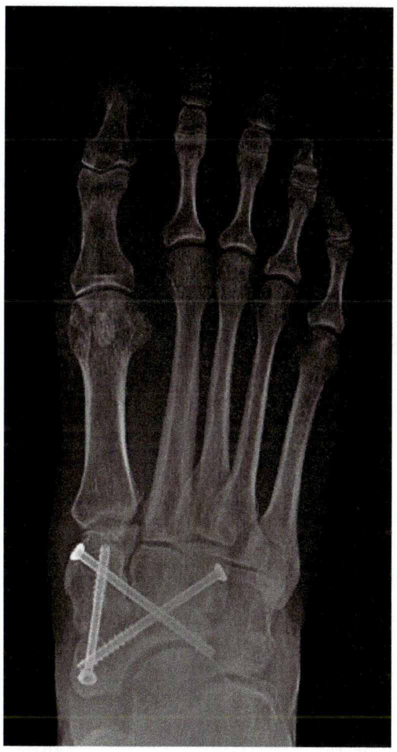

Fig. 23.46 Screw fixation with fixation of medial NC joint

cuboid. It is important that a truncated wedge not be made during this process. The removal of a pie-shaped wedge, not a truncated one, will prevent shortening of the foot (Fig. 23.45). If screw fixation is being utilized, which is the preferred method, then less bone should be removed from the navicular to allow for adequate space for the screws and/or plate placement.

One of the pitfalls with a dorsal incision is adequate fixation of the medial cuneiform to the navicular. For screw fixation, we have not only employed crossed screws but employ a screw from the navicular tuberosity to the medial cuneiform to directly compress these two bones (Fig. 23.46). This has resulted in more reproducible results of this part of the fusion.

A distinct wedge is removed from the navicular and cuneiforms, but not the cuboid. This is critical since excessive bone removal from the cuboid will dorsiflex the lateral column creating a very prominent and painful fifth metatarsal base. Understanding that the cuboid is lower than the medial column in the transverse arch results in a much smaller wedge of bone being removed from the cuboid.

Management of Complications

Complications related to the Cole osteotomy can be attributed to poor incision placement, osteotomy configuration (over-/undercorrection), nonunions, and osteotomy fixation. Overcorrection with excessive bone resection results in a painful bony prominence subfifth metatarsal or even a rocker bottom-type foot structure. A lesion most often will develop subfifth metatarsal base as a result of loss of the declination angle to the fifth metatarsal. Assessment must be done at the time of surgery and if necessary insertion of bone graft within the osteotomy is required to restore the lateral column arch. If this overcorrection is missed or ignored than resection of the plantar aspect of the fifth metatarsal, base may be required. Accommodative orthotics are also employed to help offload this area if symptomatic.

Undercorrection can occur with minimal wedge resection; however, this is not very common. Additional bone can be resected at the time of surgery if the cavus foot is not resolved. If the apex is distal after performing the Cole osteotomy, then dorsiflexory wedge osteotomies may be performed to the metatarsals to further lower the arch [57].

The most common complication with the Cole osteotomy is a nonunion, typically of the medial naviculocuneiform joint (Figs. 23.47 and 23.48). From the central incision, this joint is the most difficult to visualize. The typical crossed-screw technique doesn't afford enough compression and stability at

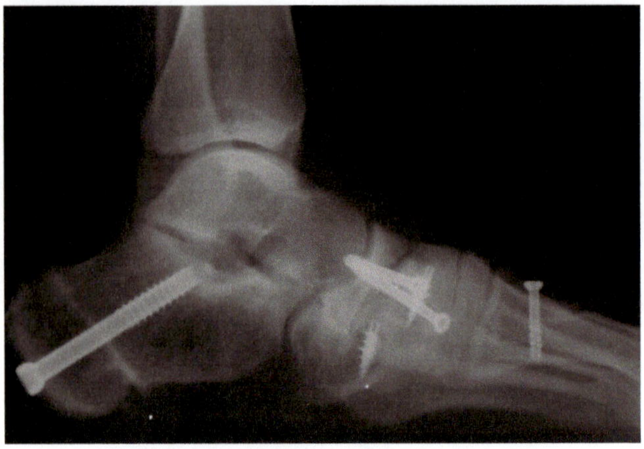

Fig. 23.47 Nonunion to NC joint

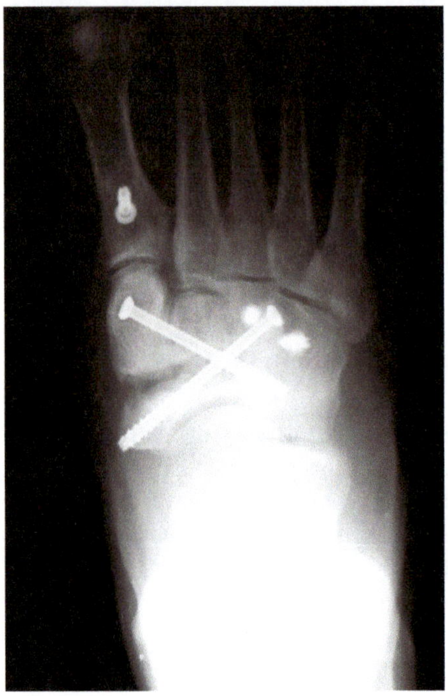

Fig. 23.48 Nonunion to NC joint. Notice that no screw from navicular tuberosity to cuneiform

this fusion location. To combat this potential complication, we have employed an additional screw from the navicular into the cuneiform to stabilize this joint. Treatment of the nonunion includes resection of the nonunion and insertion of bone graft and plate and screw fixation. This typically resolves the nonunion symptoms once healed.

In the past, complications included arthrosis of the midfoot postoperatively and change of shape of the foot into a more cube appearance. These complications are rare since we have employed screw fixation and stopped the use of large-size Steinmann pin fixation. Large pins crossing multiple joints easily can create arthrosis and have been abandoned due to more current options for fixation.

Reading the original article by Dr. Cole, he noted a triangular wedge of the bone resected from the NC joint, not a trapezoidal-shaped bone [57]. When done correctly, there is no significant shortening noted to the foot structure. Only if exuberant amount of the bone is resected will you note a shortening of the foot itself. Boxing of the hinge at the naviculocuneiform joint will require additional bone to be removed from the cuboid and the resultant shortened foot. In reality, lowering the arch with minimal plantar wedge resection of bone will actually cause lengthening of the foot.

Dwyer Calcaneal Osteotomy

Indications

Lateral closing wedge osteotomy of the calcaneus is the most common procedure used today to correct hindfoot varus deformity seen in pes cavus. Dwyer first described this procedure in 1959 in which the medial cortex remained intact [60]. This procedure is performed when a rigid rearfoot varus with a varus position of the calcaneus is present along with a mobile subtalar joint that does not display arthritic changes. It is important to evaluate the mobility of the subtalar joint. If there is subtalar arthritis, an arthrodesis of that joint with lateral wedge resection would be a more appropriate procedure choice [61, 62].

Technique, Pearls and Pitfalls

An incision is usually placed from the anterior aspect of the Achilles tendon at the dorsal aspect of the calcaneus toward to plantar cortex of the calcaneus at a 45° angle. Dissection is carried down to the bone with the sural nerve and peroneal tendons being anterior to the incision and not a factor in dissection (Figs. 23.49 and 23.50). The proximal cut for the osteotomy is performed perpendicular to the lateral surface of the calcaneus, parallel with the incision line. A sagittal saw is utilized and care is taken to not violate the medial cortex.

The second cut is placed 5 mm distal to the proximal cut and angle approximately 20° toward the medial hinge. The angle of the cut can be modified pending the amount of correction needed. Once again, the medial hinge is left intact. Following removal of the wedge, the osteotomy is manually reduced into valgus. If the osteotomy will not reduce, osteotome is utilized to release the medial hinge and mobilize the posterior tuber of the calcaneus. The surfaces are reciprocally planed to ensure excellent apposition of the osteotomy after the shift. With the osteotomy held in place, percutaneous screw fixation is achieved from the posterior-plantar heel

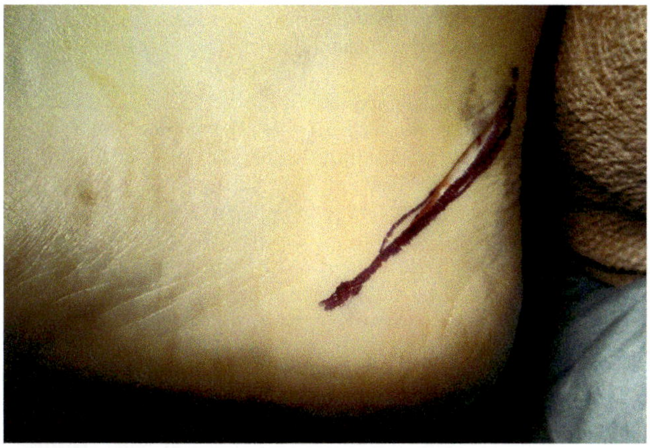

Fig. 23.49 Incision placement for Dwyer Calcaneal osteotomy

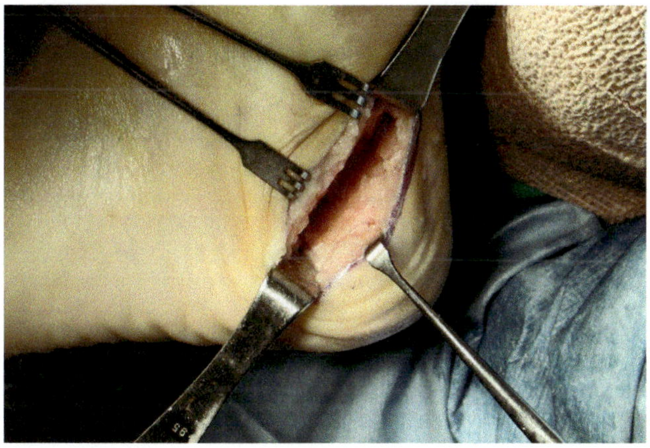

Fig. 23.50 Wedge removal for Dwyer Calcaneal osteotomy

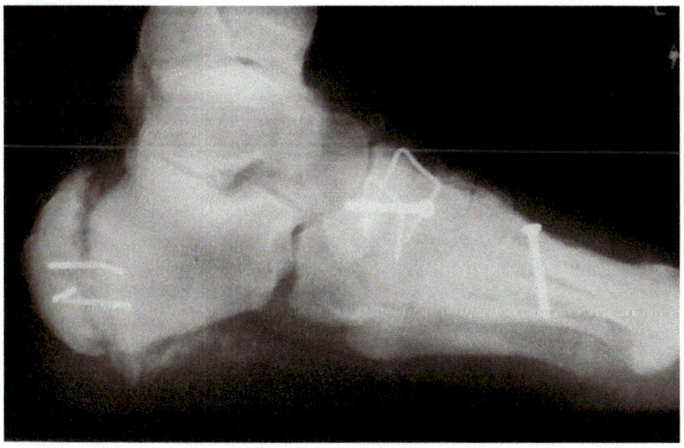

Fig. 23.51 Nonunion of a Dwyer Calcaneal osteotomy

perpendicular to the osteotomy. Different fixation techniques can be performed based on surgeon preference.

The Dwyer Calcaneal osteotomy can be used for multiplane correction of the calcaneus. After removal of the lateral wedge, the medial hinge can be broken or cut through. This will allow you to translate the posterior tuber lateral and dorsal to change the calcaneal inclination and heel alignment. A Steindler stripping should be performed prior to calcaneal osteotomy, as the contractures of the fascia and musculature can prevent plantar movement of the tuber [60, 63]. As discussed previously, this can be performed through the incision for the Dwyer by simply slightly elongating the incision plantarly.

There are many options for fixation of the Dwyer calcaneal osteotomy. Screw fixation starting at the tuberosity is the most common method, but plating and staples have been used successfully. Two points of fixation may be considered to prevent frontal plane motion of the tuberosity.

To avoid hematoma formation due to the vascular nature of the calcaneus, a subcutaneous drain should be placed in this incision. Lastly, incision closure can be an issue with skin-edge necrosis. A traumatic technique should be performed with minimal soft tissue handling. An absorbable suture results in minimal necrosis with the Dwyer skin incision.

Management of Complications

Incision complications such as dehiscence and necrosis are the majority of issues associated with a Dwyer Calcaneal osteotomy. The incision placement needs to be carefully planned prior to surgery. Often the Dwyer Calcaneal osteotomy will be associated with other procedures on the lateral side of the foot and ankle such as Steindler stripping, peroneal tendon repair/tenodesis, and also subtalar joint arthrodesis. If one is to encounter incision complications, then simple wound care with close follow-up is often all that is needed.

Sural nerve entrapment as well as peroneal tendon injury is rarely seen if careful dissection is performed. Proper incision placement is paramount to prevent the soft tissue complications. If a slide is performed with the wedge resection, then tamping the overhanging bone to the osteotomy site may prevent this irritation.

Nonunion, although very rare, is a major complication that is seen with a Dwyer Calcaneal osteotomy (Fig. 23.51). If a nonunion is encountered, then the patient should undergo conservative treatment including immobilization, possible external bone stimulator, and non-weight bearing. Displacement of the tuber fragment will necessitate surgical intervention as well as failure of conservative management. The hardware will need to be removed as well as all necrotic/sclerotic tissue from the osteotomy site. Two screws should be used at this time for rigid fixation and to prevent frontal plane motion.

Conclusion

The cavovarus foot deformity can be a daunting task to successfully resolve due to the complexity of the disorder. One must fully understand the neurologic etiology and determine the progressive or static nature of the deformity. This is critical in choosing the correct surgical procedure in order to obtain the best potential outcome and minimize complications. Typically all three planes of the foot are involved, which may require a combination of soft tissue and osseous procedures. Management of the complications for the more common surgical procedures for the cavovarus foot deformity is presented. Following these recommendations will help minimize the occurrence of complications and aid in treatment.

References

1. Kroon M, Faber FW, van der Linden M. Joint preservation surgery for correction of flexible pes cavovarus in adults. Foot Ankle Int. 2010;31:24–9.
2. Aminian A, Sangeorzan BJ. The anatomy of cavus foot deformity. Foot Ankle Clin. 2008;13(2):191–8.
3. Statler TK, Tullis BL. Pes cavus. J Am Podiatr Med Assoc. 2005;95(1):42–52.
4. Smith T, Green D. Pes Cavus. In: Banks AS, Downey MS, Martin DE, et al., editors. McGlamry's comprehensive textbook of foot and ankle surgery, vol. 1. 3rd ed. Philadelphia: Lippincott Williams & Wilkins; 2001. p. 761–98.
5. Smith T, Sapp M, Jobanpldtra R. Pes Cavus: an update of classification and management. PI Update Chapter. 2006;2:7–16.
6. Krause FG, Guyton GP. Pes Cavus. In: Mann RA, Coughlin MJ, editors. Surgery of the foot and ankle. 9th ed. St Louis (MO): Mosby; 2011. p. 1361–82.
7. McCluskey WP, Lovell WW, Cummings RJ. The cavovarus foot deformity. Etiology and management. Clin Orthop Relat Res. 1989;248:27–37.
8. Silver RL, de la Garza J, Rang M. The myth of muscle balance. A study of relative strengths and excursions of normal muscles about the foot and ankle. J Bone Joint Surg (Br). 1985;67(3):432–7.
9. Deben SE, Pomeroy GC. Subtle cavus foot: diagnosis and management. J Am Acad Orthop Surg. 2014;22(8):512–20.
10. Maskill MP, Maskill JD, Pomeroy GC. Surgical management and treatment algorithm for the subtle cavovarus foot. Foot Ankle Int. 2010;31(12):1057–63.
11. Watanabe RS. Metatarsal osteotomy for the cavus foot. Clin Orthop Relat Res. 1990;252:217–30.
12. Leeuwesteijn AE, de Visser E, Louwerens JW. Flexible cavovarus feet in Charcot-Marie-Tooth disease treated with first ray proximal dorsiflexion osteotomy combined with soft tissue surgery: a short-term to mid-term outcome study. Foot Ankle Surg. 2010;16(3):142–7.
13. DeVries JG, McAlister JE. Corrective osteotomies used in cavus reconstruction. Clin Podiatr Med Surg. 2015;32(3):375–87.
14. Sammarco GJ, Taylor R. Cavovarus foot treated with combined calcaneus and metatarsal osteotomies. Foot Ankle Int. 2001;22(1):19–30.
15. Conti SF, Kirchner JS, VanSickle D. Midfoot osteotomies. Foot Ankle Clin. 2001;6(3):519–32.
16. Sammarco GJ, Taylor R. Combined calcaneal and metatarsal osteotomies for the treatment of cavus foot. Foot Ankle Clin. 2001;6(3):533–43.
17. Zanolli DH, Glisson RR, Utturkar GM, Eckel TT, JK DO. Calcaneal "Z" osteotomy effect on hindfoot varus after triple arthrodesis in a cadaver model. Foot Ankle Int. 2014;35(12):1350–7.
18. Mandracchia VJ, Mandi DM, Nickles WA, Barp EA, Sanders SM. Pantalar arthrodesis. Clin Podiatr Med Surg. 2004;21(3):461–70.
19. Provelengios S, Papavasiliou KA, Kyrkos MJ, Kirkos JM, Kapetanos GA. The role of pantalar arthrodesis in the treatment of paralytic foot deformities. A long-term follow-up study. J Bone Joint Surg Am. 2009;91(3):575–83.
20. Provelengios S, Papavasiliou KA, Kyrkos MJ, Sayegh FE, Kirkos JM, Kapetanos GA. The role of pantalar arthrodesis in the treatment of paralytic foot deformities. Surgical technique. J Bone Joint Surg Am. 2010;92(Suppl 1 Pt 1):44–54.
21. Wapner KL. Triple arthrodesis in adults. J Am Acad Orthop Surg. 1998;6(3):188–96.
22. Steindler A. Operative treatment of pes cavus. Surg Gynecol Obstet. 1917;24:612–5.
23. Steindler A. Stripping of the os calcis. Am J Orthop Surg. 1920;2:8–12.
24. Wapner K. Pes Cavus. In: Myerson MS, editor. Foot and ankle disorders. Philadelphia: WB Saunders; 2000. p. 919–41.
25. Mann R. Pes Cavus. In: Mann RA, Coughlin MJ, editors. Surgery of the foot and ankle. St Louis (MO): Mosby; 1993. p. 785–801.
26. Schuberth JM, Babu-Spencer N. The impact of the first ray in the cavovarus foot. Clin Podiatr Med Surg. 2009;26(3):385–93.
27. Azmaipairashvili Z, Riddle EC, Scavina M, Kumar SJ. Correction of cavovarus foot deformity in Charcot-Marie-Tooth disease. J Pediatr Orthop. 2005;25(3):360–5.
28. Berg EE. Percutaneous Achilles tendon lengthening complicated by inadvertent tenotomy. J Pediatr Orthop. 1992;12(3):341–3.
29. Kay RM, Rethlefsen SA, Ryan JA, Wren TA. Outcome of gastrocnemius recession and tendo-achilles lengthening in ambulatory children with cerebral palsy. J Pediatr Orthop B. 2004;13(2):92–8.
30. Thompson GH, Hoyen HA, Barthel T. Tibialis anterior tendon transfer after clubfoot surgery. Clin Orthop Relat Res. 2009;467(5):1306–13.
31. Gray K, Burns J, Little D, Bellemore M, Gibbons P. Is tibialis anterior tendon transfer effective for recurrent clubfoot? Clin Orthop Relat Res. 2014;472(2):750–8.
32. Shapiro F, Bresnan MJ. Orthopaedic management of childhood neuromuscular disease. Part II: peripheral neuropathies, Friedreich's ataxia and arthrogryposis multiplex congenital. J Bone Joint Surg. 1982;64A:949–53.
33. Lampasi M, Bettuzzi C, Palmonari M, et al. Transfer of the tendon of tibialis anterior in relapsed congenital clubfoot: long-term results in 38 feet. J Bone Joint Surg (Br). 2010;92:277–83.
34. Bluman E, Dowd T. The basics and science of tendon transfers. Foot Ankle Clin. 2011;16:385–99.
35. Ezra E, Hayek S, Gilai AN, et al. Tibialis anterior tendon transfer for residual dynamic supination deformity in treated club feet. J Pediatr Orthop B. 2000;9:207–11.
36. Reilly CM. Principles of muscle-tendon surgery and tendon transfers. In: Banks AS, Downey MS, Martin DE, et al., editors. McGlamry's comprehensive textbook of foot and ankle surgery. 3rd ed. Philadelphia: Lippincott Williams & Wilkins; 2001. p. 1523–66.
37. Younger AS, Hansen Jr ST. Adult cavovarus foot. J Am Acad Orthop Surg. 2005;13(5):302–15.
38. Ward CM, Dolan LA, Bennett DL, et al. Long-term results of reconstruction for treatment of a flexible cavovarus foot in Charcot-Marie- Tooth disease. J Bone Joint Surg Am. 2008;90:2631–42.

39. Jay, Richard. Anatomic, mechanical, and surgical considerations in myeloblastic maneuvers about the foot and ankle. Current therapy in podiatric surgery. 1989.
40. Myerson MS. Paralytic disorders of the lower extremity. In: Myerson MS, editor. Foot and ankle disorders. Philadelphia: WB Saunders; 2000. p. 883–99.
41. Mann RA. Tendon transfers and electromyography. Clin Orthop Relat Res. 1972;85:64–6.
42. Hsu J, Hoffer M. Posterior tibial tendon transfer anteriorly through the interosseous membrane: a modification of the technique. Clin Orthop Relat Res. 1978;131:202–4.
43. Miller GM, Hsu JD, Hoffer MM, Rentfro R. Posterior tibial tendon transfer: a review of the literature and analysis of 74 procedures. J Pediatr Orthop. 1982;2(4):363–70.
44. DiDomenico LD, Cane LD. Key insights on tendon transfers for drop foot. Podiatry Today. 2009;22(5)
45. Williams PF. Restoration of muscle balance of the foot by transfer of the tibialis posterior. J Bone Joint Surg (Br). 1976;56:217–9.
46. Goecker RM, Banks AS, Downey MS, et al. Charcot-Marie-tooth disease. In: Bobery JT, Downey MS, Nakra A, et al., editors. McGlamry's comprehensive textbook of foot and ankle surgery, vol. 2. 4th ed. Philadelphia: Lippincott Williams & Wilkins; 2013. p. 761–98.
47. Beals TC, Nickisch F. Charcot-Marie-tooth disease and the cavovarus foot. Foot Ankle Clin. 2008;13(2):259–74.
48. Gould N. Surgery in advanced Charcot-Marie-tooth disease. Foot Ankle Clin. 1984;4(5):267–73.
49. Molloy R, Tisdel C. Failed treatment of peroneal tendon injuries. Foot Ankle Clin. 2003;8(1):115–29.
50. Squires N, Myerson MS, Gamba C. Surgical treatment of peroneal tendon tears. Foot Ankle Clin. 2007;12(4):675–95.
51. Mook WR, Parekh SG, Nunley JA. Allograft reconstruction of peroneal tendons: operative technique and clinical outcomes. Foot Ankle Int. 2013;34(9):1212–20.
52. Olson SL, Ledoux WR, Ching RP, et al. Muscular imbalances resulting in a clawed hallux. Foot Ankle Int. 2003;24:477–85.
53. Breusch SJ, Wenz W, Döderlein L. Function after correction of a clawed great toe by a modified Robert Jones transfer. J Bone Joint Surg (Br). 2000;82(2):250–4.
54. Abousayed M, Kwon JY. Hallux claw toe. Foot Ankle Clin. 2014;19:59–63.
55. Shaffer LW. Osteotomy of the metatarsals for pes cavus. South Med J. 1977;70:77–9.
56. Cole WH. The classic. The treatment of claw-foot. By Wallace H. Cole. 1940. Clin Orthop Relat Res. 1983;181:3–6.
57. Tullis BL, Mendicino RW, Catanzariti AR, et al. The Cole midfoot osteotomy: a retrospective review of 11 procedures in 8 patients. J Foot Ankle Surg. 2004;43:160–5.
58. Groner TW, DiDomenico LA. Midfoot osteotomies for the cavus foot. Clin Podiatr Med Surg. 2005;22:247–6.
59. Wülker N, Hurschler C. Cavus foot correction in adults by dorsal closing wedge osteotomy. Foot Ankle Int. 2002;23:344–34.
60. Dwyer FC. Osteotomy of the calcaneum for pes cavus. J Bone Joint Surg (Br). 1959;41-B(1):80–6.
61. Robinson DS, Clark Jr B, Prigoff MM. Dwyer Calcaneal osteotomy for treatment of calcaneal varus. J Foot Surg. 1988;27:541–4.
62. Bariteau JT, Blankenhorn BD, Tofte JN, DiGiovanni CW. What is the role and limit of calcaneal osteotomy in the cavovarus foot? Foot Ankle Clin. 2013;18(4):697–714.
63. Dekel S, Weissman SL. Osteotomy of the calcaneus and concomitant plantar stripping in children with talipes cavo-varus. J Bone Joint Surg (Br). 1973;55(4):802–8.

24 The Charcot Foot

Naohiro Shibuya

Introduction

Pathogenesis of neuroarthropathy is debatable. A number of theories have been proposed, but it is conceivable that sensorimotor along with autonomic neuropathy of any origin can potentially result in development of the disease. Although poliomyelitis, folate deficiency, spinal cord lesions, meningomyelocele, syringomyelia, leprosy, and peripheral nerve injuries are reported as causes of neuroarthropathy in the literature [1–7], most of the Charcot arthropathies in the foot and ankle manifest in a diabetic population [8, 9]. This may be due to the sequelae of diabetic neuroarthropathy being far more detrimental than those of nondiabetics.

In the lower limbs, development of micro- and macrovascular diseases, along with peripheral neuropathy, makes wound and bone healings extremely difficult [10, 11]. This results in the incidence of amputation being more than ten times higher in diabetics than in nondiabetics [12, 13]. Diabetic patients with Charcot disease can also be less compliant, more obese and more immunocompromised; and these characteristics can complicate the pre- and postoperative managements. While Addolorato et al. showed significantly lower body mass index in alcoholics comparing to social drinkers [14], Pinzur et al. observed a large proportion of obesity in patients with midfoot Charcot deformity [15].

Due to these reasons, people with symptomatic neuroarthropathy are categorized in one of the highest-risk groups that foot and ankle surgeons can encounter. Surgeons who treat these patients therefore need to be familiar with common complications associated with neuropathy, noncompliance, obesity, poor glycemic control, and any other underlying medical and social conditions that are common in this population.

N. Shibuya (✉)
Texas A&M University, Health Science Center, College of Medicine, Temple, TX 76504, USA

Surgical Services, Central Texas VA Health Care System, Veterans Hospital, Temple, TX, USA

Department of Surgery, Baylor Scott and White Health Care System, 2401 S. 31st St., Temple, TX 76504, USA
e-mail: shibuya@medicine.tamhsc.edu

Indication for Procedure

Due to a high complication rate, indication of such reconstructive surgery, especially in revision surgery, should be carefully evaluated. While primary Charcot reconstruction is indicated in patients who can otherwise lose his/her limb, in a revision surgery one has to reconsider the benefit of amputation as well. Charcot arthropathy represents an end spectrum of the diabetic disease process along with cardiovascular, neurological, and immunological problems; therefore, even a perfectly executed reconstructive surgery may result in major complications. If a patient is doomed to fail reconstruction, primary amputation reduces patients' burden and healthcare cost significantly.

In the arena of vascular reconstruction in critical limb ischemia, there are guidelines to assist surgeons decide whether to salvage or amputate. These guidelines are based on numerous studies evaluating quality of life and cost effectiveness of amputation versus vascular reconstruction [16–27]. These guidelines are developed to reduce futile reconstructions.

Trans-Atlantic Inter-Society Consensus have suggested that primary amputation in critical limb ischemia is indicated when (1) it is non-reconstructable, (2) there is significant necrosis on weight-bearing surface, (3) there is flexion contracture of the leg, or (4) the patient is terminal ill/limited in life expectancy [28]. Further, European Consensus Document states, "a reconstructive procedure should be attempted if there is a 25% chance of saving a useful limb for more than one year" [29].

On the other hand, there is no consensus or guidelines for Charcot reconstructive surgery though these patients may be classified in the same health-risk category. The 5-year survival rates in these critical limb ischemia patients having a major amputation and Charcot patients are similar [30, 31].

M.S. Lee, J.P. Grossman (eds.), *Complications in Foot and Ankle Surgery*, DOI 10.1007/978-3-319-53686-6_24

Lack of guidelines in Charcot reconstruction therefore demands foot and ankle surgeons to methodically evaluate the patients' medical and social conditions prior to considering extensive reconstructive works. The surgeons need to be able to evaluate the patient's practicality to rehabilitate and likelihood of saving a functional limb for a decent period of time.

For example, high-risk patients, such as ones with end-stage renal disease (ESRD) on dialysis, are known to have poor prognosis. According to US renal data system, life expectancy of dialysis patient between 65 to 69 years old is 3.2 years, and 2-year survival rate in those patients who undergo vascular reconstruction is approximately 50% [20–22, 32, 33]. When compared to a longitudinal study by Lavery et al. [34], the 2-year survival in those dialysis patients who underwent various lower extremity amputations was comparable or even superior. This may suggest that amputation may not necessary accelerate mortality in these high-risk patients.

As reconstruction requires substantial time to recover, it demands a considerable fraction of his/her remaining lifetime. These patients undergo burden of office visits and prolonged non-weight-bearing status, which may worsen their quality of life significantly. It should also be noted that a failed reconstruction resulting in amputation is significantly more debilitating to the patient when compared to primary amputation.

Therefore, only a small proportion of patients may truely benefit from these extensive procedures. These procedures may best benefit selected relatively young, compliant patients with longer remaining life expectancy, who is less likely to be deconditioned from a long recovery process, and also those who can improve underlying biology or medical conditions.

Contraindications/Limitations

Because of the reasons indicated above, many patients who are in this category are poor candidates for surgical revisions. Therefore, risk factor assessment via evaluation of medical conditions, socioeconomic state, and psychology is necessary to avoid further complications. While many surgeons may be familiar with the medical-risk factors, the patient's socioeconomic state and psychology are often overlooked.

It can be impractical for some patients to stay off-weight-bearing completely, acquire an expensive brace, and obtain family support or even to make it to the postoperative office visits frequently. A surgeon needs to be an excellent social worker to understand every aspect of perioperative socioeconomic needs for the patients.

Similarly, psychology of the patient is very important when assessing these individuals. Compliance, expectations, and intelligence of the patient and availability of his/her family need to be evaluated thoroughly. It is not uncommon that the patient's initial office visit is the surgical consultation visit, as the referring physician may have already tried conservative measures. Therefore, the surgeon may spend a little time with the patient before scheduling for surgery.

Many of these patients can have a high hope and expectations. A full comprehension of the disease process, risks, and benefits of the surgical management, postoperative convalescence, and reasonable surgical outcomes may take a long time or even several office visits for those patients. During these visits, a surgeon may gain a better understanding of the patient's and his/her family's personality, perspective, intelligence level, and expectations.

There is overwhelming evidence that a high glycated hemoglobin level is associated with poor outcomes in foot and ankle surgery. Both wound and bone healings are independently associated with poor glycemic control [35–37]. Many use a cutoff level of 7% to categorize good versus poor surgical candidates, based on the American Diabetes Association (ADA) recommendation. The ADA recommendation is derived from several studies assessing intensive glycemic control therapy in reducing long-term complications associated with diabetes. However, under glycated hemoglobin of 7%, the benefits seem to diminish, and there is also a risk of adverse events including death, weight gain, and hypoglycemic episodes from a rapid drop in the glucose level.

However, what constitutes an "acceptable" or "ideal" glycated hemoglobin level for foot and ankle Charcot surgery is still unclear. An "acceptable" upper glycated hemoglobin limit for foot and ankle surgery can be interpreted as a level from where the rate of complication spikes significantly. Alternately, the "acceptable" cutoff line can be defined as the level at which the risks associated with surgery become greater than those associated with nonsurgical treatment. Regardless, the "acceptable" level may vary depending on the procedure. For example, incision and drainage for infection may have a higher "acceptable" glycated hemoglobin level than an elective reconstructive surgery.

Most studies in foot and ankle surgery to date are comparisons of glycated hemoglobin levels between groups with or without complications. As recommended by many, including the American Diabetes Association, glycated hemoglobin of 7% is known to be a relatively good reference point, at least in terms of general health. However, there are no Charcot-specific guidelines. Jupiter et al. have shown the trend in complication rate in accordance of perioperative glycated hemoglobin [36]. They have found that the rate of complication quickly elevates after approximately 7.4%. However, at this level the soft tissue complication rate was already over 20%.

Because the patients with a Charcot foot are high risk, modifiable factors should be optimized. Smoking and morbid obesity may be relative contraindications to some surgeons in non-Charcot elective surgeries. The adverse effects of these factors are accentuated when coexisting with other uncontrollable risk factors in Charcot patients.

There are many other medical factors in these high-risk patients that are considered contraindications for a surgical management. Those other medical factors will be discussed under each specific complication section.

Technique Pearls and Pitfalls

Surgical management of Charcot foot is mostly presented in low-level studies [38]. The relative paucity of this group of patients precludes any well-controlled studies to show statistically meaningful results. Although there is no consensus on the "best" approach for primary Charcot reconstruction, some intraoperative factors are known to affect surgical outcomes. Avoiding complications is difficult in Charcot surgery since many variables besides surgical execution play a role in the poor outcomes. As mentioned earlier, underlying medical condition, psychology, and socioeconomic states of the patients are as or more important than surgical techniques themselves.

Midfoot Charcot deformity may be reconstructed with dorsal, planter, medial, lateral, or combination of those incisional approaches. Although most of these patients are insensate, a careful dissection is still paramount to preserve remaining neurological structures, as they are still important for bone and soft tissue metabolism for healing. Arthroscopic preparation of ankle or rearfoot joints or any other minimally invasive approach would also help increase the bone and wound healing potential in these high-risk patients.

Soft tissue dissection is followed by resection of necrotic or infected bone. Similar to revision surgery in nonunion patients, good bleeding cancellous bone is needed for a successful fusion. Aggressive resection is often needed to achieve this goal. It should be noted that the density of the Charcot bone might not necessarily be lower than a healthy bone. In fact, the density of chronic neuroarthropathic bone can be increased as the quality of trabecular pattern worsens [39]. Therefore, after resection of the brittle soft bone, one has to also make sure that sclerotic, chronic neuropathic bone margin is also resected. Preoperative radiographic examinations, such as plain X-rays or MRI can reveal the extent of infected or necrotic bone (Fig. 24.1).

Aggressive resection of the necrotic bone can result in shortening of the foot. Though it may not be visually appealing to the patient, biomechanically this can be advantageous. A shortened foot results in a smaller moment lever arm during the stance to propulsion phases of the gait and reduces the forefoot pressure. Though the maximum involvement in neuroarthropathy may be in the midfoot, Armstrong et al. have found that the peak pressure was in the forefoot [40]; therefore, reducing this pressure by shortening the foot may be biomechanically beneficial. It may also indirectly reduce the mechanical stress applied to the midfoot, contributing to the survival of the internal fixation devices. Though the patient needs to be aware of this potential shortening of the foot, because the reconstruction straightens the overlapped midfoot, the foot may not appear significantly shorter than preoperative length to many patients (Fig. 24.2). The patients should however be notified about digital deformities or non-purchasing digits that it may cause (Fig. 24.3).

It is not advisable to use nonviable osteobiologics to replace the necrotic Charcot bone. Not only the evidence for use of such products are lacking, replacing such a large defect and to achieve stable union is difficult even in healthy individuals. Because pathophysiology of neuroarthropathy involves inhibited anti-inflammatory process (Fig. 24.4), introduction of reactive foreign materials, excessive inflammatory cytokines, and growth factors may result in a vicious, uncontrolled, inflammatory cycle.

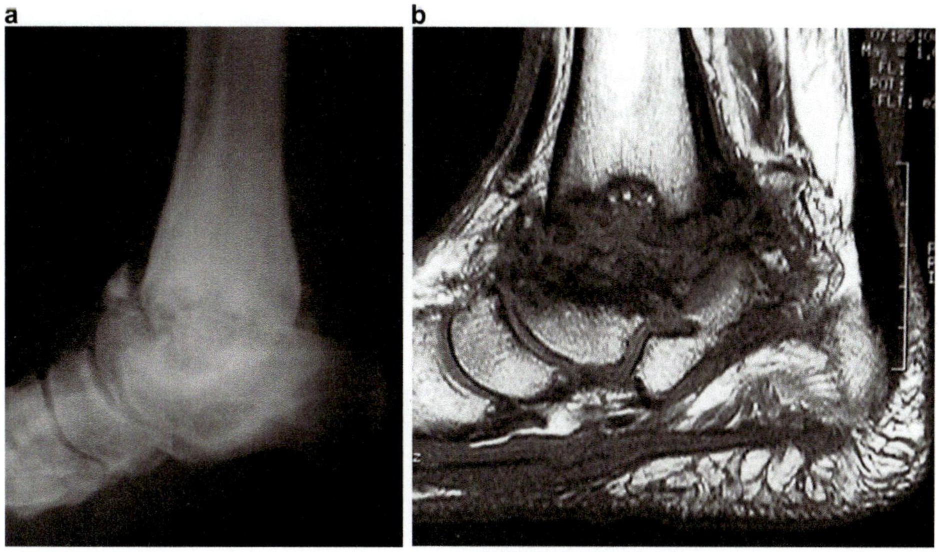

Fig. 24.1 While the extent of the diseased bone may not be clear in a plain X-ray, it may be clear in an MRI

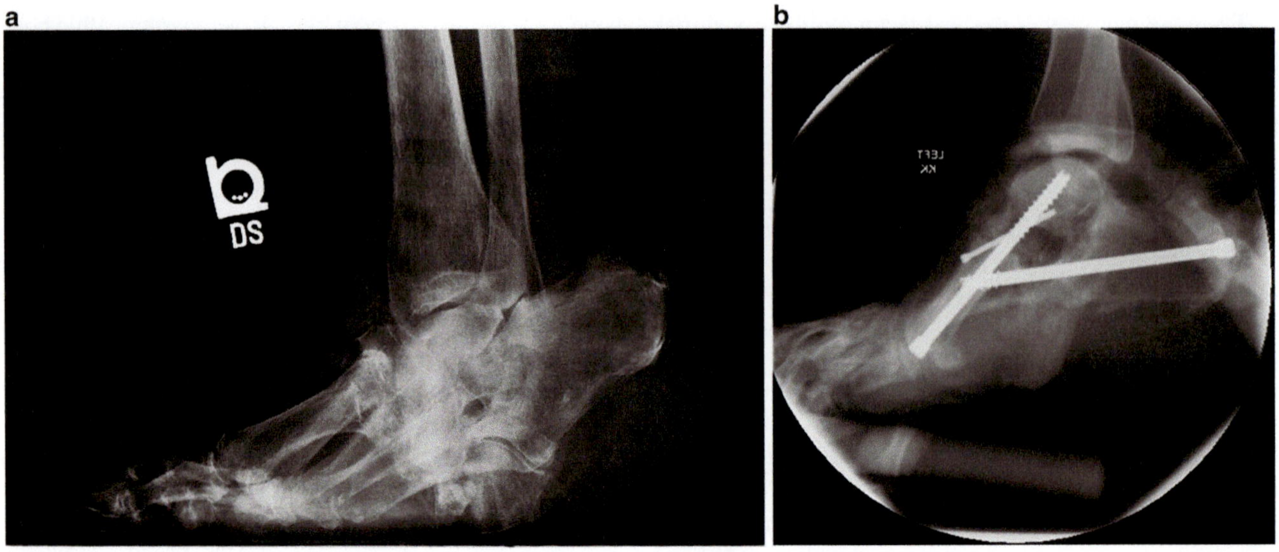

Fig. 24.2 (a) A Charcot foot may already appear shortened due to the overlapping of the midfoot. (b) Aggressive resection of the diseased midfoot bones may not necessarily result in a shorter appearing foot

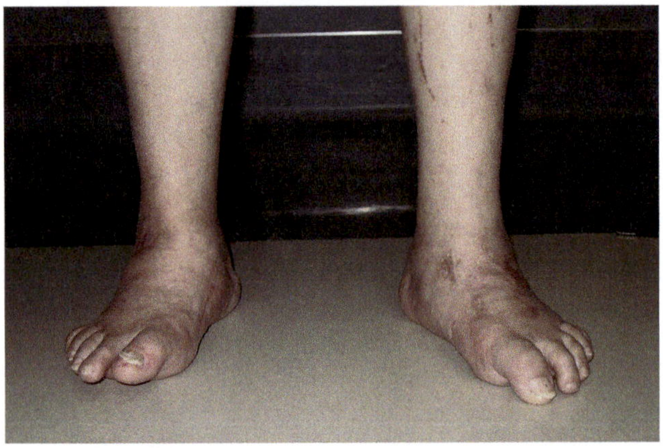

Fig. 24.3 Shortening of the midfoot can lead to non-purchasing digits due to loss of extensor and flexor stabilization

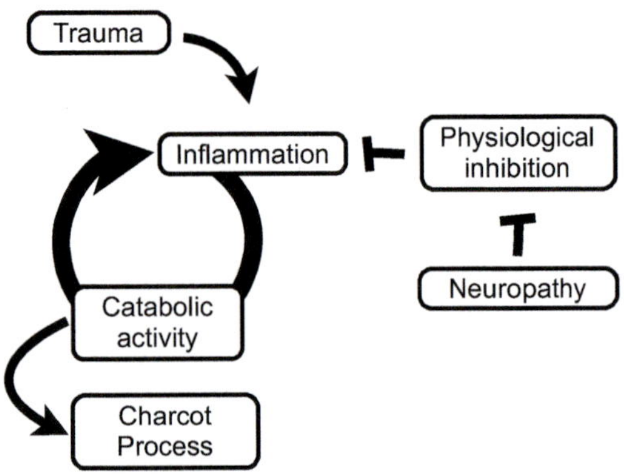

Fig. 24.4 Inhibition of the physiological anti-inflammatory feedback system due to neuropathy can result in excessive catabolic activities and a Charcot process

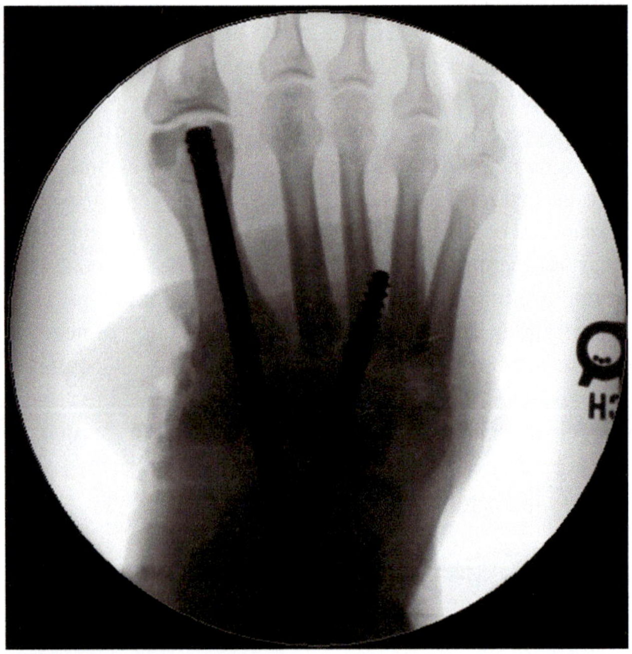

Fig. 24.5 Resection of cuneiforms and distal cuboid resulting in the fifth metatarsal not articulating with the rearfoot when the medial column is aligned due to the wider forefoot to the narrower rearfoot

A minimal amount of nonreactive material may be indicated to fill a small void given that most of the arthrodesis sites are in close proximity. Some mesenchymal cell-based products are thought to have anti-inflammatory effect in the local tissue via paracrine signaling [41–43] though this phenomenon is yet to be tested in a Charcot clinical study. Research in this area is lacking understandably due to its relatively low prevalence of the disease.

Another caveat to aggressive resection of the necrotic tissue is that it often results in mismatching of the forefoot to the rearfoot. Because forefoot is wider than the rearfoot, it may not be possible to align both medial and lateral columns onto the remaining rearfoot (Fig. 24.5). If needs to be chosen, aligning the medial column is far more critical than the lateral column. It is advisable to align the first ray with the long axis of the talus even though the lateral column alignment may be compromised.

When resecting the midfoot, it is also important to avoid severe abduction or adduction. The midfoot often needs to be resected uniformly across from medial to lateral even when Charcot is affecting one side. When neuroarthropathy affects mainly the medial side and only the medial necrotic bone is aggressively resected, the significant shortening of the medial column can result in excessive forefoot adduction. This is biomechanically intolerable; therefore, resection of the healthy lateral column may be necessary to achieve balanced medial and lateral columns.

After arthrodesis sites are prepared, the forefoot is impacted onto the rearfoot and fixations are applied. Though it is a surgeon's preference, some fundamental of fixation should be reviewed.

Many of the screws are positioning and beaming in nature in Charcot reconstruction rather than compression. It is more critical for the screws to be strong and resistant to bending. Unlike elective arthrodesis surgeries in non-neuroarthropathic patients, bone healing is expected to be prolonged, and patients are less likely to be able to off-load the operative foot effectively. It should be noted that stainless steel, solid screws are far stronger than titanium and cannulated screws given the same size. Additionally, the core diameter, rather than the outer diameter, of the screw determines the overall shearing and bending resistance.

One also needs to remember that fatigue property and ductility of the screws play a role in the long-term stability. Because of the cold-working process in stainless steel, the ductility is significantly compromised when compared to titanium. Therefore, once the metal is bent or contoured, it becomes more brittle. This concept is particularly important when considering plate fixation.

Pullout strength is significantly better with titanium since the friction is greater due to its osseointegration. Though it is a useful property for a rigid, long-term fixation, removal of such screws is more difficult. Biocompatibility is superior with titanium, yet that of stainless steel is still sufficient, and nickel allergy is rare. When a patient needs an MRI in the future, titanium avoids signal void effects.

For plate fixation, abovementioned metallurgy is still relevant. The plate fixation, however, requires more molding to a contour of the osseous structures; therefore, ductility of the metal cannot be over-emphasized.

External fixation has been popular in Charcot reconstruction [44–47]. It can provide extra stability, dynamic compression if necessary, potential earlier weight-bearing, postoperative deformity correction, and bypassing of an infected area via spanning/bridging (Fig. 24.6). One always however needs to remember that the use of such fixation, especially with combination of other internal fixations and osteobiologics, is very expensive. Cost effectiveness of such construct has not been thoroughly studied. In addition, when it is used as a sole fixation, one has to remember that the external fixation may need to be removed prematurely to avoid pin tract infection prior to bone healing. In combination with internal fixation, it may add extra stability, but a long-term clinical benefit is in question [48]. Pin tract infection is also common [49], yet for a more salvage-type procedure where internal fixation is already attempted or not feasible, external fixation may be the only option (Fig. 24.7).

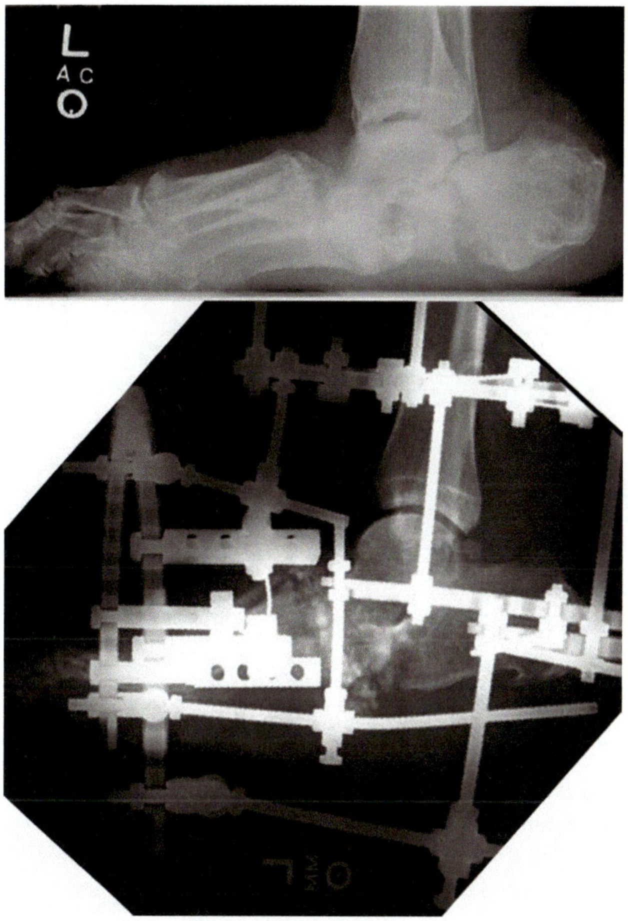

Fig. 24.6 After resection of infected midfoot bones, antibiotic impregnated bone substitute was packed in the dead space. External fixation was utilized to stabilize the foot while managing the infection and also to gradually reduce the deformity while compressing the forefoot onto the rearfoot to prepare for future arthrodesis with internal fixation

Gradual correction with dynamic multiplanar external fixation may be another option (Fig. 24.8); however, pin tract infection can be even more prevalent in these immunocompromised patients, especially with the motion and potential loosening of the transfixation wires. Internal fixation can be applied in the second stage with a minimally invasive approach after deformity is corrected [46].

Besides types of fixation, orientation of fixation is also important. The weakest point of fixation will be at the level of Charcot bone or the fusion site. The purpose of fixation is

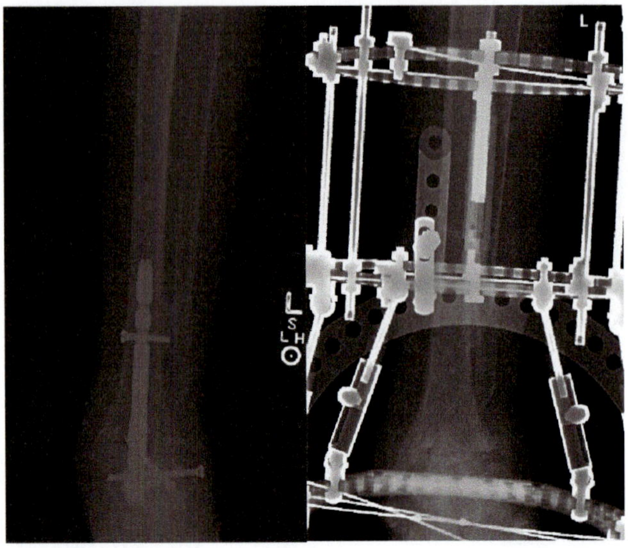

Fig. 24.7 After an infected retrograde intramedullary nail was removed, a multiplanar external fixation was utilized to maintain stability

normally to stabilize the area until union. However, in Charcot patients, pseudoarthrosis or nonunion is not uncommon. Therefore, fixations need to withstand the weight-bearing force for a long period of time. A long-term structural support may be more important than short-term rigidity in this population.

For midfoot neuroarthropathy, it is important to establish a stable medial column. An unstable medial column can result in a recurrent collapse and/or abduction or adduction of the forefoot. There are several ways to establish long-term stabilization of the medial column. The most common methods are the beaming techniques that are established by an intramedullary screw or a plate-screw construct. An intramedullary screw is inserted in the first ray through the first metatarsal phalangeal joint, through the posterior aspect of the talus or base of the first metatarsal (Fig. 24.9). While a cannulated screw will allow much easier and precise insertion, such a screw is significantly weaker than a solid one. A solid, large core diameter screw is recommended for a stronger construct. If inserted in a retrograding fashion through the first metatarsophalangeal joint, a headless screw is needed. An approximately 3 cm incision can be made plantar to the first metatarsophalangeal joint longitudinally. The joint is then dorsiflexed, and the plantar plate and capsule are incised to expose the head of the first metatarsal bone from the plantar surgical wound. Once exposed, the midfoot is reduced to the plantigrade orientation, and a guide wire is inserted though the first ray before reaming. The reaming can be performed over the guide wire utilizing cannulated instruments that are appropriate for the solid screw size. A good reaming is necessary to insert a large diameter screw without fracturing the first metatarsal.

In order to achieve stability, the beaming screw often needs to reach all the way to the talus even if the talonavicular joint is not affected by neuroarthropathy nor prepared for arthrodesis (Fig. 24.10). The navicular or medial cuneiform is not robust enough to hold the beaming screw in a Charcot patient (Fig. 24.10). As mentioned earlier, when extensive resection of the midfoot is done, the first metatarsal may not align with the long axis of the talus as the first metatarsal may sit medial to the talus in the transverse plane. The first ray may need to be translated laterally or angulated medially to capture the talus.

Alternatively, a plate fixation can be utilized to "beam" the medial column. Often a locking plate-screw construct is utilized for this purpose as it can achieve stronger angular stability at the plate-screw interface. A locking plate-screw construct does not rely on friction created on the plate-bone interface; therefore, preservation of periosteal vascular supply can be managed. With minimally invasive dissection technique, this theoretically aids in bone healing. Yet, clinical benefit of locking plate in Charcot surgery is not extensively studied.

An additional interfragmentary screw may aid more rigidity by achieving absolute stability via compression across the fusion site rather than relying solely on locking plate-screw construct, often used for relative stability. Relative stability, with flexible fixation without compression, in theory can result in secondary bone healing via more biological fixation. However, this needs to rely on natural bone callus formation. In these high-risk neuropathic patients with abnormal biology, this may be difficult. It is unknown at this point which of the healing process, between primary and secondary bone healing, is better in Charcot patients. Yet, it should be reminded that bone healing in neuropathic patients is significantly prolonged, and the fixation devices may fail prior to bone callus formation. On the other hand, excessive rigidity may transfer the stress or strain to other areas and can cause a fracture or acute Charcot process (Fig. 24.11).

Orientation of the plate significantly changes the strength of the beam. A plate applied to the dorsal aspect of the first ray is more subject to bending and fatiguing than one placed on the medial aspect (Fig. 24.12). When the plate is placed in a vertical orientation, like a floor joist, it is much harder to fail with weight-bearing.

Application of the plate more plantarly can result in conversion of the weight-bearing force into compression force via tension banding (Fig. 24.12). However, in order for tension banding to work, the bones must have a strong dorsal cortex. Many Charcot bones are fragile; therefore, a care must be taken to inspect the quality of the bone before attempting this technique.

For transfixation screws, longer screws with multiple cortical purchases are always more stable than unicortical purchases.

For the central rays and the lateral columns, the same principles are applied. While alignment of the lesser rays are

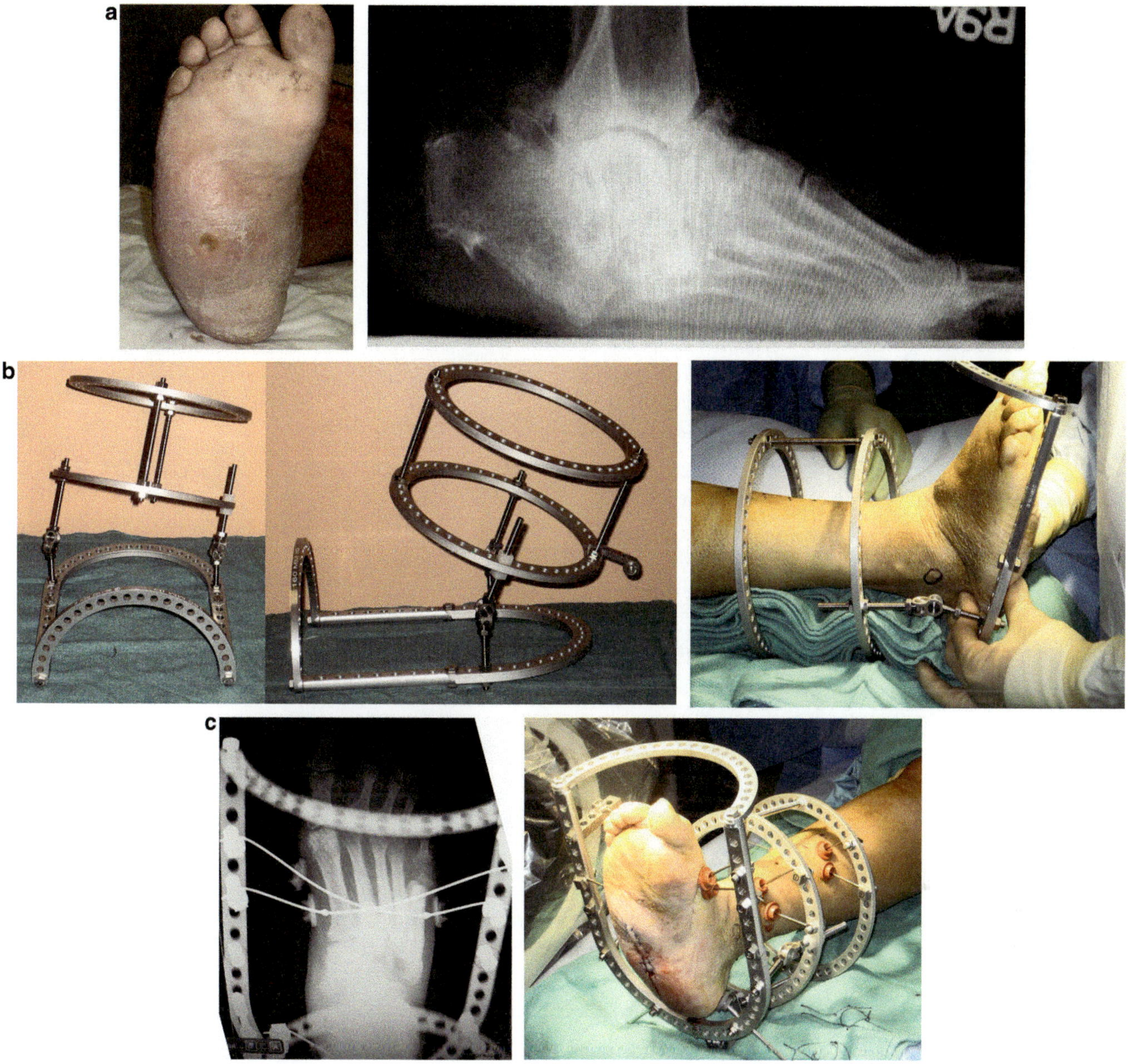

Fig. 24.8 (**a**) A patient with midfoot osteomyelitis underwent excision of the osteomyelitic bone and gradual correction of the deformity prior to a second-stage internal fixation. (**b**) The patient needed a deformity correction in the frontal and sagittal planes. The hinges of the multiplanar external fixation device were placed over the apices of the deformity. (**c**) The forefoot transfixation wires are also "walked" distally to distract the forefoot

not as critical in the transverse plane once the medial column is established, a patient will not be able to tolerate the malalignment in the frontal or sagittal planes. It can result in forefoot plantar ulceration secondary to increase in focal pressure or a fixation failure if bone healing is delayed.

In the ankle, fixation and deformity correction are little more forgiving. The larger structures with more parallel orientation of the joint to the ground surface afford more stable construct via fixations, such as retrograding intramedullary nail, multiplanar external fixation, and more robust plating systems.

Unlike the midfoot, shortening in the ankle is not beneficial however. Though a permanent brace, such as CROW or AFO, may add some height, a significantly shortened limb may not be any more functional than a proximally amputated extremity with a good prosthesis (Fig. 24.13).

Talectomy with tibiocalcaneal fusion (Boyd's procedure) is often utilized for a severe ankle neuroarthropathy (Fig. 24.14).

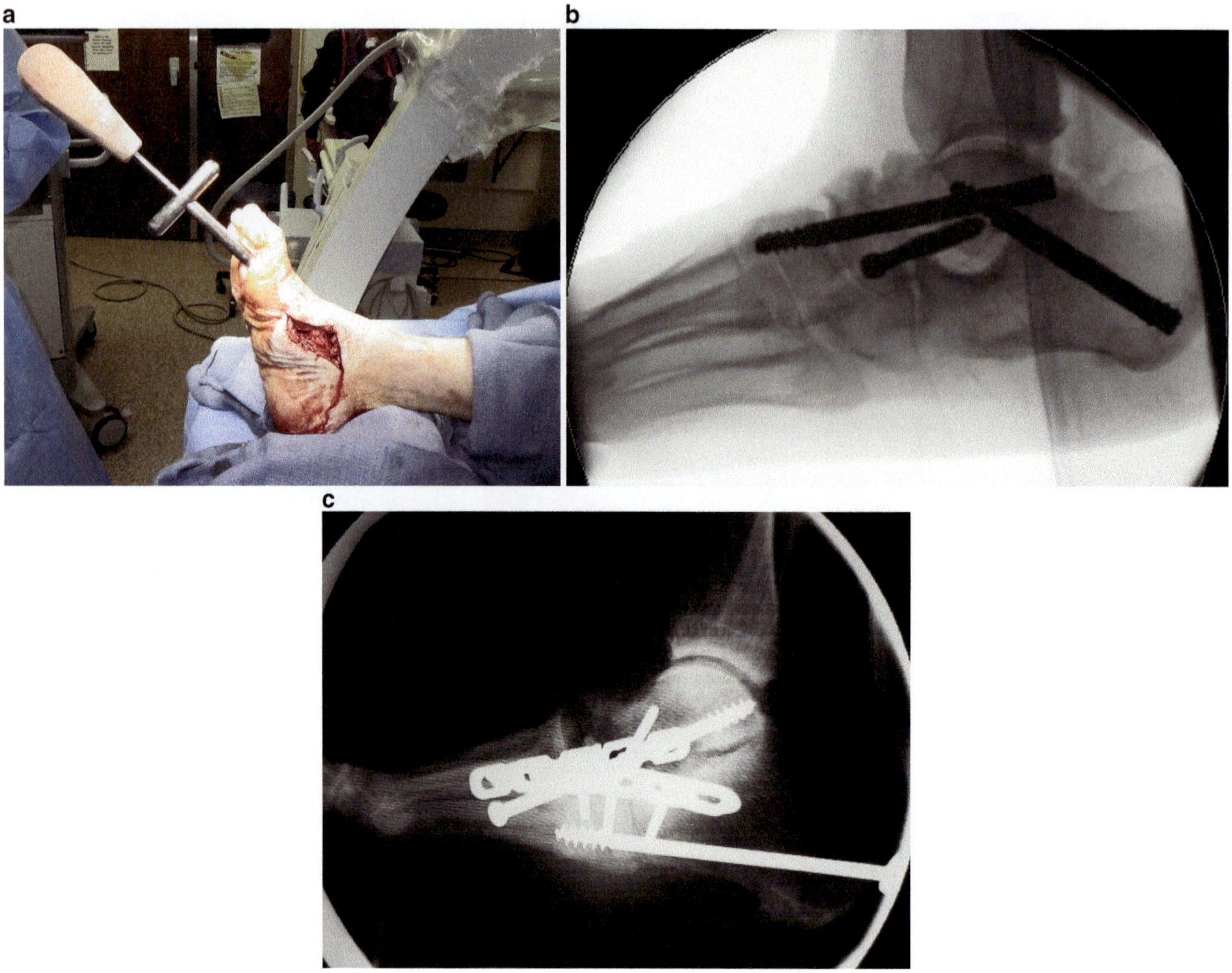

Fig. 24.9 (**a**) A beaming intramedullary screw is inserted through the plantar incision placed over the first metatarsophalangeal joint. The hallux is dorsiflexed to allow the screw to be in the long axis of the first metatarsal. Alternatively, a screw can be inserted from (**b**) the posterior aspect of the talus or (**c**) plantar aspect of the first metatarsal base

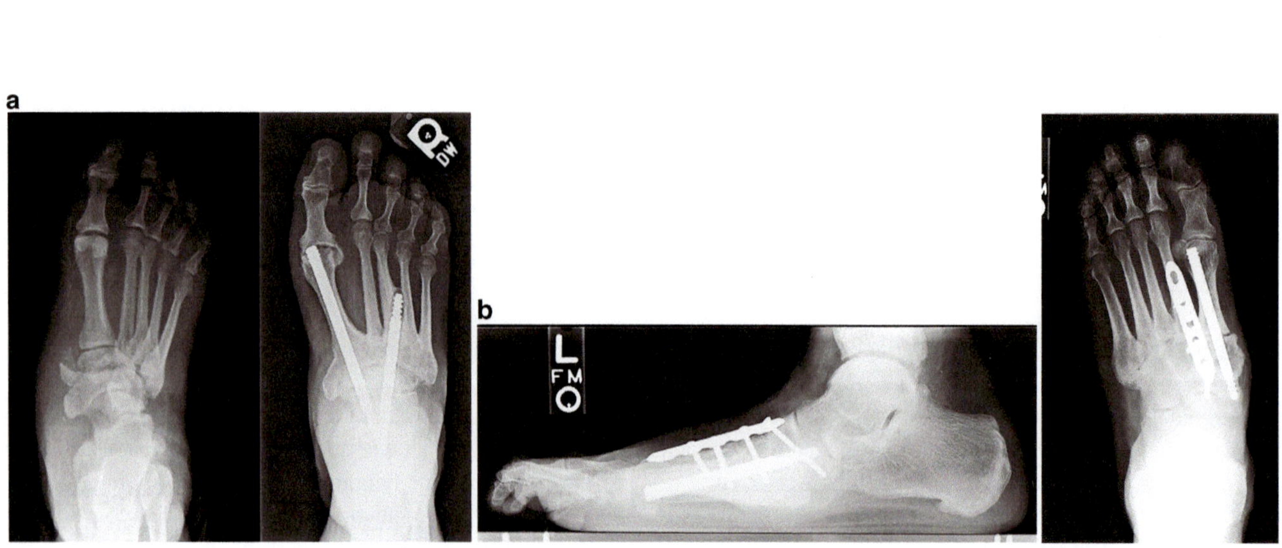

Fig. 24.10 (**a**) Even though the talonavicular joint was not affected by neuroarthropathy, the beaming intramedullary screw was inserted all the way to the talus for additional stability. (**b**) Without talar purchase, the navicular is not robust enough to maintain the medial column beam

The procedure however results in significant shortening and operative trauma in the extremity. Despite, this can be the only option in many patients short of major amputation. For those with severe, chronic deformity, this may be the

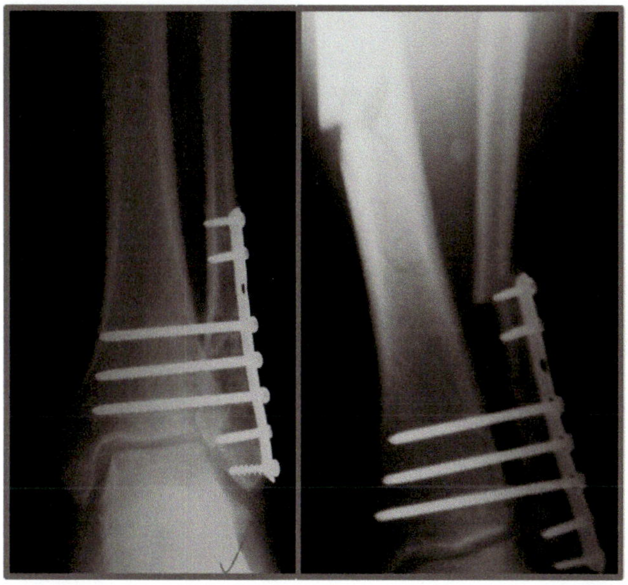

Fig. 24.11 Though this diabetic patient with severe neuropathy up to the level of the midleg did not develop a Charcot ankle after open reduction and internal fixation, the rigid construct resulted in transfer of the stress and a fracture proximally

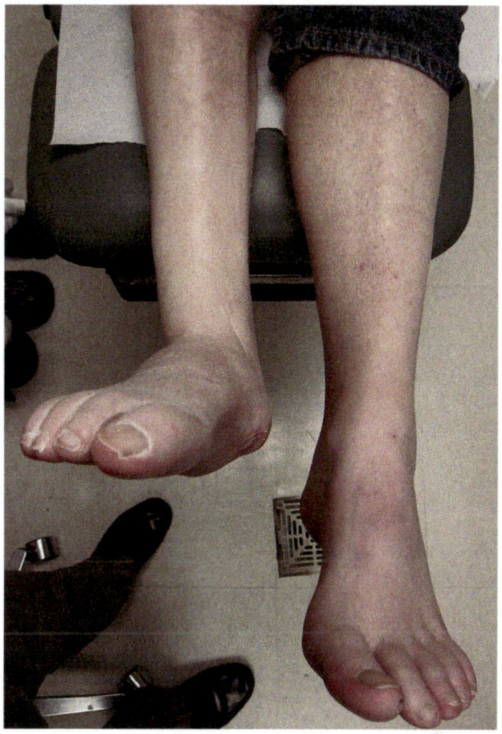

Fig. 24.13 After 6 years from an index talectomy with tibiocalcaneal fusion with external fixation, bony union never took place. Without internal fixation, it resulted in a recurrent dislocation and subsequent below the knee amputation

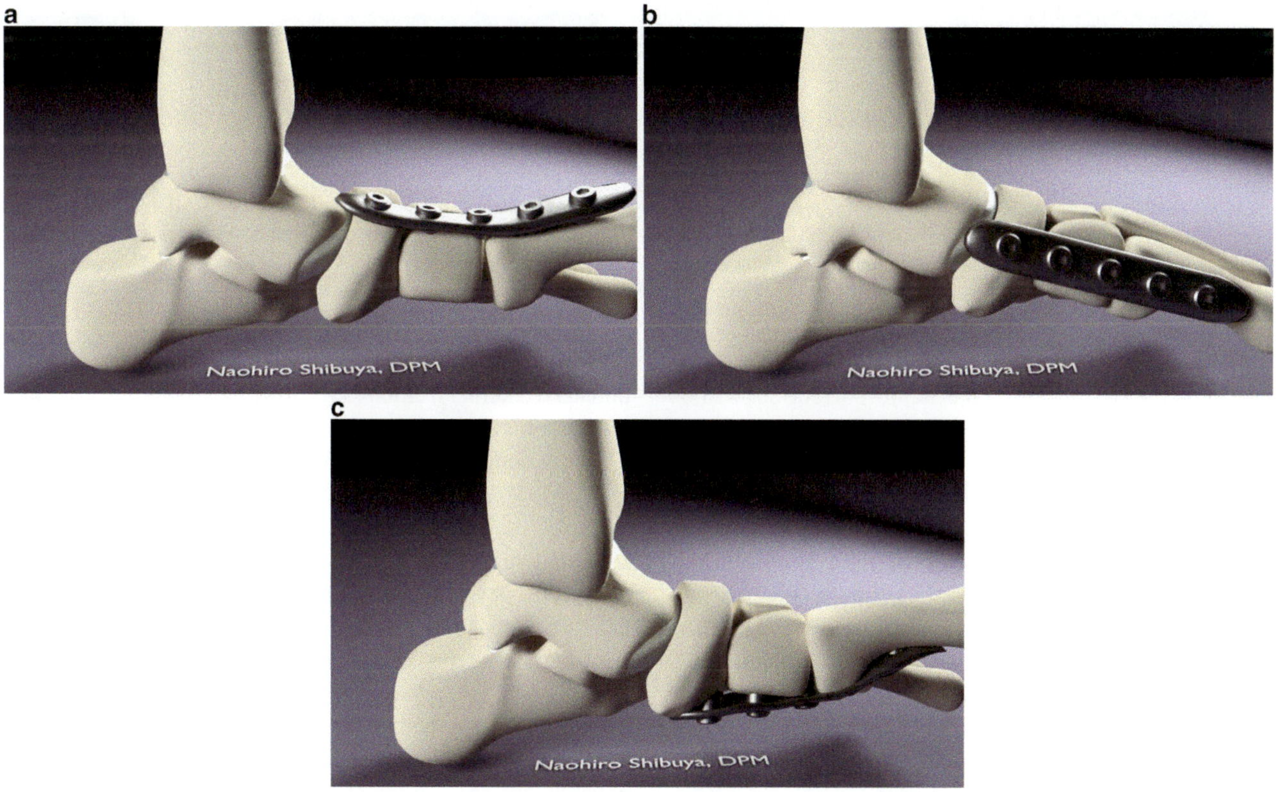

Fig. 24.12 (**a**) A dorsal plate may fail with weight-bearing force. (**b**) A medial beaming plate is stronger under weight-bearing force due to its vertical orientation. (**c**) A plantar tension banding plate may not work with fragile dorsal cortices

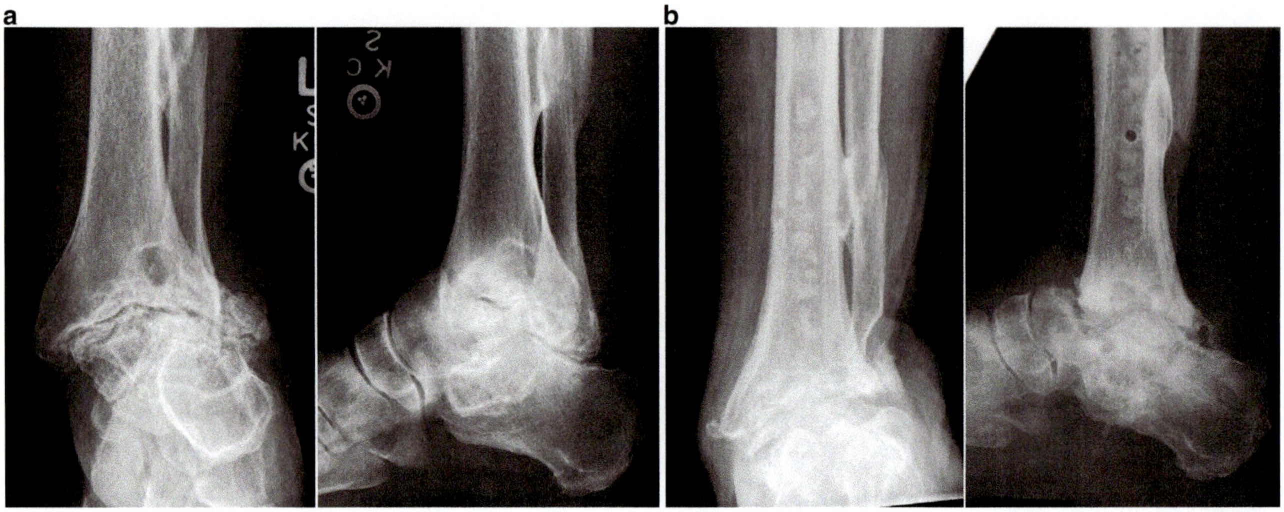

Fig. 24.14 Acute correction of (**a**) severe, chronic deformity may be possible with (**b**) a simultaneous talectomy and shortening of the limb

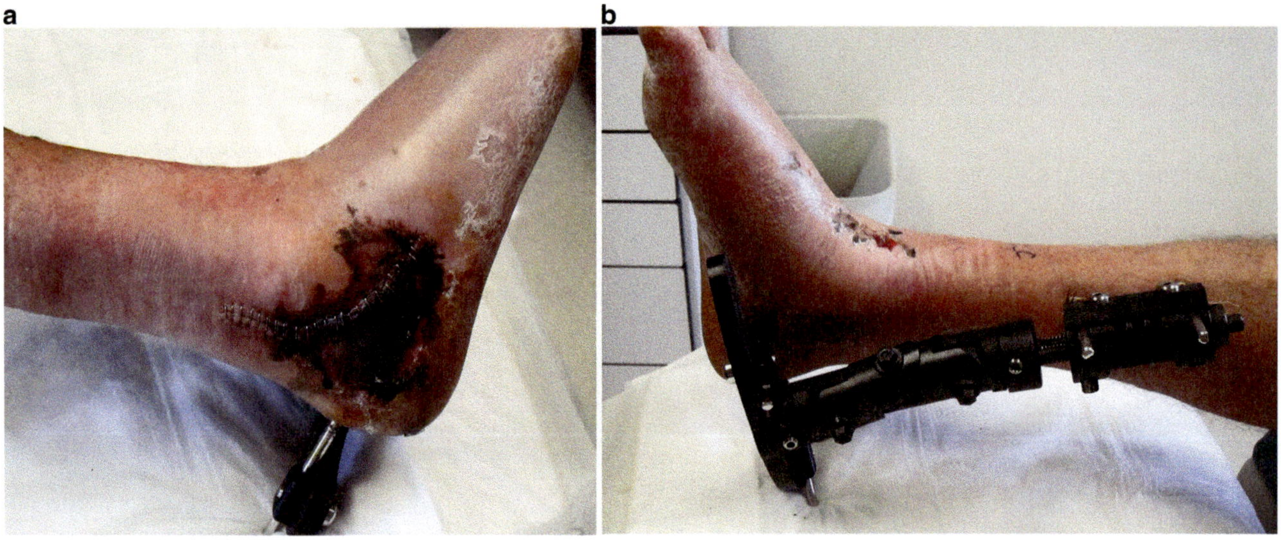

Fig. 24.15 An acute correction of chronic deformity may result in necrosis due to overstretching of the neurovascular structures

only feasible procedure since acute correction without significant shortening may compromise neurovascular structures (Fig. 24.15).

Addition of bone graft material even with osteobiologic supplementation is not advisable for the same reasons discussed earlier. Surgical trauma itself will "reactivate" the vicious inflammatory cycle (Fig. 24.4), and the bone substitute may be resorbed or "washed out" in the process (Fig. 24.16). An off-label use of bisphosphonates has been suggested to be useful in inhibiting the neuroarthropathic inflammatory process, but the clinical results are inconsistent [50–52].

For fixation in ankle Charcot reconstruction, an intramedullary nail can provide tremendous stability without needing to have significant foreign material underneath the surgical incision. Shah and De demonstrated that the union rate with a retrograde intramedullary nail was higher than that with a unilateral external fixation [53]. However, if infected, a salvage procedure is more difficult.

On the other hand, plate fixation may be better managed in a case of infection because intramedullary tracking of infection may be less likely. However, having the fixations right underneath the incision can be problematic, as postoperative dehiscence of the incision is not uncommon in a Charcot reconstructive surgery. Screw fixation is least stable. Yet, in cases of arthroscopic or minimal incision approach of the ankle arthrodesis, screw fixation can be executed via stab incisions, minimizing operative trauma.

A use of bone stimulator has been studied in Charcot patients [54, 55], yet the effectiveness of bone stimulator in this population is still questionable. Again, having meaningful statistics in a clinical study in this relatively rare disease is challenging.

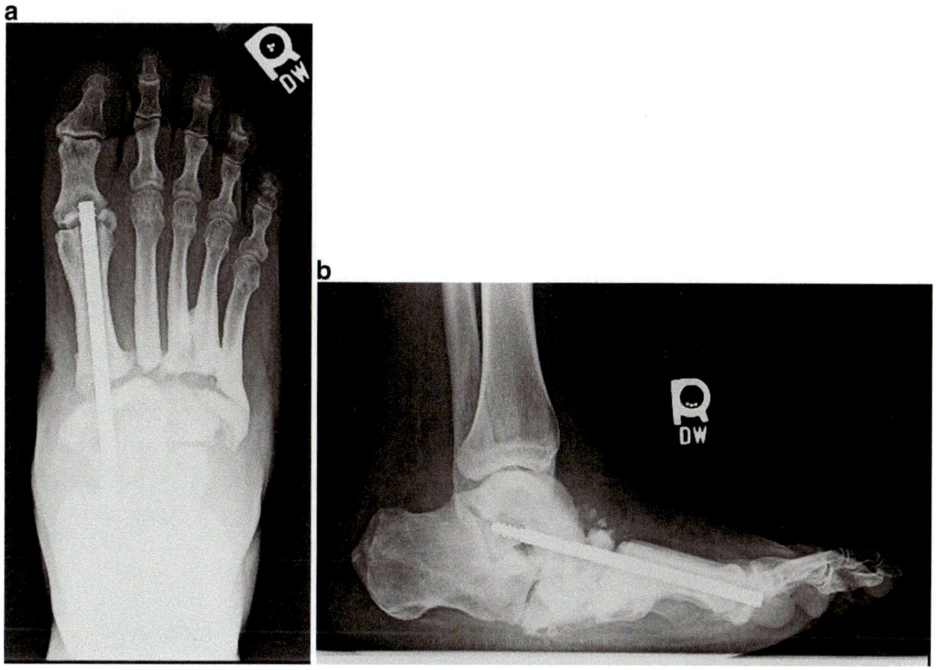

Fig. 24.16 Bone morphogenetic protein (BMP7) with demineralized bone matrix (DBM) was utilized in attempt to assist the midfoot fusion. However, (**a**) the osteobiologics were completely dissolved along with the postoperative inflammation, and (**b**) the correction was lost

There is no good evidence for use of prophylactic antibiotics in elective foot and ankle surgeries; however, in other areas, especially when hardware is utilized, a routine use of preoperative antibiotics is recommended [56]. There is no evidence for using antibiotics past 24 h after surgery. The Surgical Care Improvement Program (SCIP) guideline recommends against use of antibiotics for more than 24 h after the surgery [57]. Though the guideline was not derived from data in Charcot reconstructive surgeries, a justification to deviate from the guideline may be difficult.

Minimizing hematoma in the surgical site is highly recommended. Charcot reconstructive surgery can traumatic, and many patients often possess major bleeding disorders and/or calcified vessels. Coupled with prolonged surgery and creation of a dead space from extensive resection of necrotic soft tissue and bones, these patients are in high risk for developing hematoma. Hematoma can be minimized by utilizing a drain, releasing the tourniquet prior to closure to identify and eliminate major bleeding, managing medically for a bleeding disorder, adjusting pharmacological agents preoperatively, and applying a compressive dressing and cryotherapy.

Application of compressive dressing and cryotherapy should be done with caution since most of these patients have a significant sensory loss (Fig. 24.17). They are not able to detect abnormal pressure or extreme temperature even after the postoperative block wears off. Education regarding bandaging and cryotherapy and instruction for discontinuation or reporting adverse events are important. Frequent skin inspection and simple vascular examination should also be encouraged. Application of cryotherapy is not indicated at the level of sensory loss [58]. It needs to be proximal enough that the patient is able to feel any discomfort when too cold.

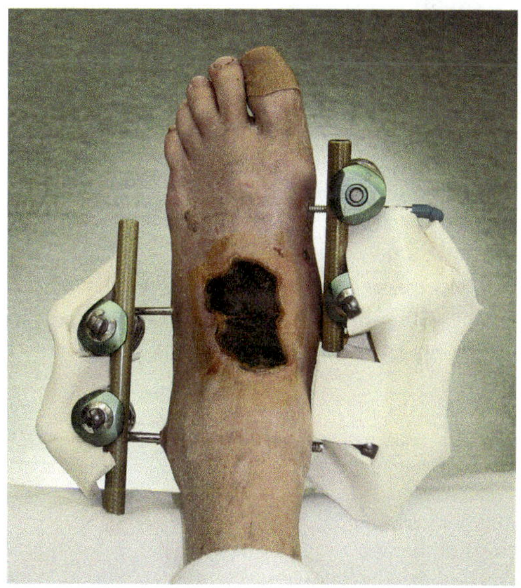

Fig. 24.17 A tight bandage in a neuropathic patient can result in necrosis of the skin

Management of Specific Complications

Hardware Failure

Hardware failure is common in Charcot reconstructive surgeries. When hardware fails, there are a couple of options, including explantation. However, before deciding on a treatment plan, one must investigate the reason for the failure. The reasons can include: infection, inadequate fixation from the previous procedure, high BMI, prolonged bone healing, and unreasonably early weight-bearing.

Charcot reconstruction requires sturdier fixation than most of other reconstructions. When evaluating plain radiographs, one can evaluate the size and orientation of the previous hardware. If the size and orientation of the fixations are adequate in the previous surgery, one can reason that the cause of the failure was due to one or more of other reasons mentioned above. If the size and orientation of the fixations were inadequate, it can be due to the surgical error but still cannot automatically rule out other causes, as more than one cause can be responsible for the failure.

A careful history and physical examination is useful to rule out most of the above-mentioned reasons for the failure. High BMI and excessively early weight-bearing can be ruled out from physical examination and careful history taking, respectively. Infection, however, is more difficult to evaluate (see *infected hardware*) since acute Charcot process can mimic an infectious process.

In most of the cases, prolonged bone healing due to underlying poor biology is responsible for the hardware fatigue and failure. If this is the case, a surgeon has to decide if a revision surgery would be of any benefit when these underlying medical conditions still exist (Fig. 24.18).

Many failed fixation devices may not be symptomatic. However, when fixation devices are protruding and/or prohibiting wound healing, removal of such implant may be necessary (Fig. 24.19). A prolonged wound closure may lead to colonization and infection. If not infected, an off-label use of a vacuum-assisted wound closure system may be used to grow granulation tissue over the hardware. Hardware removal is necessary to close the wound otherwise.

Some superficial screws can be removed from the open wound in a clinic. When rigid and deep, the patient may need to go to the operating room for removal. Even if stability is compromised, exposed hardware, when resulting in wound complication or infection, may need to be removed. Less foreign material in the open wound can result in better granulation and wound healing. In general, closed soft tissue envelope should be prioritized over stability of the fixation in this high-risk immunocompromised group of patients. A hardware removal may be coupled with application of negative pressure wound therapy to speed up granulation.

Deeper hardware, such as an intramedullary screw or nail, is much more difficult to manage when it fails. Infection and correction of malunion are the few indications for the removal of such deep hardware, as the additional procedure can be very traumatic for the patient (see *malunion, nonunion, infected hardware*).

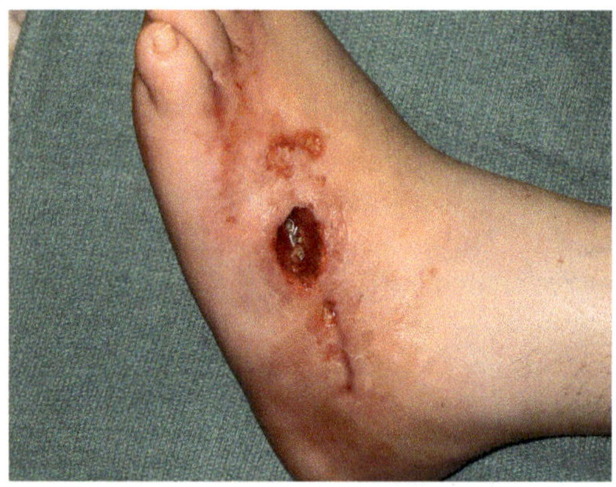

Fig. 24.19 The underlying plate and screws are prohibiting wound healing

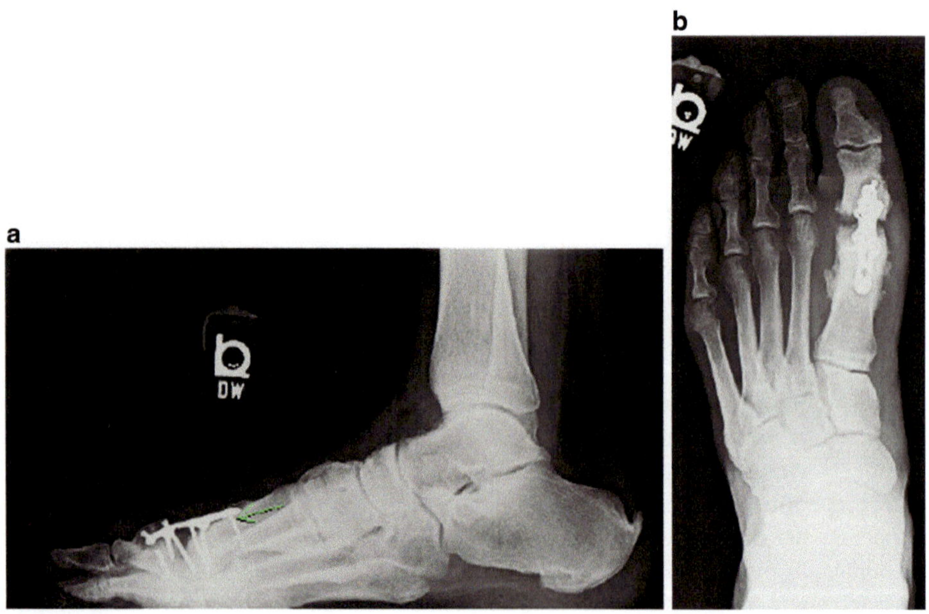

Fig. 24.18 When severe neuropathy resulting in osteolysis and hardware failure, revision surgery without modification of underlying medical condition will most likely fail again. This particular patient was non-symptomatic and did not require removal of hardware or revision surgery

Non-Healing Wound

Unlike a typical neurotrophic ulcer from pressure, wound healing complication in Charcot reconstruction may be subject to a larger problem. Assessing causes of the wound healing complication is necessary before management. Infection, hematoma, lack of biology, and extensive trauma from surgery can all lead to such a complication.

After adjusting for covariates (age, gender, race, BMI, any comorbidity, glycated hemoglobin, and serum glucose), Humphers et al. found that the significant factors associated with postoperative wound healing complication among the diabetics were elevated glycated hemoglobin and the presence of more than one comorbidity. With each % of glycated hemoglobin, the odds of wound healing complication increased by a factor of 1.28. On the other hand, the presence of any comorbidity increased the odds of the complication by a factor of 1.97. Within the comorbidities, neuropathy, high BMI, and smoking history were the ones associated with wound healing complication.

For orthopedic trauma, it has been demonstrated that obesity is a risk factor for wound healing complication [36–41]. Increased tension on the fascial edges at the time of closure with associated increased tissue pressure may reduce microperfusion and oxygen to cause surgical dehiscence [42, 43]. Hematoma and seroma formation are also more common in obese patients and can result in decreased tissue oxygenation and delayed healing [44].

The impact of smoking on wound healing complications has been well studied. Adverse effects of smoking on wound healing include: a temporary reduction in tissue perfusion and oxygenation, impairment of inflammatory cell functions and oxidative bactericidal mechanisms, and attenuation of reparative cell functions including synthesis and deposition of collagen [45]. Smoking cessation therefore is important prior to any revision surgeries. Initiation of smoking cession program 4 weeks prior to elective surgery has been shown to reduce postoperative complications significantly [59]. However, immediate postoperative cessation in orthopedic trauma did not show clinically significantly detectable benefits [60].

While a long-term glycemic control, measured in glycated hemoglobin, have obvious benefit in wound healing, tight management of perioperative serum glucose level may not. While in general perioperative serum glucose control has been believed to be an important factor [1, 2, 7, 13, 17, 23, 25–28], it did not have any statistically significant association with postoperative wound healing complication in foot and ankle procedures [35]. In addition, perioperative serum glucose level can significantly fluctuate. While some literature support tight perioperative glycemic control [29, 30], it remains a controversial topic, as a randomized trial did not demonstrate any added benefit [31].

Nutrient supplementation may be also beneficial in this patient group. Multivitamins, protein, and immune-enhancing supplementation are suggested to be effective [61–70]. Optimizing nutritional requirement is needed prior to considering surgical management.

Besides biology of the patient, biomechanics, ill-fitting brace/shoe, and infection (see *osteomyelitis*) can be responsible for non-healing open wounds. If available, pedobarograph is useful in assessing the degree and location of the planter pressure (Fig. 24.20). Without significant focal pressure present in the pedobarograph, one can deduce that the cause of the open wound can be due to lack of biology, compliance, or underlying infection.

Conservatively, these open wounds can be treated with any advanced wound care modalities; however, in many situations, aggressive off-loading may be necessary in this population. Off-loading can be achieved by reducing both focal pressure and activity level. Therefore, a cumbersome total contact cast, rather than off-loading boots or shoes, is more effective in healing wounds, as it also reduces the activity level significantly [71].

Though many of the focal pressures can be accommodated with a brace or shoes, some do not respond to orthotic management. Exostectomy or planing should be attempted if indicated prior to considering reconstructive surgery. With a general rule, a rigid Charcot foot is more manageable with exostectomy or planing (Fig. 24.21), while more flexible Charcot foot can result in further collapse. Ligamentous structures, which stabilize osseous structures, are often disrupted even with a simple exostectomy (Fig. 24.22). Simultaneous internal or external fixation without arthrodesis may be considered, but the long-term benefit of this is unclear (Fig. 24.23).

It should be reminded that the simple exostectomy could also initiate the viscous inflammatory process and potentially result in a recurrent acute Charcot process. This may propagate the rocker bottom foot and may worsen the biomechanics. Prolonged immobilization, tight glucose control, and possibly the off-label use of bisphosphonates may be helpful to prevent the occurrence of a neuropathic inflammatory process. Off-loading external fixation has been suggested by a few, but the cost utility is unclear in this situation.

Transfer lesions to the forefoot (from plantarflexed forefoot in malunion or under-corrected equinus) or subcalcaneal area (from over correction of equinus) can also be common. Percutaneous osteotomy with or without fixation can raise the corresponding metatarsal bone to off-load the metatarsal head in those with submetatarsal ulceration. A flexor hallucis longus tendon transfer may reduce enough pressure to heal the subcalcaneal lesion (Fig. 24.20).

Primary closure, skin grafting, and local flaps are other options for treatment of the open wound [72–74]. Evaluation

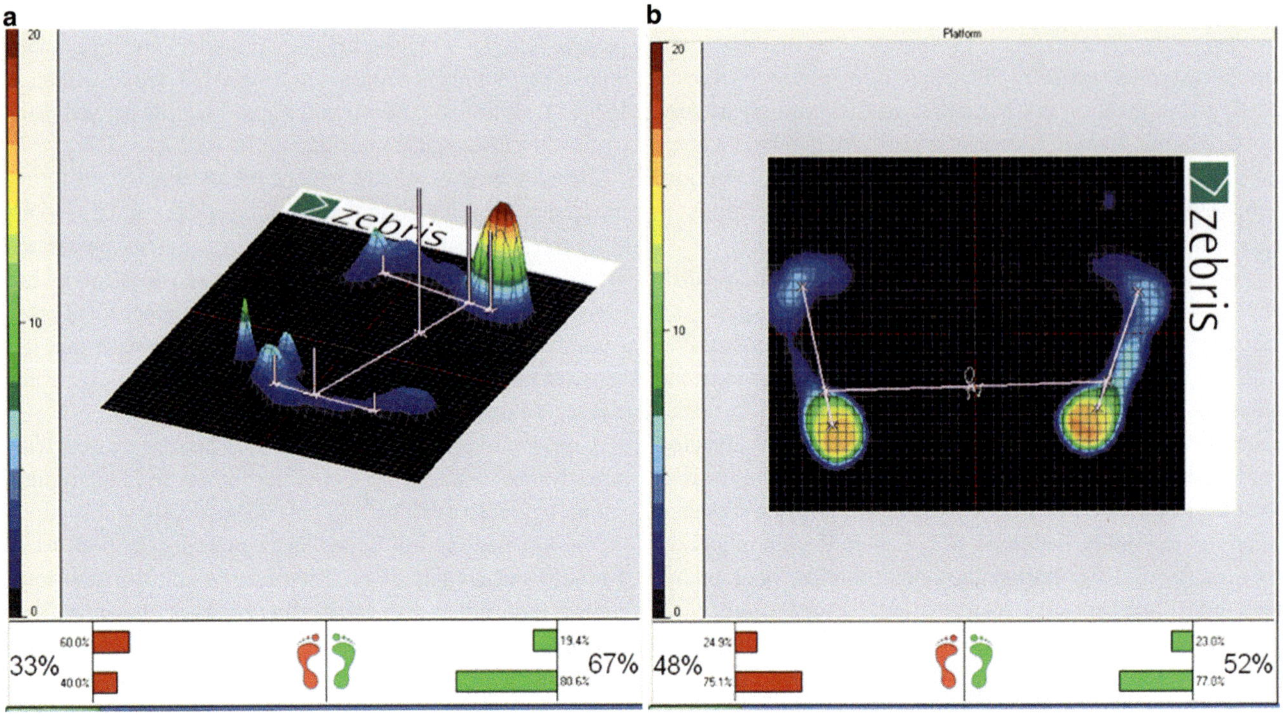

Fig. 24.20 (**a**) The pedobarograph shows an obvious increase in plantar calcaneal pressure in this patient with a plantar heel ulcer secondary to overlengthening of the Achilles tendon. (**b**) After flexor hallucis longus tendon transfer, the plantar pressure is reduced and the ulcer is healed

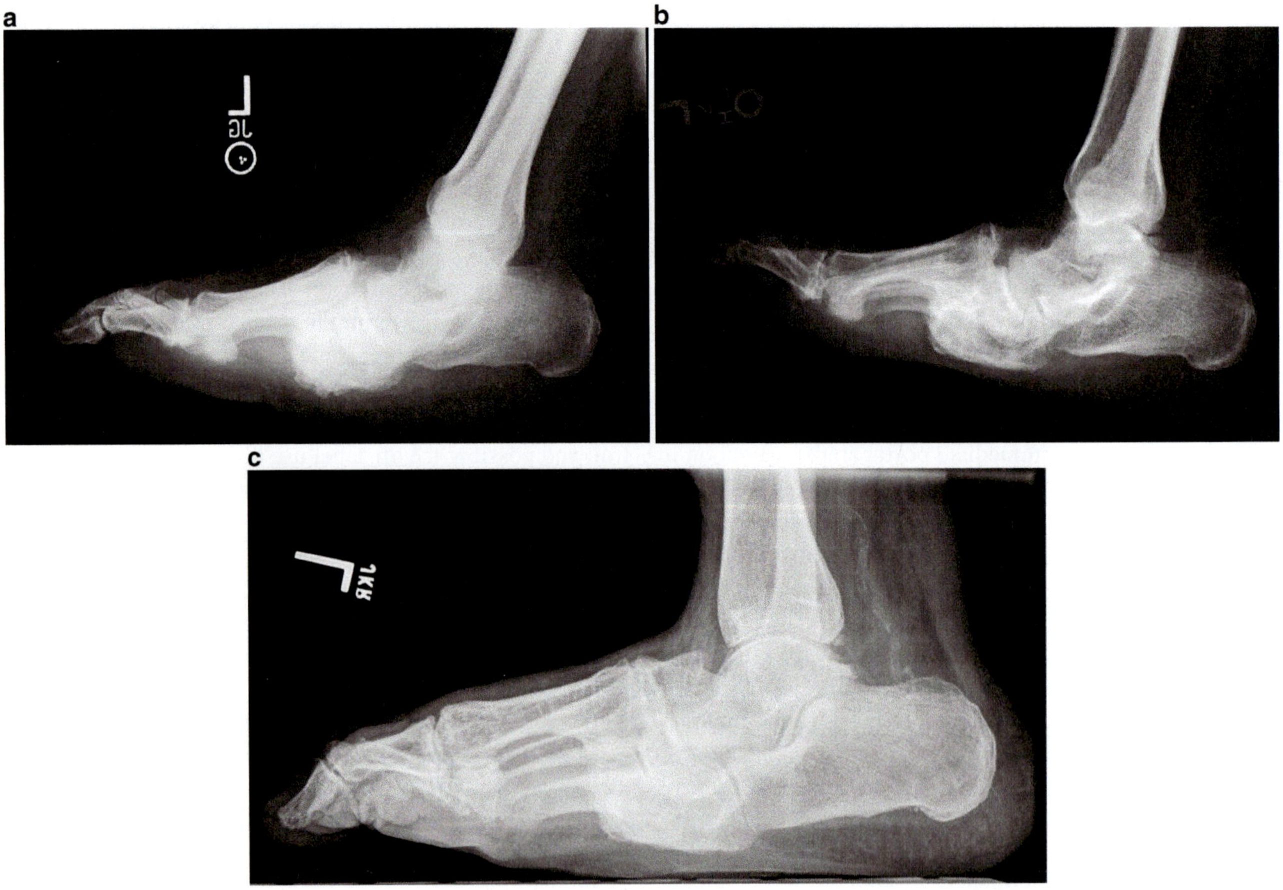

Fig. 24.21 (**a**) The patient developed a chronic plantar wound secondary to the rocker bottom foot type. (**b**) This chronic rigid Charcot foot was treated with plantar exostectomy. (**c**) Though normal foot architecture is not restored, the patient has not needed reconstructive surgery

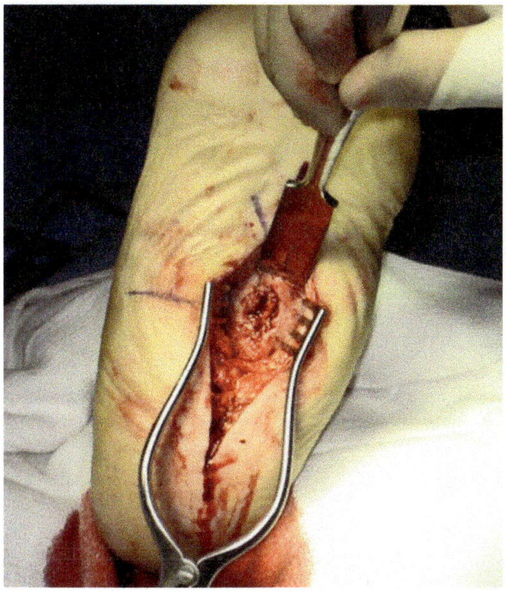

Fig. 24.22 To reach the bony prominence, plantar soft tissues including ligamentous structures are violated

of healing potential in these high-risk patients is again paramount, especially when more aggressive and traumatic soft tissue reconstruction is considered.

Malunion

Definition of malunion may be significantly different in a Charcot population than other foot and ankle conditions. In many Charcot cases, restoration of anatomical architecture of the foot and ankle may not be necessary, practical, or even beneficial. A "plantigrade" foot is the term often used to describe the final, acceptable result in diabetic Charcot reconstruction. This often means a reasonably functional and "brace-able" foot that can withstand the activities of daily living. The functional foot does not necessarily always provide a propulsive gait.

One of the most important aspects of Charcot reconstruction is to achieve the plantigrade foot without focal pressure

a b c d

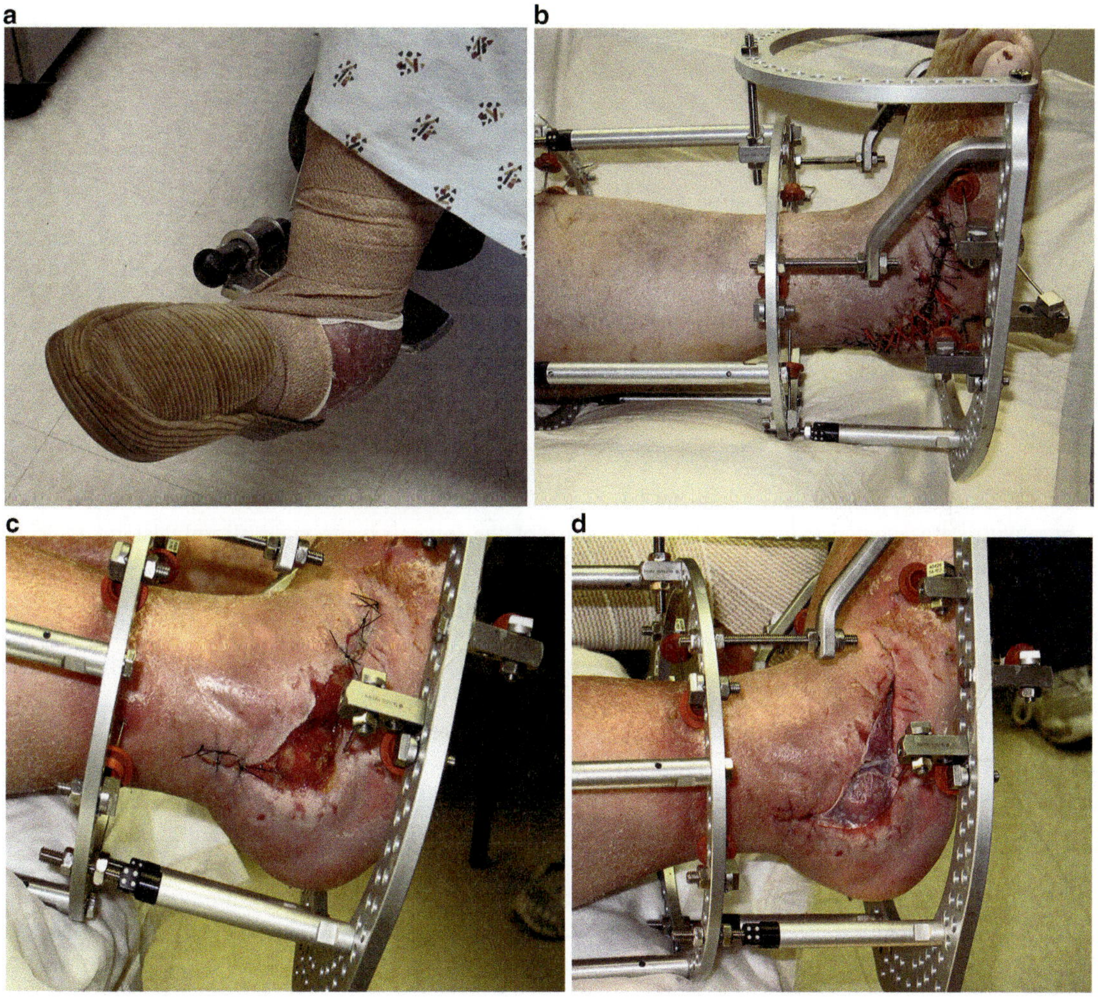

Fig. 24.23 An acute Charcot dislocation with chronic lateral ankle wound was stabilized without arthrodesis, followed by advanced wound care modalities

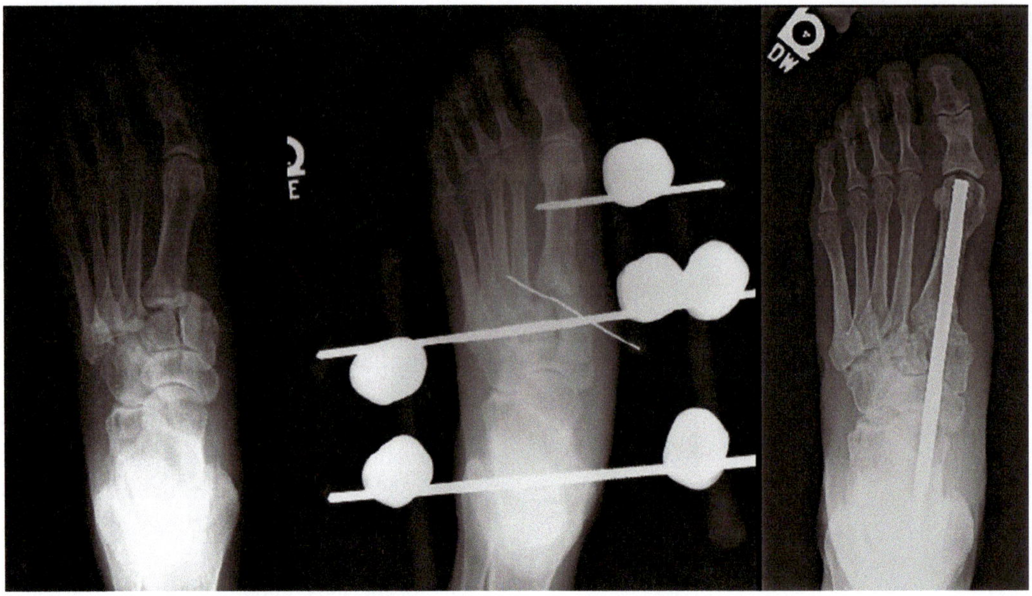

Fig. 24.24 While the close reduction with external fixation did not reduce the deformity fully, a subsequent minimally invasive open reduction and internal fixation with 3 cm incision over the tarsometatarsal joint, performed after the acute Charcot phase, provided an adequate reduction of the deformity and permanent fixation. Though naviculocuneiform and talonavicular joints were not prepared for arthrodesis, the beaming screw was inserted all the way down to the talus for additional stability

points that predispose to future neuropathic ulcerations. Severe malunion may lead to biomechanical problems that result in increased plantar, medial, lateral, and even dorsal pressure in a brace. When underlying arthrodesis is solidly fused, one may want to consider exostectomy, partial resection, or amputation before reconstruction to minimize operative trauma. It is difficult for a patient to go through multiple rehabilitation processes in a short period of time from multiple reconstructive surgeries. Inactivity and deconditioning in these patients significantly affect their mortality and quality of life. A long, thorough discussion with a patient and his/her family is critical before deciding to revise the malunion.

Pain is usually not a symptom from malunion in a neuropathic patient. When painful, there may be an underlying nonunion. In a subtle case, evaluation with a CT scan can aid identifying nonunions.

Malunion can be resulted from a previous poor surgery, infection, progressive deformity before union, and/or newly onset of acute Charcot arthropathy. If the reason is due to progression of deformity before union, then the cause of the delay union should be investigated (see *nonunion*). If a recurrent acute neuroarthropathy is not resulting in severe deformity, then the patient should be treated conservatively with protected weight-bearing with a total contact cast or complete off-loading with a wheelchair if practical. If the main cause of the nonunion was due to poor previous surgery and the patient is relatively healthy and undisturbed (still possessing adequate vascular supply, non-compromised skin and bone stock), revision reconstructive surgery may be indicated.

Some of those general pearls used for primary Charcot reconstruction can be applied for a revision surgery. However, one needs to remember that neurovascular structure is further compromised, and these patients may be significantly deconditioned from the previous surgery.

Understanding location of previous incisions is extremely important. It can help predict the status of the remaining functional neurovascular structures. These surviving neurovascular structures should be preserved at all cost. Less invasive technique is often needed to preserve those neurovascular supplies (Fig. 24.24).

To start planning for a revisional reconstructive surgery, the rearfoot alignment to the leg should be evaluated first. The calcaneus should be directly under the mechanical axis of the lower extremity or slightly lateral to it, as a varus ankle and foot is extremely difficult to brace. In some instances, a simple calcaneal slide osteotomy is enough to shift the center of pressure to relieve the symptoms, such as ulceration or progression of the deformity. Similarly, presence of equinus should also be inspected. Often, these patients have some type of posterior muscle group lengthening procedures in the past. Overlengthening of the previously lengthened posterior soft tissue structures should be avoided, as a excessively dorsiflexed calcaneus is significantly more difficult to manage than equinus.

Once the ankle level is thoroughly evaluated, one can look at the foot deformity. Many malunions result in a collapse in the sagittal plane with severe abduction or adduction of the forefoot to the rearfoot. The same principle as flatfoot reconstruction may be applied to regain the "tripod" in

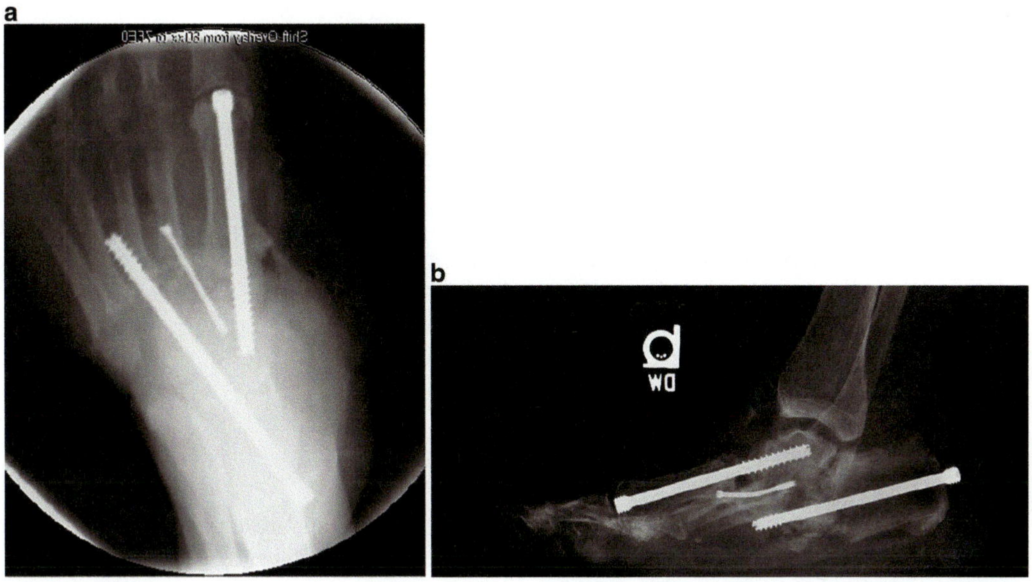

Fig. 24.25 (**a**) The medial column was shortened significantly more than the lateral column, and this resulted in an inadequate "tripod" of the foot. (**b**) The future consequences include a collapse of the medial arch from compensation of the iatrogenic forefoot varus deformity

the foot. Though it is not necessary to create a high "tripod," the concept is still important to avoid a future collapse. When the forefoot is in a varus position, the rearfoot or ankle can go into valgus to compensate for the forefoot deformity, especially when the midfoot is rigid from the previous arthrodesis. Similarly, an excessively short medial or lateral column can result in an inadequate "tripod" and can result in a future collapse (Fig. 24.25)

For correction of the foot deformity, further resection rather than bone block distraction osteotomy is suggested for the same reasons discussed earlier. Fixation can be more difficult in the revision surgery as less bone stock is available. Combination of internal and external fixation may be necessary to achieve a solid reconstruct without disturbance of both the endosteal and periosteal vasculature.

Nonunion

The main reason for nonunion in Charcot patient is stemming from the underlying medical conditions. Therefore, revision surgery in those patients may not be indicated. If the previous reconstruction was done by an experienced surgeon, yet resulted in nonunion, the chances of the second surgery resulting in union are minimal unless there are modifiable medical/social factors that can be adressed.

Diabetic bone healing complication in particular has been extensively studied in animal models [75–99]. In humans, incidence of bone healing complication in diabetic patients is believed to be high in foot and ankle surgeries as well [100–107]. Within a diabetic population, the association of hyperglycemia with bone healing complication has been well documented [76, 82, 83, 90, 91, 93, 97, 100, 108, 109], yet little clinical information is available regarding other diabetes-related comorbidities or conditions directly affecting bone healing. In diabetic animal models, there have been many theories suggesting the causes of bone metabolism disturbance, yet translational research is lacking to link the significance of those theories in a clinical practice.

In a case-control study of diabetic patients, approximately one out of four patients had one or more bone healing complications [110]. The study showed that a patient with glycated hemoglobin level of more than 7% had roughly three times greater odds of getting a bone healing complication. However, the most significant factor associated with bone healing complication in this diabetic cohort was presence of neuropathy. The diabetic patients with neuropathy had four times the odds of having bone healing complication than diabetics without neuropathy. This result coincides with many animal studies as well as clinical reports that indicate that bone healing complication can be due to malfunctions of bone metabolism resulting from neuropathy [104, 111–114]. Lack of adequate neuropeptide release in these patients may upregulate osteoclastogenesis while downregulating osteoblastic activities [111, 115–117]. Unfortunately, all Charcot patients fit into this category.

The same study also showed that every 10 min of operative time was associated with diabetic bone healing complications by the factor of 1.15. While a longer surgery may confound more complex cases or an inexperienced surgeon, this finding makes us rethink the need for an extensive surgery in this high-risk population.

If the nonunion was mainly due to poor surgical technique or noncompliance, then a revision surgery may still be beneficial. Yet, pseudoarthrosis with a "brace-able" foot does not have to be surgically managed. Conservative approach should be exhausted before attempting a surgical reconstruction.

Generous resection of nonviable bone is paramount to a successful fusion. Also, sturdy fixation without requiring significant operative trauma is important (Fig. 24.26).

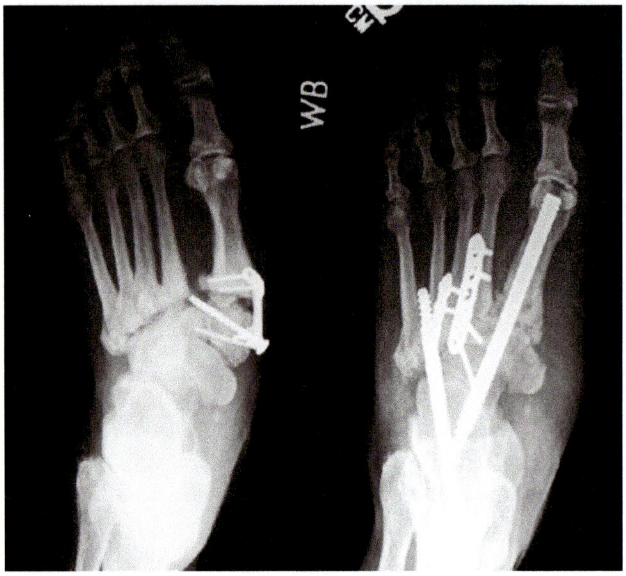

Fig. 24.26 This patient with nonunion and recurrent deformity was considered to have inadequate fixation. Sturdier fixation was utilized to achieve union in the revision surgery

The same principles for surgical reconstruction described in the previous section still apply to this revision surgery. More prolonged non-weight-bearing status may be necessary to achieve union in the revision surgery. However, the surgeon has to account for potential deconditioning and decline in quality of life when deciding to go through another prolonged rehabilitation process. A patellar tendon bearing ankle-foot orthoses or Charcot restraint orthotic walker may be needed to get the patient back in activities earlier without significant weight-bearing force applied to the surgical site (Fig. 24.27).

Infected Hardware/Soft Tissue Infection

When a patient with previous Charcot surgery presents with a red, hot, swollen foot/ankle, the differentials should include infection, recurrent neuroarthropathy, and DVT. It is important to remember that the infection may not present in a typical fashion. Often, the patient may not have any systemic symptoms or leukocytosis.

In trauma, when hardware is infected, the general rule is to leave the implant until union. However, because many Charcot reconstructive surgeries result in delay/nonunion or pseudoarthrosis, waiting for union may not be desirable. In addition, the patient is often immunocompromised; therefore, the same principle should not be applied to Charcot patients. Immediate and aggressive pharmacological and surgical treatment of the postoperative infection is warranted (Fig. 24.28).

Fig. 24.27 (**a**) Charcot restraint orthotic walker and (**b**) patellar tendon bearing brace shortens the duration of inactivity. Especially when a patient is undergoing revision procedures, deconditioning of the patient needs to be minimized

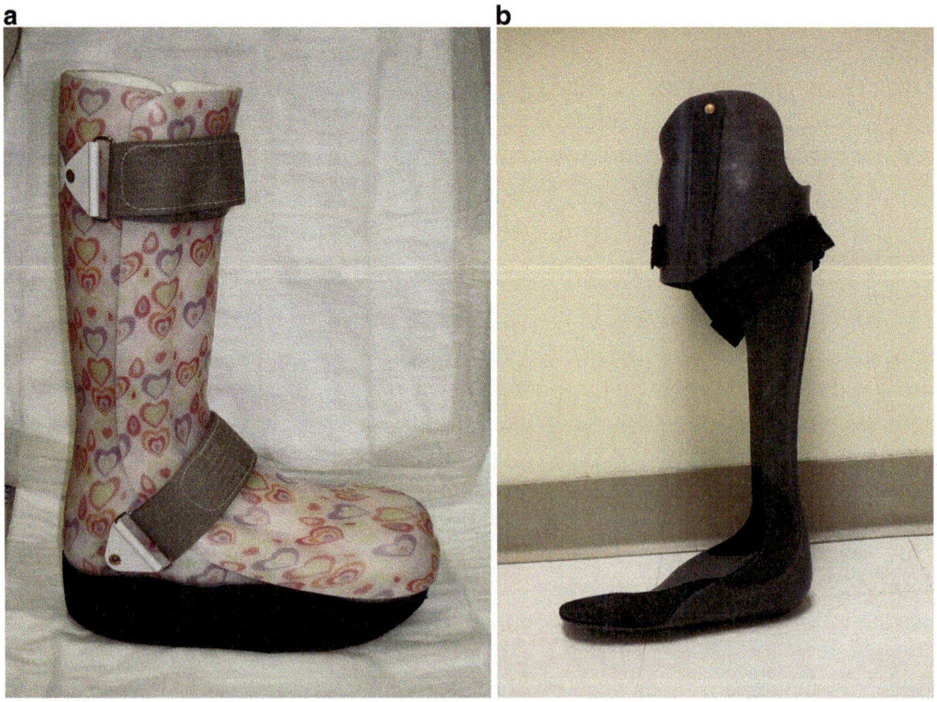

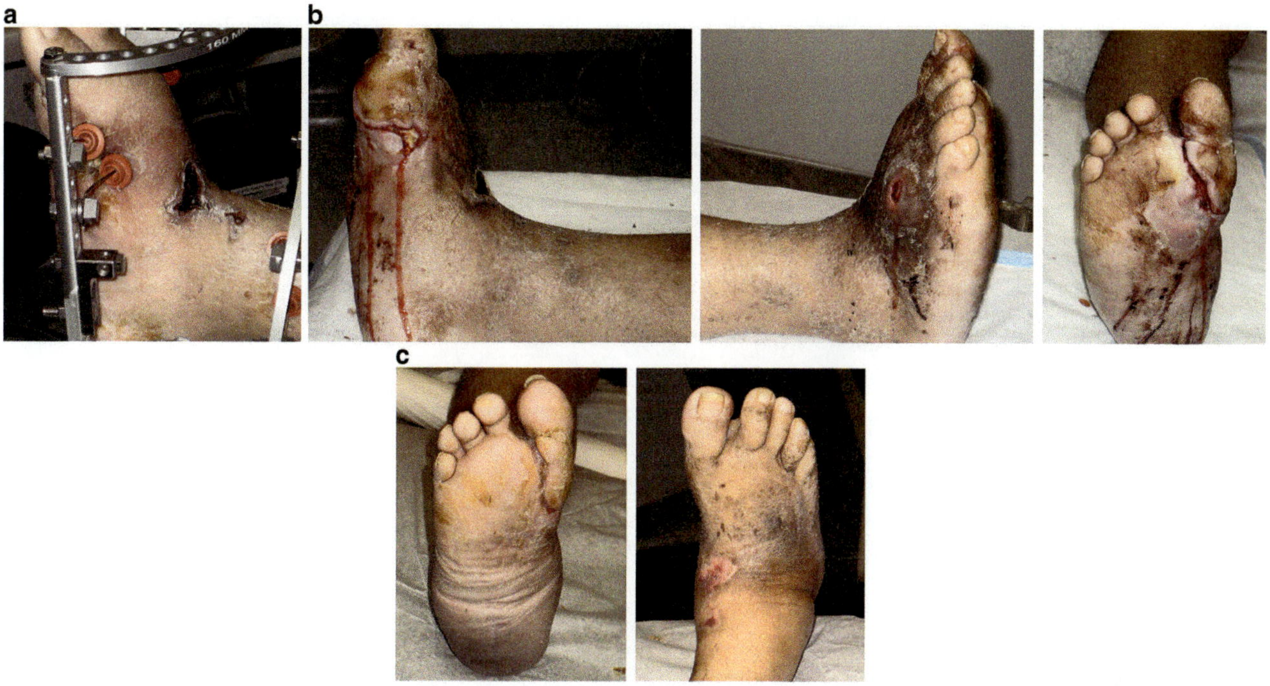

Fig. 24.28 (**a**) Deep pin tract infection extending to the dorsal and plantar foot was immediately treated with (**b**) removal of external fixation, incision and drainage, and aggressive wound care. (**c**) The infection was eradicated

Once hardware is removed, reaming or curettage of the area may be necessary to debride the adjacent bone to remove infection. In a case of intramedullary screw or nail, the reamer that is slightly larger than the one used in the previous surgery can remove the thin layer cancellous bone that may be infected. The dead space now should be replaced with antibiotic impregnated cement or bone substitute (Fig. 24.29). The cement rod or spacer can be replaced with bone graft in 2–4 weeks. It is also important to evaluate the extent of infection in the bone, as it may be necessary to debride more than the thin layer adjacent to the fixation device (see *osteomyelitis*).

Within a diabetic population, it has been demonstrated that elevation in glycated hemoglobin and having more than one comorbidities were statistically significantly associated with postoperative infection in diabetics [35]. However, adjusting for all the relevant covariates (age, gender, race, BMI, presence of any comorbidity, glycated hemoglobin, serum glucose, and type of procedure (osseous vs. soft tissue)), only glycated hemoglobin was significantly associated. Each 1% in glycated hemoglobin increased the odds of infection by a factor of 1.59. Therefore, tight long-term control of glucose in diabetic patient is once again the important factor. With a *post hoc* analysis, neuropathy was the only factor among the comorbidities that was associated with the postoperative infection in diabetics. This is in agreement with other authors, who show that peripheral neuropathy is the risk factor for postoperative infection [13, 32–35].

Treatment of soft tissue infection can be initiated with antibiotics and surgical debridement. Aggressive debridement is needed for eradication of the infection without multiple trips to the operating room. A staged, delayed primary closure after subsidence of inflammation and infection, as opposed to a one-stage procedure, minimizes further wound dehiscence or separation. Appropriate consultations, such as infectious disease, are also recommended. A multidisciplinary approach to treat complications in these high-risk patients cannot be overemphasized.

Osteomyelitis

Differentiating an acute, surgically induced neuroarthropathy process from bone infection is often difficult; therefore, keen diagnostic skills are needed to treat these complications correctly in a timely manner. Often both radiographic and laboratory workups are necessary. Though bone biopsy is considered the gold standard, a negative result may not necessarily rule out osteomyelitis. Multiple biopsies taken from different sites may be needed to capture osteomyelitic specimen if present.

American College of Radiology Appropriateness Criteria suggests that only plain X-rays or MRI have an evidence-based indication for detecting osteomyelitis in diabetic patients with neuropathic arthropathy [118]. An MRI can show tracking of osteomyelitis along the medullary canal in

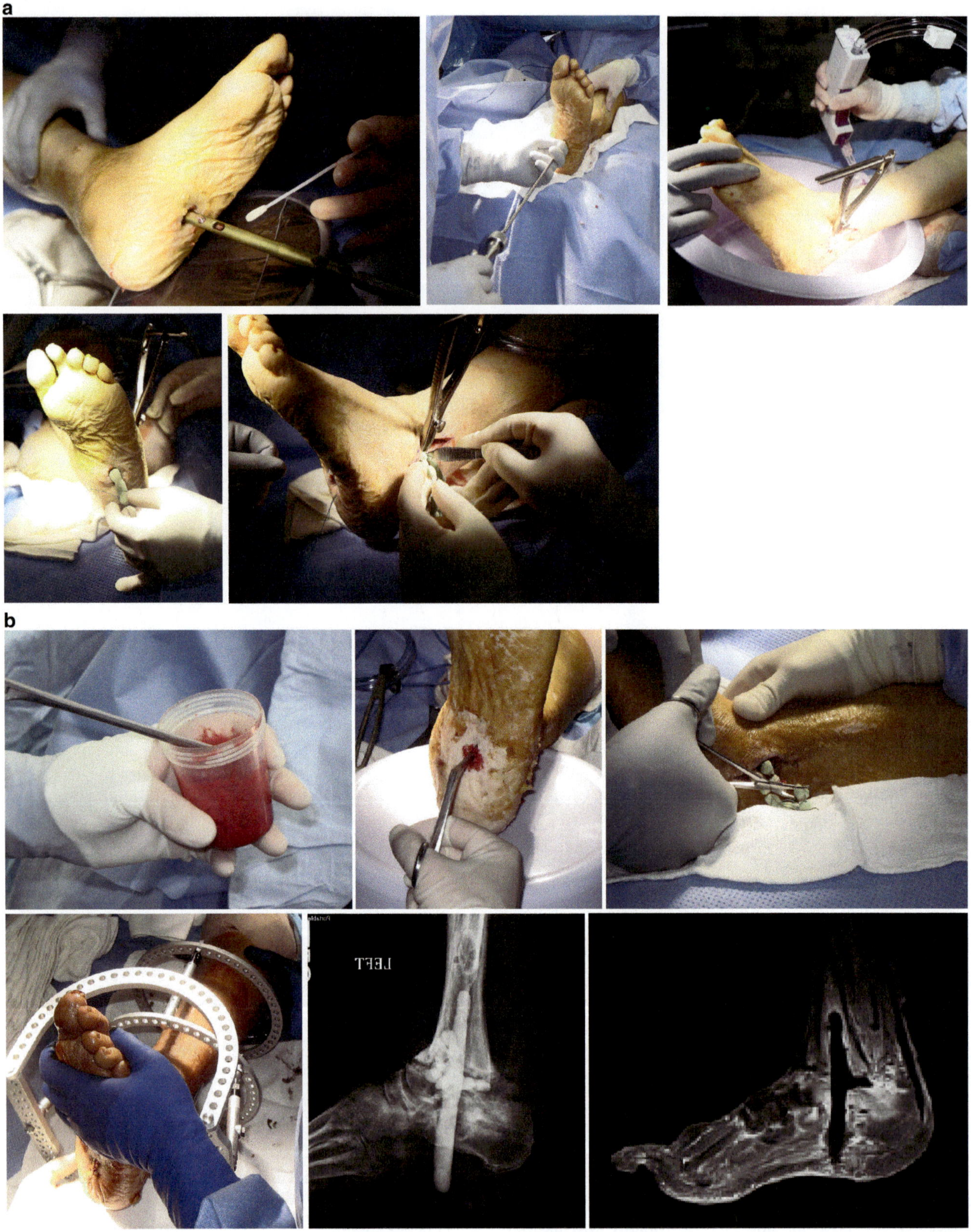

Fig. 24.29 (**a**) The infected intramedullary nail was removed and cultured, and the medullary canal was reamed. The medullary canal was then irrigated and filled with antibiotic impregnated cement nail and beads. (**b**) After infection subsided, the antibiotic impregnated cement was replaced with autograft, and external fixation was applied for stabilization and dynamic compression, by passing the area of infection

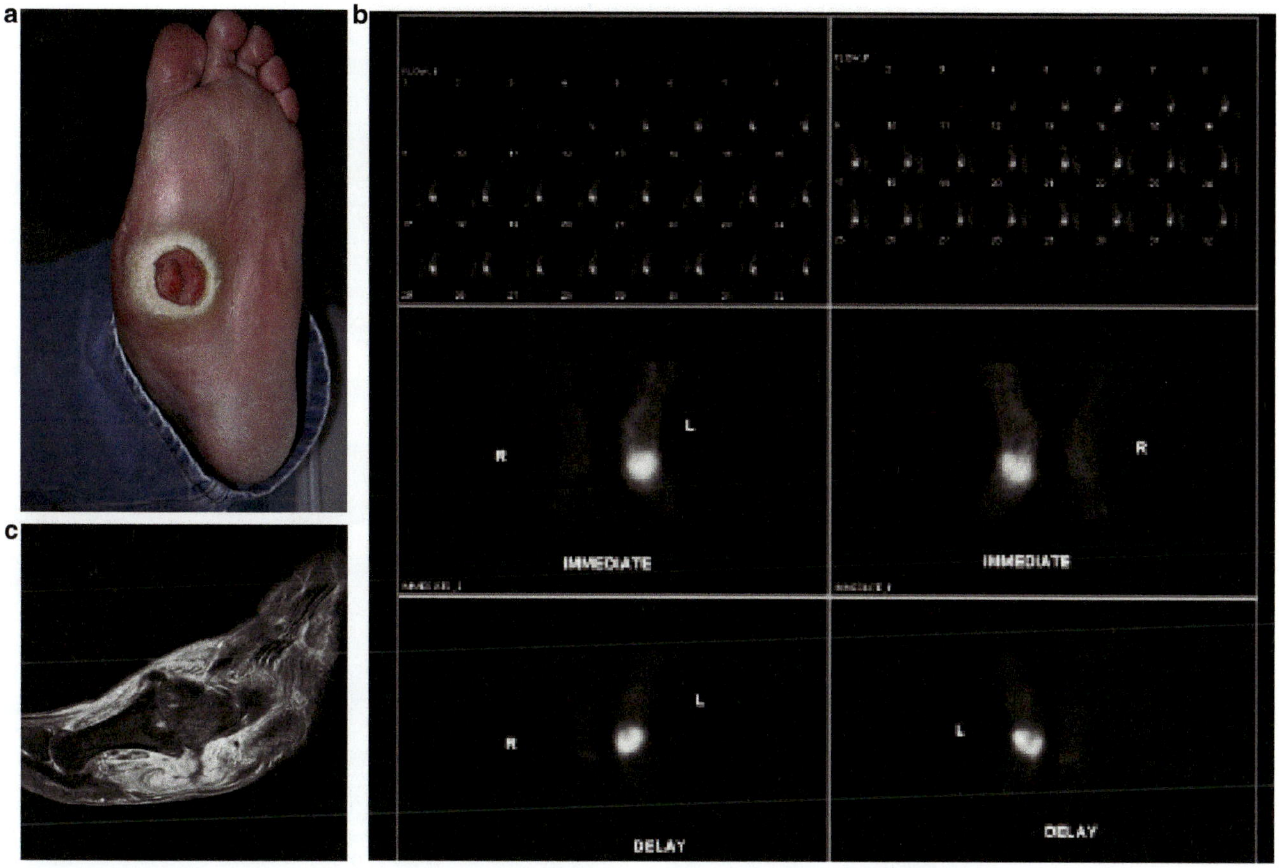

Fig. 24.30 (**a**) While the open wound probes deep and (**b**) a technetium scan shows significant uptake in the midfoot, (**c**) the MRI shows diffuse marrow edema adjacent to the tarsometatarsal joint with subchondral cysts and without medullary tracking, suggestive of an acute Charcot process rather than osteomyelitis

a long bone. In Charcot arthropathy, diffused marrow edema is found in periarticular areas of multiple bones (Fig. 24.30). Contrast may be used to show clear extent of the infected or necrotic bone and for surgical planning. Other studies such as nuclear scans (including technetium-99, labeled leukocyte scan, indium-111, and sulfur colloid), ultrasound, CT scan, and PET/CT do not have good ratings to be used for this situation according to the guideline.

Inflammatory markers may also be useful in diagnosing osteomyelitis. Use of sedimentation rate, C-reactive protein, and procalcitonin have been studied and considered useful [119, 120]. Serial laboratory examination of these markers is also useful after surgical debridement for a monitoring purpose.

The "probe-to-bone" test is popular, yet its effectiveness is greatly dependent on a situation [121–125]. Positive and negative predictive values of this test are affected by a population in which the test is utilized. This is also true for abovementioned laboratory tests for inflammatory markers. In a higher-risk patient population, positive predictive value suffers, as prevalence of a deep wound is higher. Especially in the postoperative patient population, probing through the dehisced surgical wound does not necessarily mean osteomyelitis.

Once determined osteomyelitis, resection of the infected bone, unless proximal amputation is indicated, should be planned. Long-term antibiotic treatment of osteomyelitis has also been shown effective [126]. However, it is unclear to which type of patients can be treated effectively with the non-surgical approach, as a thorough risk factor assessment has not yet to be conducted in a clinical research. Patients with minor non-symptomatic osteomyelitis or high anesthesia risk, who are no longer a surgical candidate, may be benefitted from a long-term or lifetime antibiotic suppression therapy. Again, consulting an infectious disease specialist is recommended.

Typically, aggressive excisional debridement of osteomyelitic bone is needed. Again, an MRI with contrast may be effective in showing the extent of the necrotic bone. Once extent of the excision is determined preoperatively, the surgeon has to determine if the resultant foot will be stable. If not, one should reconsider amputation and its advantages over local debridement and staged reconstruction (Fig. 24.31).

For staged procedures, the priority of the initial surgery is to resect the osteomyelitic bone. Enough bone needs to be resected to limit the number of operations. One may supplement it with antibiotic impregnated beads or spacer to eradicate the infection. Postoperatively a surgeon can follow

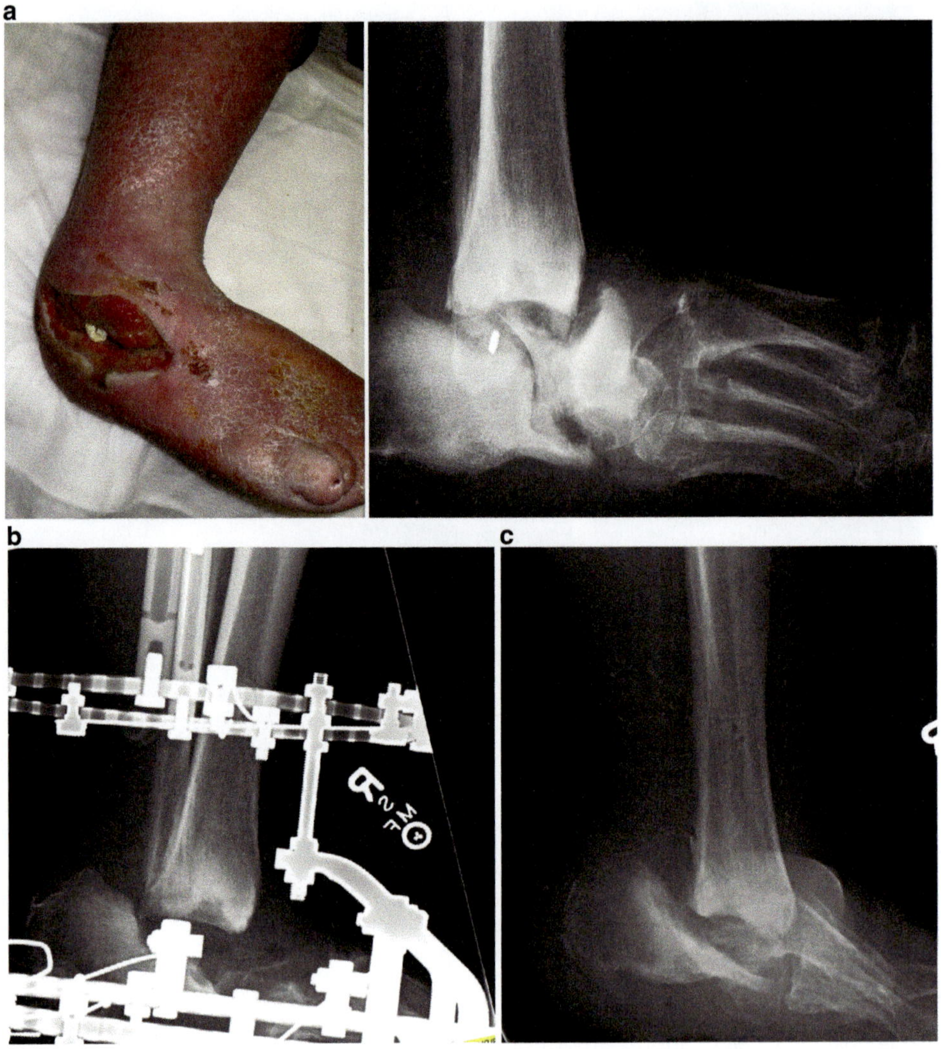

Fig. 24.31 (**a**) The patient developed osteomyelitis in the remaining talus. The talus was resected along with the infected soft tissue and (**b**) stabilized. Though the infection was eradicated, (**c**) the resultant foot was not functional. The patient ended up with a below the knee amputation

these patients with serial serum inflammatory markers to monitor the progress, and once the markers are normalized and soft tissue inflammation is resolved, a delayed arthrodesis may be attempted.

Alternatively, some may use antibiotic impregnated bone graft substitutes to attempt arthrodesis in a one-stage procedure. However, a care must be taken, as the bone substitutes can act as a foreign material once the efficacy of the antibiotics wears off, and it may result in further inflammatory processes. Also, soft tissue is often compromised from the infection, and wound healing can be difficult in a one-stage approach.

Minor Amputation

We often assume that a patient is more satisfied with a limb salvage attempt, yet this may not be true in many situations. The patient may have a better quality of life with minor amputation than having to deal with a chronic wound [127]. The burden of dressing changes; long-term non-weight-bearing status and office visits can all account for lower quality of life. In Charcot patients, the deformity decreases the patients' function, but it has been documented that mental status of the patients may not be any different when compared to patients with neurotrophic ulceration without Charcot arthropathy [128, 129]. Again, this would question the need for reconstruction in many of these patients. Considering their high mortality rate and low 5-year survival rate [31], amputation over salvage should be a part of discussion in treating these patients.

Besides eliminating infection, the purpose of amputation can also be to reduce the biomechanical stress. We often think of amputation as a last resort, non-salvage procedure, which does not require good surgical skills; however, a successful amputation that can withstand a long-term biomechanical stress can be as challenging as reconstructive procedures. Especially at the foot and ankle levels, a surgeon must have a good understanding of biomechanics to limit recurrent/transfer lesions or further amputation.

Location and level of minor amputation depends on the reason for the amputation and the current neurovascular status. Transmetatarsal amputation over ray resections has been more accepted for long-term biomechanical stability. Transmetatarsal amputation is also superior to Chopart's amputation because many of the tendon insertions are spared in transmetatarsal amputation: Both peroneals and tibialis anterior can still function after tramsmetatarsal amputation.

Both Chopart's and Syme's amputations are more difficult to brace. An experienced prosthetist is required to minimize recurrent ulceration and to maximize function.

Proximal Amputation

Salvage versus amputation has been evaluated extensively for years. In trauma patients, the studies fail to support salvage over amputation in terms of length of stay in the hospital, pain level, quality of life, function, and time to go back to work [130, 131]. In trauma, it has been found that male gender, occurrence of confounding injury, presence of a fracture, and an open wound are associated with occurrence of lower extremity amputation [132]. Similarly, in a high-risk diabetic population, male gender, having more comorbidities, history of open wounds are more susceptible to amputation [30]. Patients with neuroarthropathy possess many of these characteristics.

Major amputations, such as below the knee amputation, may be indicated when the patient's medical condition inhibits healing despite limb salvage efforts. Further, it is also dependent on a patient's preference based on his/her lifestyle, quality of life, and natural disinclination to lose a body part. It is important to remember in a revision surgery, especially in those with neurovascular diseases, that the previous surgery has insulted already-compromised neurovascular structures. Many of the complications are stemming from the patient's underlying medical/metabolic condition, compliance, and incapacity to rehabilitate. Therefore, a well-executed surgical revision may still not be sufficient to ameliorate the situation.

Depending on severity of the complication, proximal amputation above the level of area that is not affected by severe peripheral neuropathy may be the best option for the patient, who has been battling with this condition for a long time. As discussed earlier, neuropathy is the single most important risk factor that is associated with bone and soft tissue complications. Therefore, going above the level of neuropathy is often necessary to avoid further complications.

A popular belief in our community is that lower extremity amputation is a proximal cause of death [133], and many consider that limb salvage efforts are critical. However, the evidence on this phenomenon is not conclusive [134–136]. Although it is known that amputation does have an impact on vascular dynamics [137–139], it is difficult to find direct evidence that amputation leads directly to death. Underlying disease may play a larger role in eventual mortality than the amputation itself.

References

1. Barber DB, Janus RB, Wade WH. Neuroarthropathy: an overuse injury of the shoulder in quadriplegia. J Spinal Cord Med. 1996;19(1):9–11.
2. Crim JR, Bassett LW, Gold RH, Mirra JM, Mikulics M, Dawson EG, et al. Spinal neuroarthropathy after traumatic paraplegia. AJNR Am J Neuroradiol. 1988;9(2):359–62.
3. Heylen Y. Neuropathic arthropathy of the shoulder secondary to syringomyelia. J Belg Radiol. 1993;76(4):232–3.
4. Nagano J, Tada K, Masatomi T, Horibe S. Arthropathy of the wrist in leprosy--what changes are caused by long-standing peripheral nerve palsy? Arch Orthop Trauma Surg. 1989;108(4):210–7.
5. Radhakrishnan K, Vijayan VP, Ashok PP, Sridharan R, Mousa ME. Syphilitic spinal neuroarthropathy with paraplegia. Clin Neurol Neurosurg. 1985;87(1):61–4.
6. Shibata T, Tada K, Hashizume C. The results of arthrodesis of the ankle for leprotic neuroarthropathy. J Bone Joint Surg Am. 1990;72(5):749–56.
7. Trepman E, Nihal A, Pinzur MS. Current topics review: Charcot neuroarthropathy of the foot and ankle. Foot Ankle Int. 2005; 26(1):46–63.
8. Brodsky JW, Rouse AM. Exostectomy for symptomatic bony prominences in diabetic Charcot feet. Clin Orthop Relat Res. 1993;296:21–6.
9. Frykberg RG. Osteoarthropathy. Clin Podiatr Med Surg. 1987;4(2):351–9.
10. Falanga V. Wound healing and its impairment in the diabetic foot. Lancet. 2005;366(9498):1736–43.
11. Rosenberg CS. Wound healing in the patient with diabetes mellitus. Nurs Clin North Am. 1990;25(1):247–61.
12. Siitonen OI, Niskanen LK, Laakso M, Siitonen JT, Pyorala K. Lower-extremity amputations in diabetic and nondiabetic patients. A population-based study in eastern Finland. Diabetes Care. 1993;16(1):16–20.
13. Van Damme H, Limet R. Amputation in diabetic patients. Clin Podiatr Med Surg. 2007;24(3):569–82.
14. Addolorato G, Capristo E, Greco AV, Stefanini GF, Gasbarrini G. Influence of chronic alcohol abuse on body weight and energy metabolism: is excess ethanol consumption a risk factor for obesity or malnutrition? J Intern Med. 1998;244(5):387–95.
15. Pinzur MS, Sage R, Stuck R, Kaminsky S, Zmuda A. A treatment algorithm for neuropathic (Charcot) midfoot deformity. Foot Ankle. 1993;14(4):189–97.
16. Beard JD. Should we save critically ischaemic legs at any cost? Acta Chir Belg. 2008;108(6):651–5.
17. Cheshire NJ, Wolfe JH, Noone MA, Davies L, Drummond M. The economics of femorocrural reconstruction for critical leg ischemia with and without autologous vein. J Vasc Surg. 1992;15(1):167–74. discussion 74-5
18. Driver VR, Fabbi M, Lavery LA, Gibbons G. The costs of diabetic foot: the economic case for the limb salvage team. J Vasc Surg. 2010;52(3 Suppl):17S–22S.
19. Gupta SK, Veith FJ, Ascer E, Flores SA, Gliedman ML. Cost factors in limb-threatening ischaemia due to infrainguinal arteriosclerosis. Eur J Vasc Surg. 1988;2(3):151–4.
20. Harrington EB, Harrington ME, Schanzer H, Haimov M. End-stage renal disease--is infrainguinal limb revascularization justified? J Vasc Surg. 1990;12(6):691–5. discussion 5–6

21. Johnson BL, Glickman MH, Bandyk DF, Esses GE. Failure of foot salvage in patients with end-stage renal disease after surgical revascularization. J Vasc Surg. 1995;22(3):280–5. discussion 5–6
22. Korn P, Hoenig SJ, Skillman JJ, Kent KC. Is lower extremity revascularization worthwhile in patients with end-stage renal disease? Surgery. 2000;128(3):472–9.
23. Panayiotopoulos YP, Tyrrell MR, Arnold FJ, Korzon-Burakowska A, Amiel SA, Taylor PR. Results and cost analysis of distal [crural/pedal] arterial revascularisation for limb salvage in diabetic and non-diabetic patients. Diabet Med. 1997;14(3):214–20.
24. Perler BA. Cost-efficacy issues in the treatment of peripheral vascular disease: primary amputation or revascularization for limb-threatening ischemia. J Vasc Interv Radiol. 1995;6(6 Pt 2 Suppl):111S–5S.
25. Raviola CA, Nichter LS, Baker JD, Busuttil RW, Machleder HI, Moore WS. Cost of treating advanced leg ischemia. Bypass graft vs primary amputation. Arch Surg. 1988;123(4):495–6.
26. Singh S, Evans L, Datta D, Gaines P, Beard JD. The costs of managing lower limb-threatening ischaemia. Eur J Vasc Endovasc Surg. 1996;12(3):359–62.
27. Taylor Jr LM, Hamre D, Dalman RL, Porter JM. Limb salvage vs amputation for critical ischemia. The role of vascular surgery. Arch Surg. 1991;126(10):1251–7. discussion 7–8
28. Shigematsu H. Epidemiology from the Trans Atlantic Inter-Society Consensus Group Guidelines II. Nihon Geka Gakkai zasshi. 2007;108(4):171–5.
29. Second European Consensus Document on chronic critical leg ischemia. Circulation. 1991;84(4 Suppl):IV1–26.
30. Jupiter DC, Thorud JC, Buckley CJ, Shibuya N. The impact of foot ulceration and amputation on mortality in diabetic patients. I: from ulceration to death, a systematic review. Int Wound J. 2015;13(5):892–903.
31. Gazis A, Pound N, Macfarlane R, Treece K, Game F, Jeffcoate W. Mortality in patients with diabetic neuropathic osteoarthropathy (Charcot foot). Diabet Med. 2004;21(11):1243–6.
32. Baele HR, Piotrowski JJ, Yuhas J, Anderson C, Alexander JJ. Infrainguinal bypass in patients with end-stage renal disease. Surgery. 1995;117(3):319–24.
33. Sanchez LA, Goldsmith J, Rivers SP, Panetta TF, Wengerter KR, Veith FJ. Limb salvage surgery in end stage renal disease: is it worthwhile? J Cardiovasc Surg. 1992;33(3):344–8.
34. Lavery LA, Hunt NA, Ndip A, Lavery DC, Van Houtum W, Boulton AJ. Impact of chronic kidney disease on survival after amputation in individuals with diabetes. Diabetes Care. 2010;33(11):2365–9.
35. Humphers J, Shibuya N, Fluhman BL, Jupiter D. The impact of glycosylated hemoglobin and diabetes mellitus on postoperative wound healing complications and infection following foot and ankle surgery. J Am Podiatr Med Assoc. 2014;104(4):320–9.
36. Jupiter DC, Humphers JM, Shibuya N. Trends in postoperative infection rates and their relationship to glycosylated hemoglobin levels in diabetic patients undergoing foot and ankle surgery. J Foot Ankle Surg. 2014;53(3):307–11.
37. Shibuya N, Humphers JM, Fluhman BL, Jupiter DC. Factors associated with nonunion, delayed union, and malunion in foot and ankle surgery in diabetic patients. J Foot Ankle Surg. 2013;52(2):207–11.
38. Lowery NJ, Woods JB, Armstrong DG, Wukich DK. Surgical management of Charcot neuroarthropathy of the foot and ankle: a systematic review. Foot Ankle Int. 2012;33(2):113–21.
39. La Fontaine J, Shibuya N, Sampson HW, Valderrama P. Trabecular quality and cellular characteristics of normal, diabetic, and charcot bone. J Foot Ankle Surg. 2011;50(6):648–53.
40. Armstrong DG, Lavery LA. Elevated peak plantar pressures in patients who have Charcot arthropathy. J Bone Joint Surg Am. 1998;80(3):365–9.
41. Manferdini C, Maumus M, Gabusi E, Piacentini A, Filardo G, Peyrafitte JA, et al. Adipose-derived mesenchymal stem cells exert antiinflammatory effects on chondrocytes and synoviocytes from osteoarthritis patients through prostaglandin E2. Arthritis Rheum. 2013;65(5):1271–81.
42. Bao XJ, Liu FY, Lu S, Han Q, Feng M, Wei JJ, et al. Transplantation of Flk-1+ human bone marrow-derived mesenchymal stem cells promotes behavioral recovery and anti-inflammatory and angiogenesis effects in an intracerebral hemorrhage rat model. Int J Mol Med. 2013;31(5):1087–96.
43. Canzi L, Castellaneta V, Navone S, Nava S, Dossena M, Zucca I, et al. Human skeletal muscle stem cell antiinflammatory activity ameliorates clinical outcome in amyotrophic lateral sclerosis models. Mol Med. 2012;18:401–11.
44. Roukis TS, Zgonis T. The management of acute Charcot fracture-dislocations with the Taylor's spatial external fixation system. Clin Podiatr Med Surg. 2006;23(2):467–83.
45. Illgner U, Budny T, Frohne I, Osada N, Siewe J, Wetz HH. Clinical benefit and improvement of activity level after reconstruction surgery of Charcot feet using external fixation: 24-months results of 292 feet. BMC Musculoskelet Disord. 2014;15:392.
46. Lamm BM, Gottlieb HD, Paley D. A two-stage percutaneous approach to charcot diabetic foot reconstruction. J Foot Ankle Surg. 2010;49(6):517–22.
47. Pinzur MS. Neutral ring fixation for high-risk nonplantigrade Charcot midfoot deformity. Foot Ankle Int. 2007;28(9):961–6.
48. DeVries JG, Berlet GC, Hyer CF. A retrospective comparative analysis of Charcot ankle stabilization using an intramedullary rod with or without application of circular external fixator–utilization of the Retrograde Arthrodesis Intramedullary Nail database. J Foot Ankle Surg. 2012;51(4):420–5.
49. Wukich DK, Belczyk RJ, Burns PR, Frykberg RG. Complications encountered with circular ring fixation in persons with diabetes mellitus. Foot Ankle Int. 2008;29(10):994–1000.
50. Jude EB, Selby PL, Burgess J, Lilleystone P, Mawer EB, Page SR, et al. Bisphosphonates in the treatment of Charcot neuroarthropathy: a double-blind randomised controlled trial. Diabetologia. 2001;44(11):2032–7.
51. Pakarinen TK, Laine HJ, Maenpaa H, Mattila P, Lahtela J. The effect of zoledronic acid on the clinical resolution of Charcot neuroarthropathy: a pilot randomized controlled trial. Diabetes Care. 2011;34(7):1514–6.
52. Pitocco D, Ruotolo V, Caputo S, Mancini L, Collina CM, Manto A, et al. Six-month treatment with alendronate in acute Charcot neuroarthropathy: a randomized controlled trial. Diabetes Care. 2005;28(5):1214–5.
53. Shah NS, De SD. Comparative analysis of uniplanar external fixator and retrograde intramedullary nailing for ankle arthrodesis in diabetic Charcot's neuroarthropathy. Indian J Orthop. 2011;45(4):359–64.
54. Hockenbury RT, Gruttadauria M, McKinney I. Use of implantable bone growth stimulation in Charcot ankle arthrodesis. Foot Ankle Int. 2007;28(9):971–6.
55. Hanft JR, Goggin JP, Landsman A, Surprenant M. The role of combined magnetic field bone growth stimulation as an adjunct in the treatment of neuroarthropathy/Charcot joint: an expanded pilot study. J Foot Ankle Surg. 1998;37(6):510–5. discussion 50–51
56. Dayton P, DeVries JG, Landsman A, Meyr A, Schweinberger M. American college of foot and ankle surgeons' clinical consensus statement: perioperative prophylactic antibiotic use in clean elective foot surgery. J Foot Ankle Surg. 2015;54(2):273–9.
57. Cataife G, Weinberg DA, Wong HH, Kahn KL. The effect of Surgical Care Improvement Project (SCIP) compliance on surgical site infections (SSI). Med Care. 2014;52(2 Suppl 1): S66–73.

58. Shibuya N, Schinke TL, Canales MB, Yu GV. Effect of cryotherapy devices in the postoperative setting. J Am Podiatr Med Assoc. 2007;97(6):439–46.
59. Lindstrom D, Sadr Azodi O, Wladis A, Tonnesen H, Linder S, Nasell H, et al. Effects of a perioperative smoking cessation intervention on postoperative complications: a randomized trial. Ann Surg. 2008;248(5):739–45.
60. Nasell H, Adami J, Samnegard E, Tonnesen H, Ponzer S. Effect of smoking cessation intervention on results of acute fracture surgery: a randomized controlled trial. J Bone Joint Surg Am. 2010;92(6):1335–42.
61. Burkiewicz CJ, Guadagnin FA, Skare TL, do Nascimento MM, Servin SC, de Souza GD. Vitamin D and skin repair: a prospective, double-blind and placebo controlled study in the healing of leg ulcers. Rev Col Brasileiro de Cirurgioes. 2012;39(5):401–7.
62. Blass SC, Goost H, Tolba RH, Stoffel-Wagner B, Kabir K, Burger C, et al. Time to wound closure in trauma patients with disorders in wound healing is shortened by supplements containing antioxidant micronutrients and glutamine: a PRCT. Clin Nutr. 2012; 31(4):469–75.
63. Desneves KJ, Todorovic BE, Cassar A, Crowe TC. Treatment with supplementary arginine, vitamin C and zinc in patients with pressure ulcers: a randomised controlled trial. Clin Nutr. 2005;24(6):979–87.
64. Neiva RF, Al-Shammari K, Nociti Jr FH, Soehren S, Wang HL. Effects of vitamin-B complex supplementation on periodontal wound healing. J Periodontol. 2005;76(7):1084–91.
65. Frias Soriano L, Lage Vazquez MA, Maristany CP, Xandri Graupera JM, Wouters-Wesseling W, Wagenaar L. The effectiveness of oral nutritional supplementation in the healing of pressure ulcers. J Wound Care. 2004;13(8):319–22.
66. Lischer Ch J, Koller U, Geyer H, Mulling C, Schulze J, Ossent P. Effect of therapeutic dietary biotin on the healing of uncomplicated sole ulcers in dairy cattle–a double blinded controlled study. Vet J. 2002;163(1):51–60.
67. van Anholt RD, Sobotka L, Meijer EP, Heyman H, Groen HW, Topinkova E, et al. Specific nutritional support accelerates pressure ulcer healing and reduces wound care intensity in non-malnourished patients. Nutrition. 2010;26(9):867–72.
68. Lee SK, Posthauer ME, Dorner B, Redovian V, Maloney MJ. Pressure ulcer healing with a concentrated, fortified, collagen protein hydrolysate supplement: a randomized controlled trial. Adv Skin Wound Care. 2006;19(2):92–6.
69. Collins CE, Kershaw J, Brockington S. Effect of nutritional supplements on wound healing in home-nursed elderly: a randomized trial. Nutrition. 2005;21(2):147–55.
70. Snyderman CH, Kachman K, Molseed L, Wagner R, D'Amico F, Bumpous J, et al. Reduced postoperative infections with an immune-enhancing nutritional supplement. Laryngoscope. 1999;109(6):915–21.
71. Lavery LA, Higgins KR, La Fontaine J, Zamorano RG, Constantinides GP, Kim PJ. Randomised clinical trial to compare total contact casts, healing sandals and a shear-reducing removable boot to heal diabetic foot ulcers. Int Wound J. 2014;12(6):710–5.
72. Ramanujam CL, Zgonis T. Versatility of intrinsic muscle flaps for the diabetic Charcot foot. Clin Podiatr Med Surg. 2012;29(2):323–6.
73. Ramanujam CL, Stapleton JJ, Kilpadi KL, Rodriguez RH, Jeffries LC, Zgonis T. Split-thickness skin grafts for closure of diabetic foot and ankle wounds: a retrospective review of 83 patients. Foot Ankle Spec. 2010;3(5):231–40.
74. Rosenblum BI, Giurini JM, Miller LB, Chrzan JS, Habershaw GM. Neuropathic ulcerations plantar to the lateral column in patients with Charcot foot deformity: a flexible approach to limb salvage. J Foot Ankle Surg. 1997;36(5):360–3.
75. Alblowi J, Kayal RA, Siqueira M, McKenzie E, Krothapalli N, McLean J, et al. High levels of tumor necrosis factor-alpha contribute to accelerated loss of cartilage in diabetic fracture healing. Am J Pathol. 2009;175(4):1574–85.
76. Beam HA, Parsons JR, Lin SS. The effects of blood glucose control upon fracture healing in the BB Wistar rat with diabetes mellitus. J Orthop Res. 2002;20(6):1210–6.
77. Black CT, Hennessey PJ, Ford EG, Andrassy RJ. Protein glycosylation and collagen metabolism in normal and diabetic rats. J Surg Res. 1989;47(3):200–2.
78. Coords M, Breitbart E, Paglia D, Kappy N, Gandhi A, Cottrell J, et al. The effects of low-intensity pulsed ultrasound upon diabetic fracture healing. J Orthop Res. 2011;29(2):181–8.
79. Follak N, Kloting I, Merk H. Influence of diabetic metabolic state on fracture healing in spontaneously diabetic rats. Diabetes Metab Res Rev. 2005;21(3):288–96.
80. Follak N, Kloting I, Wolf E, Merk H. Improving metabolic control reverses the histomorphometric and biomechanical abnormalities of an experimentally induced bone defect in spontaneously diabetic rats. Calcif Tissue Int. 2004;74(6):551–60.
81. Follak N, Kloting I, Wolf E, Merk H. Histomorphometric evaluation of the influence of the diabetic metabolic state on bone defect healing depending on the defect size in spontaneously diabetic BB/OK rats. Bone. 2004;35(1):144–52.
82. Follak N, Kloting L, Wolf E, Merk H. Delayed remodeling in the early period of fracture healing in spontaneously diabetic BB/OK rats depending on the diabetic metabolic state. Histol Histopathol. 2004;19(2):473–86.
83. Gandhi A, Beam HA, O'Connor JP, Parsons JR, Lin SS. The effects of local insulin delivery on diabetic fracture healing. Bone. 2005;37(4):482–90.
84. Gandhi A, Doumas C, O'Connor JP, Parsons JR, Lin SS. The effects of local platelet rich plasma delivery on diabetic fracture healing. Bone. 2006;38(4):540–6.
85. Gandhi A, Liporace F, Azad V, Mattie J, Lin SS. Diabetic fracture healing. Foot Ankle Clin. 2006;11(4):805–24.
86. Gebauer GP, Lin SS, Beam HA, Vieira P, Parsons JR. Low-intensity pulsed ultrasound increases the fracture callus strength in diabetic BB Wistar rats but does not affect cellular proliferation. J Orthop Res. 2002;20(3):587–92.
87. Goto S, Fujii H, Kono K, Nakai K, Hamada Y, Yamato H, et al. Carvedilol ameliorates low-turnover bone disease in non-obese type 2 diabetes. Am J Nephrol. 2011;34(3):281–90.
88. Hamada Y, Kitazawa S, Kitazawa R, Fujii H, Kasuga M, Fukagawa M. Histomorphometric analysis of diabetic osteopenia in streptozotocin-induced diabetic mice: a possible role of oxidative stress. Bone. 2007;40(5):1408–14.
89. Hamada Y, Kitazawa S, Kitazawa R, Kono K, Goto S, Komaba H, et al. The effects of the receptor for advanced glycation end products (RAGE) on bone metabolism under physiological and diabetic conditions. Endocrine. 2010;38(3):369–76.
90. Kayal RA, Alblowi J, McKenzie E, Krothapalli N, Silkman L, Gerstenfeld L, et al. Diabetes causes the accelerated loss of cartilage during fracture repair which is reversed by insulin treatment. Bone. 2009;44(2):357–63.
91. Kayal RA, Tsatsas D, Bauer MA, Allen B, Al-Sebaei MO, Kakar S, et al. Diminished bone formation during diabetic fracture healing is related to the premature resorption of cartilage associated with increased osteoclast activity. J Bone Miner Res. 2007;22(4):560–8.
92. Lange J, Barz T, Ekkernkamp A, Kloting I, Follak N. Gene expression profile in bone of diabetes-prone BB/OK rats fed a high-fat diet. Genes Nutr. 2012;8(1):99–104.
93. Lu H, Kraut D, Gerstenfeld LC, Graves DT. Diabetes interferes with the bone formation by affecting the expression of transcrip-

tion factors that regulate osteoblast differentiation. Endocrinology. 2003;144(1):346–52.
94. Macey LR, Kana SM, Jingushi S, Terek RM, Borretos J, Bolander ME. Defects of early fracture-healing in experimental diabetes. J Bone Joint Surg Am. 1989;71(5):722–33.
95. Mathey J, Horcajada-Molteni MN, Chanteranne B, Picherit C, Puel C, Lebecque P, et al. Bone mass in obese diabetic Zucker rats: influence of treadmill running. Calcif Tissue Int. 2002; 70(4):305–11.
96. Ogasawara A, Nakajima A, Nakajima F, Goto K, Yamazaki M. Molecular basis for affected cartilage formation and bone union in fracture healing of the streptozotocin-induced diabetic rat. Bone. 2008;43(5):832–9.
97. Santana RB, Xu L, Chase HB, Amar S, Graves DT, Trackman PC. A role for advanced glycation end products in diminished bone healing in type 1 diabetes. Diabetes. 2003;52(6):1502–10.
98. Topping RE, Bolander ME, Balian G. Type X collagen in fracture callus and the effects of experimental diabetes. Clin Orthop Relat Res. 1994;308:220–8.
99. Tyndall WA, Beam HA, Zarro C, O'Connor JP, Lin SS. Decreased platelet derived growth factor expression during fracture healing in diabetic animals. Clin Orthop Relat Res. 2003;408:319–30.
100. Perlman MH, Thordarson DB. Ankle fusion in a high risk population: an assessment of nonunion risk factors. Foot Ankle Int. 1999;20(8):491–6.
101. Bibbo C, Lin SS, Beam HA, Behrens FF. Complications of ankle fractures in diabetic patients. Orthop Clin North Am. 2001; 32(1):113–33.
102. Blotter RH, Connolly E, Wasan A, Chapman MW. Acute complications in the operative treatment of isolated ankle fractures in patients with diabetes mellitus. Foot Ankle Int. 1999;20(11): 687–94.
103. Connolly JF, Csencsitz TA. Limb threatening neuropathic complications from ankle fractures in patients with diabetes. Clin Orthop Relat Res. 1998;348:212–9.
104. Costigan W, Thordarson DB, Debnath UK. Operative management of ankle fractures in patients with diabetes mellitus. Foot Ankle Int. 2007;28(1):32–7.
105. Jones KB, Maiers-Yelden KA, Marsh JL, Zimmerman MB, Estin M, Saltzman CL. Ankle fractures in patients with diabetes mellitus. J Bone Joint Surg (Br). 2005;87(4):489–95.
106. Kristiansen B. Ankle and foot fractures in diabetics provoking neuropathic joint changes. Acta Orthop Scand. 1980;51(6):975–9.
107. Prisk VR, Wukich DK. Ankle fractures in diabetics. Foot Ankle Clin. 2006;11(4):849–63.
108. Tang SY, Vashishth D. Non-enzymatic glycation alters microdamage formation in human cancellous bone. Bone. 2010;46(1): 148–54.
109. Mehta SK, Breitbart EA, Berberian WS, Liporace FA, Lin SS. Bone and wound healing in the diabetic patient. Foot Ankle Clin. 2010;15(3):411–37.
110. Shibuya N, Humphers JM, Fluhman BL, Jupiter DC. Factors associated with nonunion, delayed union, and malunion in foot and ankle surgery in diabetic patients. J Foot Ankle Surg. 2013; 52(2):207–11.
111. La Fontaine J, Harkless LB, Sylvia VL, Carnes D, Heim-Hall J, Jude E. Levels of endothelial nitric oxide synthase and calcitonin gene-related peptide in the Charcot foot: a pilot study. J Foot Ankle Surg. 2008;47(5):424–9.
112. Shibuya N, La Fontaine J, Frania SJ. Alcohol-induced neuroarthropathy in the foot: a case series and review of literature. J Foot Ankle Surg. 2008;47(2):118–24.
113. Jeffcoate WJ. Theories concerning the pathogenesis of the acute charcot foot suggest future therapy. Curr Diab Rep. 2005;5(6): 430–5.
114. Sinacore DR, Hastings MK, Bohnert KL, Fielder FA, Villareal DT, Blair 3rd VP, et al. Inflammatory osteolysis in diabetic neuropathic (Charcot) arthropathies of the foot. Phys Ther. 2008;88(11):1399–407.
115. Zaidi M. Neural surveillance of skeletal homeostasis. Cell Metab. 2005;1(4):219–21.
116. Irie K, Hara-Irie F, Ozawa H, Yajima T. Calcitonin gene-related peptide (CGRP)-containing nerve fibers in bone tissue and their involvement in bone remodeling. Microsc Res Tech. 2002; 58(2):85–90.
117. Young MJ, Marshall A, Adams JE, Selby PL, Boulton AJ. Osteopenia, neurological dysfunction, and the development of Charcot neuroarthropathy. Diabetes Care. 1995;18(1):34–8.
118. Alazraki N, Dalinka MK, Berquist TH, Daffner RJ, De Smet AA, El-Khoury GY, et al. Imaging diagnosis of osteomyelitis in patients with diabetes mellitus. American College of Radiology. ACR Appropriateness Criteria. Radiology. 2000;215:303–10.
119. Michail M, Jude E, Liaskos C, Karamagiolis S, Makrilakis K, Dimitroulis D, et al. The performance of serum inflammatory markers for the diagnosis and follow-up of patients with osteomyelitis. Int J Low Extrem Wounds. 2013;12(2):94–9.
120. Shen CJ, Wu MS, Lin KH, Lin WL, Chen HC, Wu JY, et al. The use of procalcitonin in the diagnosis of bone and joint infection: a systemic review and meta-analysis. Eur J Clin Microbiol Infect Dis. 2013;32(6):807–14.
121. Alvaro-Afonso FJ, Lazaro-Martinez JL, Aragon-Sanchez FJ, Garcia-Morales E, Carabantes-Alarcon D, Molines-Barroso RJ. Does the location of the ulcer affect the interpretation of the probe-to-bone test in the diagnosis of osteomyelitis in diabetic foot ulcers? Diabet Med. 2014;31(1):112–3.
122. Mutluoglu M, Uzun G, Sildiroglu O, Turhan V, Mutlu H, Yildiz S. Performance of the probe-to-bone test in a population suspected of having osteomyelitis of the foot in diabetes. J Am Podiatr Med Assoc. 2012;102(5):369–73.
123. Aragon-Sanchez J, Lipsky BA, Lazaro-Martinez JL. Diagnosing diabetic foot osteomyelitis: is the combination of probe-to-bone test and plain radiography sufficient for high-risk inpatients? Diabet Med. 2011;28(2):191–4.
124. Lavery LA, Armstrong DG, Peters EJ, Lipsky BA. Probe-to-bone test for diagnosing diabetic foot osteomyelitis: reliable or relic? Diabetes Care. 2007;30(2):270–4.
125. Grayson ML, Gibbons GW, Balogh K, Levin E, Karchmer AW. Probing to bone in infected pedal ulcers. A clinical sign of underlying osteomyelitis in diabetic patients. JAMA. 1995;273(9): 721–3.
126. Lazaro-Martinez JL, Aragon-Sanchez J, Garcia-Morales E. Antibiotics versus conservative surgery for treating diabetic foot osteomyelitis: a randomized comparative trial. Diabetes Care. 2014;37(3):789–95.
127. Ragnarson Tennvall G, Apelqvist J. Health-related quality of life in patients with diabetes mellitus and foot ulcers. J Diabetes Complicat. 2000;14(5):235–41.
128. Pakarinen TK, Laine HJ, Maenpaa H, Mattila P, Lahtela J. Long-term outcome and quality of life in patients with Charcot foot. Foot Ankle Surg. 2009;15(4):187–91.
129. Sochocki MP, Verity S, Atherton PJ, Huntington JL, Sloan JA, Embil JM, et al. Health related quality of life in patients with Charcot arthropathy of the foot and ankle. Foot Ankle Surg. 2008;14(1):11–5.
130. Busse JW, Jacobs CL, Swiontkowski MF, Bosse MJ, Bhandari M. Complex limb salvage or early amputation for severe lower-limb injury: a meta-analysis of observational studies. J Orthop Trauma. 2007;21(1):70–6.
131. Saddawi-Konefka D, Kim HM, Chung KC. A systematic review of outcomes and complications of reconstruction and amputation

for type IIIB and IIIC fractures of the tibia. Plast Reconstr Surg. 2008;122(6):1796–805.
132. Jupiter DC, Shibuya N, Clawson LD, Davis ML. Incidence and risk factors for amputation in foot and ankle trauma. J Foot Ankle Surg. 2012;51(3):317–22.
133. Gailey R, Allen K, Castles J, Kucharik J, Roeder M. Review of secondary physical conditions associated with lower-limb amputation and long-term prosthesis use. J Rehabil Res Dev. 2008;45(1):15–29.
134. Boutoille D, Feraille A, Maulaz D, Krempf M. Quality of life with diabetes-associated foot complications: comparison between lower-limb amputation and chronic foot ulceration. Foot Ankle Int. 2008;29(11):1074–8.
135. Harness N, Pinzur MS. Health related quality of life in patients with dysvascular transtibial amputation. Clin Orthop Relat Res. 2001;383:204–7.
136. Tennvall GR, Apelqvist J, Eneroth M. Costs of deep foot infections in patients with diabetes mellitus. PharmacoEconomics. 2000;18(3):225–38.
137. Pinzur MS. Gait analysis in peripheral vascular insufficiency through-knee amputation. J Rehabil Res Dev. 1993;30(4):388–92.
138. Pinzur MS. The metabolic cost of lower extremity amputation. Clin Podiatr Med Surg. 1997;14(4):599–602.
139. Pinzur MS, Gold J, Schwartz D, Gross N. Energy demands for walking in dysvascular amputees as related to the level of amputation. Orthopedics. 1992;15(9):1033–6. discussion 6–7

Part V

Ankle

Complications Associated with Ankle Arthroscopy

25

Graham A. Hamilton and Lawrence A. Ford

Introduction

Despite a late start within the realm of arthroscopy, foot and ankle arthroscopy has proven to be an important diagnostic and therapeutic tool for the foot and ankle surgeon. As the indications for foot and ankle arthroscopy increase the complications associated with the procedure must be revisited.

Prior to the 1980s, the narrow anatomical confines of the ankle joint were found to be highly challenging to approach with an arthroscope. Burman, in 1931, stated the ankle was unsuitable for arthroscopy because of the narrow joint space and the large sized nature of the instrumentation [1]. As technology improved, so did our ability to gain access to smaller joints, using an arthroscope. In 1989, prior to the joint distraction era, Sprauge had a high complication rate of 24.6% [2]. In the mid-1980s invasive joint distraction was popularized leading to a decline in complications. Guhl looked at 131 ankle arthroscopies and noted a complication rate of 10% [3]. Martin and associates found a 15% complication rate in their long-term follow-up on a series of 101 ankles [4, 5]. Barber reported an incidence of 17% in 53 cases [6]. Ferkel in 1996 reported an overall complication rate of 9.8% in 612 cases [7]. Deng and colleagues retrospectively reviewed 405 arthroscopic surgeries of the foot and ankle performed by four surgeons over 3 years. Their overall complication rate was 7.69% [8].The average of published complications is 10.5% [2–4, 6–11] (Table 25.1). Given a 1 in 10 chance of a potential complication, extreme caution and close scrutiny of indications and surgical technique is important.

G.A. Hamilton (✉)
Department of Orthopedics and Podiatric Surgery, Kaiser Permanente Medical Center,
4501 Sand Creek Road, Antioch, CA 94531, USA

Kaiser San Francisco Bay Area Foot and Ankle Residency Program, Oakland, CA, USA
e-mail: graham_hamilton@mac.com

L.A. Ford
Department of Orthopedics and Podiatric Surgery, Kaiser Permanente Medical Center,
3600 Broadway Blvd, Oakland, CA 94611, USA

Kaiser San Francisco Bay Area Foot and Ankle Residency Program, Oakland, CA, USA

Indications

The most frequent indications for ankle arthroscopy can be broken down to those procedures that are approached from the anterior aspect of the joint and those that are approached posteriorly. A summary of both is listed below (Table 25.2).

Types of Complications

Complications can be broken down into various categories: systemic, preoperative, and procedure-related (Tables 25.3, 25.4, and 25.5). Most complications are related to the procedure itself.

Neurological Injury

The most common complication in foot and ankle arthroscopy is injury to one of the nerves that traverses the ankle joint secondary to improper portal placement or equipment handling. This usually involves a transient neuritis of one of the superficial nerves, but on occasion, it can be associated with permanent paresthesias or paresis. Neuromas can also form from injury to the nerve during the surgical procedure. A thorough understanding of the foot and ankle anatomy is paramount when performing placing portals so as not to iatrogenically injure neurovascular structures. At the ankle level, five nerves cross the joint from the leg to the foot. Two of them are deep: the posterior tibial nerve and deep peroneal nerve. Three are superficial: the superficial peroneal nerve, the saphenous nerve, and the sural nerve.

M.S. Lee, J.P. Grossman (eds.), *Complications in Foot and Ankle Surgery*, DOI 10.1007/978-3-319-53686-6_25

Table 25.1 Summary of current articles and the complications rates in foot & ankle arthroscopy

Author	Year	Journal	No. of patients	% Complications
Guhl	1986	Orthopedics	62	8
Guhl	1988	Arthroscopy	131	10
Sprague et al.	1989	Book	201	17.4
Martin et al.	1989	Am J Sports Med	58	15
Barber et al.	1990	Foot Ankle	53	17
Ferkel et al.	1996	Arthroscopy	612	9
Amendola	1996	Arthroscopy	79	7.6
Unger et al.	2000	Unfallchirurg	155	9
Zengerick and Van Dijk	2012	Knee Surg Sports Traumatol Arthrosc	1305	3.5
Deng et al.	2012	J Foot Ankle Surg	405	7.7
Total		10		10.4

Table 25.2 Indications for anterior & posterior ankle arthroscopy

Anterior ankle arthroscopy
Anterior ankle impingement (bone spurs, ossicles, as well as soft tissue)
Osteochondral defects
Loose bodies
Synovectomy
Treatment for ankle instability
Arthroscopic assisted fracture reduction
Arthroscopic ankle arthrodesis
Posterior ankle arthroscopy
Posterior ankle impingement
Osteochondral defects
Loose bodies
Synovectomy

Table 25.3 Systemic complications in foot & ankle arthroscopy

Systemic complications: related to illness, stress of injury, anesthesia, surgery
Atelectasis
Pulmonary embolism
Myocardial infarction
Other cardiopulmonary event
Loss of limb
Loss of life

Table 25.4 Pre-operative complications in foot & ankle arthroscopy

Preoperative complications
Lack of preoperative planning
Failure to obtain appropriate preoperative diagnostic studies
Operating for the wrong diagnosis

Ten portals have been described to gain access to the ankle (Figs. 25.1, 25.2, and 25.3a–c), but for nearly all cases typically only two or three are used. These include the anteromedial, anterolateral, and posterolateral portals.

Table 25.5 Procedure-related complications in foot & ankle arthroscopy

Procedure related complications
Operating on the incorrect extremity
Tourniquet complications
Neurovascular injury
Tendon injury
Ligament injury
Wound complications
Infection
Articular cartilage damage
Compartment syndrome
Hemarthrosis
Postoperative effusion
Complex regional pain syndrome
Fluid management complications
Distraction-related complications
Postoperative stress fracture
Instrument breakage

Nerve injury can be minimized by marking out the surface anatomy around the anterior and posterior ankle joint before committing to portal placement. Vertical incisions through the skin are preferred, as opposed to transverse ones. This serves two purposes. First there is less likelihood that with vertical incisions the cutaneous nerves could be injured, and if necessary, the incision can be extended for joint access. Once the skin incision has been made, the surgeon is advised to spread with a blunt hemostat before penetrating the joint capsule. This is followed by cannula insertion. Once the cannula is inserted, all instruments should then be passed through the cannula.

The safest portal is the anteromedial ankle portal. When creating this portal, care must be taken to avoid the saphenous nerve and great saphenous vein and its branches. Using the medial edge of the tibialis anterior tendon, with the joint dorsiflexed using the surgeon's abdomen, the

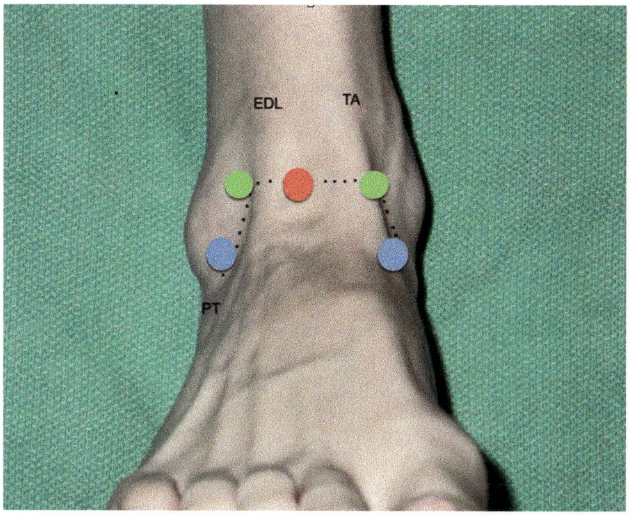

Fig. 25.1 Anterior ankle portals. The most commonly utilized anteromedial and antero lateral portals are labeled in *green*. The anterocentral given its proximity to the neurovascular bundle should be avoided and is labeled *red*. The accessory portals are labeled in *blue*. *TA* tibialis anterior tendon, *EDL* extensor digitorum longus tendon, *PT* peroneus tertius; *dotted line* is the ankle joint line

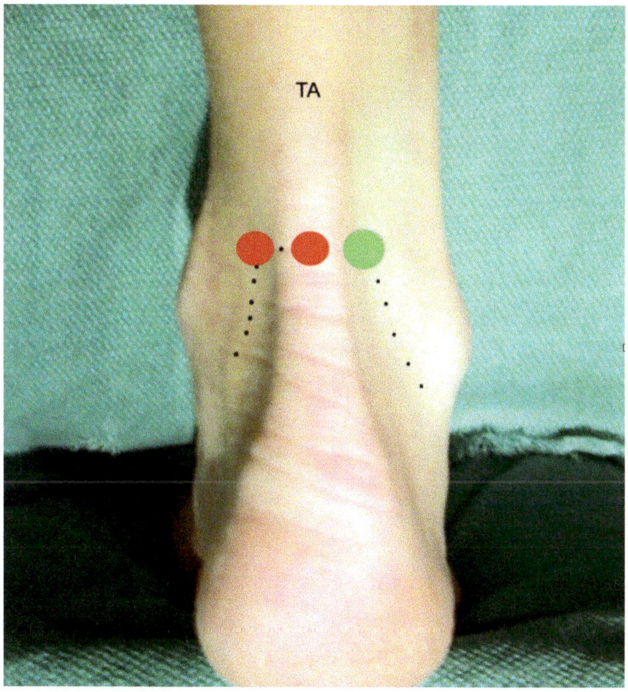

Fig. 25.2 Posterior ankle portals. The commonly utilized posterolateral portal is labeled in *green*. This is best established using a switching stick, so as to avoid injury to the sural nerve. The trans-achilles and posteromedial portal should be avoided and are labeled *red*

distal tibia is palpated with the index finger. It is followed distally to the joint line and the "soft spot" of the medial tibiotalar joint is palpated. Portal placement in this location avoids nerve injury.

The anterolateral portal has the greatest risk of nerve injury to the intermediate dorsal cutaneous nerve (the lateral branch of the superficial peroneal nerve). It is always advisable to identify this superficial nerve prior to portal placement. By plantarflexing and inverting the foot, this nerve can often be identified and marked. In patients with greater adiposity, this is not always achievable (Fig. 25.4). Another arthroscopic technique that decreases the likelihood of injury is creating this portal under direct transillumination with the arthroscope. Occasionally the surgeon may elect to establish a posterolateral portal. Care must be taken with this entry point, as damage to the sural nerve has been reported. The incidence of nerve injury can be as high as 22% in some studies [6]. There is less likelihood of nerve injury, when the portal is established using an inside out switching stick. For this method, the arthroscope is placed in the anterolateral portal. A blunt 4 mm switching stick is placed in the anteromedial portal and directed through the anatomic notch of Harty postero-laterally. It should exit through the posterior–inferior tibiofibular ligaments. Once it tents the skin, a small stab incision is made and a cannula sleeve can then be inserted over the switching stick and followed back into the joint. Care must also be taken to avoid aggressive debridement of the anterior capsule. Inadvertent suction of the capsule can incarcerate the deep peroneal nerve and/or the dorsalis pedis vessels.

Vascular Injury

Vascular injury and pseudoaneurysms, while rare, can occur at the portal sites. The use of the anterocentral portal has been associated with injury to the dorsalis pedis artery. Given the potential high risk of this portal it is typically avoided [12–14].

Tourniquet

Although the use of a tourniquet is often unnecessary in ankle arthroscopy, there are instances where it can aid in visualization. Excessive cuff times and pressures can cause thigh paresthesias resulting in pain and paresis. Sherman and colleagues reported on 2646 knee scopes that there were no complications with a tourniquet, unless the time exceeded 60 min [14]. The authors have found when performing ankle arthroscopy, that insufflation of the joint with lidocaine and epinephrine (1:100,000) provides chemical hemostasis and excellent visualization obviating the need for a tourniquet. If a thigh cuff is used, it is typically inflated at 250 mmHg pressure and released after 1 h during the procedure.

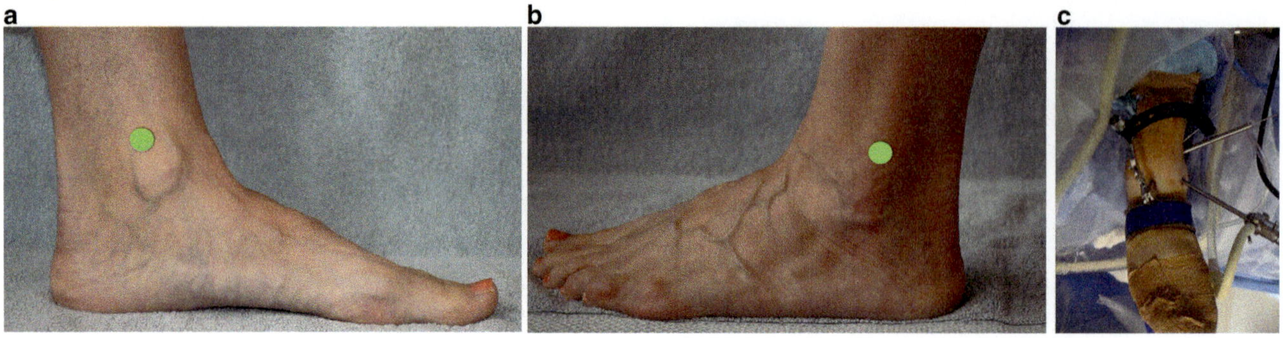

Fig. 25.3 (**a–c**) Malleolar portals (medial and lateral malleolus). Occasionally trans-fibular and trans-tibial pin insertion is used for drilling of osteochondral defects. This is typically performed with an aiming device as is shown here (**c**)

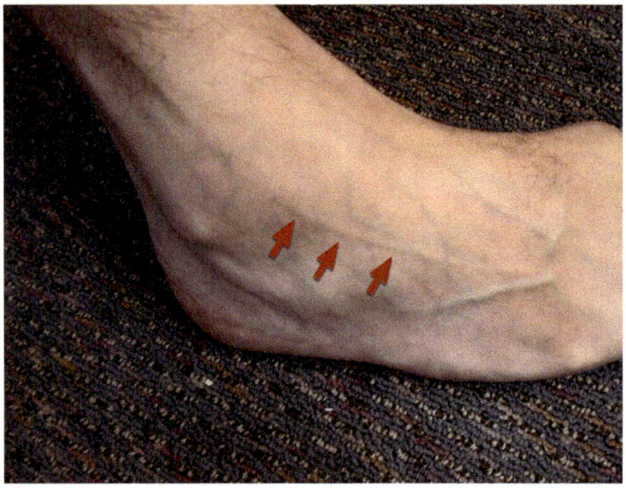

Fig. 25.4 The intermediate dorsal cutaneous nerve is marked by the *red arrows*. Prior to creating the anterolateral portal, this nerve should be identified and marked so as to avoid potential injury. This is best identified by plantarflexing and inverting the foot. In patients with greater adiposity, this nerve is not always identifiable

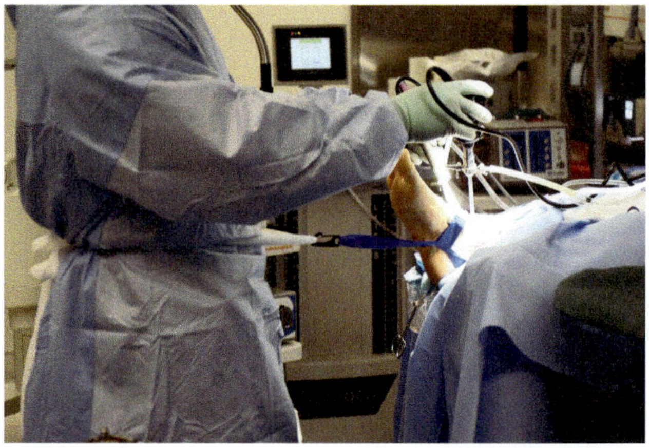

Fig. 25.5 Non-invasive ankle distraction using a commercially available strap and Kerlix roll

Tendon/Ligament Injuries

Ten tendons cross the ankle joint from the leg to the foot. One of these described is the trans-achilles portal. This has been abandoned by most surgeons due to the high risk of tendinopathy and possible rupture. Injury to ligaments about the ankle can occur through improper portal placement. Injury can occur with over aggressive debridement during the procedure and excessive distraction. In cases where accessory portals are used, such as the anterolateral or anteromedial accessory portal, a spinal needle should be inserted and visualized with the arthroscope, at the planned portal site, prior to committing to a cannula. This ensures accuracy of placement and minimizes potential damage to the lateral collateral or deltoid ligaments. Excessive traction can also potentially place the ankle ligaments at risk. In most ankle arthroscopy cases, the pathology is anterior and nearly all work can be done without distraction. In cases where traction is needed, such as for a postero-medial osteochondral lesions, the authors prefer using a Kerlix roll along with a non-invasive ankle strap (Fig. 25.5). This provides excellent distraction when needed and the surgeon can relax distraction as he or she sees fit. It also facilitates intermittent distraction versus a constant distraction that comes with other non-invasive distractors.

Articular Cartilage Injury

One must be careful when performing ankle arthroscopy to not cause iatrogenic injury to the articular surface. The cartilage is susceptible to injury at the time of initial instrument insertion. For the novice arthroscopist it is preferable to use the small joint 2.7 mm arthroscope to decrease risk to the articular surface. This has a smaller lever arm compared to the 4.0 mm arthroscope. This size differential decreases the likelihood of iatrogenic articular damage. Deng and colleagues, in their retrospective review on complications, found no statistical significance between a large joint scope and small. However, all arthroscopists were experienced surgeons. Sharp trochars with cannula insertion should be avoided at all costs; as they increase the likelihood of iatrogenic injury. The blunt obturator is preferable. Another key point to protecting the cartilage from instrument damage is to maximally dorsiflex the ankle joint during instrument insertion. In so doing, the talar dome is covered by the tibial plafond. This ensures the instrumentation is placed into the anterior pouch of the ankle and does not skive across the joint surface.

Broken Instrument Complications

The small equipment used in ankle arthroscopy is more fragile and prone to breaking. Instruments prior to insertion into the joint; joint should always be checked to ensure they are intact. If an instrument does break inside the joint, then the fluid inflow and outflow should be stopped immediately and the arthroscope should be fixed on the broken piece. A small joint grasper is then typically used to retrieve the foreign body (Fig. 25.6). In some cases the fragment can migrate into the gutters in particular the posterior recess. A useful tool to have is a small-joint suction magnet (Golden retriever). If the broken instrument cannot be retrieved, then an image intensifier should be used and an arthrotomy made to remove the foreign body.

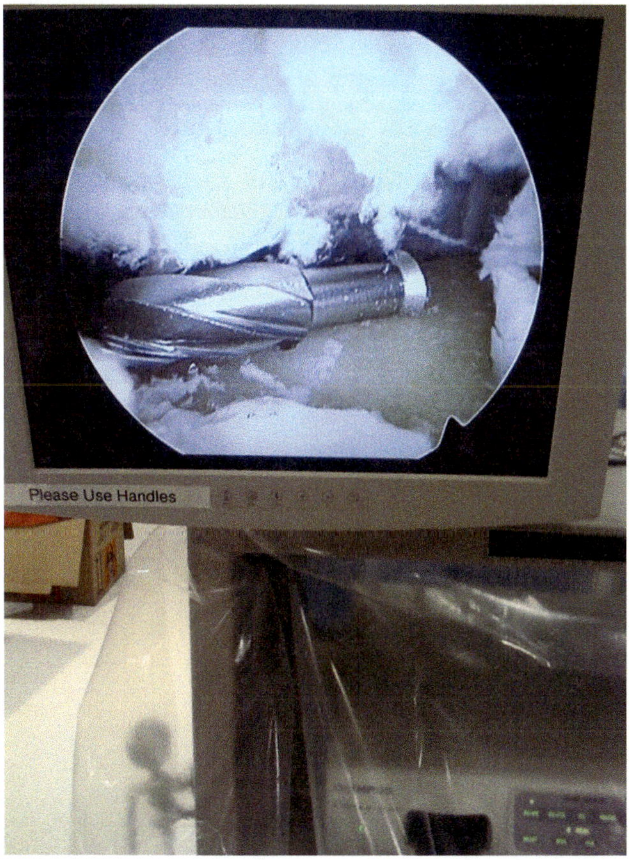

Fig. 25.6 Broken burr in the ankle joint. This was retrieved with a grasper and by stopping fluid inflow

Fluid Management Complications

Problems with fluid management can be broken down to challenges with joint distention, visualization, and extravasation. Use of a separate inflow and outflow portal solves the problem of distention and visualization. The authors recommend gravity inflow. 3–4 L bags of lactated ringers solution at about 3 feet above the joint and large diameter high-flow Y-tubing offer adequate distention and visualization.

Pump technology has greatly improved over the last decade, but they carry the potential risk of compartment ischemia and syndrome. If the cannula slips into a subcutaneous space and no outflow is measured, the pump can dramatically increase pressure.

Wound Complications

It is well documented that the anatomy of the ankle joint differs greatly from joints located more proximally. The ankle lies at the base of the body and has far less subcutaneous fat compared to other joints. As a result, the potential for wound problems (seromas, hematomas, sloughs, and sinus tracts) is far greater. Synovial fistulas are thankfully rare, but can be very challenging to manage. Persistent drainage from a standard portal should raise the suspicion of a synovial fistula. If a fistula is identified, then as a first line approach, the drainage should be cultured, oral antibiotics started empirically, and the joint immobilized. If at 7–10 days, the wound remains open, then the patient should be taken back to the operating room, the sinus tract excised, and the wound re-sutured and the joint immobilized.

Infection

Surgical procedures involving the foot and ankle have higher infection rates than other areas of the body [15]. This is due to a lower amount of subcutaneous fat and the unique resident organisms that colonize this region of the body. Given the higher risk region of anatomy, it is incumbent upon the surgeon to minimize skin flora and maximize prophylaxis.

Reducing post-op infection rates starts with the surgical preparation.

Ostrander in 2005 compared various antiseptics. They prospectively looked at 125 patients undergoing foot and ankle surgery and randomized the surgical prep, to either 0.7% Iodine and 74% isopropyl alcohol (Duraprep); 3% Chloroxylenol (techni-care); Chloraprep (2% chlorhexidine and 74% isopropyl alcohol). All patients received 1 g of cefazolin for prophylaxis. Cultures were then taken from the anterior ankle (control), the hallux nail fold (hallux), and third and fourth web space (toes).

The most common bacteria cultured in all areas was *Staphylococcus epidermidis*. Alcohol plus chlorhexidine was the most effective antiseptic [16].

Despite vigilant skin preparation and antibiotic prophylaxis, infections can manifest. Infections are broken down into superficial and deep. Ferkel's retrospective review published in Arthroscopy in 1996 on 612 arthroscopes had an incidence of 1.3% [6]. Deng had an incidence 3.5% (1 deep, 7 superficial) [7]. Ferkel in his review noted there was an increase in superficial wound infections when steri-strips were used for wound closure versus skin [6]. For infection control, the authors recommend a surgical preparation with Alcohol then hibiclens. Antibiotic prophylaxis with a first generation cephalosporin, or clindamycin or Vancomycin for allergic patients is recommended. This should be given 30–60 min before the incision is made. Portal sites should be sutured. The surgical limb should be splinted for about 7–10 days.

Conclusion

Although arthroscopic surgery of the ankle is minimally invasive, there is still the potential for complications. As with all surgery, understanding the risks is the first step in mitigating this potential. Careful preparation, meticulous technique, and early detection and intervention are paramount in optimizing outcomes following ankle arthroscopy.

References

1. Burman MS. Arthroscopy of direct visualization of joints. An experimental cadaver study. J Bone Joint Surg. 1931;13:669–95.
2. Sprague III NF, Guhl JF, Olson DW. Specific complications: elbow, wrist, hip, and ankle. In: Spraque III NF, editor. Complications in arthroscopy, vol. 1. New York: Raven Press; 1989. p. 199–224.
3. Guhl JF. New concepts (distraction) in ankle arthroscopy. Arthroscopy. 1988;4(3):160–7.
4. Martin DF, Baker CL, Curl WW, Andrews JR, Robie DB, Haas AF. Operative ankle arthroscopy. Long-term followup. Am J Sports Med. 1989;17:16–23.
5. Barber FA, Click J, Britt BT. Complications of ankle arthroscopy. Foot Ankle. 1990;l0:263–6.
6. Ferkel RD, Heath DD, Guhl JF. Neurological complications of ankle arthroscopy. Arthroscopy. 1996;12(2):200–8.
7. Deng DF, Hamilton GA, Lee M, Rush S, Ford LA, Patel S. Complications associated with foot and ankle arthroscopy. J Foot Ankle Surg. 2012;51(3):281–4.
8. Guhl JF. New techniques for arthroscopic surgery of the ankle: preliminary report. Orthopedics. 1986;9(2):261–9.
9. Arnendola A, Petriik J, Webster-Bogaert S. Ankle arthroscopy: outcome in 79 consecutive patients. Arthroscopy. 1996;12:565–73.
10. Unger F, Lajtai G, et al. Arthroscopy of the upper ankle joint. A retrospective analysis of complications. Unfallchirurg. 2000;103:858–63.
11. Zengerick M, Van Dijk CN. Complications in ankle arthroscopy. Knee Surg Sports Traumatol Arthrosc. 2012;20(8):1420–31.
12. Darwish A, Ehsan O, Marynissen H, Al-Khaffaf H. Pseudoaneurysm of the anterior tibial artery after ankle arthroscopy. Arthroscopy. 2004;20(6):e63–4.
13. Mariani PP, Mancini L, et al. Pseudoaneurysm as a complication of ankle arthroscopy. Arthroscopy. 2001;17:400–2.
14. Sherman OH, Fox JM, Snyder SJ, Del Pizzo W, Friedman MJ, Ferkel RD, Lawley MJ. Arthroscopy—"no-problem surgery". An analysis of complications in two thousand six hundred and forty cases. J Bone Joint Surg Am. 1986;68(2):256–65.
15. Miller WA. Postoperative wound infection in foot and ankle surgery. Foot Ankle Int. 1983;4(2):102–4.
16. Ostrander RV, Botte MJ, Brage ME. Efficacy of surgical preparation solutions in foot and ankle surgery. J Bone Joint Surg Am. 2005;87(5):980–5.

Osteochondral Lesions of the Talus

26

Kyle S. Peterson and Christopher F. Hyer

Abbreviations

ACI	autologous chondrocyte implantation
CT	computerized tomography
MACI	matrix-induced autologous chondrocyte implantation
MRI	magnetic resonance imaging
OATS	osteochondral autograft or allograft transfer system
OCD	osteochondritis dissecans
OLT	osteochondral lesion of the talus

Introduction

An osteochondral lesion of the talus (OLT) or osteochondritis dissecans (OCD) is a debilitating disorder of the articular cartilage characterized by loose body formation or subchondral bone fracture. Kappis originally described this process involving the ankle joint in 1922 [1]. Lesions of the talus account for 4% of all osteochondral lesions in the body [2]. The primary etiology is associated with traumatic injuries to the ankle involving up to 70% of sprains and fractures [3, 4]. Nontraumatic causes of OLTs have also been described and include congenital factors, ligamentous laxity, spontaneous necrosis, steroid treatment, and endocrine abnormalities [5, 6].

A primary ischemic event in the talus has often been implicated in the development of an osteochondral lesion [7]. Whether by direct insult to the vasculature of the talus or repetitive articular microtrauma, both can lead to cellular death by disruption of the collagen fibrils and thickening of the subchondral bone [8].

K.S. Peterson
Suburban Orthopaedics,
1110 W Schick Rd, Bartlett, IL 60103, USA

C.F. Hyer (✉)
Orthopedic Foot and Ankle Center,
300 Polaris Parkway, Suite 2000, Westerville, OH 43082, USA
e-mail: ofacresearch@orthofootankle.com

In 1959, Berndt and Harty created a classification system based on radiographic and surgical parameters, which has become one of the most widely utilized staging systems for describing OLTs [9]. Stages of the classification system are described in Table 26.1. Numerous other classification systems utilizing advancements in computerized tomography (CT), magnetic resonance imaging (MRI), and arthroscopy have also been developed to improve on treatment protocols and outcomes [10–13].

The mechanism of injury to the ankle can often describe the location of the osteochondral lesion of the talus. An inverted and dorsiflexed position of the ankle causes damage to the anterolateral portion of the talar dome. A shearing force is created with the talus impacting the fibula creating a shallow, wafer-shaped lesion [14]. When the ankle is inverted and plantarflexed, a posteromedial lesion most often occurs. Talar inversion and rotation result in the medial talar dome impacting against the medial malleolus or the posterior aspect of the tibia [14]. Post-traumatic medial lesions are characteristically described as a deep, cup-shaped appearance.

The goals of treating an OLT are symptomatic pain relief and returning patients to work, sports, and activities of daily living. This can be accomplished through various conservative and surgical methods. Initial treatment options for OLTs often begin with conservative therapy, such as immobilization in a cast or prefabricated boot, nonsteroidal anti-inflammatory medications, bracing, corticosteroid injections, and activity modification [15]. Although nonoperative treatment methods initially alleviate pain in the short term, OLTs often recur due to inadequate healing of the lesion [16]. Therefore, surgical treatment is often indicated to restore the articular cartilage anatomy.

Surgical Treatment for Primary Talar Osteochondral Lesions

Operative treatment is indicated in those patients with symptomatic OLTs that have failed initial conservative treatment efforts and those with acute, displaced fragments. Reparative

M.S. Lee, J.P. Grossman (eds.), *Complications in Foot and Ankle Surgery*, DOI 10.1007/978-3-319-53686-6_26

Table 26.1 One of the most widely used staging systems for describing OLTs based on radiographic and surgical parameters

Berndt and Harty classification system for OLTs [9]	
Stage 1	Small subchondral compression fracture
Stage 2	Partially detached fragment of the cartilage
Stage 3	Completely detached fragment of the cartilage without displacement
Stage 4	Completely detached and displaced fragment of the cartilage floating in the joint space

methods focus on bone marrow stimulation (microfracture), tissue transplantation with autograft or allograft transfer system, autologous chondrocyte implantation, hyaline cartilage grafts, and biologic augmentation.

Bone marrow stimulation techniques include debridement, microfracture, antegrade drilling, or retrograde drilling. These techniques are often considered first-line treatment for primary osteochondral lesions up to 15 mm in diameter [17–24]. This treatment is primarily performed arthroscopically and involves excision of the OLT to a stable cartilage border. Multiple drill holes in the subchondral bone spaced 3–4 mm apart then allow mesenchymal stem cells and growth factors to form a fibrocartilage cap comprised primarily of type I collagen [25, 26]. Native hyaline cartilage, however, is primarily comprised of type II collagen, while type I collagen contains different mechanical and biological properties that have been shown to degenerate over time [27]. This can be one of the primary reasons for a patient to have a failure of a primary microfracture procedure.

Outcomes of marrow stimulation techniques have been reported, with good to excellent results, in 65–90% of patients [15, 18, 22, 28–34]. Many clinical factors have been described to be predictive of patient outcome. These factors include size of lesion, patient age, bony edema on MRI, and cystic nature of lesion [35]. Size of talar lesions less than 15 mm in diameter has shown to have superior clinical outcomes. Patient aged less than 18 years old also has shown better outcomes than older patients with microfracture and drilling. Lastly, improved clinical symptoms postoperatively correlate when patients exhibit a lower intensity of bony edema on MRI.

Osteochondral autologous or allograft transplantation systems (OATS) are indicated in large primary lesions or failed secondary lesions [17, 36–39]. In the OATS procedure, the OLT is replaced with a single osteochondral plug or multiple plugs (mosaicplasty) with an intact hyaline cartilage surface. The graft can be harvested from the ipsilateral knee or from a fresh allograft talus. The advantages of this system include replacing the defect with hyaline cartilage rather than the formation of fibrocartilage with microfracture. Disadvantages, though, include an increase in donor site morbidity from an ipsilateral knee, healing of the host to graft interface, and the need for a malleolar osteotomy.

Favorable outcomes have also been reported with OATS, although most reports are retrospective studies. Hangody et al. reported a large case series of 1097 patients who received autologous osteochondral mosaicplasty, with 98 receiving the procedure in the talus [40]. Ninety-three percent of patients had good to excellent clinical results in the talus at a mean follow-up of 7 years.

Autologous chondrocyte implantation (ACI) is a two-stage procedure involving the transplantation of cultured chondrocytes into a defect and sealed with a periosteal patch. The first procedure harvests hyaline cartilage cells from the talus or the knee, while the second procedure involves injection of the cell suspension under a sutured periosteal flap harvested from the distal end of the tibia [41]. Recent advances to the technique include a procedure using matrix-induced ACI (MACI). This utilizes a porcine collagen membrane carrier for chondrocytes, which is injected into a defect and secured with fibrin glue. Reduced operative times, elimination of a periosteal patch, and an even distribution of cells are potential advantages of the MACI technique, although this is not available in the United States [42].

Particulated juvenile articular cartilage graft (DeNovo® NT Natural Tissue Graft, Zimmer, Warsaw, IN) is a new technique that was first published which is used in the patella in 2007 [43]. This novel product uses scaffold-free allogenic juvenile cartilage that can be implanted into a lesion with a fibrin sealant. The cartilage graft has shown the ability to migrate, multiply, and form new hyaline-like cartilage tissue matrix that integrates with the surrounding host tissue [44]. The largest study to date for use in the foot and ankle was published by Coetzee et al. and demonstrated 78% of patients with good to excellent functional results with an average postoperative AOFAS scores of 85 at mean follow-up of 16.2 months in patients with lesions greater than 125 mm^2 [45].

Management of Specific Complications

Failed Microfracture

Tol and colleagues provided one of the largest systematic reviews of osteochondral lesions of the talus [15]. They demonstrated an 85% success rate when excision, curettage, and drilling were performed on primary osteochondral lesions of the talus. However, when this technique fails, the surgeon is faced with a difficult situation for appropriate second-line treatment. A variety of reasons have been implicated for the failure of microfracture, including age, gender, size of the lesion, body mass index, location, the presence of subchondral cysts or marrow edema, and other intra-articular pathologies [35, 46]. A study that evaluated cartilage repair after microfracture by second-look arthroscopy revealed that 40% of lesions remained abnormal at 1 year postoperatively with incomplete healing [47]. However, this study did show that all patients had an improvement in clinical outcomes despite the arthroscopic findings at 1 year postoperative.

Surgical options for the symptomatic, failed microfracture patient include repeat marrow stimulation and microfracture technique, cell transplanting, or direct grafting of the lesion. Savva et al. revealed that repeat arthroscopy and marrow stimulation with microfracture do lead to improved clinical results in 12 patients who failed a primary microfracture procedure [48]. One recent study also demonstrated an improvement in clinical outcomes in ten ankles that underwent an open osteochondral autograft procedure following a failed primary arthroscopic microfracture [49]. Additionally, Kreuz et al. found a significant clinical improvement in patients undergoing an osteochondral autograft mosaicplasty procedure to treat recurrent OCD lesions of the talus that previously underwent primary arthroscopic microfracture [50].

Moreover, a comparison study of osteochondral autograft transplant (OAT) to repeat arthroscopy and microfracture in patients with failed primary osteochondral lesions found clinical improvement with the OAT procedure [51]. These authors found that both repeat arthroscopy and OAT both give promising results early within the first year of follow-up; however, OAT was significantly superior to repeat arthroscopy and microfracture at long-term follow-up of 4 years. They also found that the size of osteochondral lesion affected the surgical outcome between the OAT procedure and repeat arthroscopy. Among patients with >150 mm^2 lesions, 25% resulted in failure for the OAT group, while 100% of patients exhibited clinical failure with repeat arthroscopy and microfracture with large lesions.

When large lesions (greater than 1.5 cm^2) are encountered in patients who have failed a primary microfracture surgery, fresh structural osteochondral bulk allografts can also be utilized. The benefit of this system provides a large surface area of intact hyaline cartilage with attached subchondral bone, the ability to match anatomic contour of the talus, and the avoidance of donor site morbidity in the knee. Recent studies have found encouraging patient outcomes when utilized for large talar defects, uncontained talar lesions, and large talar cysts and in revision patients who failed a primary arthroscopic microfracture procedure [52, 53].

Autologous chondrocyte implantation remains a viable option for a patient with a symptomatic, chronic osteochondral lesion of the talus. Since the introduction of ACI in 1994, the majority of literature has focused on chondral defects in the knee. Though, a recent meta-analysis for ACI use in the talus revealed a clinical success rate of 89% in 16 reviewed studies [54]. The mean defect size in the analysis was on considerably larger lesions of the talus at 2.3 cm^2. The majority of the included studies evaluated patients undergoing surgery for failed primary microfracture lesions. The data available suggests an improvement in patient outcomes can be achieved with the use of ACI as a second-line treatment option for patients with chronic pain following primary microfracture surgery. Consideration should be taken into account, however, with increased time and cost with the procedure.

Additional surgical options for patients with a failed primary arthroscopic microfracture technique include the use of particulated juvenile cartilage grafting. The largest study in the foot and ankle, performed by Coetzee et al., found a 78% success rate of good to excellent outcome scores in 24 ankles treated with particulated juvenile cartilage grafts in symptomatic osteochondral lesions, with 14 (58%) of the ankles having a previous arthroscopic bone marrow stimulation procedure performed [45].

Biological adjuncts, such as platelet-rich plasma and bone marrow aspirate concentrate, have also been investigated to improve cartilage regeneration for osteochondral lesions of the talus [55]. Early studies with biological augmentation are promising because they exhibit high chromogenic activity as well as display anti-inflammatory properties that may improve poor cartilage healing in a patient with an osteochondral lesion with a failed primary microfracture procedure. An equine model demonstrated the benefit of performing microfracture with the use of concentrated bone marrow aspirate for the treatment of full-thickness cartilage defects [56]. They found an increased filling of the defects and improved integration of repair tissue into surrounding native cartilage when concentrated bone marrow aspirate was used compared to microfracture alone. Additionally, a greater amount of type II collagen content and a significant increase in the amount of glycosaminoglycan were found in lesions treated with bone marrow aspirate.

Case Reports

A 43-year-old male presented with chronic ankle pain over 1 year postoperatively following an arthroscopic microfracture procedure for a medial osteochondral lesion measuring approximately 10 mm in diameter at the initial surgery. After failing previous microfracture surgery and continuing to have pain with activities, a second surgery was planned. Repeat arthroscopy demonstrated an unhealed osteochondral lesion of the medial talus with a loose piece of cartilage present overlying the lesion (Fig. 26.1). Repeat arthroscopic microfracture was performed; however, additional grafting with particulated juvenile hyaline cartilage graft and bone marrow aspirate from the ipsilateral calcaneus were also utilized with success (Figs. 26.2 and 26.3).

A 50-year-old male presented with a large, chronic osteochondral lesion of the talus measuring over 2.5 cm^2 in posteromedial aspect of his talus. He had also failed a microfracture procedure over 5 years prior. Due to the chronicity and size of

Fig. 26.1 Repeat arthroscopy demonstrating an unhealed osteochondral lesion of the talus following primary microfracture procedure over 1 year prior

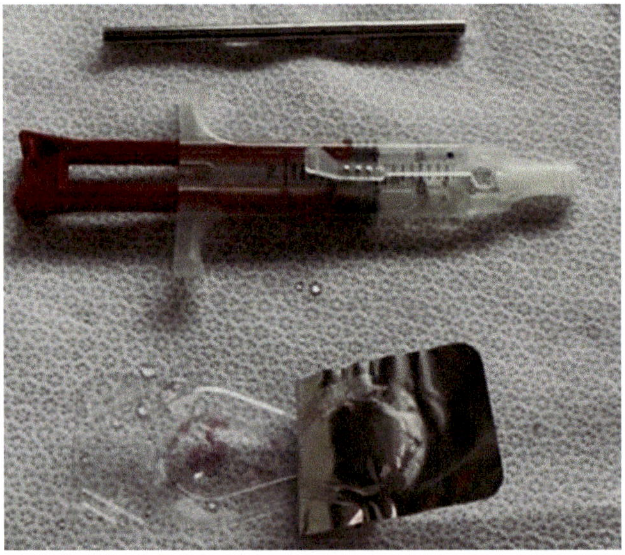

Fig. 26.2 Particulate juvenile hyaline cartilage graft with a fibrin glue and an arthroscopic cannula for delivery of graft

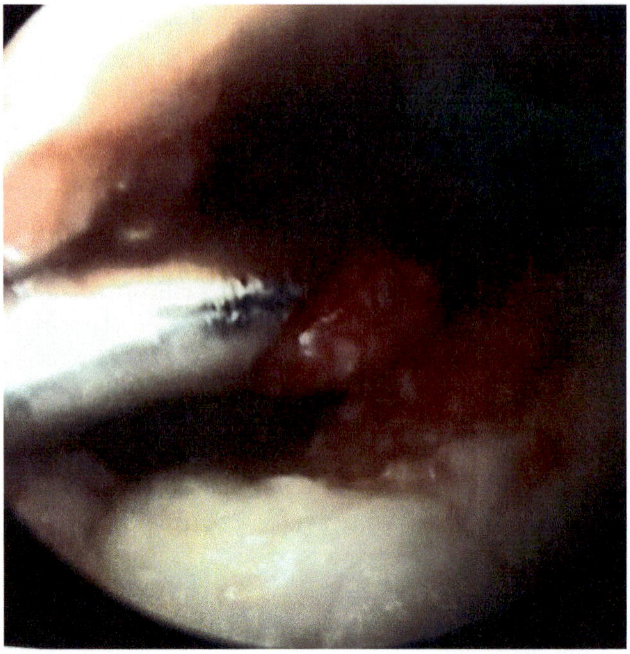

Fig. 26.3 Repeat arthroscopy and microfracture with additional grafting with particulated juvenile graft and bone marrow aspirate

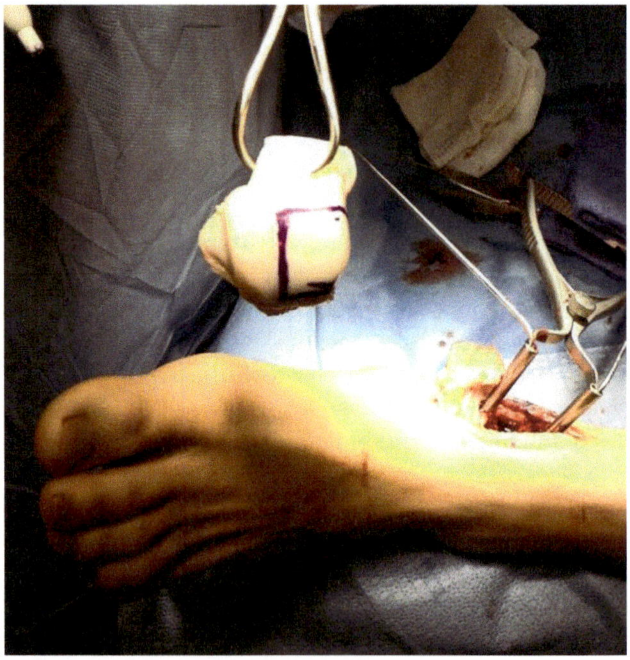

Fig. 26.4 Fresh structural osteochondral allograft transfer for a chronic and failed lesion of the talus

his lesion, the decision was made to perform an open debridement and grafting with fresh osteochondral allograft talus (Fig. 26.4). A chevron-shaped malleolar osteotomy was performed, and a fresh donor-matched bulk allograft talus was transferred and fixated with bio-absorbable pins (Fig. 26.5).

Osteochondral Autograft and Allograft Failure

Osteochondral autograft and allograft procedures raise concern over the viability of the transplanted cartilage and the ability to incorporate a large graft-host bone interface. A considerable risk of graft collapse, graft resorption, and joint space narrowing exists when performing these procedures. If this procedure fails, chronic pain and debilitation leave both the surgeon and patient with few options for salvage. Surgical reconstruction options for an osteochondral autograft or allograft failure include conversion to a total ankle replacement, ankle arthrodesis, or bipolar total ankle allograft.

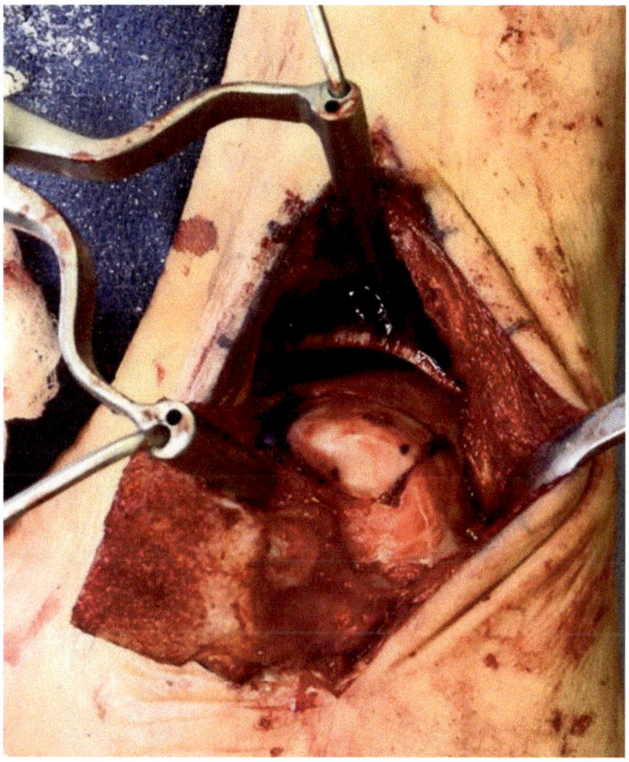

Fig. 26.5 Final placement of the fresh structural osteochondral allograft

When autograft and allograft transfer procedures are performed, long-term monitoring of the graft should be employed. Gross et al. reported a case series of nine patients who underwent fresh talar osteochondral allograft transplantation with a mean follow-up of 11 years [57]. Three of the nine grafts demonstrated radiographic evidence of fragmentation and resorption of over 50% of the graft with secondary osteoarthritic changes at an average of 58.3 months postoperatively. The three patients with graft failure required conversion to an ankle arthrodesis.

In 2009, Raikin reported his results on 15 patients who underwent bulk fresh osteochondral allograft transplantation for cystic talar defects [58]. Two of fifteen patients required ankle arthrodesis procedures following graft resorption and joint space narrowing at 32 and 76 months postoperatively.

Additionally, Adams et al. reported midterm results on talar shoulder lesions treated with fresh osteochondral allograft transplantation in eight patients [52]. They observed radiographic lucency at the interface of the allograft and host bone in five of the eight patients at an average follow-up of 2 years. No patients, however, were converted to an ankle arthrodesis, but one required two arthroscopic debridement surgeries. They also concluded that long-term monitoring of the grafts is required, and perhaps the radiographic lucency seen in their patients was due to early resorption.

Lastly, El-Rashidy et al. found graft failure in four of forty-two patients who underwent fresh osteochondral allograft transplantation for chronic talar lesions with an average follow-up of 37.7 months [59]. This resulted in two patients undergoing total ankle replacement, one ankle arthrodesis, and one bipolar total ankle allograft.

Malleolar Complications

Open exposure of the talus requires the use of a medial malleolar osteotomy or anterior plafond bone block. The medial malleolus typically heals well with a low incidence of nonunion; however, care must be taken to place the osteotomy in the correct position with protection of the adjacent neurovascular structures and tendons. Kim et al. revealed decreased patient outcomes on second-look arthroscopy when the tibial plafond at the malleolar osteotomy site was uneven [49]. Alternatively, an anterior access bone block window may be utilized; however, this limits the access to posterior talar lesions [60]. If a malleolar nonunion or malunion is encountered, revision surgery with anatomic alignment and bone grafting is often necessary. In these cases, additional medial anti-glide plate should also be employed for added stability.

Technique Pearls and Pitfalls to Avoid Complications

Debridement and microfracture of an OLT is a successful procedure; however, intraoperative technique may play a role in obtaining a favorable result. Enhanced arthroscopic equipment and instrumentation allow the talar dome to have increased visualization. At our institution, general inhalation anesthesia with a regional nerve block and a thigh tourniquet is used routinely. Noninvasive ankle distraction is also utilized for easy arthroscopic access to accomplish a proper microfracture technique (Fig. 26.6). Additionally, a cystoscopy thigh holder allows the ankle to be suspended for easy use with distraction (Fig. 26.7). Standard anteromedial and anterolateral portals are utilized with a 2.7- or 4.0-mm diameter and 30° or 70° arthroscope. Plantarflexion aids in exposure of posterior lesions; however, this maneuver requires caution to avoid damaging the branches of the superficial peroneal nerve. In cases with extreme posterior lesions, a posterolateral accessory portal can also be used. For most medial-based talar dome lesions, the arthroscope and inflow enter through the anterolateral portal, while the instrumentation for debridement is through the anteromedial portal. Lateral talar dome lesions are best approached with the arthroscope and camera in the anteromedial portal with instrumentation through the anterolateral portal. Instruments available to debride osteochondral lesions include blunt-tipped probes, pituitary graspers, gouges, full-radius shavers, ring curettes, and high-speed burrs (Fig. 26.8). Appropriate angled microfracture chondral awls or Kirschner wires should be used to ensure a stable drill is performed with the proper depth (Fig. 26.9). The surgeon should also be sure not to skive off the talus and cause damage to healthy cartilage with the chondral awl. Multiple drill holes of the talar lesion should be performed with a minimum of 3- to 4-mm intervals [61]. Additionally, the inflow pump can be reduced in order to visualize fat droplets and blood return out of microfracture holes to ensure adequate depth into the subchondral bone has been reached with the awl (Fig. 26.10).

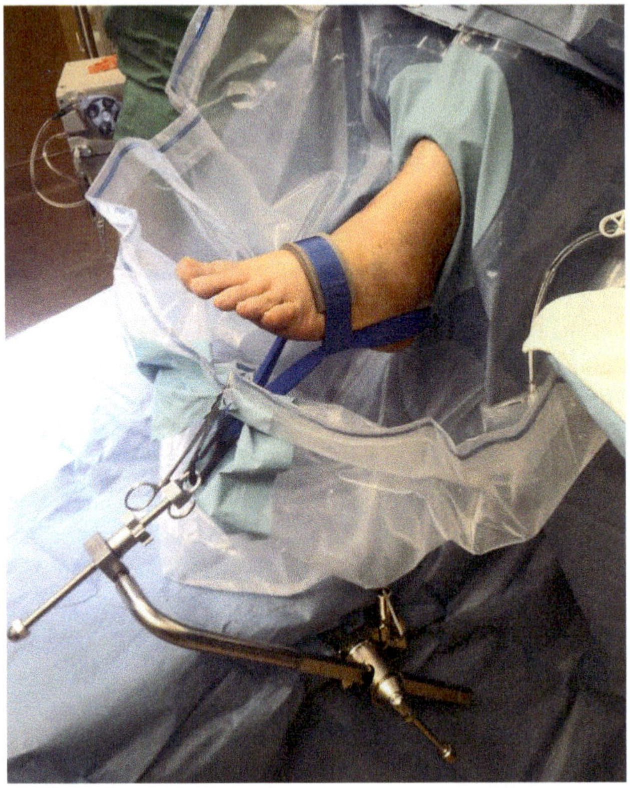

Fig. 26.6 Noninvasive ankle distraction utilized for easy access into the ankle portals

If a cystic talar dome lesion with an intact cartilage surface is encountered during arthroscopy, then retrograde or trans-talar drilling can be performed to enable revascularization of the fragment (Fig. 26.11) [22]. The primary aim is to induce subchondral bone revascularization and subsequently develop new bone formation to fill the cyst [17]. If needed, a cancellous graft can also be used to fill defects. Posteromedial lesions are accessed through a sinus tarsi approach into the talus, while lateral lesions are approached from the anteromedial to the cyst. Fluoroscopic guidance should be utilized to ensure proper localization of the cyst.

When large posterior and medial lesions are encountered, open treatment with a malleolar osteotomy should be performed. Osteotomies of the medial malleolus have been previously described using an oblique, step cut, crescentic, or chevron shape [4, 62–65]. The author's preferred technique for increased exposure of the medial talar dome is the biplane chevron-shaped medial malleolus osteotomy (Fig. 26.12). The chevron-shaped cut is inherently stable when compared to the oblique or transverse osteotomies. A sagittal saw is used to

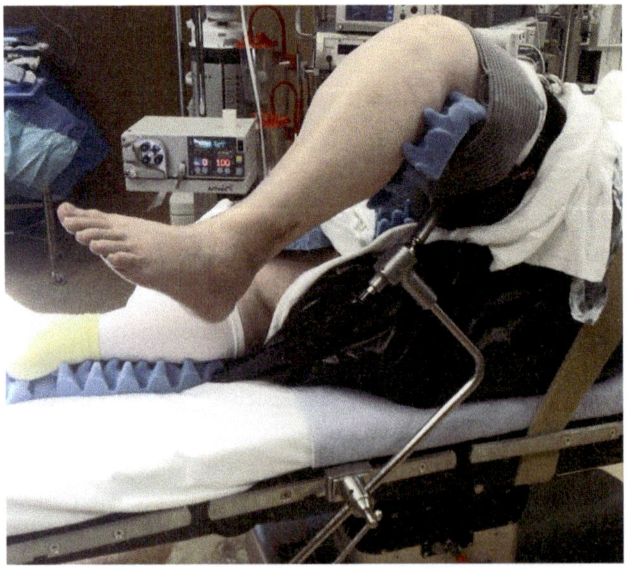

Fig. 26.7 Cystoscopy thigh holder used to suspend the leg and allow the ankle to be placed in a noninvasive distractor

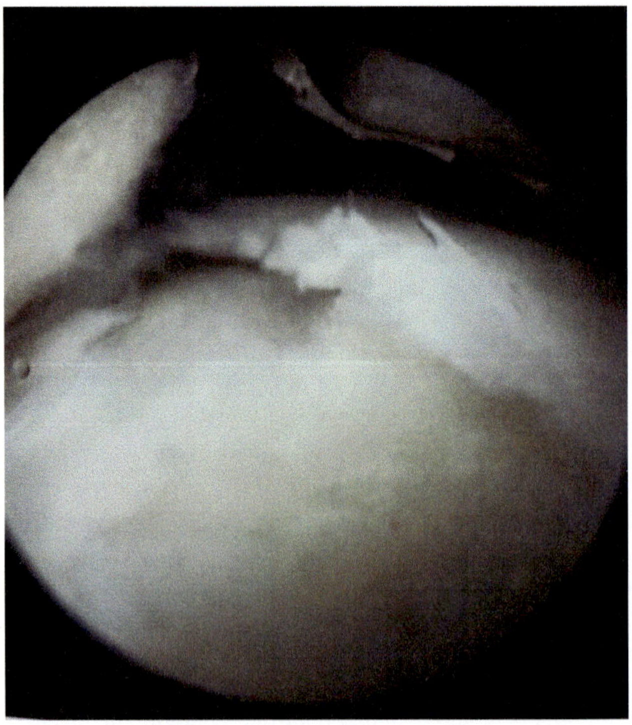

Fig. 26.8 Arthroscopic view of a shaver utilized for debridement to a stable border of an osteochondral lesion of the talus

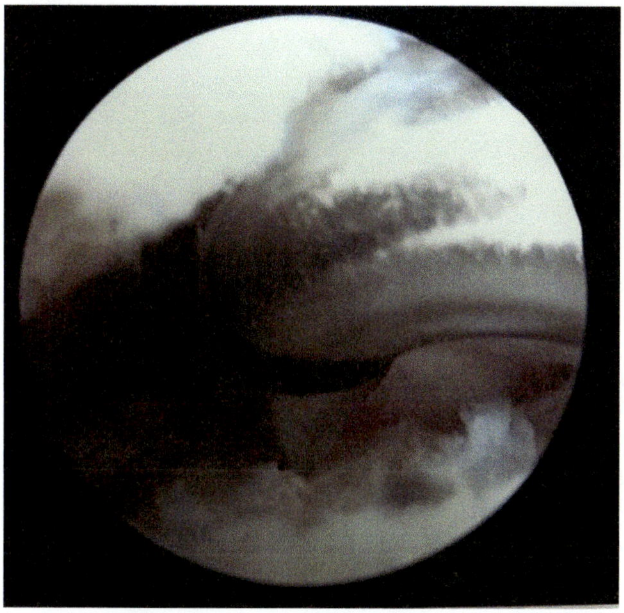

Fig. 26.9 Arthroscopic awl utilized to perform microfracture to an appropriate depth

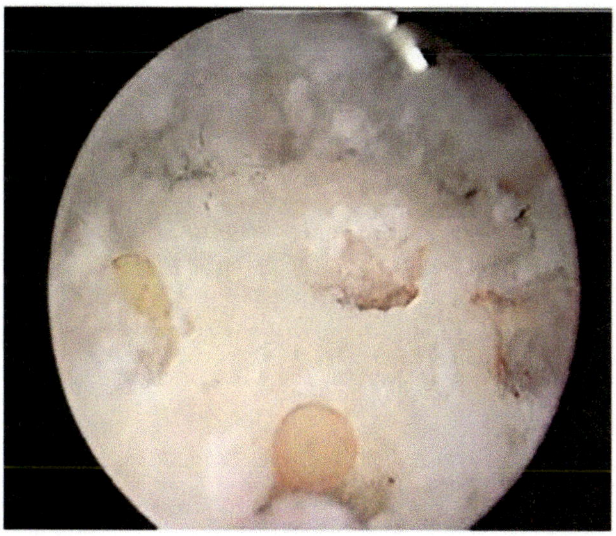

Fig. 26.10 Arthroscopic view of microfracture technique with fat droplets present to confirm adequate depth has been reached into the talus

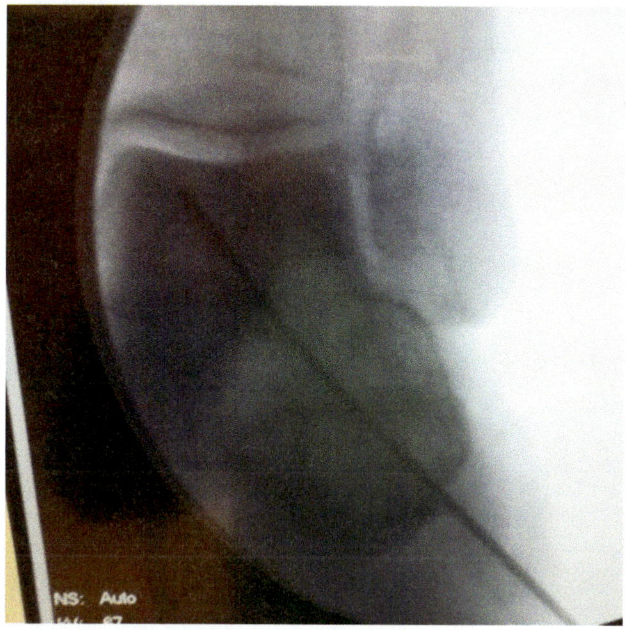

Fig. 26.11 Retrograde drilling from the sinus tarsi to a posterior medial cystic lesion in the talus with the use of intraoperative fluoroscopy

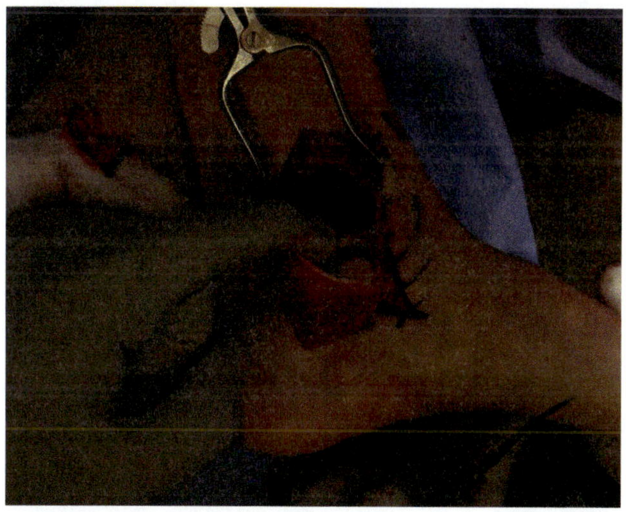

Fig. 26.12 Chevron-shaped medial malleolar osteotomy is performed for access to the complete medial aspect of the talus

initiate the osteotomy with the apex inverted V proximal in the midline of the tibia. The angle of the saw blade will allow for a larger or smaller amount of exposure to the talus. Once the saw meets resistance to the cortex, the osteotomy should be completed with an osteotome to create greater interdigitation between the fragments while also protecting the tibia plafond from damage with the saw (Fig. 26.13). Extra care should be taken to avoid damage to the articular surface of the tibial plafond as this can lead to inferior clinical outcomes. If additional exposure is needed after performing the medial malleolar osteotomy, a pin-based distractor can also be utilized to aid in visualization (Fig. 26.14). Fixation should be performed with two lag screws, although with larger osteotomies, a medial anti-glide plate can also be utilized for added rigidity (Figs. 26.15 and 26.16). Pre-drilling for the path of the screws in the malleolus is often recommended prior to cutting the osteotomy to easily reduce and fixate the fragment at the end of the procedure. It is also imperative to achieve precise anatomic reduction and fixation of the osteotomy to avoid a nonunion or malunion.

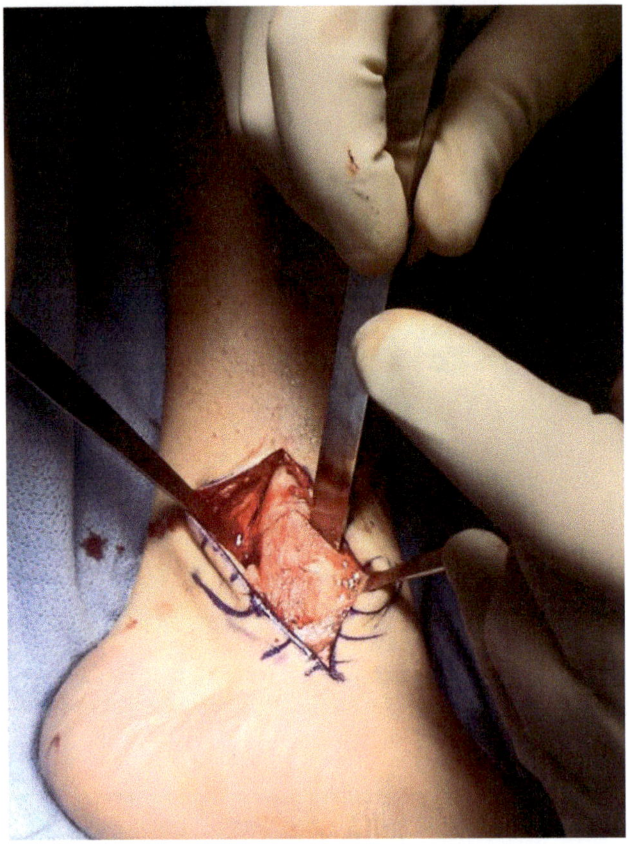

Fig. 26.13 An osteotome is utilized for the completion of the osteotomy in order to protect the articular cartilage in the ankle joint

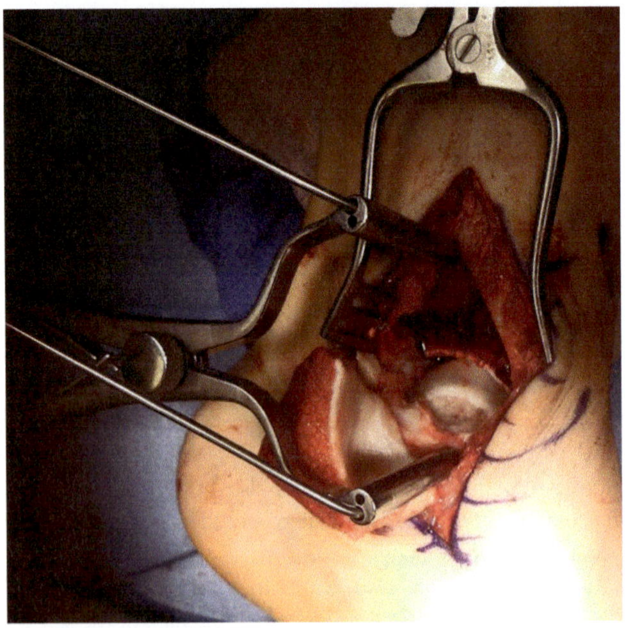

Fig. 26.14 A pin-based distractor utilized to increase visualization and exposure of the medial talus following a chevron osteotomy of the malleolus

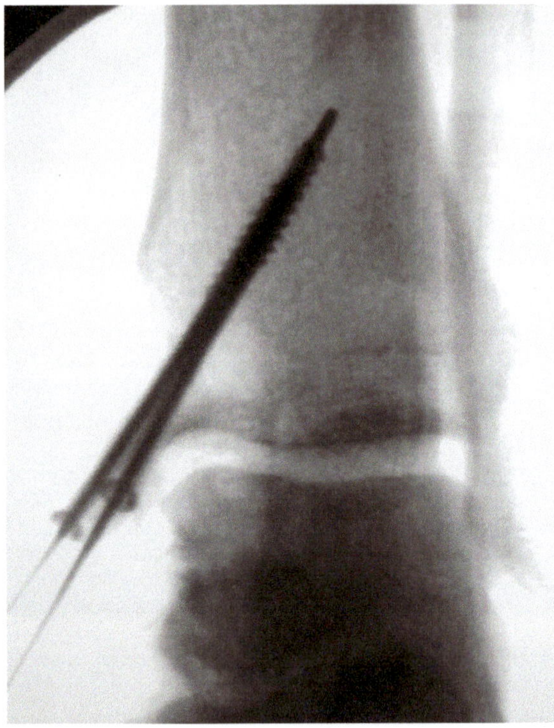

Fig. 26.15 Two-screw fixation following a chevron malleolar osteotomy with anatomic reduction of the articular plafond

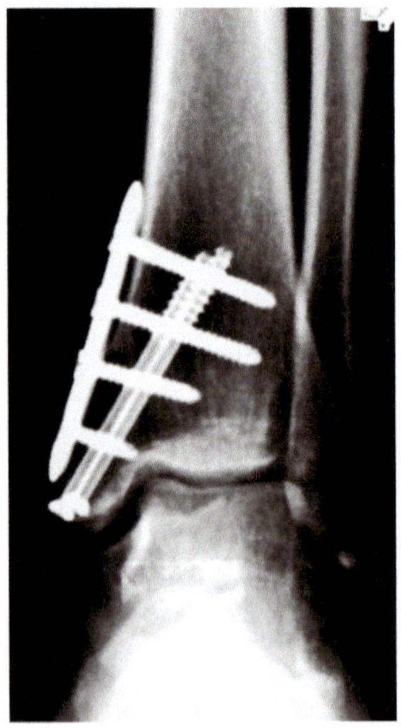

Fig. 26.16 Medial malleolar osteotomy fixated with both lag screws and anti-glide plate for added rigidity

When performing osteochondral autograft and allograft procedures, several factors may affect the outcome. When using cylindrical plugs to fill a defect, it is important to carefully match the size and shape of the graft to the corresponding defect in order to minimize the amount of fibrocartilage that forms around the grafted hyaline cartilage plug. Additionally, when using multiple plugs to fill a defect, the surgeon should take care to match both the height of each cylindrical graft and the height of the graft to the corresponding native cartilage border, in order to achieve a smooth surface.

Conclusions

Surgical treatment methods for osteochondral lesions of the talus continue to evolve as newer grafting technology is incorporated. The method for primary and revision osteochondral lesions also remains a controversial topic. Depending on patient age, activity, and size of the lesion, arthroscopic marrow stimulation techniques with microfracture are generally accepted as first-line treatment. Osteochondral autograft and allograft procedures, cellular grafting with hyaline cartilage, and biologic adjuncts should be considered carefully as second-line therapy in those patients who have failed a primary arthroscopic microfracture procedure. Future comparison studies are needed to substantiate the clinical guidelines for treatment of failed osteochondral lesions. Controversies will also continue to revolve around reducing patient morbidity and decreasing the cost of cellular grafts as healthcare changes.

References

1. Kappis M. Weitere beitrage zur traumatisch-mechanischen entstehung der "spontanen" knorpela biosungen. Dtsch Z Chir. 1922;171:13–29.
2. Alexander AH, Lichtman DM. Surgical treatment of transchondral talar-dome fractures (osteochondritis dissecans). Long-term follow-up. J Bone Joint Surg Am. 1980;62(4):646–52.
3. Hintermann B, Regazzoni P, Lampert C, Stutz G, Gachter A. Arthroscopic findings in acute fractures of the ankle. J Bone Joint Surg Br. 2000;82(3):345–51.
4. Flick AB, Gould N. Osteochondritis dissecans of the talus (transchondral fractures of the talus): review of the literature and new surgical approach for medial dome lesions. Foot Ankle. 1985;5(4):165–85.
5. O'Loughlin PF, Heyworth BE, Kennedy JG. Current concepts in the diagnosis and treatment of osteochondral lesions of the ankle. Am J Sports Med. 2010;38(2):392–404.
6. Gardiner TB. Osteochondritis dissecans in three members of one family. J Bone Joint Surg Br. 1955;37-B(1):139–41.
7. Laffenetre O. Osteochondral lesions of the talus: current concept. Orthop Traumatol Surg Res. 2010;96(5):554–66.
8. Hannon CP, Smyth NA, Murawski CD, Savage-Elliott I, Deyer TW, Calder JD, et al. Osteochondral lesions of the talus: aspects of current management. Bone Joint J. 2014;96-B(2):164–71.
9. Berndt AL, Harty M. Transchondral fractures (osteochondritis dissecans) of the talus. J Bone Joint Surg Am. 1959;41-A:988–1020.
10. Cheng MS, Ferkel RD, Applegate GR. Osteochondral lesion of the talus: a radiologic and surgical comparison. Annual meeting of the academy of orthopaedic surgeons. New Orleans, LAL; 1995.
11. Lee KB, Bai LB, Park JG, Yoon TR. A comparison of arthroscopic and MRI findings in staging of osteochondral lesions of the talus. Knee Surg Sports Traumatol Arthrosc. 2008;16(11):1047–51.
12. Ferkel RD. Articular surface defects, loose bodies, and osteophytes. Arthroscopic Surgery: the foot and ankle. Philadelphia, PA: Lippincott-Raven; 1996. p. 145.
13. Hepple S, Winson IG, Glew D. Osteochondral lesions of the talus: a revised classification. Foot Ankle Int. 1999;20(12):789–93.
14. Fallat LM, Christensen JC, Hord JA. Osteochondroses of the foot and ankle. In: Southerland JT, Boberg JS, Downey MS, Nakra A, Rabjohn LV, editors. McGlamry's comprehensive textbook of foot and ankle surgery. 4th ed. Philadelphia: Wolters Kluwer Health, Lippincott Williams and Wilkins; 2013. p. 780–800.
15. Tol JL, Struijs PA, Bossuyt PM, Verhagen RA, van Dijk CN. Treatment strategies in osteochondral defects of the talar dome: a systematic review. Foot Ankle Int. 2000;21(2):119–26.
16. Navid DO, Myerson MS. Approach alternatives for treatment of osteochondral lesions of the talus. Foot Ankle Clin. 2002;7(3):635–49.
17. Zengerink M, Struijs PA, Tol JL, van Dijk CN. Treatment of osteochondral lesions of the talus: a systematic review. Knee Surg Sports Traumatol Arthrosc. 2010;18(2):238–46.
18. Choi WJ, Park KK, Kim BS, Lee JW. Osteochondral lesion of the talus: is there a critical defect size for poor outcome? Am J Sports Med. 2009;37(10):1974–80.
19. Lahm A, Erggelet C, Steinwachs M, Reichelt A. Arthroscopic management of osteochondral lesions of the talus: results of drilling and usefulness of magnetic resonance imaging before and after treatment. Arthroscopy. 2000;16(3):299–304.
20. Chuckpaiwong B, Berkson EM, Theodore GH. Microfracture for osteochondral lesions of the ankle: outcome analysis and outcome predictors of 105 cases. Arthroscopy. 2008;24(1):106–12.
21. Choi WJ, Kim BS, Lee JW. Osteochondral lesion of the talus: could age be an indication for arthroscopic treatment? Am J Sports Med. 2012;40(2):419–24.
22. Ferkel RD, Zanotti RM, Komenda GA, Sgaglione NA, Cheng MS, Applegate GR, et al. Arthroscopic treatment of chronic osteochondral lesions of the talus: long-term results. Am J Sports Med. 2008;36(9):1750–62.
23. Murawski CD, Foo LF, Kennedy JG. A review of arthroscopic bone marrow stimulation techniques of the talus: the good, the bad, and the causes for concern. Cartilage. 2010;22:137–44.
24. van Bergen CJ, de Leeuw PA, van Dijk CN. Treatment of osteochondral defects of the talus. Rev Chir Orthop Reparatrice Appar Mot. 2008;94(8 Suppl):398–408.
25. Mankin HJ. The response of articular cartilage to mechanical injury. J Bone Joint Surg Am. 1982;64(3):460–6.
26. Alford JW, Cole BJ. Cartilage restoration, part 1: basic science, historical perspective, patient evaluation, and treatment options. Am J Sports Med. 2005;33(2):295–306.
27. Furukawa T, Eyre DR, Koide S, Glimcher MJ. Biochemical studies on repair cartilage resurfacing experimental defects in the rabbit knee. J Bone Joint Surg Am. 1980;62(1):79–89.
28. Barnes CJ, Ferkel RD. Arthroscopic debridement and drilling of osteochondral lesions of the talus. Foot Ankle Clin. 2003;8(2):243–57.
29. Becher C, Thermann H. Results of microfracture in the treatment of articular cartilage defects of the talus. Foot Ankle Int. 2005;26(8):583–9.
30. Han SH, Lee JW, Lee DY, Kang ES. Radiographic changes and clinical results of osteochondral defects of the talus with and without subchondral cysts. Foot Ankle Int. 2006;27(12):1109–14.

31. Kono M, Takao M, Naito K, Uchio Y, Ochi M. Retrograde drilling for osteochondral lesions of the talar dome. Am J Sports Med. 2006;34(9):1450–6.
32. Kumai T, Takakura Y, Higashiyama I, Tamai S. Arthroscopic drilling for the treatment of osteochondral lesions of the talus. J Bone Joint Surg Am. 1999;81(9):1229–35.
33. Robinson DE, Winson IG, Harries WJ, Kelly AJ. Arthroscopic treatment of osteochondral lesions of the talus. J Bone Joint Surg Br. 2003;85(7):989–93.
34. Schuman L, Struijs PA, van Dijk CN. Arthroscopic treatment for osteochondral defects of the talus. Results at follow-up at 2 to 11 years. J Bone Joint Surg Br. 2002;84(3):364–8.
35. Deol PP, Cuttica DJ, Smith WB, Berlet GC. Osteochondral lesions of the talus: size, age, and predictors of outcomes. Foot Ankle Clin. 2013;18(1):13–34.
36. Imhoff AB, Paul J, Ottinger B, Wortler K, Lammle L, Spang J, et al. Osteochondral transplantation of the talus: long-term clinical and magnetic resonance imaging evaluation. Am J Sports Med. 2011;39(7):1487–93.
37. Kennedy JG, Murawski CD. The treatment of osteochondral lesions of the talus with autologous osteochondral transplantation and bone marrow aspirate concentrate: surgical technique. Cartilage. 2011;2:327–36.
38. Scranton Jr PE, Frey CC, Feder KS. Outcome of osteochondral autograft transplantation for type-V cystic osteochondral lesions of the talus. J Bone Joint Surg Br. 2006;88(5):614–9.
39. Reddy S, Pedowitz DI, Parekh SG, Sennett BJ, Okereke E. The morbidity associated with osteochondral harvest from asymptomatic knees for the treatment of osteochondral lesions of the talus. Am J Sports Med. 2007;35(1):80–5.
40. Hangody L, Vasarhelyi G, Hangody LR, Sukosd Z, Tibay G, Bartha L, et al. Autologous osteochondral grafting—technique and long-term results. Injury. 2008;39(Suppl 1):S32–9.
41. Murawski CD, Kennedy JG. Operative treatment of osteochondral lesions of the talus. J Bone Joint Surg Am. 2013;95(11):1045–54.
42. Dickschas J, Welsch G, Strecker W, Schoffl V. Matrix-associated autologous chondrocyte transplantation combined with iliac crest bone graft for reconstruction of talus necrosis due to villonodular synovitis. J Foot Ankle Surg. 2012;51(1):87–90.
43. Bonner KF, Daner W, Yao JQ. 2-year postoperative evaluation of a patient with a symptomatic full-thickness patellar cartilage defect repaired with particulated juvenile cartilage tissue. J Knee Surg. 2010;23(2):109–14.
44. Cerrato R. Particulated juvenile articular cartilage allograft transplantation for osteochondral lesions of the talus. Foot Ankle Clin. 2013;18(1):79–87.
45. Coetzee JC, Giza E, Schon LC, Berlet GC, Neufeld S, Stone RM, et al. Treatment of osteochondral lesions of the talus with particulated juvenile cartilage. Foot Ankle Int. 2013;34(9):1205–11.
46. Cuttica DJ, Shockley JA, Hyer CF, Berlet GC. Correlation of MRI edema and clinical outcomes following microfracture of osteochondral lesions of the talus. Foot Ankle Spec. 2011;4(5):274–9.
47. Lee KB, Bai LB, Yoon TR, Jung ST, Seon JK. Second-look arthroscopic findings and clinical outcomes after microfracture for osteochondral lesions of the talus. Am J Sports Med. 2009;37(Suppl 1):63S–70S.
48. Savva N, Jabur M, Davies M, Saxby T. Osteochondral lesions of the talus: results of repeat arthroscopic debridement. Foot Ankle Int. 2007;28(6):669–73.
49. Kim YS, Park EH, Kim YC, Koh YG, Lee JW. Factors associated with the clinical outcomes of the osteochondral autograft transfer system in osteochondral lesions of the talus: second-look arthroscopic evaluation. Am J Sports Med. 2012;40(12):2709–19.
50. Kreuz PC, Steinwachs M, Erggelet C, Lahm A, Henle P, Niemeyer P. Mosaicplasty with autogenous talar autograft for osteochondral lesions of the talus after failed primary arthroscopic management: a prospective study with a 4-year follow-up. Am J Sports Med. 2006;34(1):55–63.
51. Yoon HS, Park YJ, Lee M, Choi WJ, Lee JW. Osteochondral autologous transplantation is superior to repeat arthroscopy for the treatment of osteochondral lesions of the talus after failed primary arthroscopic treatment. Am J Sports Med. 2014;42(8):1896–903.
52. Adams SB, Jr., Viens NA, Easley ME, Stinnett SS, Nunley JA, 2nd. Midterm results of osteochondral lesions of the talar shoulder treated with fresh osteochondral allograft transplantation. J Bone Joint Surg Am 2011;93(7):648–654.
53. Haene R, Qamirani E, Story RA, Pinsker E, Daniels TR. Intermediate outcomes of fresh talar osteochondral allografts for treatment of large osteochondral lesions of the talus. J Bone Joint Surg Am. 2012;94(12):1105–10.
54. Niemeyer P, Salzmann G, Schmal H, Mayr H, Sudkamp NP. Autologous chondrocyte implantation for the treatment of chondral and osteochondral defects of the talus: a meta-analysis of available evidence. Knee Surg Sports Traumatol Arthrosc. 2012;20(9):1696–703.
55. Smyth NA, Murawski CD, Haleem AM, Hannon CP, Savage-Elliott I, Kennedy JG. Establishing proof of concept: Platelet-rich plasma and bone marrow aspirate concentrate may improve cartilage repair following surgical treatment for osteochondral lesions of the talus. World J Orthod. 2012;3(7):101–8.
56. Fortier LA, Potter HG, Rickey EJ, Schnabel LV, Foo LF, Chong LR, et al. Concentrated bone marrow aspirate improves full-thickness cartilage repair compared with microfracture in the equine model. J Bone Joint Surg Am. 2010;92(10):1927–37.
57. Gross AE, Agnidis Z, Hutchison CR. Osteochondral defects of the talus treated with fresh osteochondral allograft transplantation. Foot Ankle Int. 2001;22(5):385–91.
58. Raikin SM. Fresh osteochondral allografts for large-volume cystic osteochondral defects of the talus. J Bone Joint Surg Am. 2009;91(12):2818–26.
59. El-Rashidy H, Villacis D, Omar I, Kelikian AS. Fresh osteochondral allograft for the treatment of cartilage defects of the talus: a retrospective review. J Bone Joint Surg Am. 2011;93(17):1634–40.
60. Sammarco GJ, Makwana NK. Treatment of talar osteochondral lesions using local osteochondral graft. Foot Ankle Int. 2002;23(8):693–8.
61. Steadman JR, Rodkey WG, Rodrigo JJ. Microfracture: surgical technique and rehabilitation to treat chondral defects. Clin Orthop Relat Res. 2001;391(Suppl):S362–9.
62. Alexander IJ, Watson JT. Step-cut osteotomy of the medial malleolus for exposure of the medial ankle joint space. Foot Ankle. 1991;11(4):242–3.
63. Wallen EA, Fallat LM. Crescentic transmalleolar osteotomy for optimal exposure of the medial talar dome. J Foot Surg. 1989;28(5):389–94.
64. Mendicino RW, Lee MS, Grossman JP, Shromoff PJ. Oblique medial malleolar osteotomy for the management of talar dome lesions. J Foot Ankle Surg. 1998;37(6):516–23.
65. Granata JD, DeCarbo WT, Hyer CF, Granata AM, Berlet GC. Exposure of the medial talar dome: bi-plane chevron medial malleolus osteotomy. Foot Ankle Spec. 2013;6(1):12–4.

Ankle Stabilization

27

Sean T. Grambart

Introduction

Chronic lateral ankle instability has continued to increase its prevalence in the United States over the years as the patient population becomes more active. There are over two million ankle sprains reported in the United States every year. The prevalence is probably even higher as the majority of low-grade injuries are treated without the intervention of a healthcare provider. It is the moderate- to high-grade injuries that are seen in the emergency room and in clinics around the country. Of these acute injuries, the majority, 80%, respond to conservative treatment. Conservative treatments consist of bracing, rehabilitation programs, rest, ice, compression, and elevation. Rehabilitation should focus on restoring proprioception and increasing inversion and eversion strength. Van Dijk did a review of different ankle supports and demonstrated that lace-up ankle braces were most effective in the subacute period after sprains [1]. Ankle braces have been shown to decrease severity and frequency of ankle sprains.

One of the biggest pitfalls in treating lateral ankle instability is the lack of a true definition. The authors' definition is the history of multiple ankle sprains that can occur on a flat surface. Stability of the ankle joint is provided by the bony congruity and syndesmotic ligaments, retinaculum, capsule, tendons, and collateral ligaments. The anterior talofibular ligament (ATFL), calcaneofibular ligament (CFL), and posterior talofibular ligament (PTFL) are the major ligamentous stabilizers of the ankle. The ATFL resists anterior ankle subluxation and inversion of the ankle when it is in a plantarflexed position. The CFL resists inversion with the ankle in neutral or dorsiflexed position. In cadaver studies the CFL requires 3.5% more load to failure than the ATFL [2–4]. The ATFL is the most commonly injured structure in an ankle during a sprain present 90% of the time. The CFL is involved 50–75% of the time. The PTFL is damaged in less than 10% of all ankle sprains [2–5].

An important item to remember is that instability by itself does not produce pain. Pain is a result of associated pathology. When pain is lateral along the fibula, the peroneal tendons should be evaluated. Ankle pain whether medial or lateral can be related to impingement syndromes, osteochondral defects, or arthritic conditions. The patient population that does not respond to conservative treatment with persistent pain and complaints of instability requires further evaluation, and possible intervention is necessary.

Indications for Procedure

In patients with chronic lateral ankle instability, a thorough history and lower extremity physical examination are necessary. One of the more overlooked underlying pathologies is the presence of generalized ligamentous laxity or connective tissue disorders (i.e., Ehler–Danlos syndrome) that would make patients more susceptible to instability and poor candidates for certain procedures such as a primary repair of the ligaments since the tissue quality may be poor.

Overall, the alignment needs to be addressed at the same time as the ligament repair. Evaluation of a varus heel, plantar flexion of the first ray, and malalignment or tibia varum requires additional procedures. Coleman block test needs to be performed on the varus heel for accurate assessment. Peroneal weakness should be evaluated for tendon tears or ruptures and consideration of tendon transfer with a peroneus longus to brevis. Anterior draw and talar tilt assessments are performed. In the examination the practitioner should evaluate the contralateral limb as well for comparison. A talar tilt greater than 10° or greater than 5° compared to the contralateral is pathologic [2, 6–8]. Anterior translation of 1 cm or 5 mm greater than the contralateral side during the anterior drawer is also pathologic (Fig. 27.1). The authors recommend lateral ankle ligament stress next with the elimination of the

S.T. Grambart (✉)
Carle Physician Group, Champaign, IL 61821, USA
e-mail: sean.grambart@carle.com

M.S. Lee, J.P. Grossman (eds.), *Complications in Foot and Ankle Surgery*, DOI 10.1007/978-3-319-53686-6_27

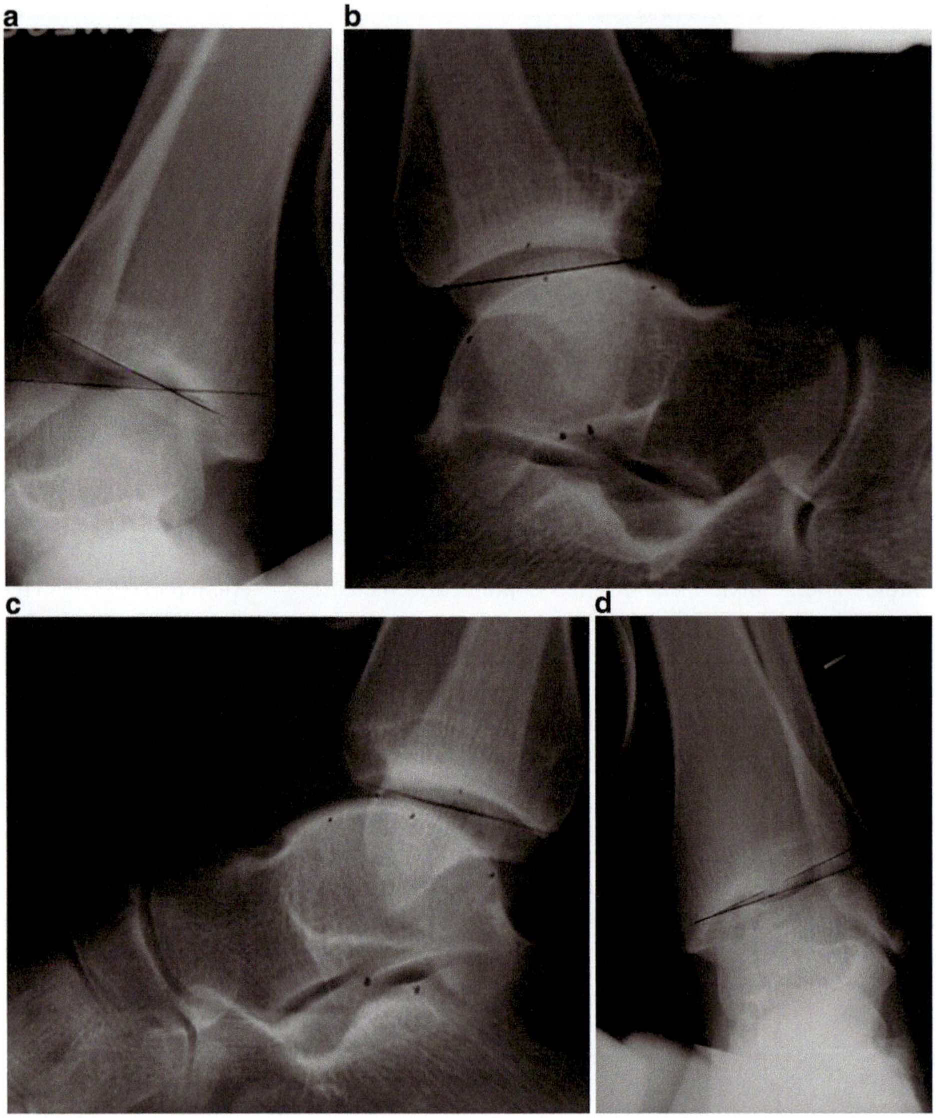

Fig. 27.1 Unstressed lateral radiograph. (**a**) Positive anterior drawer with stressed lateral radiograph showing anterior displacement of the talus on the tibia. (**b**) Unstressed AP radiograph of the ankle. (**c**) Stressed view with a positive talar tilt

pull of the peroneal tendons either through a block of the common peroneal nerve or sedation. In addition to a physical examine, standard AP and lateral radiographic evaluation is necessary for joint evaluation and positional changes.

Up to 93% of patients that suffer from chronic lateral ankle instability also have other secondary pathology such as osteochondral lesion, synovitis, or peroneal tendon pathology; therefore, an MRI can be beneficial in the workup of these patients [9]. Kibler et al. preformed 46 ankle arthroscopies prior to Brostrom procedures and found 83% had intra-articular problems, such as anterolateral soft tissue impingement, tibial talar spurring, meniscoid lesion, chondral injury, and loose bodies [9]. Digiovanni et al. found the most common corresponding pathology with chronic lateral ankle instability to be peroneal tenosynovitis, anterolateral impingement, and ankle synovitis [2]. Hu et al. found that 52.3–63.4% of patients underwent additional procedures along with the lateral ankle stabilization [7].

Indications for lateral ankle ligament reconstruction include inability to perform activities, failure of ankle bracing and therapy, and positive structural ligament rupture. Associated factors or pathology should be repaired at the same time as the ligament reconstruction.

Procedure Selection

More than 70 operative procedures have been described in the literature for treatment of chronic lateral ankle instability. These lateral ankle reconstructions can be broken down into anatomic and nonanatomic procedures. Anatomic procedures are further divided into primary repair (Brostrom) versus allograft or autograft reconstruction. Nonanatomic procedures involve tenodesis procedures with rerouting of a tendon (Watson-Jones). Anatomic procedures are beneficial because they restore as close as possible the normal anatomy and joint kinematics, as well as maintain ankle and subtalar joint range of motion. Unfortunately, primary anatomic reconstruction is not always a viable option due to poor tissue quality, and it relies on the ability to tension ligaments appropriately and the security of fixation. Anatomic reconstruction with a Brostrom procedure was first described in 1966 with repair of the anterior talofibular ligament [10–12]. Many modifications have been made to this procedure over the years, most notability the Gould modification in 1980 with the addition of repair of the calcaneofibular ligament and reinforcement with inferior extensor retinaculum [13]. The Brostrom procedure with Gould modification has become the standard for primary lateral ankle stabilization. In this technique the ATF and possibly CF ligaments are primarily repaired and reinforced with the inferior extensor retinaculum. When Brostrom first described the repair, it was a direct repair of the AFTL and CFL with imbrication of the ligaments to decrease any laxity from previous injury. The Gould modification with the reinforcement with the inferior retinaculum was adopted due to concerns of inadequate tissue quality. Multiple studies have found the Brostrom-Gould procedure to be extremely effective with good to excellent outcome in greater than 85% of patients [1, 4, 6, 8–17]. Nonanatomic repair consists of adding structural support to the ankle perpendicular to the perceived axis of instability. The first documented procedure of Watson-Jones in 1952 utilized the entire peroneus brevis tendon and routed in through the fibula from posterior to anterior and then secured in the tendon into the talar neck [18]. Multiple other nonanatomic repairs have been described utilizing allografts and autogenous grafts, most commonly the peroneus brevis tendon. These procedures should be reserved for patients with generalized ligamentous laxity and salvage procedures.

Hennrikus et al. compared anatomic to nonanatomic and found similar success rates around 85% but higher complication rate with nonanatomic, consisting of sural nerve damage, wound complications, stiffness, and residual instability [19]. Brostrom had no wound complications but did have superficial peroneal nerve paresthesias, stiffness, and one repeat rupture. Krips et al. reviewed 300 patients over 30-year follow-up and found initially no difference but nonanatomic correlated with increased rate of decreased function, increased pain, stiffness, increased reversional procedures, and increased arthritis [1].

Multiple exposure techniques have been described for the Brostrom-Gould procedure. The standard approach consists of an approximate 4 cm curvilinear incision over the distal anterior aspect of the fibula (Fig. 27.2). This incision can be utilized to visualize the course of the peroneal tendons extending anteriorly around the distal tip of the fibula. Dissection is taken down to the underlying inferior extensor retinaculum; during this part of the dissection, you may encounter a focal area of adipose tissue, especially in the female population. A moist sponge is helpful at this point to help with blunt dissection to identify the inferior retinaculum. The retinaculum should be seen parallel to the CFL and mobilize and reflect this layer (Fig. 27.3). The ATFL and CFL can be visualized at this time as thickened fibers of the capsule. Make a capsular incision along the anterior aspect of the fibula to the distal tip, leaving a few millimeters attached to the fibula to facilitate repair. Nonabsorbable suture 2-0 or larger is passed through the ATFL and CFL, and the foot and ankle are held in an everted valgus position while sutures are advanced (Fig. 27.4). The previously reflected inferior extensor retinaculum is sutured to the anterior edges of the fibula. Subcutaneous and cutaneous closure is done in standard fashion. Special care must be taken, and a good assistant is needed to maintain the foot in the everted valgus position during the remainder of the procedure and during cast or

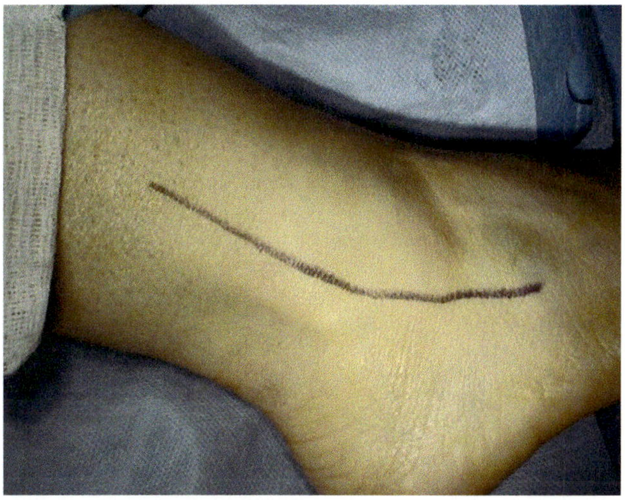

Fig. 27.2 Lateral linear incision for ligament reconstruction

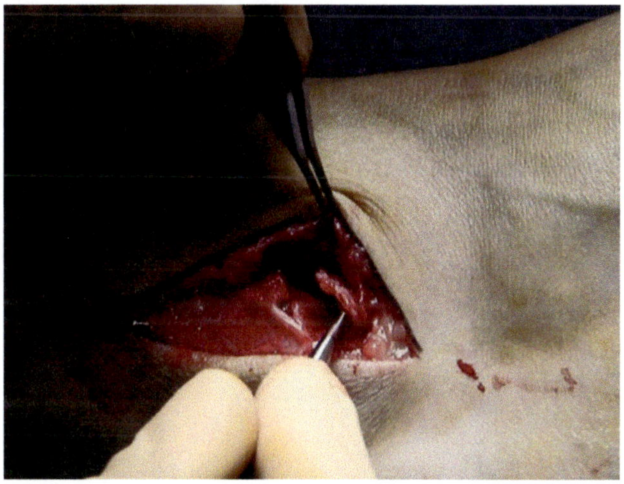

Fig. 27.3 Elevation of the retinaculum and the anterior talofibular ligament

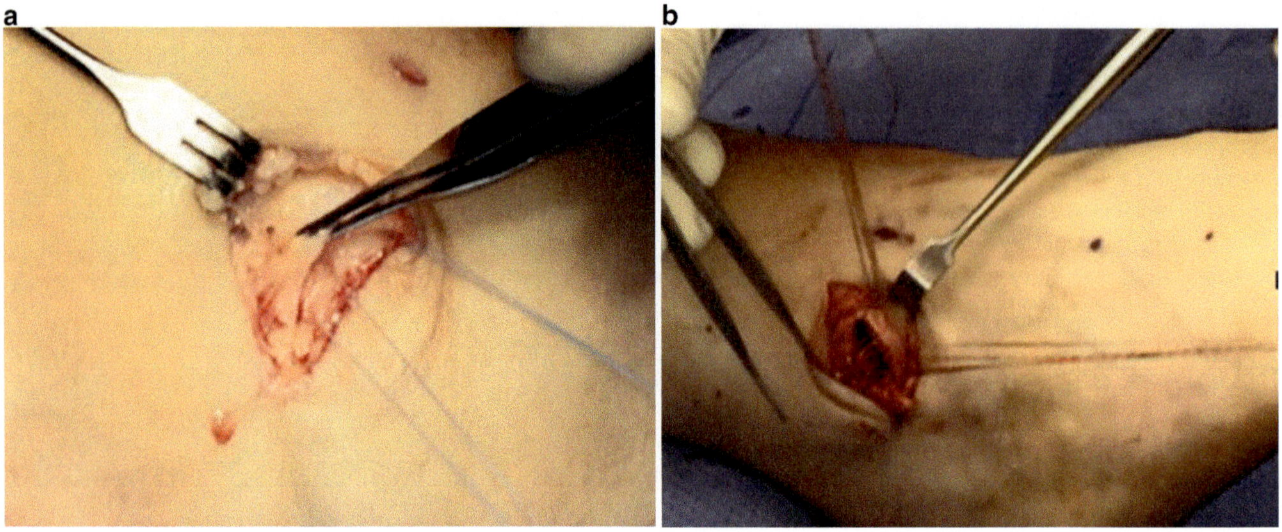

Fig. 27.4 (a) Nonabsorbable suture 2-0 or larger is passed through the ATFL and CFL, and the foot and ankle are held in an everted valgus position while sutures are placed

splint application. Standard protocol consists of non-weight bearing in cast for 6 weeks, but there is literature that supports accelerate rehabilitation protocol results in faster return to sport. Petrera et al. advocated immediate protective weight bearing in a walking boot and early range of motion to promote recovery of proprioception and decrease stiffness and muscle atrophy [4]. They found in their study a return to sport 3 weeks faster with accelerated rehabilitation protocol.

Complications of the Brostrom

As with any procedure, there is risk for complications which may occur intraoperatively, immediate postoperatively, and late onset. To help limit these complications, a thorough patient workup is necessary, and assessing other problems at the time of the procedure is imperative. The patients with long-standing instability, poor tissue quality, generalized ligamentous laxity, and structural deformity are patients that are more prone to complications. Superficial wound complications and neuritis are the most common complication which can occur in up to 7–19% of the cases [1–3, 8, 10–14, 19, 20]. In these cases meticulous surgical dissection and tissue handling are imperative. Overcorrection and undercorrection need to be taken into account, and a good assistant is beneficial to hold the foot in the corrected position during repair. Stiffness and overcorrection are common in both anatomic and nonanatomic repairs but more common in the nonanatomic group.

Recurrence and postoperative instability are normally secondary to acute injury. Petrera et al. reported a 6% failure rate with 3 out of 49 patients re-rupturing secondary to traumatic inversion ankle injuries during sporting events [4]. These patients were treated conservatively and did not require reversional surgery. If implementing an accelerated rehabilitation protocol, the patient should be protected in the initial postoperative period to help decrease risk of repeat traumatic rupture. In the case of a repeat rupture or undercorrection, salvage procedures with anatomic augmented tenodesis reconstructions are always a viable option for repair.

The first step in limiting complications is being familiar and acknowledging the contraindication and limitations of the different procedures. Limitations of these procedures start with patients with morbid obesity, previous documented arthritic changes of the subtalar or ankle joint, and subtalar joint inability and patients with collagen disorders. Contraindications consist of patients with progressive neuromuscular disorders, tarsal coalitions, and complex regional pain syndrome.

Techniques, Pearls, and Pitfalls

Most complications with the Brostrom procedure can be avoided during the preoperative assessment of the patient. When evaluating patients preoperatively, instead of looking at patient factors that would indicate a successful outcome, the authors prefer to evaluate patient factors that would lead to an unsuccessful outcome with a Brostrom. Does the patient have a large BMI, or do they have a job that requires a high amount of stress on the ankle? Do they have a varus position of their heel, a cavus foot, or have weakness of the peroneal muscles? One of the more often overlooked issues is recognizing patients with hypermobility syndromes such as Ehlers–Danlos syndrome (Fig. 27.5). These types of conditions often have poor tissue quality that will require surgical augmentation in order to be successful. If the answers to these questions are negative, then the success rate of a Brostrom procedure is high.

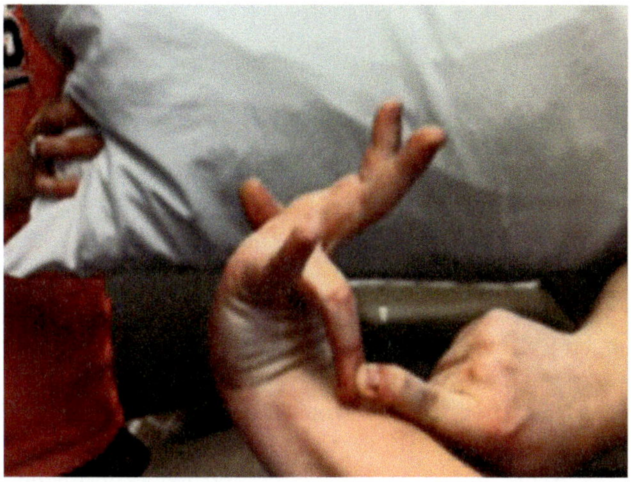

Fig. 27.5 Example of recognizing patients with hypermobility syndromes such as Ehlers–Danlos syndrome

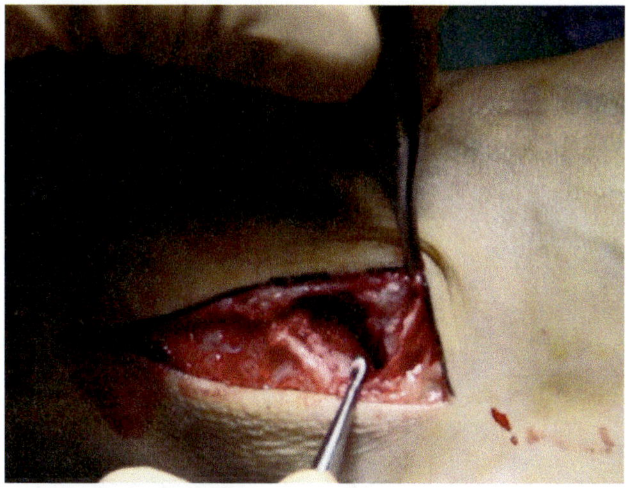

Fig. 27.6 Curettage of the periosteum around the attachment site of the ATF ligament

On physical examination, make sure that pathologic joints have been identified. Radiographic stress exam can be utilized. To improve accuracy of the stress exam, eliminate the tension on the peroneal tendons either through use of sedation or local anesthetic. Also, pay attension to any instability of the subtalar joint during the exam. Intra-articular injections of the ankle serve as a strong diagnostic tool. Evaluate both the ankle joint and subtalar joint for arthritic conditions.

As previously mentioned, there is a high correlation between chronic lateral ankle instability and intra-articular pathology, and the addition of ankle arthroscopy is often beneficial. If an arthroscopic procedure is scheduled, it is a good practice to mark out bony landmarks and incision site for the lateral ankle stabilization prior to the arthroscopic procedure, as extravasation of fluid with the arthroscopy may obscure exact boney anatomic landmarks making them difficult to palpate and therefore altering incision placement.

Intraoperatively, making an incision along the anterior aspect of the lateral malleolus will usually avoid the superficial peroneal nerve and prevent potential scarring along the fibula. Prior to reattachment of the ATF to the fibula, one should curette the periosteum around the attachment site to provide healthy bone to help ensure reattachment (Fig. 27.6). The surgeon should try to avoid exposing the subtalar joint during the operative procedure. Hold the position of the foot in a maximally everted position when reattaching and tensioning the ligament.

Postoperatively, the patient is placed in a non-weight-bearing splint for 2 weeks, then 2 weeks in a weight-bearing cast, and followed by 2 weeks in a walking boot.

Failed Brostroms

The primary reason for failed Brostroms is the failure to identify a factor that could lead to a compromised repair such as a varus heel or hypermobility syndrome. Recognizing

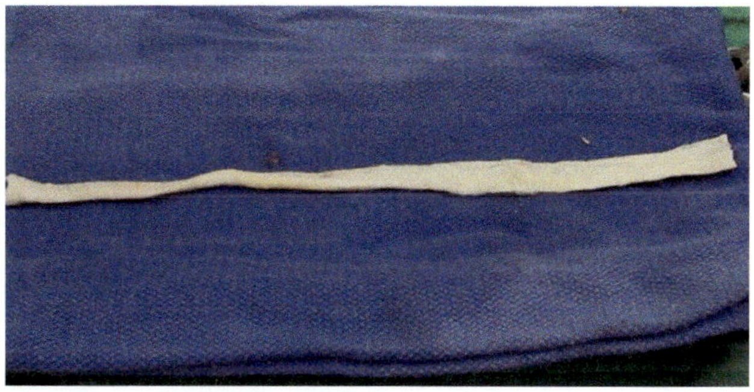

Fig. 27.7 Allograft reconstruction using a peroneus longus allograft which gives plenty of length and both a round and flat section for various types of repair

these factors preoperatively will limit many of the failures. If a Brostrom fails, MRI should be considered to evaluate for peroneal injury. The authors also recommend a stress test with sedation prior to the repair to evaluate the lateral ankle ligament complex and the lateral subtalar ligament complex.

Failed Brostrom requires reconstruction with either an autograft/allograft type of primary reconstruction or biotenodesis procedure such as a Watson-Jones. For a failed Brostrom with a stable subtalar joint, the authors' preferred method is an allograft graft reconstruction. In the presence of a combined ankle and subtalar joint instability, a biotenodesis Watson-Jones repair is utilized.

Allograft reconstruction is performed using a peroneus longus allograft which gives plenty of length and both a round and flat section for various types of repair (Fig. 27.7). An incision is placed over the anterior aspect of the lateral malleolus. The lateral malleolus is exposed at the distal tip resecting off both the ATF and CF ligaments. The lateral talus at the junction of the body and neck is then exposed. A soft tissue tunnel is created along the course of the CF ligament under the peroneal tendons. Minimizing the exposure of the

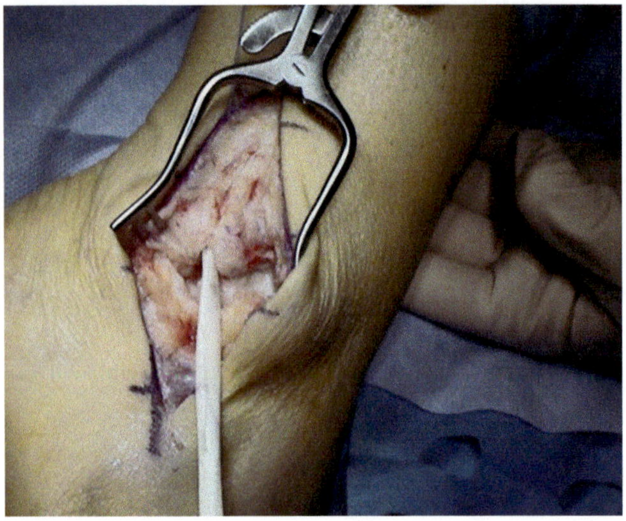

Fig. 27.8 The peroneal longus allograft is secured in place to the fibula with a biotenodesis screw

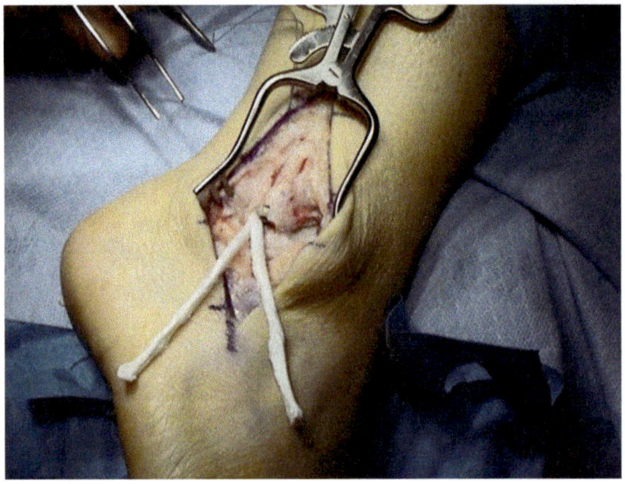

Fig. 27.9 Graft is split into anterior and posterior halves for placement into the talus and calcaneus

peroneal tendons will reduce the risk of painful adhesions. An osseous tunnel is created from the tip of the lateral malleolus oriented from distal anterior to proximal posterior. The authors limit the diameter of the osseous tunnel to a maximum of 6 mm in order to prevent fracture of the lateral malleolus. The graft needs to move smoothly through the tunnel. The graft is secured in place to the fibula with a biotenodesis screw (Fig. 27.8). With the fibular portion in place, the graft is split into anterior and posterior halves for placement into the talus and calcaneus, respectively (Fig. 27.9).

The osseous tunnel in the calcaneus is located inferior to the posterior facet of the subtalar joint approximately halfway along the joint. Care should be taken to avoid penetrating the joint. Aiming slightly inferior will help avoid violating the joint. The osseous tunnel is typically a 7 mm tunnel and the allograft diameter is 6 mm. Since the pass of the graft can be difficult to visualize, the diameter difference ensures an easy pass of the graft. The graft is not secured in place at this time.

The location of the osseous tunnel within the talus is at the junction of the body and neck. The authors prefer that the tunnel is more in the body of the talus rather than in the neck if possible. This is usually a 6 mm tunnel.

With both arms in position, the heel is held in an everted position, but not dorsiflexed. Keep the ankle in a neutral to slightly plantarflexed position. Placing the wider anterior portion of the talus with dorsiflexed position will lead to a less stable reconstruction. With the foot positioned properly, the calcaneal portion of the graft is secured followed by the talus. There should be good tension on the reconstruction since there will be some give to the graft over time.

Postoperative course is 2 weeks non-weight bearing in a splint, followed by 2 weeks weight-bearing cast, and then 2 weeks in a walking boot. When in the walking boot, the patient can begin range of motion using an ankle brace to limit inversion and eversion. At 6 weeks post-op, the patient is advanced into a shoe with an ankle brace when walking, and physical therapy is started to advance activities and begin weaning out of the brace. Ankle braces or taping is recommended with activities that have a higher risk at inversion injuries.

Fibular Fracture

With the advancement of biotenodesis screws, the use of an anterior to posterior tunnel in the fibula is not as common. If a tunnel is used, most fibular fractures can be avoided with proper placement of the osseous canal. The ideal location of the osseous tunnel is 1.5 cm proximal to the tip of the lateral malleolus and directly in the center of the fibular.

Using a cannulated screw system that will create a guide hole will ensure proper placement of the tunnel. Remembering that the guidewire is placed a little higher than the 1.5 cm location will make sure that the tunnel is not located too distal. Try to avoid an osseous tunnel of greater than 6 mm in diameter. Creating a tunnel that is too large or too low can lead to a fracture of the fibula (Figs. 27.10 and 27.11).

Fracture of the fibula should be secured with two small screws across the fracture site with purchasing both the distal and proximal cortex (Fig. 27.12). The authors also recommend X-rays at the 2 weeks post-op visit. If X-rays are stable, the patient can be started in a weight-bearing cast as tolerated. Weight-bearing cast is used until 6 weeks post-op, and if the X-rays show healing, then the patient can progress in a walking boot for an additional 2 weeks.

The ligament repair can be so stable that several months after a ligament reconstruction, avulsion fracture of the fibu-

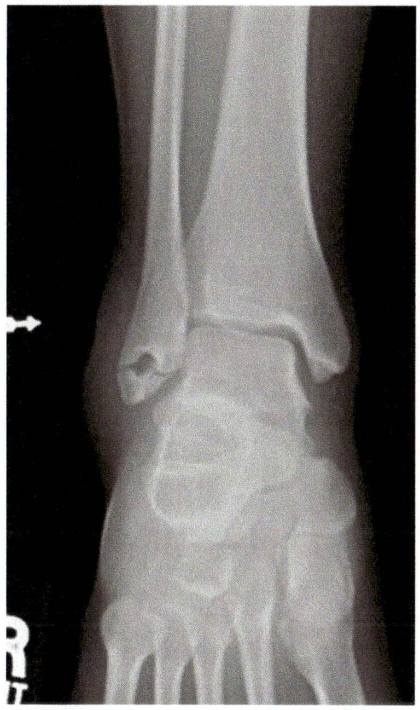

Fig. 27.10 Fracture of the distal fibula through the osseous tunnel

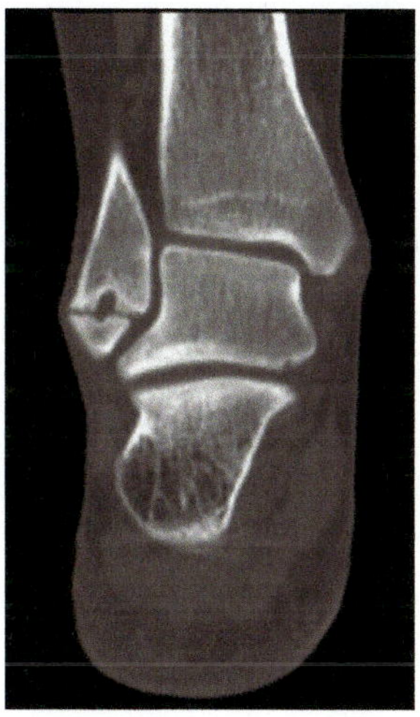

Fig. 27.11 CT scan confirming nonunion of the fibular fracture

lar can occur through the osseous tunnel with an inversion injury. These fractures, while rare, do poorly with conservative treatment due to the tethering of the ligament against the fracture site and can lead to a nonunion. The authors recommend surgical intervention with open reduction internal fixation of the fracture. These fractures often take quite a long time to heal (Fig. 27.13).

If a nonunion develops, MRI or CT is helpful to check for possible AVN of the fragment piece. If the distal piece has not developed an AVN, grafting with fixation can stabilize the ankle ligaments and salvage the repair. The authors recommend a conservative post-op management for the patient.

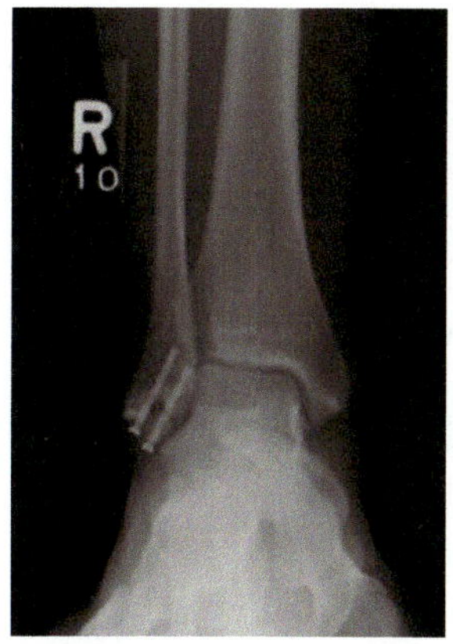

Fig. 27.12 Fracture of the fibula should be secured with two small screws across the fracture site with purchasing both the distal and proximal cortex

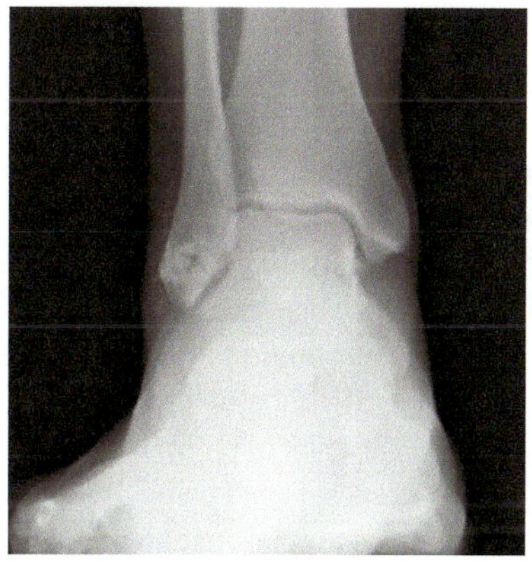

Fig. 27.13 Healed fracture of the osseous tunnel with subsequent hardware removal

This typically involves 4 weeks non-weight bearing in a cast followed by 4 weeks in a walking boot. Repeat CT scan is recommended prior to advancement of activities to ensure healing.

Tenodesed Ankle

A tenodesed or "stiff" ankle can be a debilitating complication. It is the lack of dorsiflexion and plantar flexion that the patient will complain about more than the lack of inversion and eversion. This is more commonly seen with the nonanatomic repairs for isolated ankle instability in the presence of a normal subtalar joint or with underestimated arthritis of the ankle or malposition of the ankle or tibia. The restriction of both ankle and subtalar joint motion will cause the foot to be fixed in a rigid, everted position.

Preoperative assessment should properly evaluate range of motion of the ankle as well as position of the ankle. In the presence of a rigid ankle or a fixed varus position, ligament

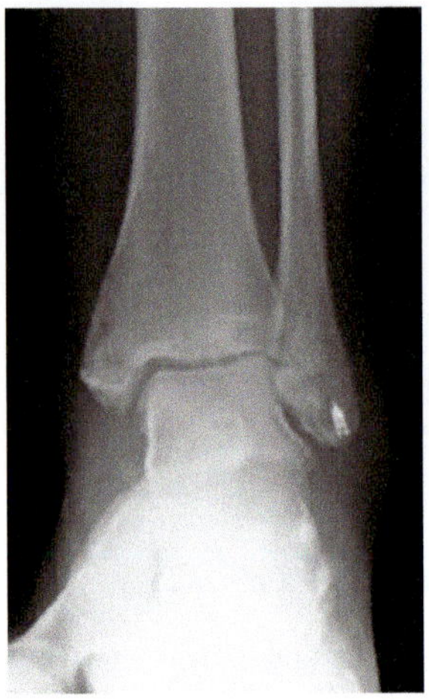

Fig. 27.14 Overtensioning of the lateral ankle ligament with narrowing of the lateral ankle mortise

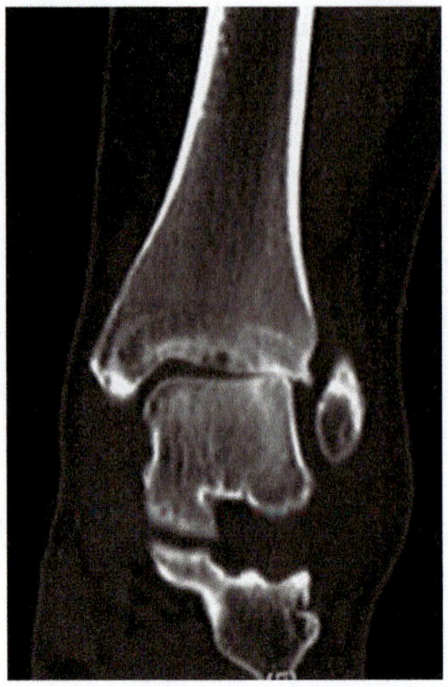

Fig. 27.15 Coronal CT scan showing arthritic changes of the lateral ankle

reconstruction would not be advised, and arthrodesis may be the better choice. Supramalleolar osteotomy or heel realignment may also be considered.

Overtensioning of the ligament reconstruction can occur (Fig. 27.14). The natural instinct is to make the ligament as tight as possible which can cause a rigid ankle or STJ. In order to prevent this, after reconstitution of the graft, the authors do not "stretch" the allograft prior to insertion and tightening. This will allow a small amount of natural lengthening to occur. Prepping the contralateral side and using this as a guide is also helpful. If the patient has normal functioning of the contralateral ligaments, then the operative side can be tightened slightly more than the "normal" side. If dealing with a patient with hypermobility on the contralateral side as well, the operative side will need to be tightened a bit more aggressively.

Protected, postoperative range of motion after 4 weeks will try to minimize the amount of adhesions. Once mentioned before, range of motion with an ankle brace to limit inversion-eversion initially will prevent both adhesions and loss of stability. The use of physical therapy begins once the patient is allowed to start to wean out of the boot at 6–8 weeks post-op.

If tenodesis of the ankle or STJ occurs with failure of conservative treatment, more invasive treatments can be beneficial. Continual passive motion (CPM) machines can be helpful, but are often expensive. Manipulation under anesthesia with injection of the ankle is a more invasive treatment option. Manipulation should try to improve plantar flexion/dorsiflexion first and inversion/eversion secondly. Injection of the ankle and/or STJ with a steroid and local anesthetic may help reduce adhesions. For the ankle joint, 1 cm^3 of a steroid and 4 cm^3 of a local anesthetic are used and 1 cm^3 of a steroid and 2 cm^3 of a local anesthetic for the STJ.

Surgical intervention may be needed to help with continued pain and limitations. Arthroscopic debridement may be of benefit especially if the patient did get some short-term improvement with the injection. Of these options, ankle and/or STJ arthrodesis may be warranted. Advanced imaging with CT scan to determine the presence of arthritic changes and diagnostic injections would be of benefit to determine the level of arthrodesis or replacement (Figs. 27.15 and 27.16).

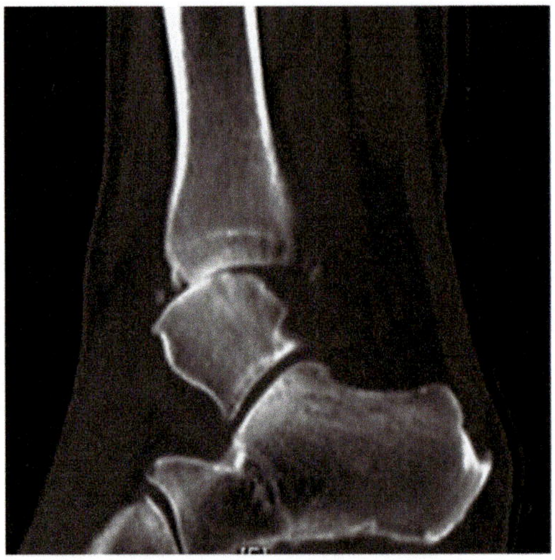

Fig. 27.16 Sagittal CT scan of narrowing of the ankle with arthritic changes

Treatment of Subtalar Joint Instability

The primary concern with subtalar joint instability is missing the diagnosis. This is often mistaken as lateral ankle instability. A high index of suspicion is needed. Often a patient has the complaint of instability with a normal ankle stress exam. Diagnostic injections of the ankle or subtalar joint can be performed, but ankle impingement and STJ instability can coexist.

When subtalar joint instability is noted independent or in conjunct with chronic lateral ankle instability, the surgeon must determine whether to perform anatomic reconstruction or to stabilize with the use of a traditional tenodesis procedure. Although the Brostrom-Gould procedure does add support to the subtalar joint, in the circumstance of increased subtalar joint instability, the addition of a tendon autograft or allograft should be implemented to further augment of the repair. Watson-Jones or Chrisman-Snook have been found to be effective in these situations, but will alter the normal kinematics.

With isolated STJ instability, primary repair or anatomic allograft/autograft can be performed. Care should be taken to avoid overzealous dissection of the lateral talus to preserve the ATFL attachment site. Postoperative course is the same for lateral ankle instability.

Conclusion

Proper diagnosis and correction of the deforming structures are the key to a successful outcome with any lateral ligament work around the ankle and foot. The use of biotenodesis screws has made anatomic reconstruction with allograft or autograft an excellent reconstruction option for patients with either a failed Brostrom or with poor native tissue. Tenodesis procedures are better suited for concurrent STJ instability.

References

1. Krips R, et al. Anatomical reconstruction and Evans tenodesis of the lateral ligaments of the ankle. Clinical and radiological findings after follow-up for 15 to 30 years. J Bone Joint Surg Br. 2002;84(2):232–6.
2. DiGiovanni CW, Brodsky A. Current concepts: lateral ankle instability. Foot Ankle Int. 2006;27(10):854–66.
3. Brown CA, et al. Biomechanical comparison of an all-soft suture anchor with a modified Brostrom-Gould suture repair for lateral ligament reconstruction. Am J Sports Med. 2014;42(2):417–22.
4. Petrera M, et al. Short- to medium-term outcomes after a modified Brostrom repair for lateral ankle instability with immediate postoperative weightbearing. Am J Sports Med. 2014;42(7):1542–8.
5. Ng ZD, Das De S. Modified Brostrom-Evans-Gould technique for recurrent lateral ankle ligament instability. J Orthop Surg (Hong Kong). 2007;15(3):306–10.
6. Messer TM, et al. Outcome of the modified Brostrom procedure for chronic lateral ankle instability using suture anchors. Foot Ankle Int. 2000;21(12):996–1003.
7. Hu CY, et al. Comparison of bone tunnel and suture anchor techniques in the modified Brostrom procedure for chronic lateral ankle instability. Am J Sports Med. 2013;41(8):1877–84.
8. Peterson KS, et al. Surgical approach for combined ankle and subtalar joint chronic mechanical instability. J Foot Ankle Surg. 2013;52(4):537–42.
9. Kibler WB. Arthroscopic findings in ankle ligament reconstruction. Clin Sports Med. 1996;15(4):799–804.
10. Brostrom L. Sprained ankles. V. Treatment and prognosis in recent ligament ruptures. Acta Chir Scand. 1966;132(5):537–50.
11. Brostrom L. Sprained ankles. VI. Surgical treatment of "chronic" ligament ruptures. Acta Chir Scand. 1966;132(5):551–65.
12. Brostrom L, Sundelin P. Sprained ankles. IV. Histologic changes in recent and "chronic" ligament ruptures. Acta Chir Scand. 1966;132(3):248–53.
13. Gould N, Seligson D, Gassman J. Early and late repair of lateral ligament of the ankle. Foot Ankle. 1980;1(2):84–9.
14. Catanzariti AR, Mendicino RW. Tenodesis for chronic lateral ankle instability. Clin Podiatr Med Surg. 2001;**18**(3):429–42.
15. Drakos M, Behrens BS, Paller D, Murphy C, Di Giovanni C. Biomechanical comparison of an open vs arthroscopic approach for lateral ankle instability. J Arthroscopic Relat Surg. 2011;27:60–1.
16. Cho BK, et al. Outcomes of the modified Brostrom procedure using suture anchors for chronic lateral ankle instability—a prospective, randomized comparison between single and double suture anchors. J Foot Ankle Surg. 2013;52(1):9–15.
17. Miyamoto W, et al. Accelerated versus traditional rehabilitation after anterior talofibular ligament reconstruction for chronic lateral instability of the ankle in athletes. Am J Sports Med. 2014;42(6):1441–7.
18. Watson-Jones R. Recurrent forward dislocation of the ankle joint. J Bone Joint Surg Br. 1952;34:519.
19. Hennrikus WL, et al. Outcomes of the Chrisman-Snook and modified-Brostrom procedures for chronic lateral ankle instability. A prospective, randomized comparison. Am J Sports Med. 1996;24(4):400–4.
20. Miyamoto W, Takao M, Matsushita T. Hindfoot endoscopy for posterior ankle impingement syndrome and flexor hallucis longus tendon disorders. Foot Ankle Clin. 2015;20(1):139–47.

Ankle Fractures

28

George Tye Liu

Introduction

Malleolar fractures of the tibiotalar joint are common fractures of the human body often caused by falls from heights or sports-related trauma and more common in young males [1, 2]. One study estimated the incidence rate in the United States to be 187 per 100,000 person-years [1].

Malleolar fracture malunions can lead to limb deformity, pain, stiffness, difficulty with gait, and posttraumatic arthritis from joint malalignment [3–5]. Though there is little published data on the rate of malleolar ankle fracture malunions, posttraumatic arthritis comprises an estimated 78% of all ankle arthritis [6].

The tibiotalar joint is a congruent joint which measures 350 mm^2 in surface area and can bear upward of five times the body weight during walking [7]. The articular geometry of the tibiotalar joint with a concave tibial plafond and convex talar dome contributes to the stability of the joint during weightbearing [8]. Malunions from malaligned malleolar fractures can lead to articular incongruity of tibiotalar joint leading to posttraumatic arthritis (Fig. 28.1). In a cadaveric study, Ramsey et al. [9] demonstrated that 1 mm lateral displacement of the talus can unload the tibiotalar joint by 42%. Thordarson et al. [10] reported that tibiotalar incongruity in their cadaveric fibular fracture malunion model with deep deltoid ligament rupture and concomitant shortening, lateral displacement, and malrotation of the fibula increased peak contact pressures to the mid-lateral quadrant of the tibiotalar joint. Clinical reports have demonstrated an association between maligned malleolar ankle fractures with clinical and radiographic outcomes. In his prospective evaluation of 306 ankle fracture cases, Lindsjö [11] identified that accuracy of ankle fracture reduction affected clinical outcomes. Rikavina et al. [12] also reported that posttraumatic arthritis was higher in malleolar fractures with short fibulas and widened ankle mortises. Additionally, ankle fractures with involvement of the posterior malleolar fracture were associated with lower patient satisfaction scores, increased rates of osteoarthritis, and need for revisional surgery compared to ankle fractures without posterior malleolar involvement [13–16].

Injury of the distal tibiofibular syndesmosis can occur concomitantly with ankle fractures. In general, the estimated rate of ankle syndesmosis injuries has been reported at 2.15 per 100,000 person-years [17]. However, up to 45% of supination external rotation ankle fractures are associated with an unstable syndesmosis disruption [18].

Syndesmosis malunions are prevalent with malreduction rates reported as high as 52% (Fig. 28.2) [19]. The high rate of malalignment has been attributed to the insensitivity of radiographic measures that allow occult syndesmosis injuries to go undetected [20–22]. One study demonstrated that syndesmosis widening evidenced by the tibiofibular clear space from radiographic imaging remained unchanged with up to 30° of external rotation the fibula (Fig. 28.3a, b) [23]. Malreduced syndesmosis disruptions associated with talar malalignment have been associated with instability, pain, and poor functional outcomes [24, 25]. Reduction and stability of the syndesmosis have also been attributed to the posterior malleolar fracture due to its attachment to the fibula via the posterior tibiofibular syndesmosis [26].

Diagnostic Workup

Bilateral weightbearing radiographs can reveal asymmetries to either identify occult malleolar and syndesmosis malalignments or be used for deformity correction planning. Tibiotalar axis which is the middiaphyseal axis of the tibia should bisect

G.T. Liu (✉)
Department of Orthopaedic Surgery, University of Texas Southwestern Medical Center, Dallas, TX 75390, USA
e-mail: george.liu@utsouthwestern.edu

M.S. Lee, J.P. Grossman (eds.), *Complications in Foot and Ankle Surgery*, DOI 10.1007/978-3-319-53686-6_28

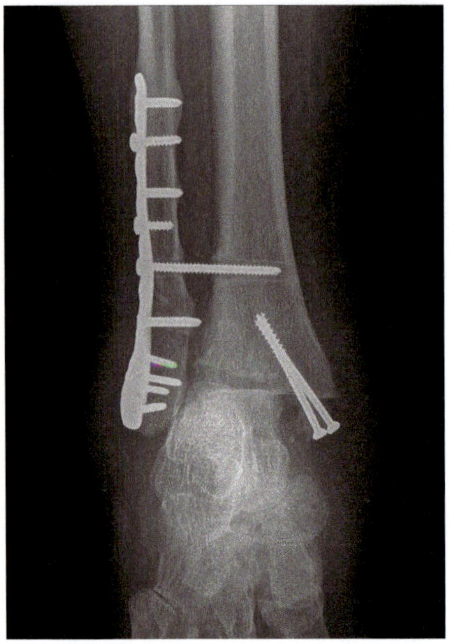

Fig. 28.1 Ankle fracture malunions often lead to posttraumatic arthritis as shown in this radiograph with medial malleolar malreduction allowing lateral subluxation of the talus

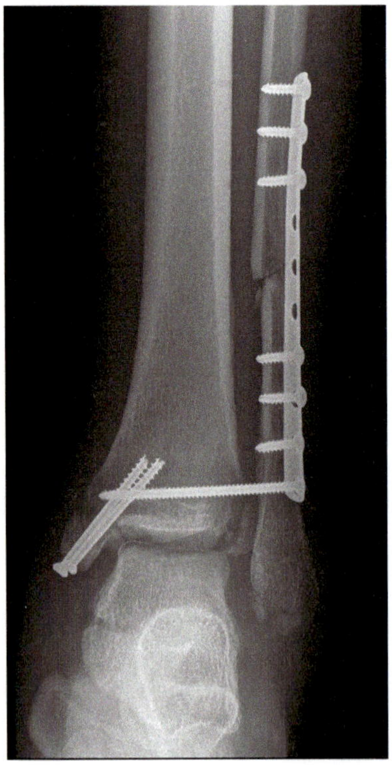

Fig. 28.2 Distal tibiofibular malunions are most apparent with frank diastasis of the tibiofibular clear space though most rotational misalignments can be undetected up to 30° of fibular external rotation

the talus. Deviation of tibiotalar axis can demonstrate malalignment of a malleolus, malleoli, or syndesmosis (Fig. 28.4). Medial, tibiotalar, and lateral spaces of the ankle mortise view should be equidistant. On the ankle AP view, the medial clear space and the tibiofibular overlap should also be symmetric. Fibular length may be assessed by comparing bilateral talocrural angles, which is the medial intersection of a perpendicular line from the tibial plafond to the intermalleolar line (Fig. 28.5) [27]. On the ankle mortise view, the tibiofibular clear space should also be symmetric (Fig. 28.6). Alternatively, fibular length may also be measured with the angle of the bimalleolar angle which is the intersection between the line parallel to the fibular shaft and the intermalleolar line. Normal variations of bimalleolar angles in contralateral ankles have been reported to be an average of 1.3° [28]. Other measures of fibular length include Shenton's line, a curved congruous subchondral bone line from Wagstaffe's tubercule projecting to the tibial plafond, and the circle sign or dime sign, a concentric curve from the lateral talar process to the fibular recess (Fig. 28.7) [29]. Computed tomography (CT) 2-dimensional images or 3-dimensional reconstructions can provide further information on planes of deformity and the presence of joint degeneration.

Radiographic measures used to evaluate the syndesmosis include the tibiofibular clear space on the mortise projection and tibiofibular overlap on the anterior-posterior projection (Fig. 28.6). On the lateral projection, the anterior border of the fibula is often midline of the tibial axis as evidenced by normative data from CT scans [30]. Because radiographic parameters are relatively insensitive for identifying syndesmosis disruptions, CT scans of bilateral ankles are often necessary to identify rotational and translational malalignments otherwise missed on plain radiographs (Fig. 28.3a, b) [30–33].

Indications of Procedure

Restoration of tibiotalar and talomalleolar articular congruity and joint stability are the primary objectives of malleolar malunion and syndesmosis repair. Articular realignment can reduce abnormal focal contact pressures that can lead to advanced cartilage degeneration. Reestablishing tibiotalar joint stability will reduce abnormal joint kinematics leading to degenerative arthrosis, pain, and dysfunction.

Contraindications/Limitations

Specific contraindications to malunion repair should be considered if manifestations of advanced degenerative changes are seen clinically and/or radiographically or if reconstruction cannot achieve joint stability or anatomic articular alignment.

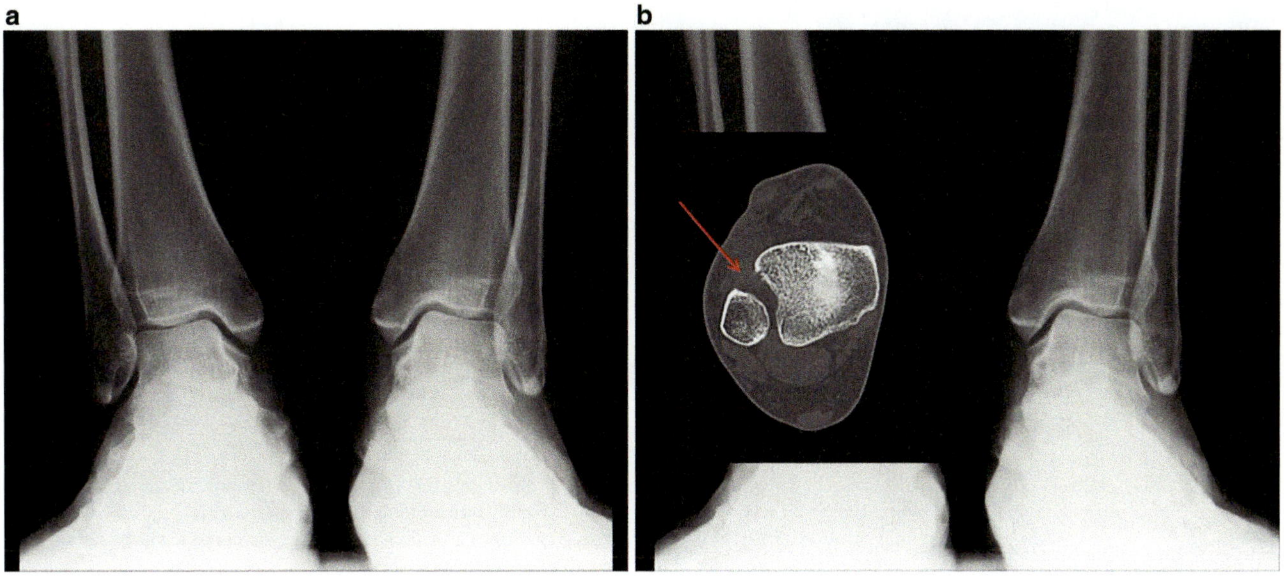

Fig. 28.3 (**a**) Radiographic studies are often insensitive in identifying rotational alignments of the fibular in the fibular incisura of the tibia as seen in this patient with chronic syndesmosis pain from external rotation injury sustained 1.5 years ago. (**b**) Computed tomography of the same patient case demonstrates widening of the syndesmosis with external rotation of the fibula in the fibular incisura of the tibia not obvious on plain radiograph

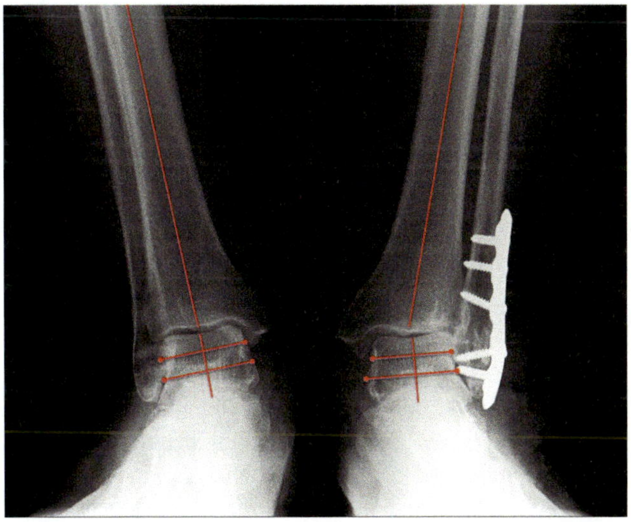

Fig. 28.4 Bilateral weightbearing ankle views can reveal asymmetries suggestive of ankle malalignments. The middiaphyseal axis of the tibia bisecting the talus denotes anatomic tibiotalar alignment as shown on the *left*. Deviation of tibiotalar axis can demonstrate malalignment of a malleolus, malleoli, or syndesmosis as shown on the *right*

Ankle Malleolar Fracture Malunion

Restoring Fibular Length and Rotation

Loss of length and malrotation of the fibula are the most common causes of talar malalignment within the tibiotalar joint. Fibular fracture displacement alone whether it is shortened, laterally displaced, and/or external rotated does not cause talar instability provided the medial malleolus and the deep deltoid ligament are intact. Lateral talar subluxation is often seen in cases of isolated fibular malleolar ankle fractures with deep deltoid ligament rupture or in bimalleolar/trimalleolar ankle fractures, which are inherently unstable. In either clinical circumstance, the medial restraint (medial malleolus and/or deep deltoid ligament), which provides talar stability, is disrupted allowing the talus to sublux. In most cases, the talus will displace in the direction of the fibula as the lateral collateral ligaments remain intact and the peroneal tendons pull will cause displacement of the fibula (Fig. 28.8a–c). Reestablishing fibular length restores the lateral buttress preventing the talus from subluxing laterally. Correcting fibular rotation restores talofibular articulation, tibiotalar alignment, and congruent range of motion of the tibiotalar joint. Secondarily, failure to restore fibular length will render difficulty with distal tibiofibular syndesmosis reduction.

Through a standard lateral longitudinal incisional approach, fibular length can be achieved by several methods (Fig. 28.9). For isolated fibular malleolar ankle fractures with medial clear space widening, a small medial incisional approach is often needed to debride the scar tissue, which interposes the articulation between the medial malleolus and medial talus preventing reduction (Fig. 28.10a, b). In chronic cases of malunion and medial clear space widening, adhesive fibrosis of the scar tissue can occur along the articular cartilage, therefore, should be debrided carefully. Fibular

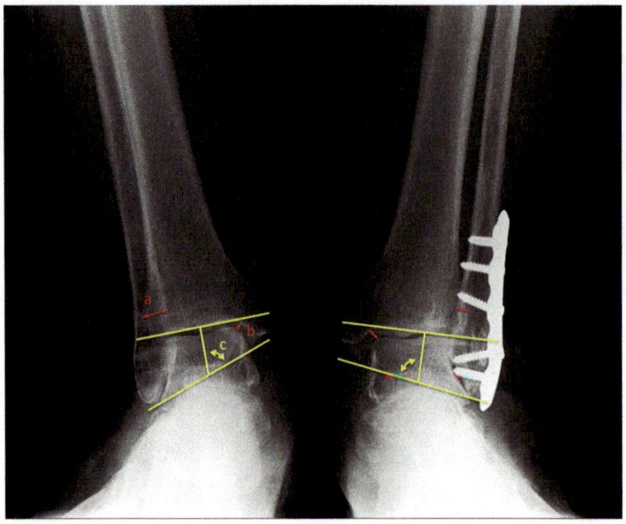

Fig. 28.5 Comparing bilateral weightbearing AP ankle views: medial clear space (**b**) and tibiofibular overlap (**a**) of the ankle mortise view should be symmetric. Fibular length may be assessed by comparing the symmetry of talocrural angles, which is the medial intersection of a perpendicular line from the tibial plafond to the intermalleolar line (**c**). All radiographic values are increased on the *right*

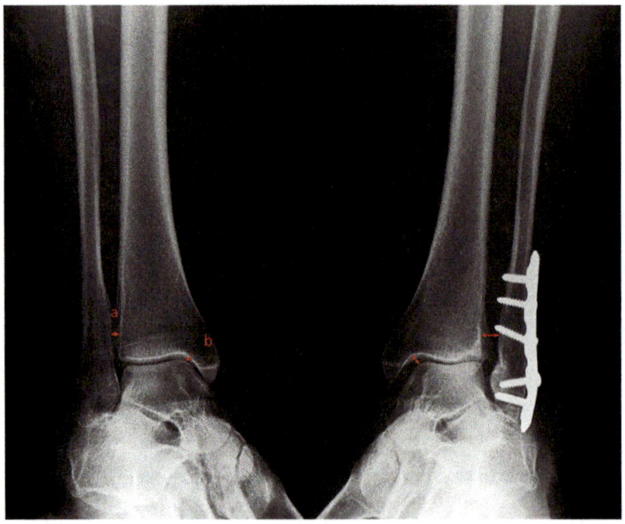

Fig. 28.6 Comparing bilateral weightbearing mortise ankle views: medial clear space (**b**) and tibiofibular clear space (**a**) should be symmetric. Both values are increased on the right and suggestive of deep deltoid and syndesmosis ligament disruption

osteotomy should be performed in the orientation of the original fracture, and the use of an intercalary bone graft should be anticipated for bony deficits encounter with deformity correction (Fig. 28.11a, b). The use of CT imaging can assist in identifying the orientation for the osteotomy. A locking plate is positioned on the lateral fibula held in place with a towel clamp along the proximal segment of the fibular fracture to ensure axial alignment of the plate. The locking plate is secured to the distal fibular fracture with locking screws

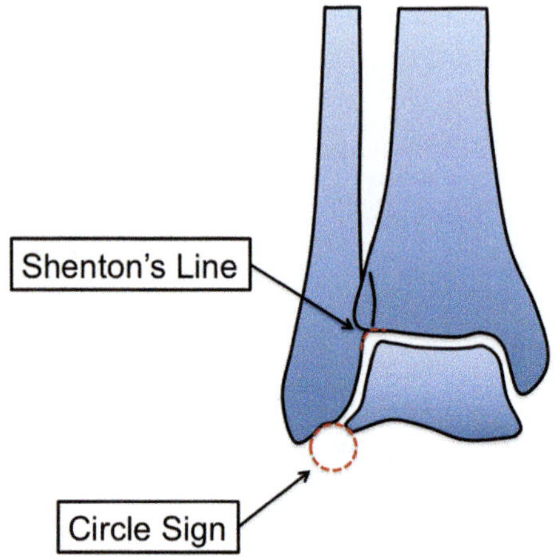

Fig. 28.7 Shenton's line is a curved congruous subchondral bone line from Wagstaffe's tubercule projecting to the tibial plafond and the circle sign or dime sign which is a concentric curve from the lateral talar process to the fibular recess

(Fig. 28.12). In the isolated fibular malleolar or bimalleolar fracture malunions, the use of a Weber reduction clamp placed along the transmalleolar axis can assist in the reduction of the talus axially beneath the tibia during the process of restoring fibular length (Fig. 28.13). Because the fibula is often bound by peripheral scar and fibrosis, achieving fibular length often requires use of an articulated distractor, which is secured to the proximal fibular segment and lengthens the distal fibula through the locking plate (Fig. 28.14). The bolt to the threaded rod is turned providing incremental distraction. The proximal towel clamp secures the position of the plate on the fibula to better resist anterior, posterior, or lateral migration of the distal fibular segment during the lengthening. Appropriate length is determined by restoring fibular symmetry with contralateral ankle radiographs, Shenton's lines, and the subfibular circle sign. A second towel clamp is applied along the distal malleolus to correct rotational malalignment of the fibula by achieving patency of the lateral talofibular articulation on the ankle mortise view (Fig. 28.15a, b). Once satisfactory fibular length has been achieved and rotation has been corrected, the reduction is stabilized with a locking screw in the proximal fibular segment (Fig. 28.16a–c). Nonlocking screws to secure the proximal portion of the plate may cause loss of rotational correction to the distal fibular segment due to contact of the plate on the irregular lateral surface of the fibula.

Restoring Medial Malleolar Rotation and Alignment

Deformity correction of medial malleolar malunions and nonunions can be complicated by resorptive bone loss and loss of cortical margins to guide anatomic reduction. For the

a b c

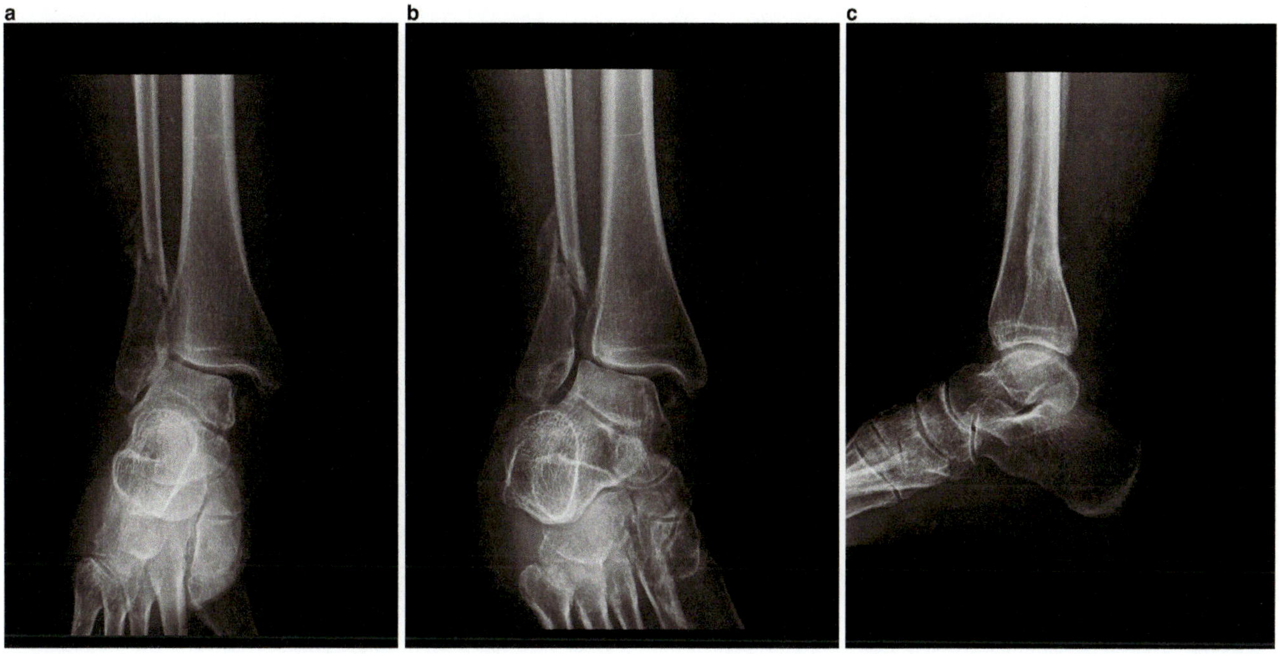

Fig. 28.8 Anterior-posterior (**a**), mortise (**b**), and lateral (**c**) ankle conventional radiographs of failed nonoperative management of Weber C fibular fracture with deep deltoid ligament disruption and lateral talar subluxation. Anterior-posterior views demonstrate a short fibula is short and wide medial clear space (**a**), while the mortise view shows both widening of medial and tibiofibular clear space (**b**)

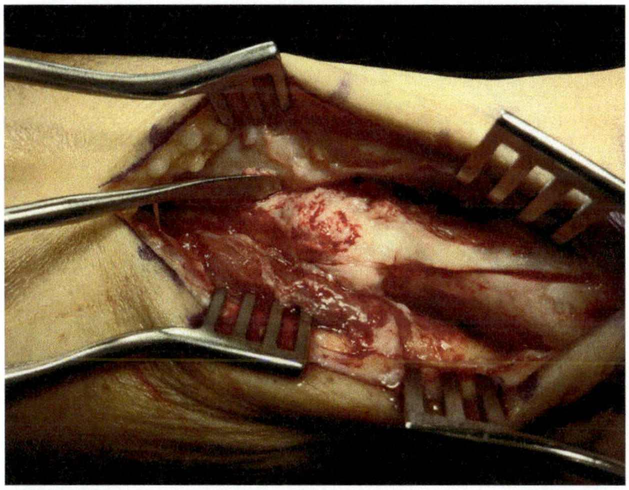

Fig. 28.9 Standard lateral approach to ankle reveals fibular malunion with woven bone callus formation the fibular shaft

medial malleolar component of ankle fracture cases, CT scan can provide the orientation of the malunion and the plane for intended osteotomy. A standard medial longitudinal or anterior medial curvilinear approach provides adequate exposure. In bimalleolar ankle fracture malunion/nonunion, medial malleolar osteotomy is often performed prior to fibular osteotomy and lengthening to ensure no malleolar obstruction to tibiotalar alignment (Figs. 28.17a–c and 28.18a, b). In cases of bimalleolar or trimalleolar ankle fracture malunions, the fibular malleolus is often fixed first because the ankle joint radiographic landmarks to guide fibular length and rotation are often preserved compared to the few landmarks available to the medial malleolus (Figs. 28.19, 28.20, and 28.21).

Because of the deformity from the malunion and subsequent bony gap that is encountered with subsequent realignment of the medial malleolus, cortical landmarks available to guide reduction may be limited. The only method of reduction to ensure anatomic congruity of the medial malleolar-talus articulation is through indirect reduction of the medial malleolus through loading of the tibiotalar joint. Once the medial malleolar osteotomy is performed, loading the ankle at 90° will allow full contact of the tibiotalar articulation stabilizing the tibiotalar joint by realigning the tibiotalar axis [8]. Secondarily, while the tibiotalar joint is loaded and axis corrected, the congruity of the medial malleolar-talus articulation allows correct rotation and alignment of the medial malleolus (Fig. 28.22). Because a bony defect is frequently encountered, in bicortical fixation fully threaded 3.5 or 4.0 mm cortical screws are used as positional screws to bridge the gap and maintain correction (Figs. 28.23a–d and 28.24a–c). Alternatively, an angled locking plate may also be used to bridge the bony defect.

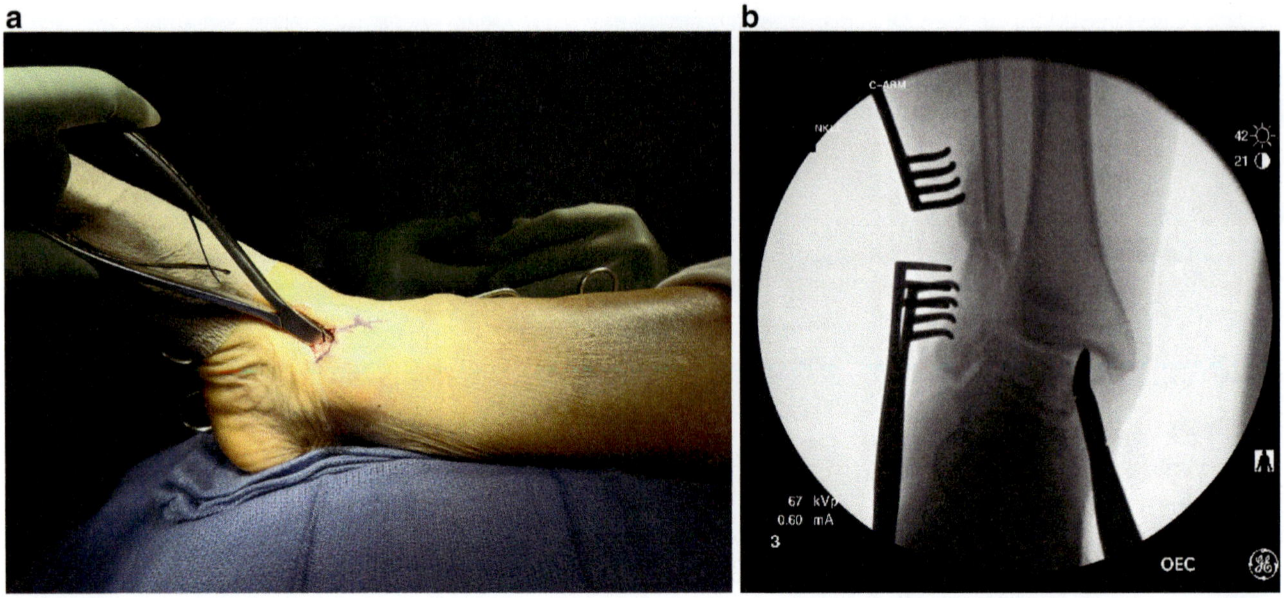

Fig. 28.10 Clinical (**a**) and intraoperative fluoroscopy (**b**) demonstrates medial clear space debridement. Anterior medial ankle arthrotomy is performed, and scar tissue interposed in the medial clear space is carefully debrided

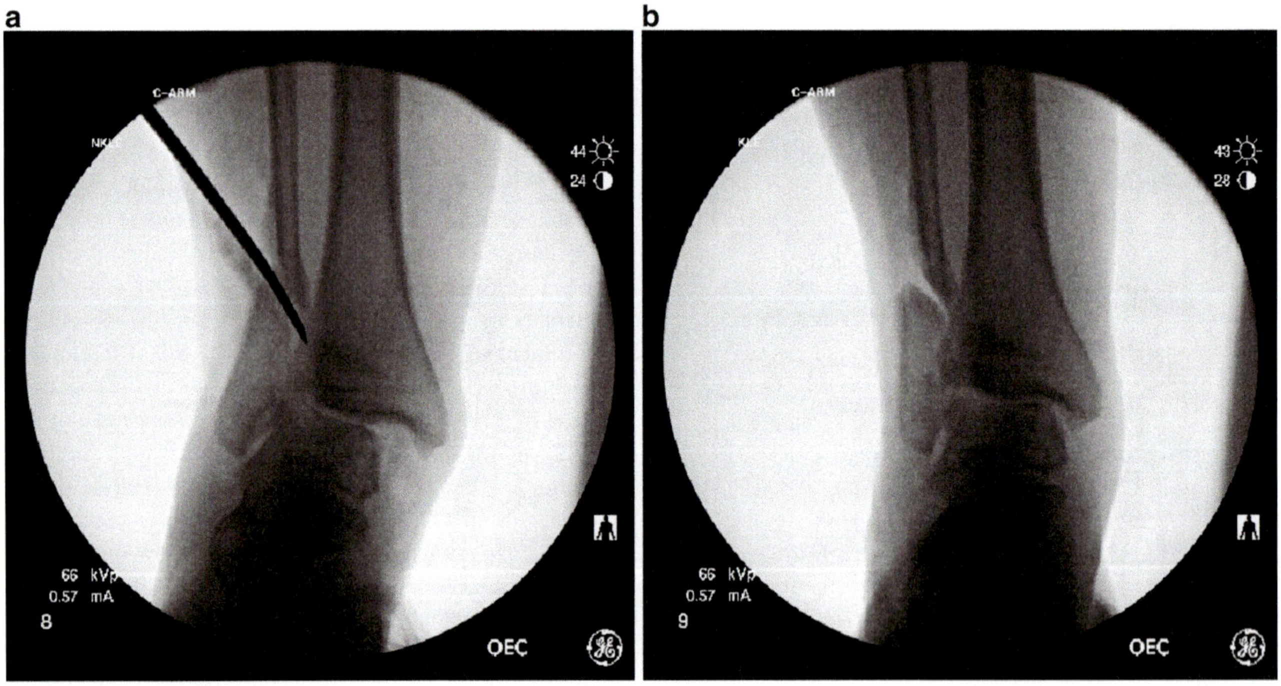

Fig. 28.11 Fibular osteotomy is performed either with sagittal saw or osteotome in the orientation of the original fracture (**a**). Once fibular malunion deformity correction is performed, spatial bone deficit is often encountered (**b**)

Restoring Posterior Malleolar Articulation

Posterior malleolar malalignments can occur in various ankle fracture patterns.

In trimalleolar ankle fractures, posterior malleolar alignment can be directly affected by reduction of fibular fractures that occur at or above the level of the syndesmosis. If fibular length is not adequately restored, the posterior malleolus will remain elevated or maligned through its interconnection with the posterior-inferior tibiofibular ligament (PITFL) (Fig. 28.25). Additionally, if the fibula is anteriorly or posteriorly translated or internally or externally rotated within the

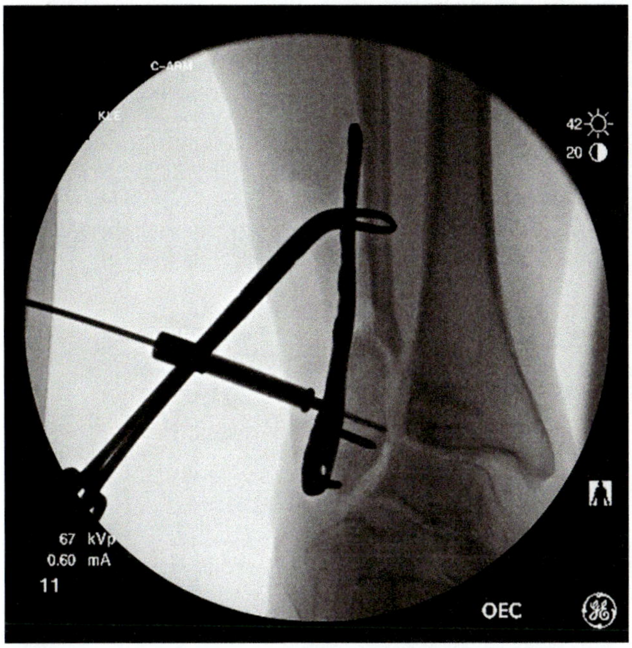

Fig. 28.12 A locking plate is held on the fibula proximally with a towel clamp to maintain axial alignment of the plate, while the distal portion of the locking plate is secured to the distal fibula with locking screws

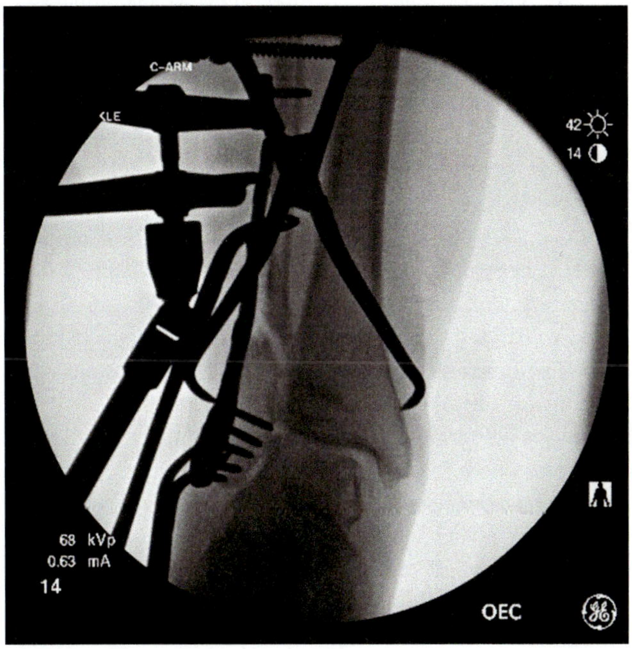

Fig. 28.13 A Weber reduction clamp placed across the transmalleolar axis to assist in the reduction of the talar dome within the ankle mortise while achieving fibular length

fibular incisura of the tibia, the posterior malleolus may be malreduced through the PITFL attachment to the fibula (Fig. 28.26a, b). Accordingly, reduction of the posterior mal-

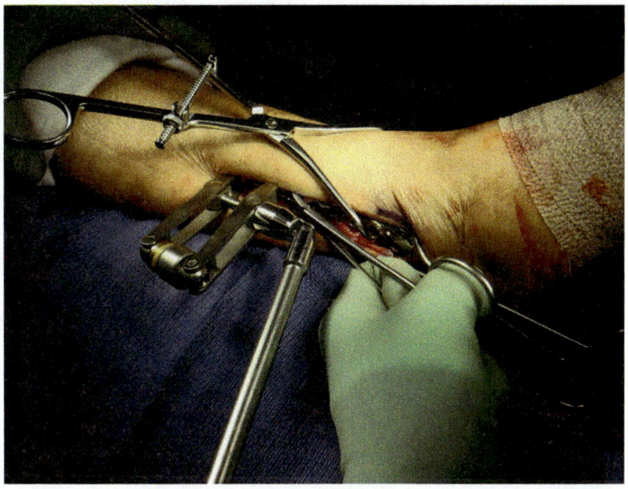

Fig. 28.14 An articulated distractor is applied to the proximal end of the fibula with a screw and lengthens the fibula through its attachment to the locking plate

leolar fracture better restores anatomic alignment of the tibiofibular syndesmosis [34].

Though larger size posterior malleolar fractures have been widely thought to be associated with posterior subluxation of the talus and abnormal articular pressure patterns of the tibiotalar joint, studies have shown that these pathologies are more associated with syndesmosis instability (Fig. 28.27a–d) [35]. If posterior malleolar malunion repair is anticipated in combination with a lateral malleolar osteotomy, a curvy linear incision posterior-lateral to the fibular malleolus extending to the fibular colliculus can provide adequate exposure for both osteotomies and subsequent fixation (Figs. 28.28 and 28.29). Patient should be positioned prone. CT scan and radiographic studies should demonstrate the plane of the posterior malleolar malunion and subsequent osteotomy. Osteotomy may be performed initially with sagittal saw, then completed with straight osteotome under fluoroscopic guidance (Fig. 28.30a–e). Fixation with a posteiror-lateral plate can function as either an antiglide or for neutralization providing optimal stability compared to only compression screw techniques [36]. A dynamic compression plate is contoured and affixed to the posterior malleolar fragment with locking screws (Fig. 28.31). Restoring length of the posterior malleolus is performed with an articulated distractor affixed to the proximal tibial articulated with the plate providing reduction under fluoroscopy until tibiotalar alignment is achieved. The use of a Weber reduction or periarticular reduction forceps will prevent posterior displacement of the posterior malleolus when achieving reduction (Figs. 28.32 and 28.33a, b). Once anatomic reduction is achieved by alignment of the lateral process of the talus with the middiaphyseal axis of the tibia, posterior malleolar reduction is stabilized with bridge plate with either positional or locking screws (Figs. 28.34a–c and 28.35a–c). Additional positional screws may be used if needed.

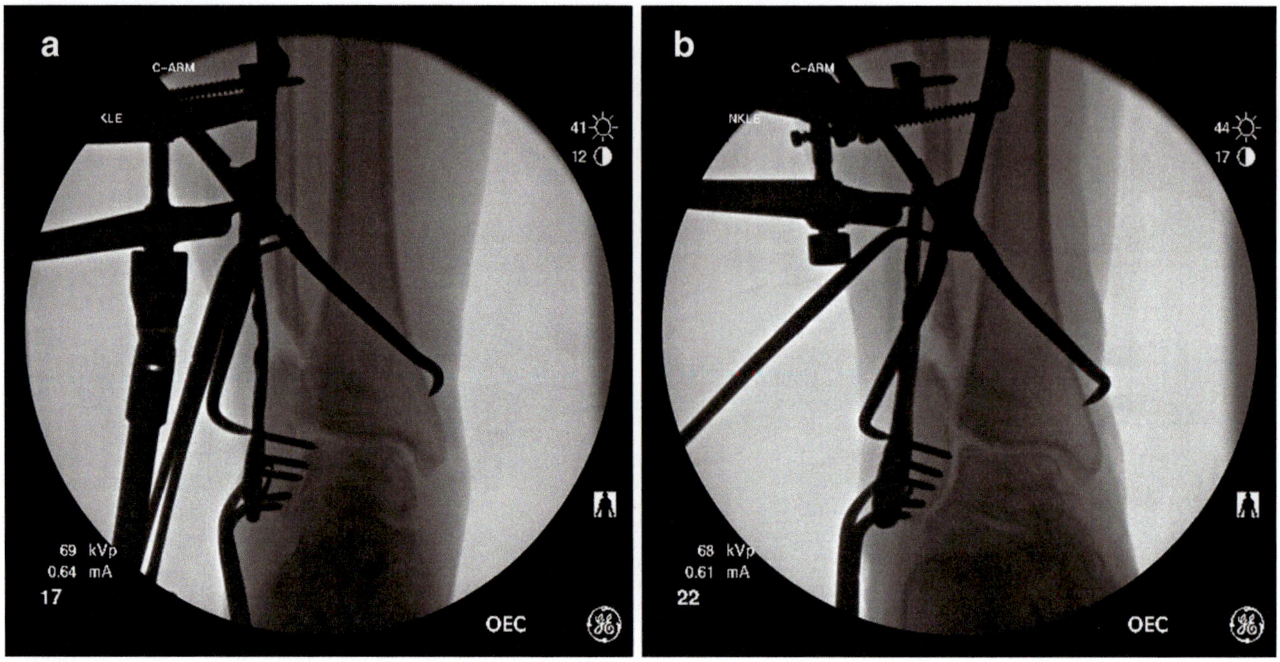

Fig. 28.15 Intraoperative fluoroscopy demonstrating application of a towel clamp along the distal malleolus (**a**). The fibula is rotated until a patent talofibular articulation on the ankle mortise view is achieved on mortise view (**b**)

Addressing Bone Loss in Ankle Nonunion and Malunion Repair

Nonunions of malleolar fractures may be encountered with open fractures, tobacco use, uncontrolled diabetes mellitus, extensive periosteal stripping with operative approach, and steroids. Bony deficits can be encountered once debridement of nonviable margins of the nonunion has been performed. Additionally, bony deficits are commonly encountered following osteotomy and correction of malunion. Intercalary bone grafting is often required to fill the spatial deficit (Fig. 28.36a–c). Autologous bone graft is often considered primary choice due to its osteoconductive, osteoinductive, osteogenic properties of bone healing. Several sites of harvest may be considered including iliac crest, proximal tibia, distal tibia, and calcaneus; however, it is based upon the size of spatial deficit and type of bone required (Fig. 28.37a, b) [37–39]. Autologous cortical cancellous graft provides both structural support and biologic stimulation.

Management of Syndesmosis Complications

Complications with the distal tibiofibular syndesmosis are seen with either malreduction or loss of reduction (Fig. 28.38). If identified within 6 weeks, revisional open reduction internal fixation may be performed, as remnant syndesmosis ligament is often present to heal through fibrosis. For chronic syndesmosis disruptions or malreductions, syndesmosis reconstruction options are based upon two factors associated with the time delay to intervention: (1) the presence of posttraumatic arthritis and (2) whether remnant syndesmosis ligament is available. Between 6 weeks and 6 months, open reduction internal fixation is performed in the same fashion with screw fixation. If remnant ligament is available, sutured repair may be performed [40]. If remnant ligament is absent, ligament reconstruction with autograft or allograft tendon may be indicated [41, 42]. Distal tibiofibular syndesmosis arthrodesis is recommended for syndesmosis malreductions or disruptions greater than 6 months old without signs of advanced posttraumatic arthritis [43].

Tendon allograft reconstruction is indicated in clinical situations where loss of reduction of syndesmosis is identified between 6 weeks and 6 months. Clinical or radiographic evidence of advanced ankle arthrosis should be considered a primary contraindication to syndesmosis ligament reconstruction. Tendon allograft reconstruction of the syndesmotic ligaments allows template for functional fibrosis of the fibula to the tibia to maintain ankle joint stability.

The syndesmosis is exposed via standard lateral longitudinal approach over the distal fibula. Disorganized scar tissue between fibular notch of the tibia and the fibula as well as the medial clear space should be debrided to allow anatomic reduction of the tibiofibular syndesmosis (Fig. 28.39). Open reduction and internal fixation of the distal tibiofibular syndesmosis should be performed in the usually standard

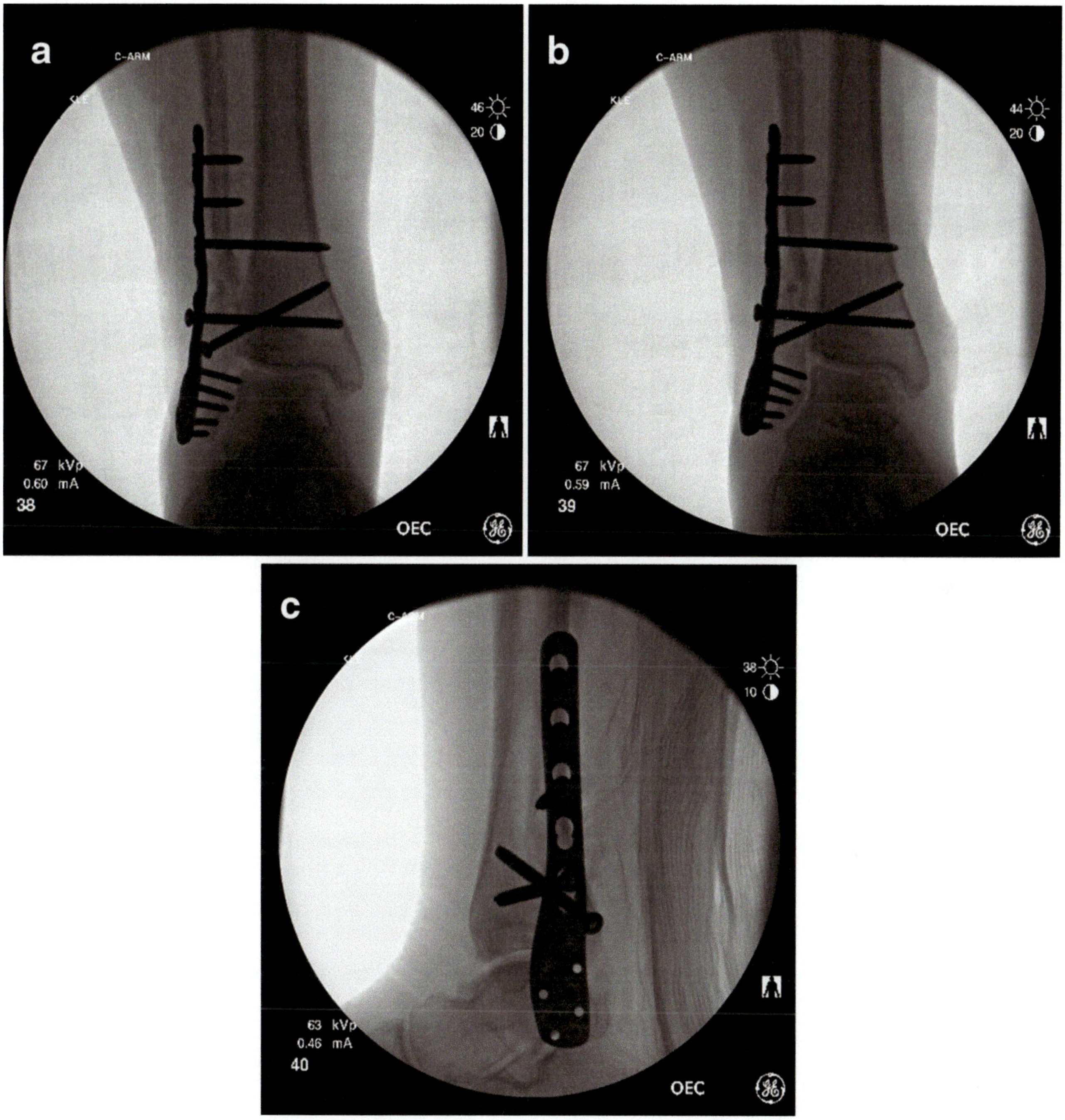

Fig. 28.16 Once fibular length and rotation has been corrected, the reduction is stabilized with a locking screw in the proximal fibular segment. Anterior-posterior view of ankle demonstrating patent medial clear space (**a**). Mortise view of ankle demonstrates equidistant medial, tibiotalar, and lateral clear spaces (**b**). Lateral view of ankle demonstrates patent tibiotalar joint with fibular positioned anatomically at the posterior ½ of the tibia (**c**)

fashion to protect the planned syndesmosis reconstruction. Reduction of the tibiofibular syndesmosis is performed with reduction tenaculums along the biomechanical axis of the ankle (Fig. 28.40). The biomechanical axis is parallel to the anterior colliculus of the medial and lateral malleoli, which is often the central to the circumference of the tibia and fibula. Length of the fibula is assessed with Shenton's lines and dime sign. Fibular rotation is assessed by the visible alignment of the subchondral bone line of the fibular articulation seen on the ankle mortise view where a symmetric medial tibiotalar and lateral fibulotalar space should be seen. A two-to-three hole 1/3 tubular plate is used to reduce torsional and shearing stress across the transyndesmotic positional screws (Fig. 28.41a, b).

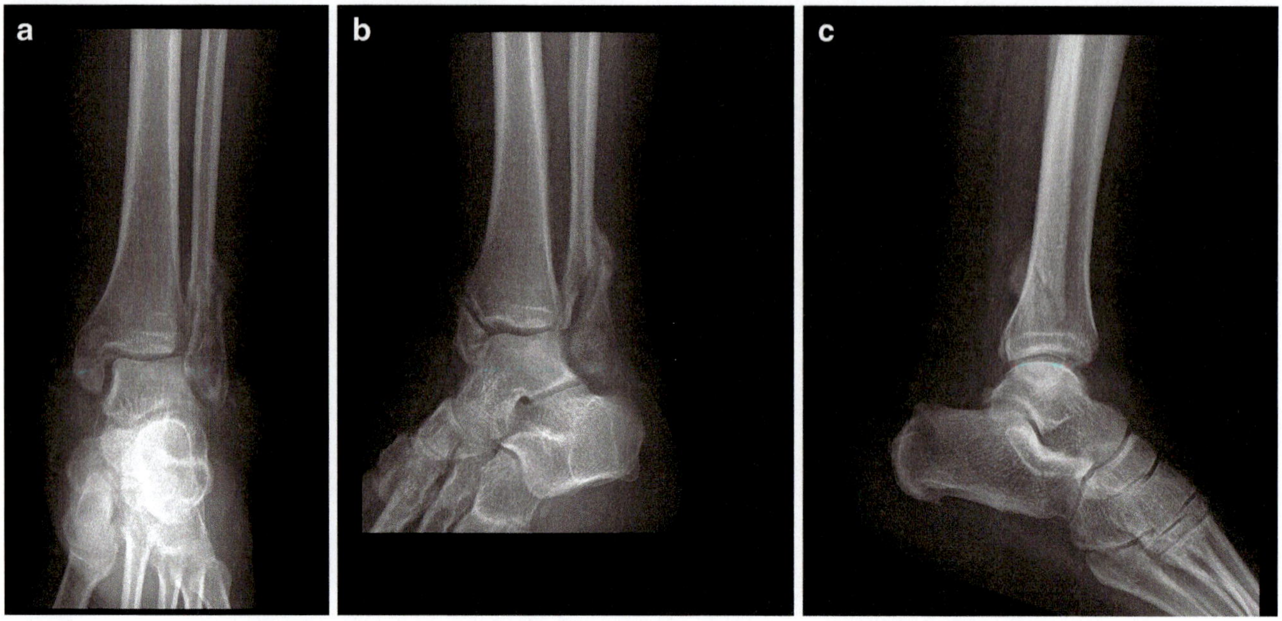

Fig. 28.17 Anterior-posterior (**a**), mortise (**b**), and lateral (**c**) ankle conventional radiographs of a 51-year-old female with a trimalleolar ankle fracture sustained 4 months prior treated nonoperatively at an outside facility presenting with resultant malunion/nonunion and pain with walking

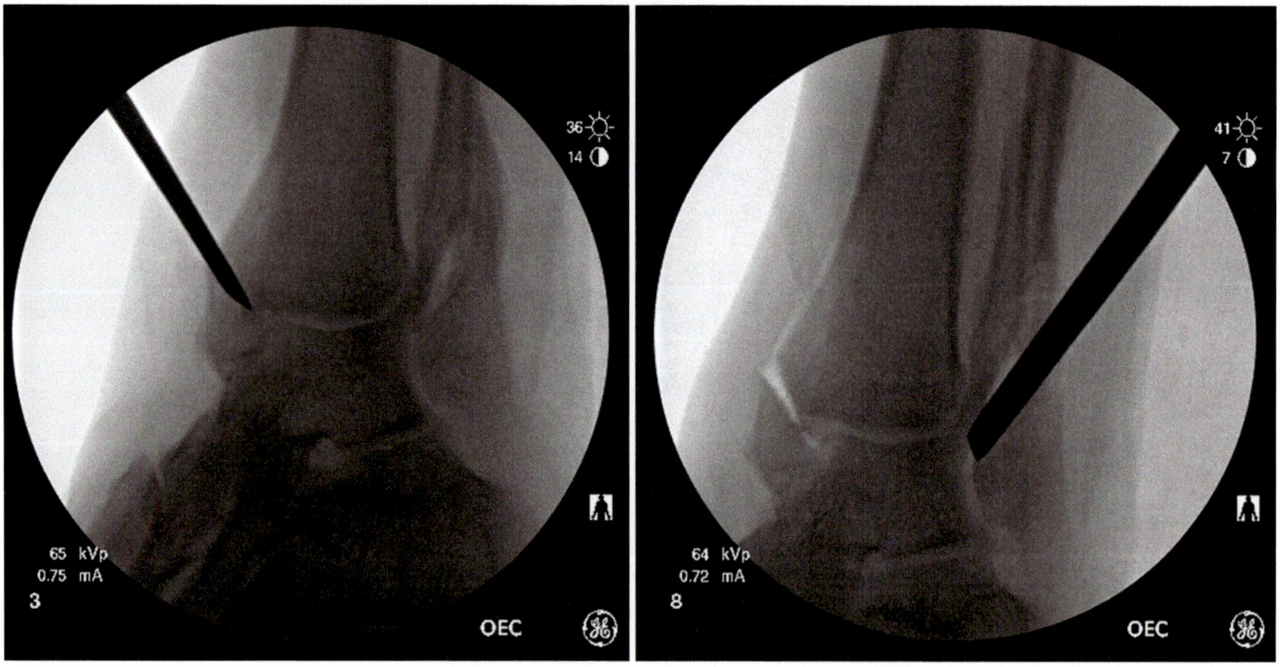

Fig. 28.18 Intraoperative fluoroscopy demonstrating medial malleolar osteotomy (**a**) and lateral malleolar osteotomy (**b**)

To reconstruct the anterior-inferior tibiofibular, interosseous, and posterior-inferior tibiofibular ligament, a 5.0 to 6.0 mm drill hole is made from anterior to posterior along the distal tibial just medial to the fibular notch (Fig. 28.42). For the interosseous ligament, a second 5.0 to 6.0 mm drill hole is placed lateral to medial from the fibula to the tibia intersecting the anterior to posterior hole (Fig. 28.43). Peroneus longus tendon allograft is secured with a whip or loop stitch using braided suture then passed from the tibial hole posteriorly through the transverse hole from medial to lateral with a

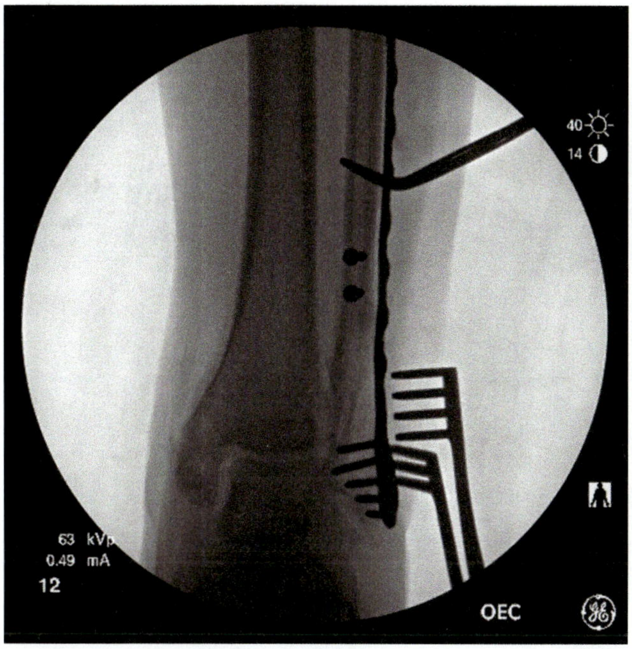

Fig. 28.19 Fibula is lengthened and stabilized with positional screws and locking plate

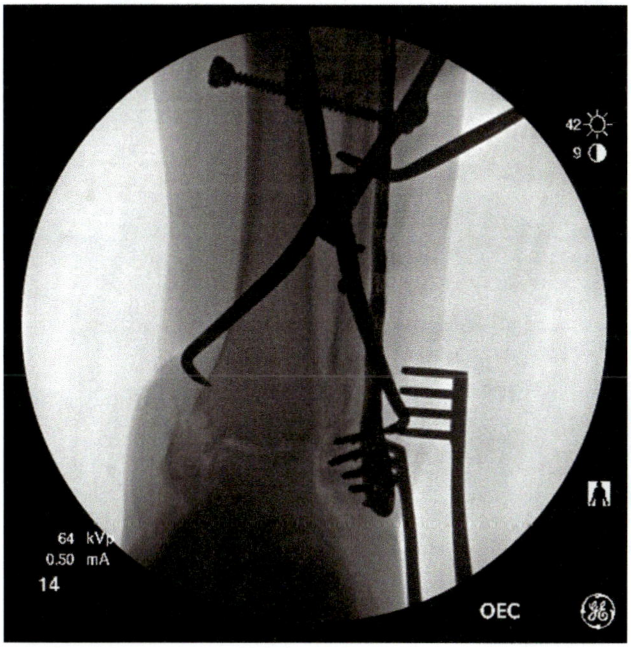

Fig. 28.20 Weber reduction forceps are used to reduce the chronic syndesmosis diastasis and allow the fibula to buttress the talus into the ankle mortise. Towel clamp is applied to the fibular malleolus to correct the talofibular articulation and concomitantly the syndesmosis

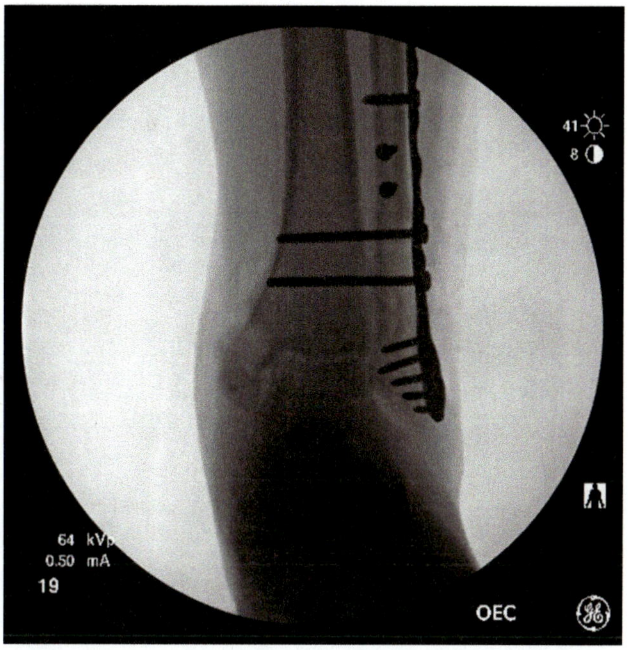

Fig. 28.21 Once fibular rotation is corrected, two-positional 3.5 mm tetracortical transyndesmotic screws are placed to maintain reduction of fibular rotation and syndesmosis

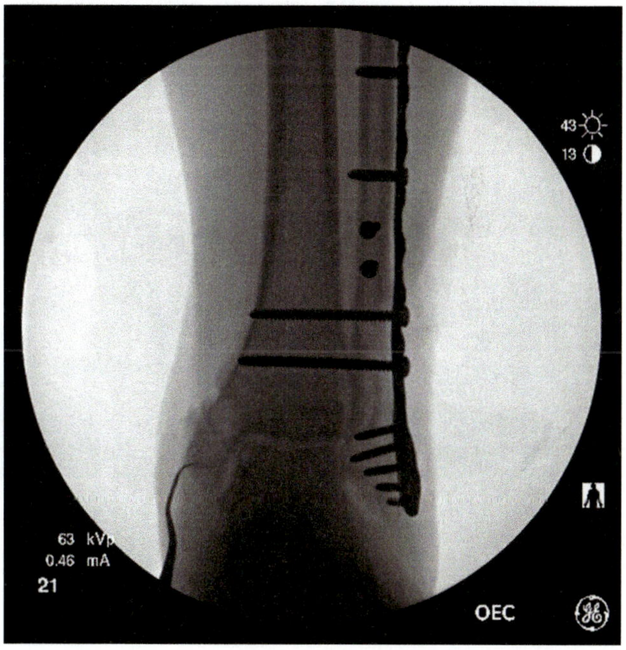

Fig. 28.22 Ankle is dorsiflexed to neutral position allowing the wider section of the talar dome to serve as an articular buttress for the talar-medial malleolar articulation reducing the medial malleolus

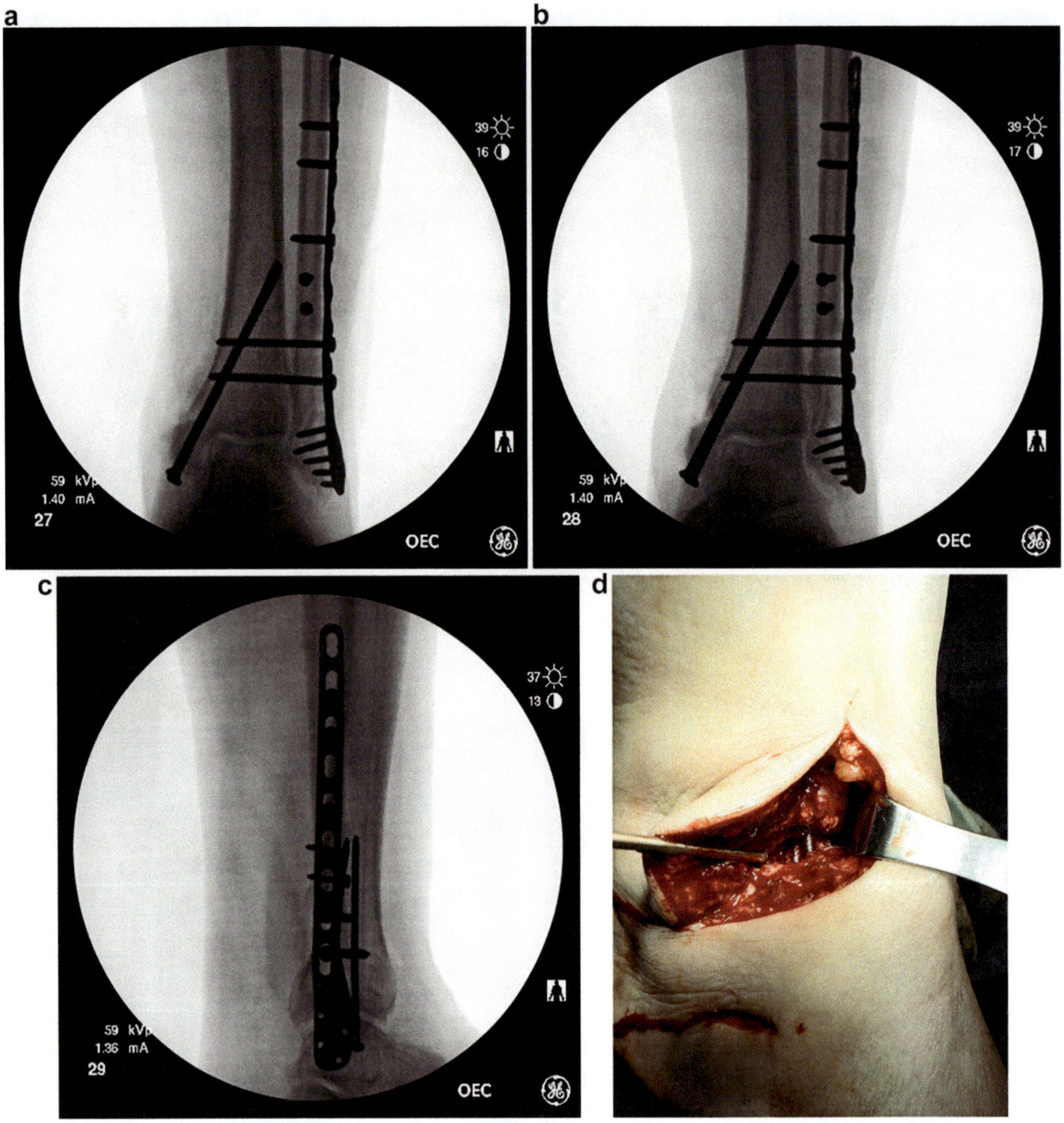

Fig. 28.23 Anterior-posterior (**a**), mortise (**b**), and lateral (**c**) ankle intraoperative fluoroscopy demonstrating restoration of radiographic parameters. Intraoperative view of medial malleolar deficit and positional screws maintaining deformity correction after medial malleolar osteotomy (**d**)

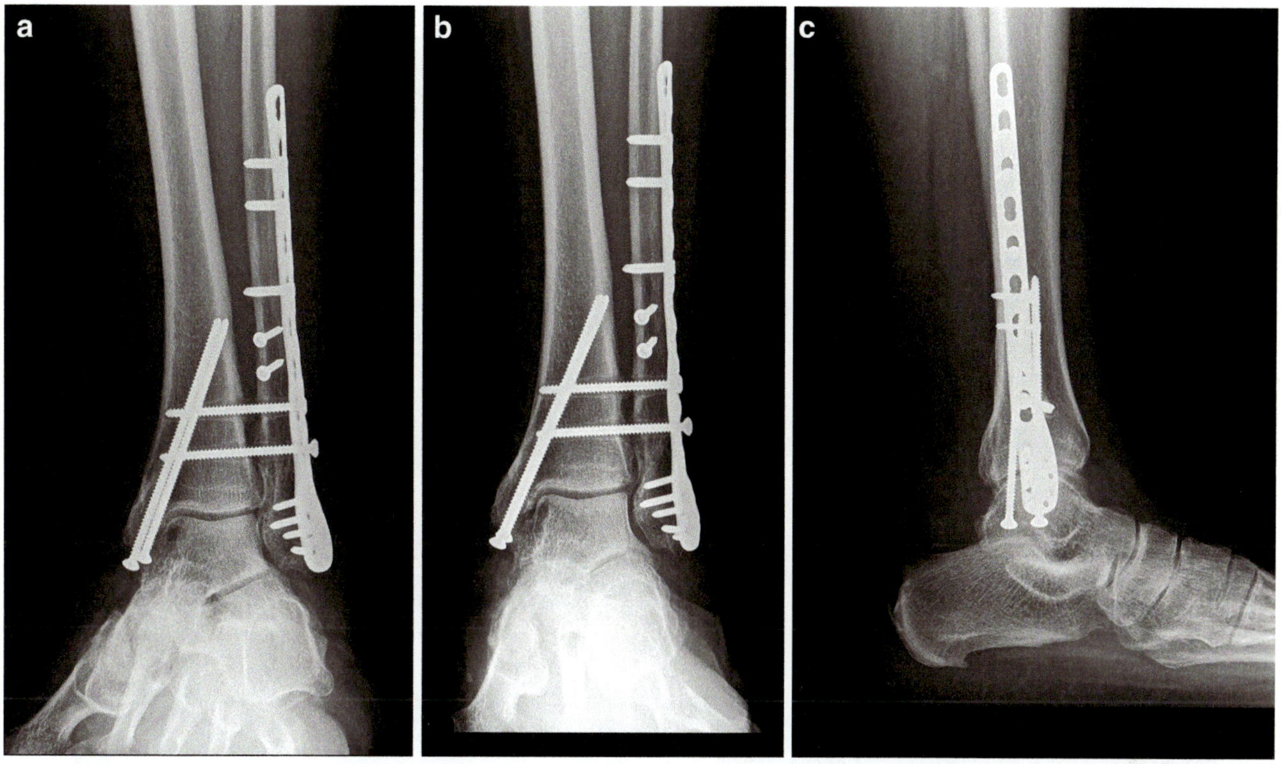

Fig. 28.24 Anterior-posterior (**a**), mortise (**b**), and lateral (**c**) ankle conventional radiographs 1-year postoperative follow-up demonstrating ankle mortise joint spaces maintained without early onset of posttraumatic arthritis

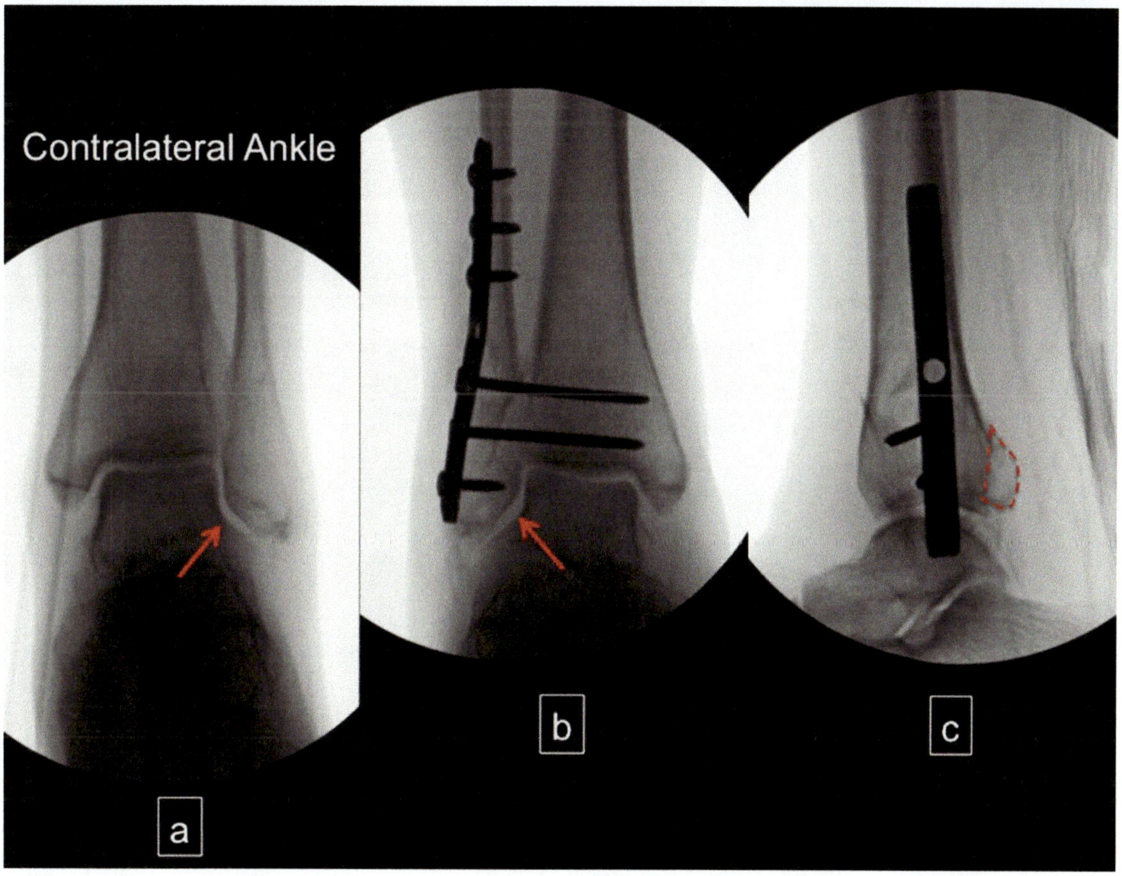

Fig. 28.25 Intraoperative fluoroscopy of an open reduction internal fixation of a comminuted fibular malleolar fracture from outside facility demonstrates a short and malrotated fibula (**b**) evidenced by widening of the fibular talar articulation at the inferior fibular flare and lateral process of talus (denoted by *red arrows*), loss of Shenton's line, and disruption of the subfibular circle when compared to contralateral ankle (**a**). Malreduction of the posterior malleolus is associated with fibular shortening or malrotation by the ligamentous attachment of both the superior and inferior fascicles PITFL. In this clinical case, the posterior malleolus follows the shortened fibula (**c**)

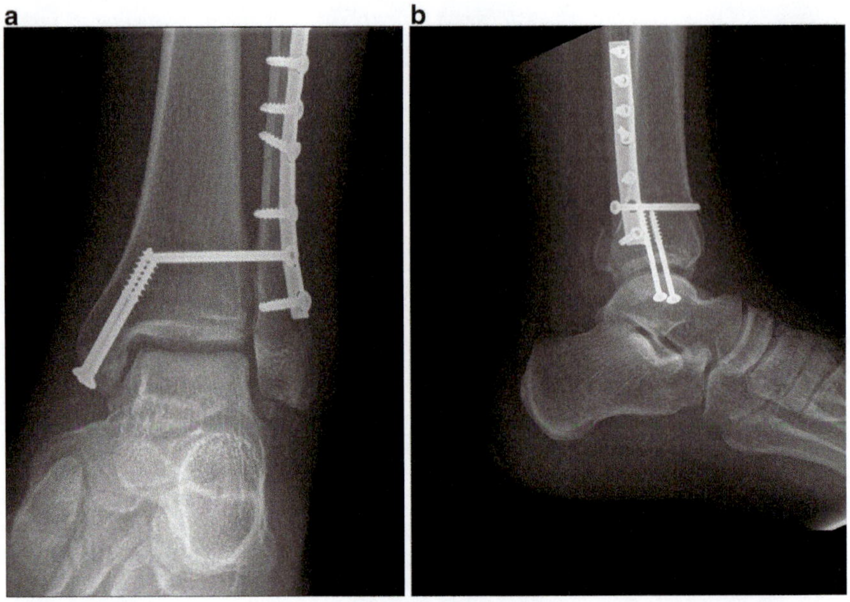

Fig. 28.26 Open reduction internal fixation of trimalleolar ankle fracture performed at outside facility presenting with anterior-posterior ankle radiograph (**a**) demonstrating a fibula appearing short but with satisfactory cortical alignment; however, lateral ankle radiograph (**b**) demonstrates posterior translation of the fibula. Posterior malleolus is concomitantly posteriorly displaced

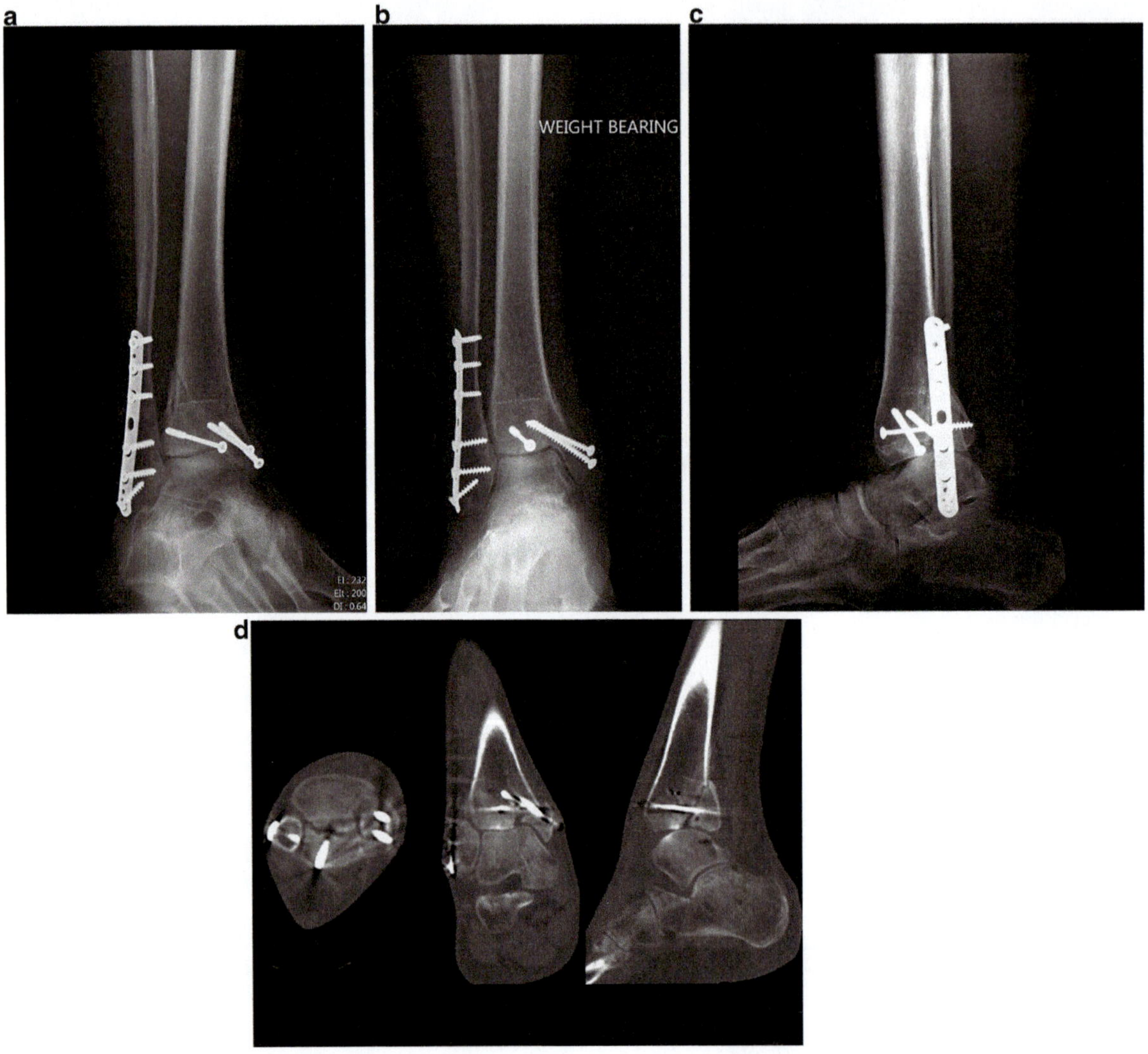

Fig. 28.27 Anterior-posterior (**a**), mortise (**b**), and lateral (**c**) ankle radiographs of a 54-year-old male 4 months' status post-open reduction internal fixation of trimalleolar ankle fracture performed at an outside facility presenting with persistent ankle pain and swelling. Radiographs demonstrate medial malleolar malunion (**a**) and posterior subluxation of the talus with posterior malleolar malunion/nonunion likely due to insufficient posterior malleolar fixation and syndesmosis instability (**c**). (**d**) CT scans demonstrates trimalleolar, posterior pilon fracture variant with medial and posterior malleolar malunion/partial nonunion

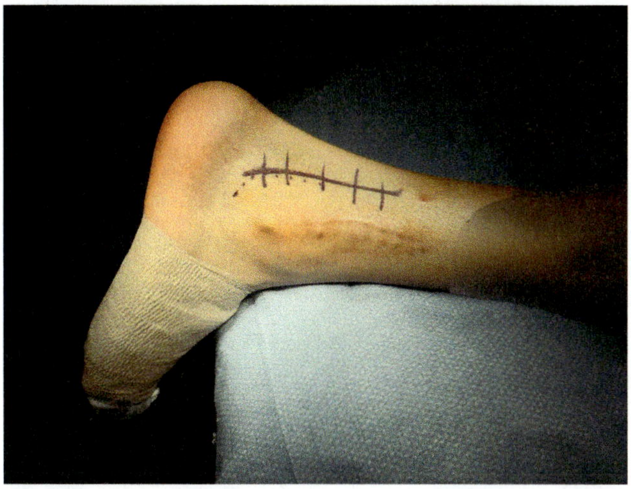

Fig. 28.28 Posterior-lateral incision is placed 1 cm posterior to the fibular malleolus

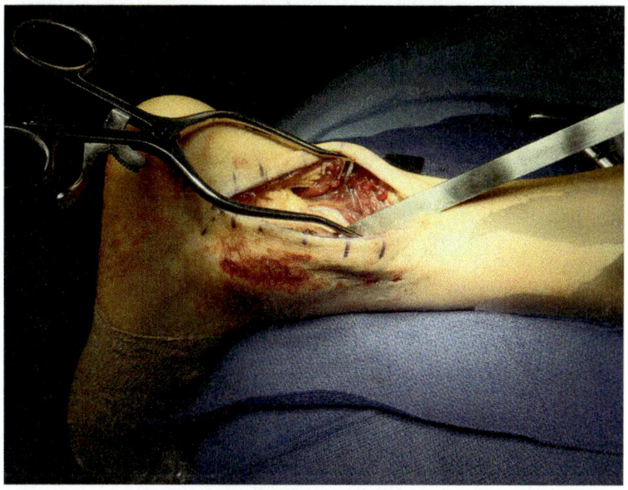

Fig. 28.29 Posterior-lateral incision provides direct exposure of the posterior malleolus. Dissection proceeds lateral to the peroneal tendons sheath; therefore, it is not necessary to disturb the peroneal tendons. Sural nerve is often seen with this exposure and gently retracted out of the surgical field

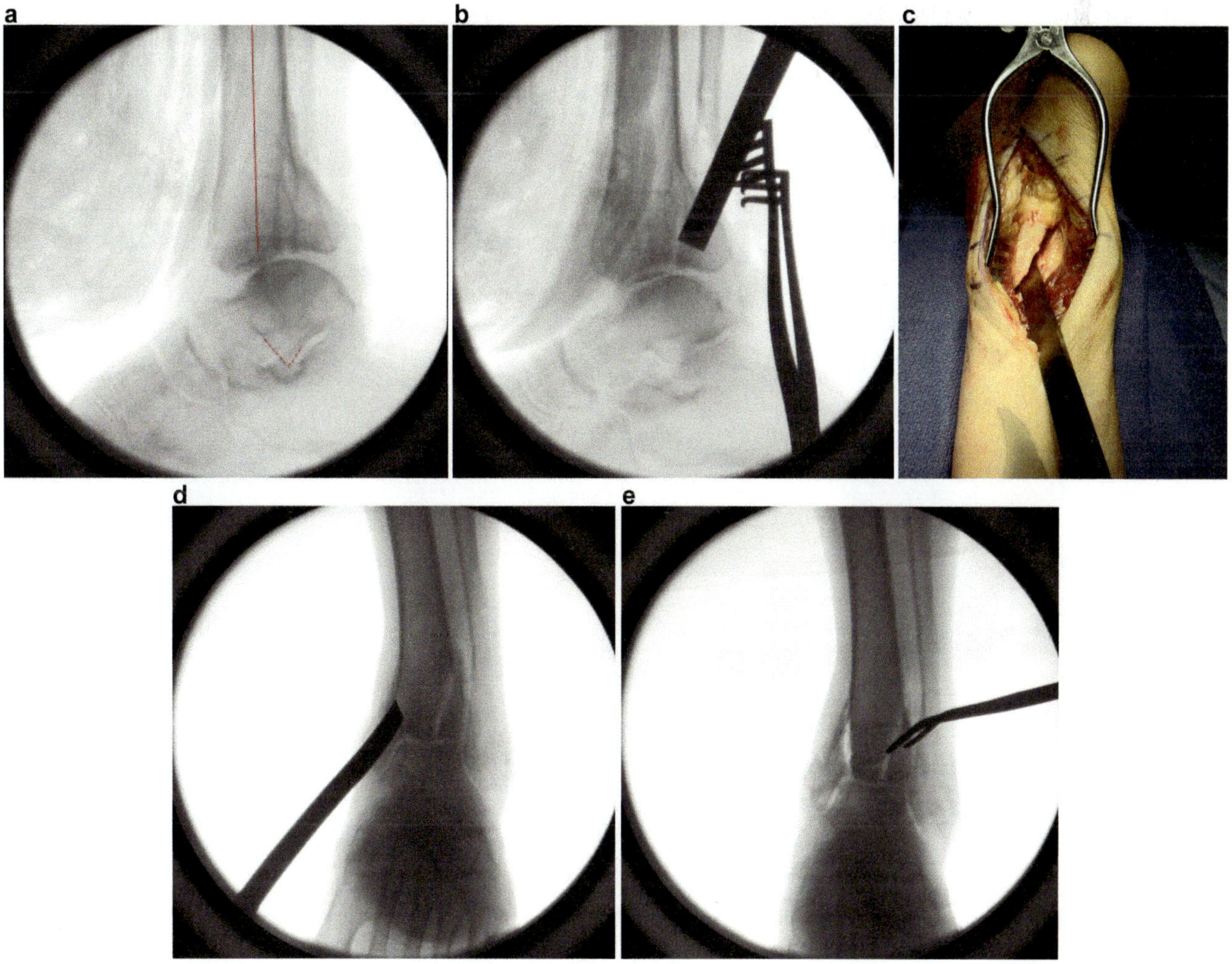

Fig. 28.30 Posterior malleolus malunion is shown after hardware removal. The talus is posteriorly subluxed shown with the lateral process of the talus (*dotted red*) and the middiaphyseal axis of the tibia (*red line*) (**a**). Posterior malleolar osteotomy performed under fluoroscopic (**b**) and intraoperative guidance (**c**). Medial malleolar osteotomy is performed under fluoroscopic guidance (**d**, **e**)

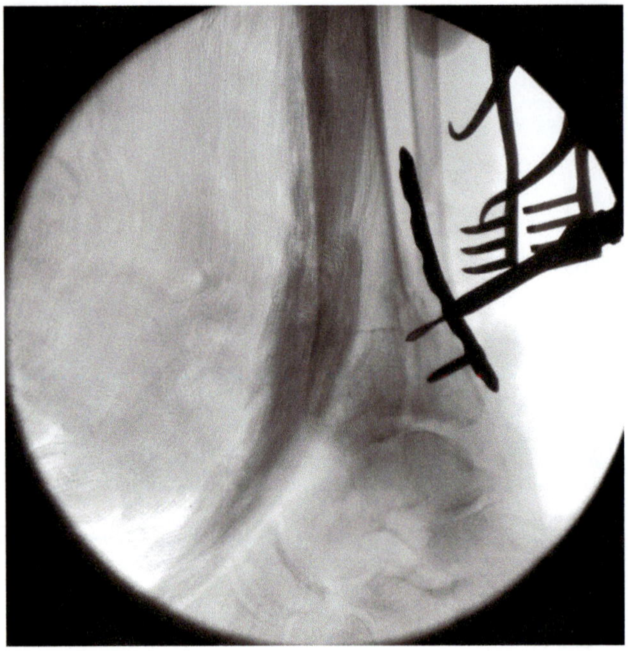

Fig. 28.31 A dynamic compression plate is contoured and affixed to the posterior malleolar fragment with locking screws

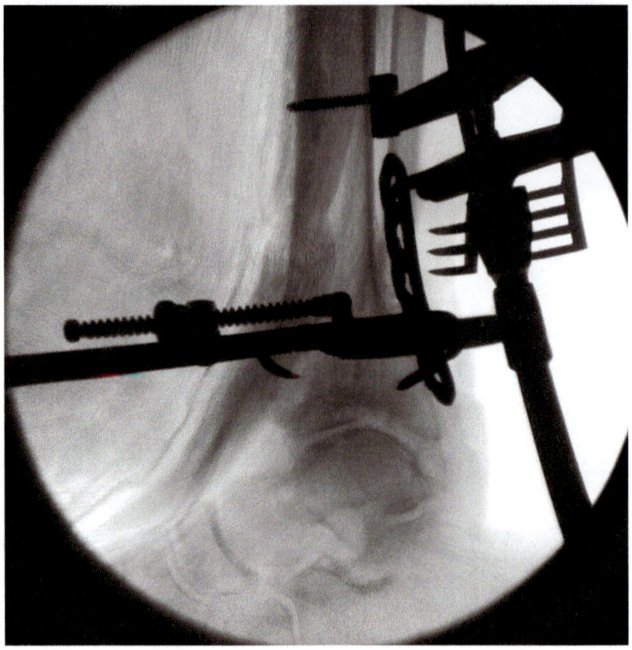

Fig. 28.32 A pair of periarticular reduction forceps is applied to prevent posterior displacement of the posterior malleolus while restoring length of the posterior malleolus. An articulated distractor is affixed to the proximal tibial articulated with the plate providing reduction under fluoroscopy until tibiotalar alignment is achieved

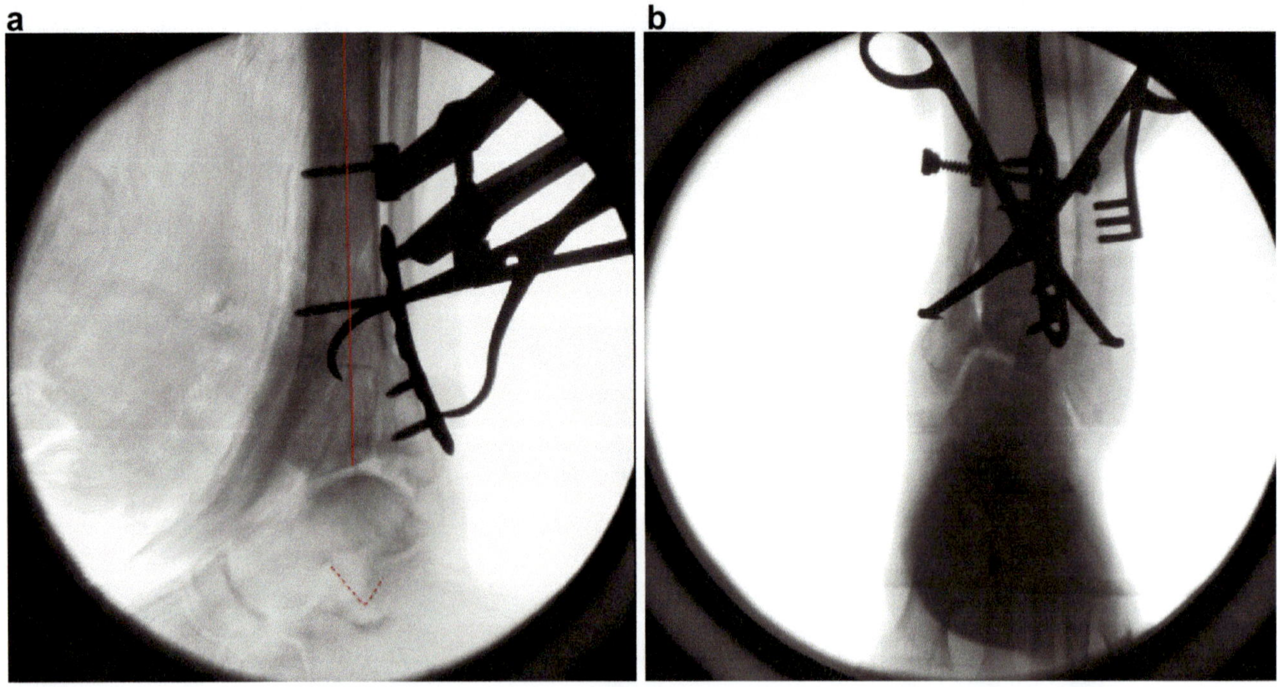

Fig. 28.33 Appropriate length of the posterior malleolus is demonstrated by alignment of the lateral process of the talus (*dotted red*) and the mid-diaphyseal axis of the tibia (*red line*) (**a**). Medial malleolus is then reduced with Weber reduction forceps

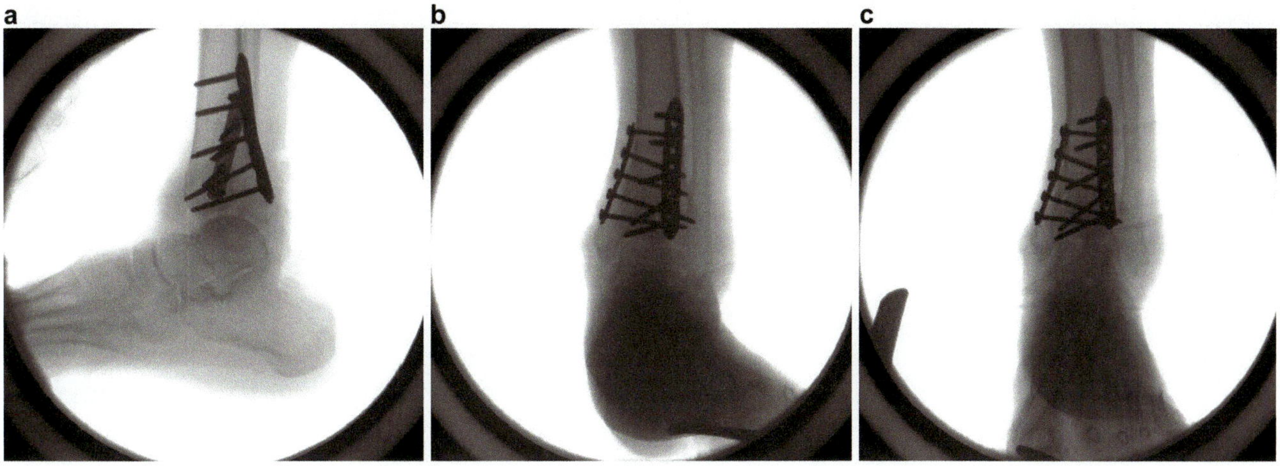

Fig. 28.34 Final fluoroscopic views of lateral (**a**), anterior-posterior (**b**), and mortise (**c**). The medial malleolus was reduced then stabilized with antiglide plate with positional screws

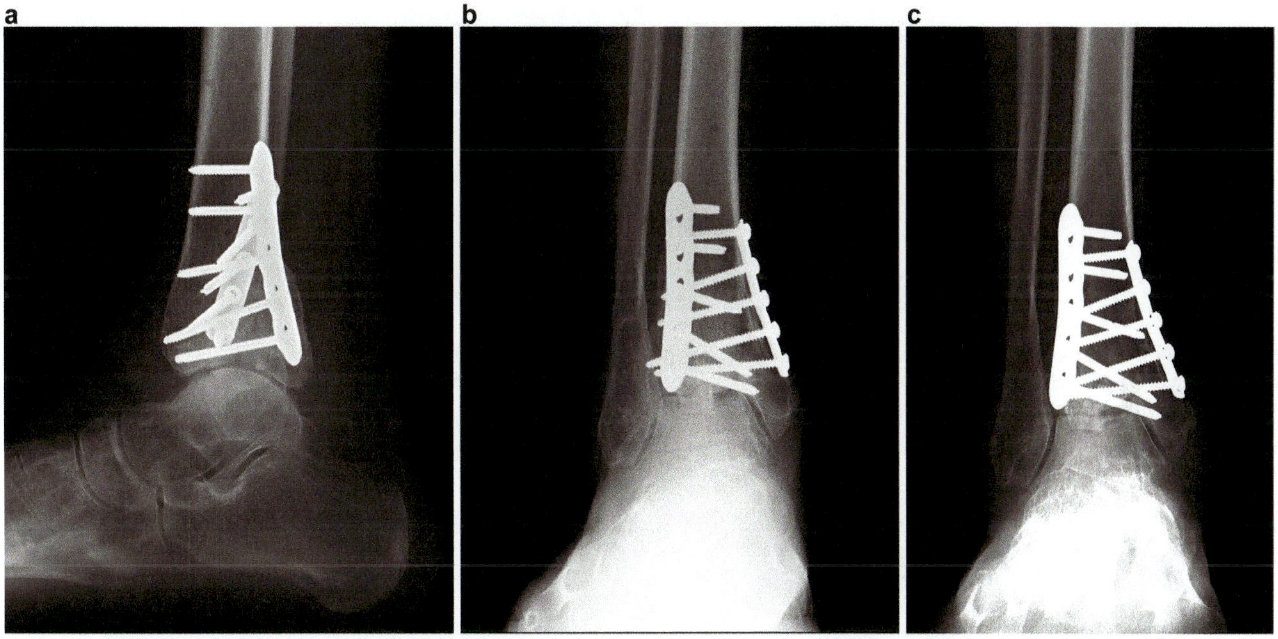

Fig. 28.35 Weightbearing radiographic views of lateral (**a**), anterior-posterior (**b**), and mortise (**c**). Patient is 9 months of postoperative weightbearing as tolerated

suture passer (Fig. 28.44a–c). The lead tendon is secured to the anterior tibial hole with an interference screw (Fig. 28.45). The posterior tail portion of the tendon allograft is pulled taut to remove any existing slack then sutured to the lead tendon (Figs. 28.46a, b, 28.47a–c, and 28.48).

Postoperative Course

Postoperative course for ankle malunion repair with spatial bony deficits or tendon allograft repair is short leg cast nonweightbearing for 10–12 weeks.

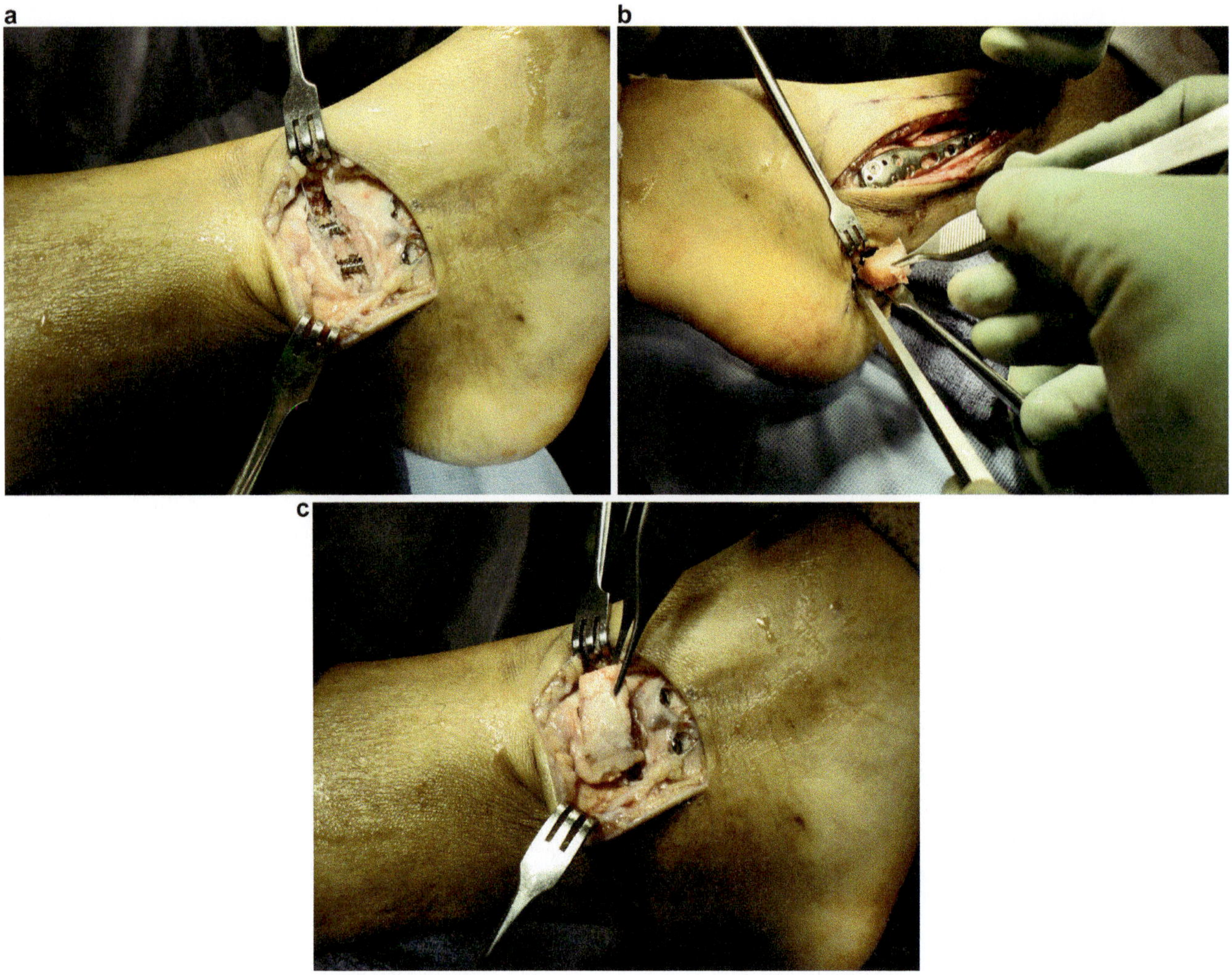

Fig. 28.36 Positional screws span across medial malleolar deficit after debridement of nonviable bone from nonunion and anatomic reduction of medial malleolus (**a**). Autogenous calcaneal bone harvest can provide cortical cancellous graft (**b**). Cortical cancellous graft is tamped press fit into the deficit (**c**)

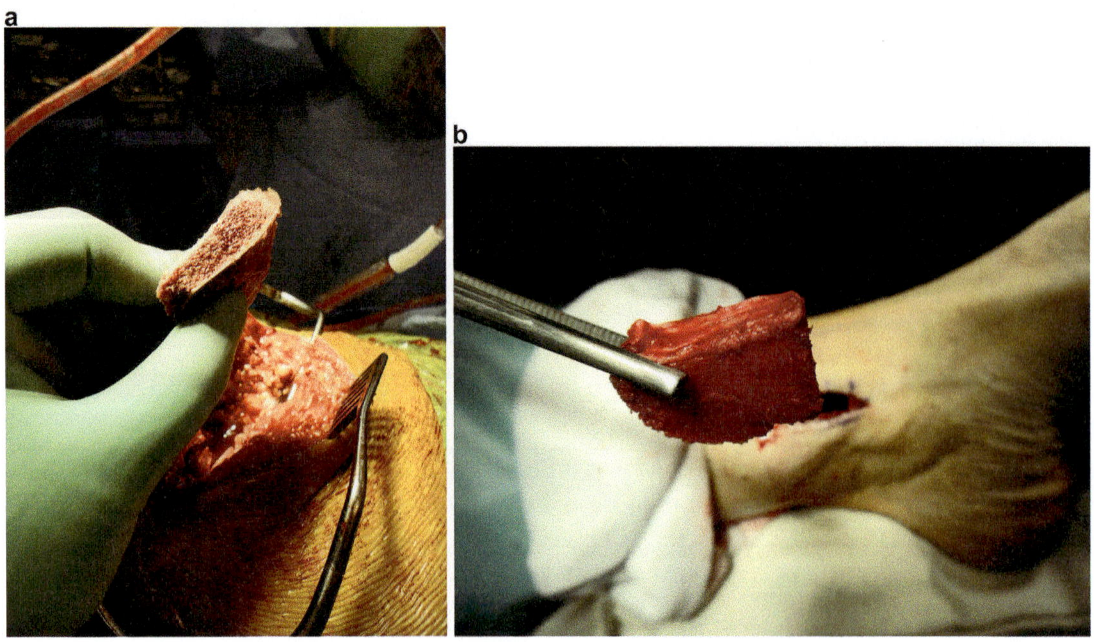

Fig. 28.37 Anterior superior iliac crest autogenous bone harvest provides the largest volume of cortical cancellous media with mesenchymal stem cells graft (**a**). Distal tibial autogenous bone harvest provides cortical cancellous sufficient for lower volume deficits

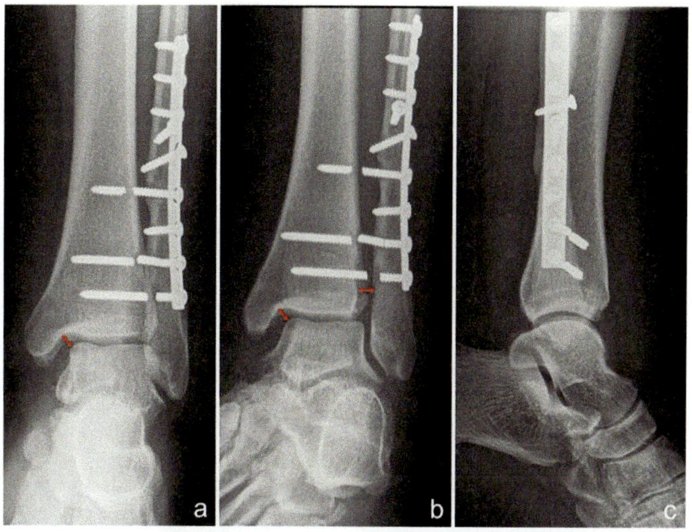

Fig. 28.38 Anterior-posterior (**a**), mortise (**b**), and lateral (**c**) ankle radiographs of a 24-year-old female 12 months' status post-open reduction internal fixation of Weber C fibular ankle fracture and syndesmosis disruption demonstrating loss of reduction at 6 months after surgery demonstrate by both medial and tibiofibular clear space widening (*red arrows*)

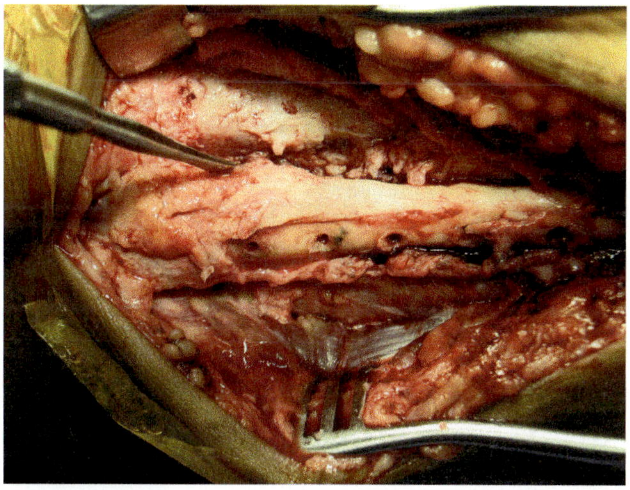

Fig. 28.39 Standard lateral approach shows no remnant syndesmotic ligament. Interval scar tissue is debrided to allow reduction of the syndesmosis

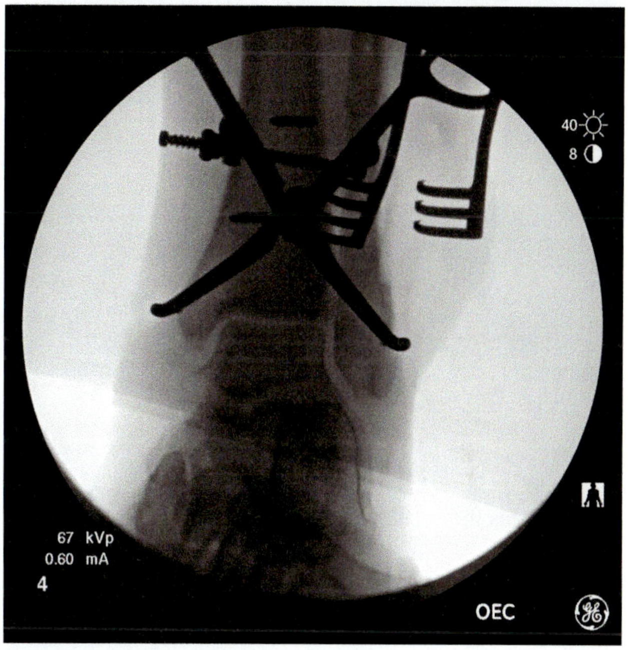

Fig. 28.40 Weber reduction forceps are placed along the biomechanical axis to reduce the syndesmosis

Nonweightbearing ankle range of motion exercise may be initiated at 4–6 weeks. Standing with progressive toe touch weightbearing is allowed at weeks 10–12 with radiographs verifying that there is no mechanical loosening of the screws. Physical therapy is ordered for balance and proprioceptive exercise, strengthening, and stretching.

References

1. Daly PJ, Fitzgerald Jr RH, Melton LJ, Ilstrup DM. Epidemiology of ankle fractures in Rochester, Minnesota. Acta Orthop Scand. 1987;58(5):539–44.
2. Jensen SL, Andresen BK, Mencke S, Nielsen PT. Epidemiology of ankle fractures. A prospective population-based study of 212 cases in Aalborg, Denmark. Acta Orthop Scand. 1998;69(1):48–50.

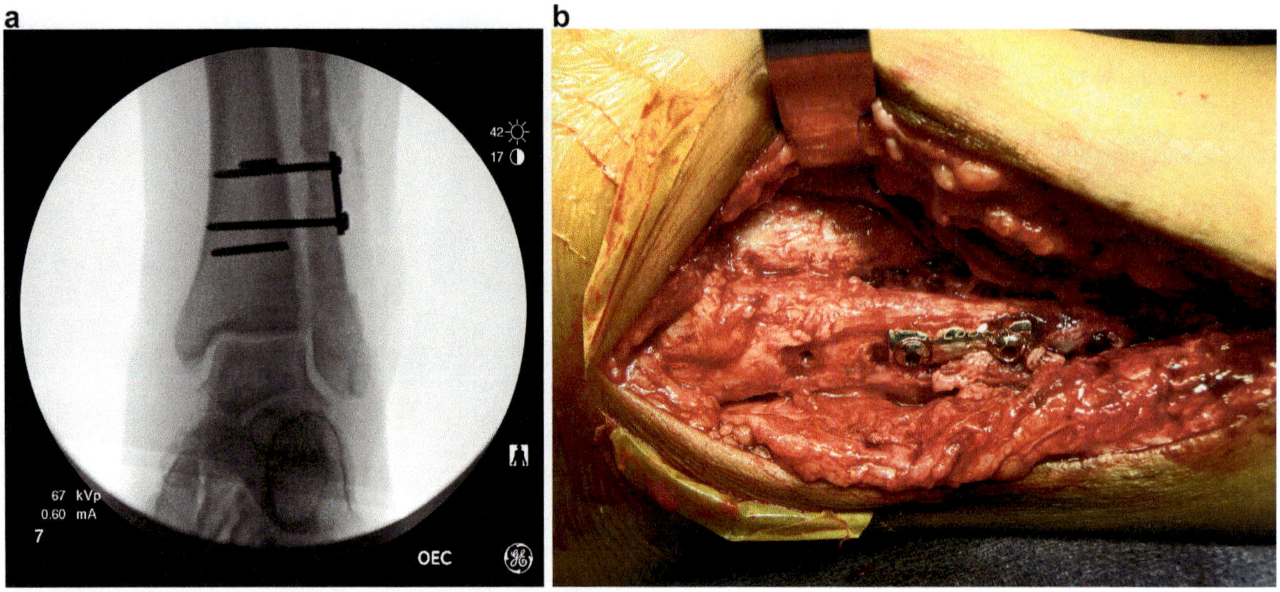

Fig. 28.41 Intraoperative fluoroscopic view of syndesmosis is stabilized with two-positional screws and two-hole 1/3 tubular plate (**a**). Intraoperative view of syndesmosis reduced without gap between the fibula and tibia (**b**)

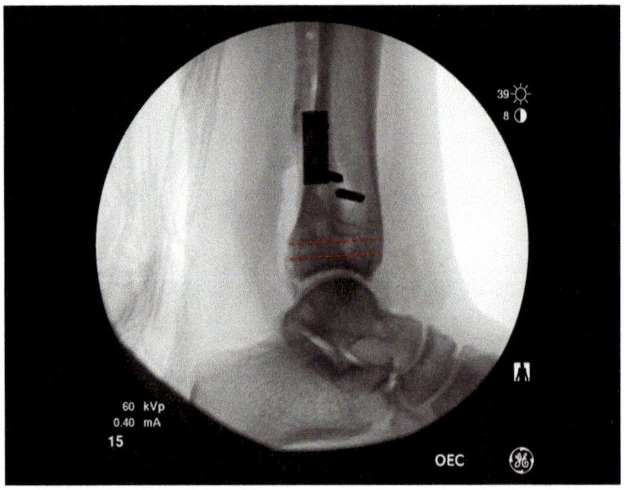

Fig. 28.42 Anterior-posterior drill hole placed along the distal tibial just medial to the fibular notch and 0.5 to 1.0 cm superior to the tibiotalar joint line

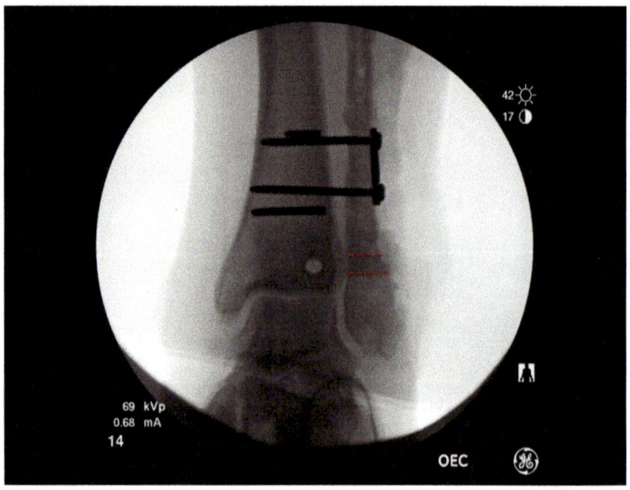

Fig. 28.43 Transverse lateral-medial drill hole from the fibula to the tibia intersecting the anterior to posterior hole seen just medial to the fibular notch

3. Davis JL, Giacopelli JA. Transfibular osteotomy in the correction of ankle joint incongruity. Journal Foot Ankle Surg : Off Publ Am Coll Foot Ankle Surg. 1995;34(4):389–99.
4. Ward AJ, Ackroyd CE, Baker AS. Late lengthening of the fibula for malaligned ankle fractures. J Bone Joint Surg Br. 1990;72(4):714–7.
5. Yablon IG, Leach RE. Reconstruction of malunited fractures of the lateral malleolus. J Bone Joint Surg Am. 1989;71(4):521–7.
6. Valderrabano V, Horisberger M, Russell I, Dougall H, Hintermann B. Etiology of ankle osteoarthritis. Clin Orthop Relat Res. 2009;467(7):1800–6.
7. Kimizuka M, Kurosawa H, Fukubayashi T. Load-bearing pattern of the ankle joint. Contact area and pressure distribution. Arch Orthop Trauma Surg Arch Orthop Unfall-Chir. 1980;96(1):45–9.
8. Tochigi Y, Rudert MJ, Saltzman CL, Amendola A, Brown TD. Contribution of articular surface geometry to ankle stabilization. J Bone Joint Surg Am. 2006;88(12):2704–13.
9. Ramsey PL, Hamilton W. Changes in tibiotalar area of contact caused by lateral talar shift. J Bone Joint Surg Am. 1976;58(3):356–7.
10. Thordarson DB, Motamed S, Hedman T, Ebramzadeh E, Bakshian S. The effect of fibular malreduction on contact pres-

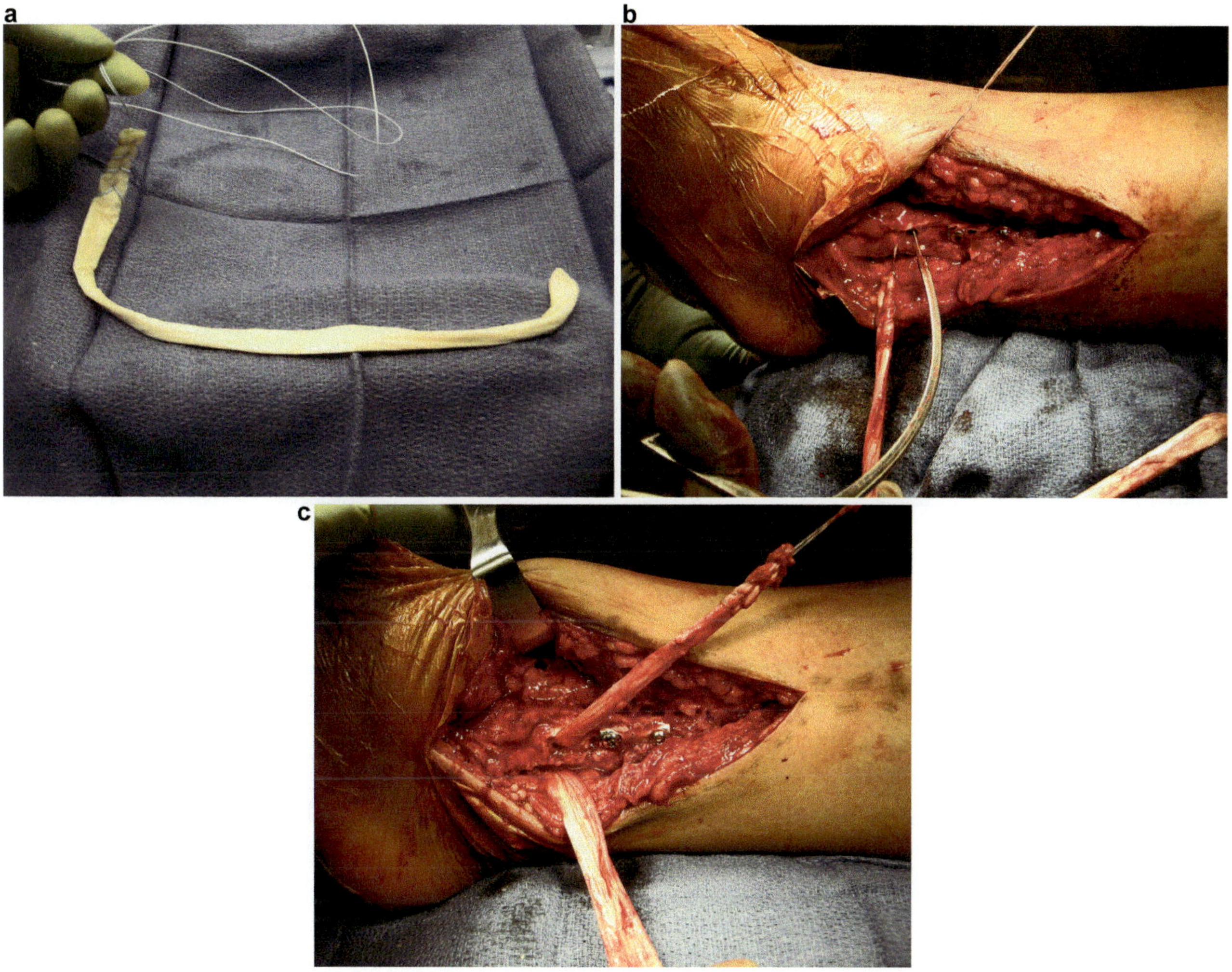

Fig. 28.44 Peroneus longus tendon allograft is secured with a whip or loop stitch using braided suture (**a**) then passed from the posterior hole through the transverse hole with a suture passer (**b**, **c**)

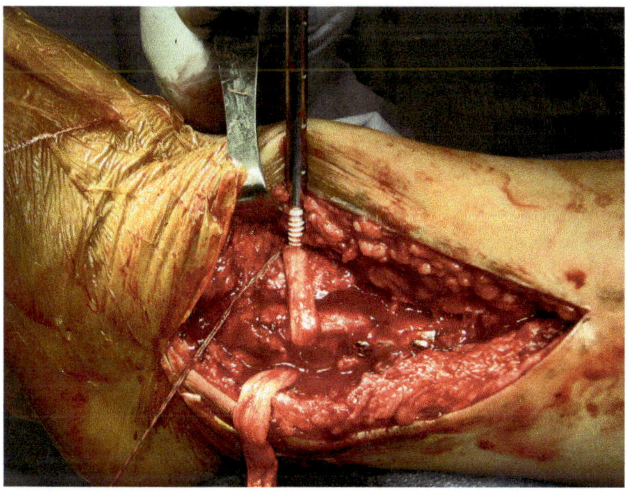

Fig. 28.45 The lead tendon is shown secured to the anterior hole with an interference screw

sures in an ankle fracture malunion model. J Bone Joint Surg Am. 1997;79(12):1809–15.

11. Lindsjo U. Operative treatment of ankle fracture-dislocations. A follow-up study of 306/321 consecutive cases. Clin Orthop Relat Res. 1985;199:28–38.
12. Rukavina A. The role of fibular length and the width of the ankle mortise in post-traumatic osteoarthrosis after malleolar fracture. Int Orthop. 1998;22(6):357–60.
13. De Vries JS, Wijgman AJ, Sierevelt IN, Schaap GR. Long-term results of ankle fractures with a posterior malleolar fragment. J Foot Ankle Surg: Off Publ Am Coll Foot Ankle Surg. 2005;44(3):211–7.
14. Jaskulka RA, Ittner G, Schedl R. Fractures of the posterior tibial margin: their role in the prognosis of malleolar fractures. J Trauma. 1989;29(11):1565–70.
15. Ovaska MT, Makinen TJ, Madanat R, Kiljunen V, Lindahl J. A comprehensive analysis of patients with malreduced ankle fractures undergoing re-operation. Int Orthop. 2014;38(1):83–8.
16. Stufkens SA, van den Bekerom MP, Kerkhoffs GM, Hintermann B, van Dijk CN. Long-term outcome after 1822 operatively treated ankle fractures: a systematic review of the literature. Injury. 2011;42(2):119–27.

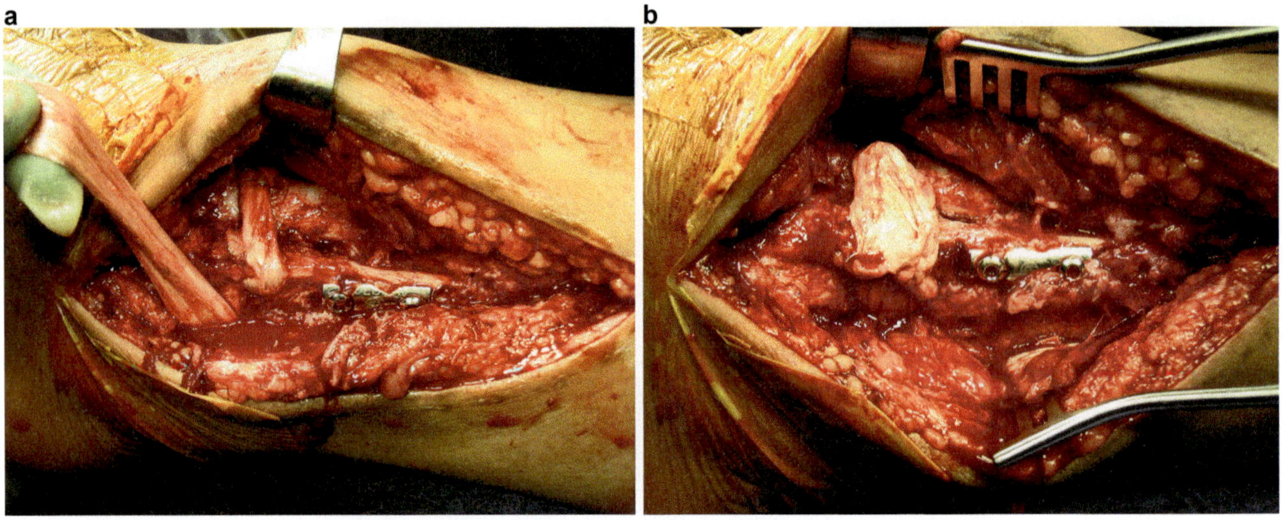

Fig. 28.46 The posterior tail portion of the tendon allograft is pulled taut to remove any existing slack (**a**) then sutured to the lead tendon (**b**)

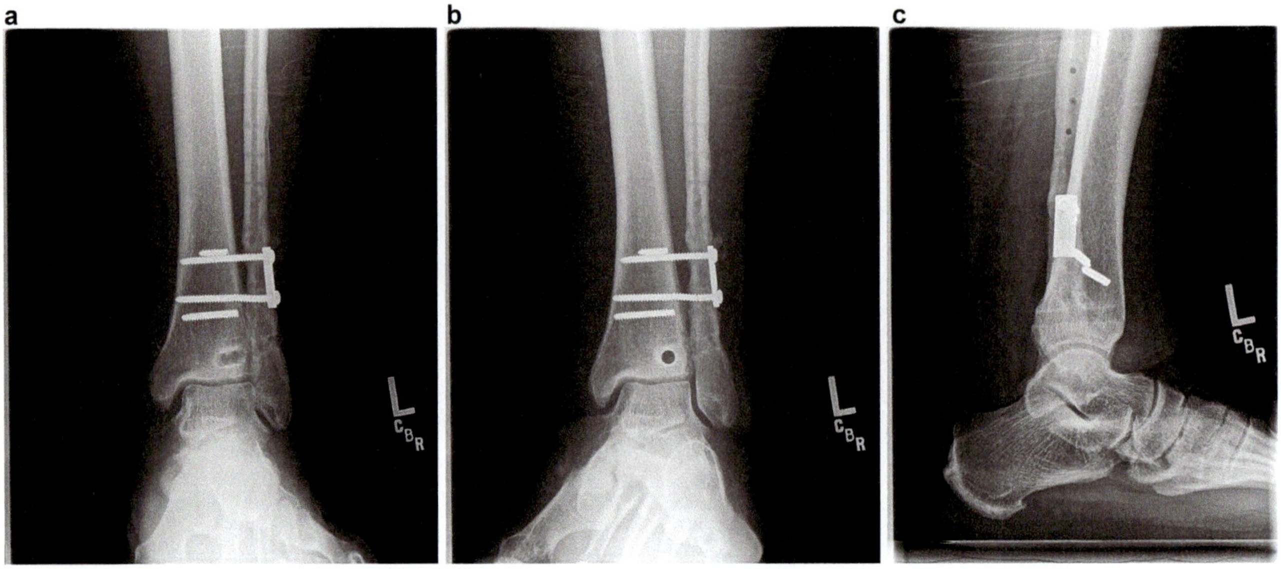

Fig. 28.47 Anterior-posterior (**a**), mortise (**b**), and lateral (**c**) ankle radiographs. Patient with 1-year status post-syndesmosis reconstruction with tendon allograft

17. Vosseller JT, Karl JW, Greisberg JK. Incidence of syndesmotic injury. Orthopedics. 2014;37(3):e226–9.
18. Tornetta III P, Axelrad TW, Sibai TA, Creevy WR. Treatment of the stress positive ligamentous SE4 ankle fracture: incidence of syndesmotic injury and clinical decision making. J Orthop Trauma. 2012;26(11):659–61.
19. Gardner MJ, Demetrakopoulos D, Briggs SM, Helfet DL, Lorich DG. Malreduction of the tibiofibular syndesmosis in ankle fractures. Foot Ankle Int. 2006;27(10):788–92.
20. Beumer A, van Hemert WL, Niesing R, Entius CA, Ginai AZ, Mulder PG, et al. Radiographic measurement of the distal tibiofibular syndesmosis has limited use. Clin Orthop Relat Res. 2004;423:227–34.
21. Ebraheim NA, Lu J, Yang H, Mekhail AO, Yeasting RA. Radiographic and CT evaluation of tibiofibular syndesmotic diastasis: a cadaver study. Foot Ankle Int. 1997;18(11):693–8.
22. Nielson JH, Gardner MJ, Peterson MG, Sallis JG, Potter HG, Helfet DL, et al. Radiographic measurements do not predict syndesmotic injury in ankle fractures: an MRI study. Clin Orthop Relat Res. 2005;436:216–21.
23. Marmor M, Hansen E, Han HK, Buckley J, Matityahu A. Limitations of standard fluoroscopy in detecting rotational malreduction of the syndesmosis in an ankle fracture model. Foot Ankle Int. 2011;32(6):616–22.
24. Sagi HC, Shah AR, Sanders RW. The functional consequence of syndesmotic joint malreduction at a minimum 2-year follow-up. J Orthop Trauma. 2012;26(7):439–43.

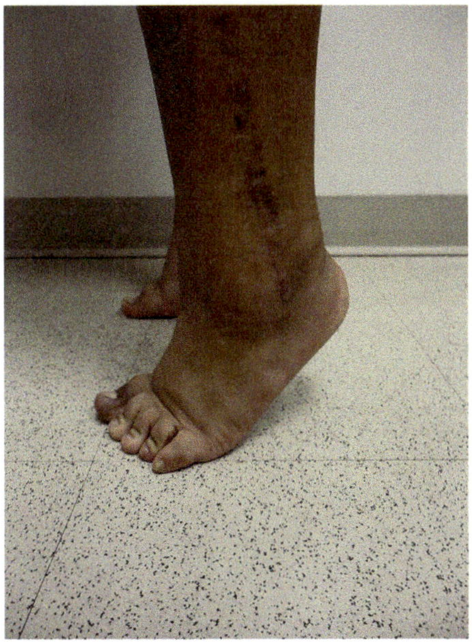

Fig. 28.48 Clinical photo shows patient with greater than 1-year status post-syndesmosis reconstruction with tendon allograft without pain nor stiffness able to perform heel rise and hop test

25. Weening B, Bhandari M. Predictors of functional outcome following transsyndesmotic screw fixation of ankle fractures. J Orthop Trauma. 2005;19(2):102–8.
26. Miller AN, Carroll EA, Parker RJ, Helfet DL, Lorich DG. Posterior malleolar stabilization of syndesmotic injuries is equivalent to screw fixation. Clin Orthop Relat Res. 2010;468(4):1129–35.
27. Sarkisian JS, Cody GW. Closed treatment of ankle fractures: a new criterion for evaluation - a review of 250 cases. J Trauma. 1976;16(4):323–6.
28. Rolfe B, Nordt W, Sallis JG, Distefano M. Assessing fibular length using bimalleolar angular measurements. Foot Ankle. 1989;10(2):104–9.
29. Weber BG, Simpson LA. Corrective lengthening osteotomy of the fibula. Clin Orthop Relat Res. 1985;199:61–7.
30. Lepojarvi S, Pakarinen H, Savola O, Haapea M, Sequeiros RB, Niinimaki J. Posterior translation of the fibula may indicate malreduction: CT study of normal variation in uninjured ankles. J Orthop Trauma. 2014;28(4):205–9.
31. Knops SP, Kohn MA, Hansen EN, Matityahu A, Marmor M. Rotational malreduction of the syndesmosis: reliability and accuracy of computed tomography measurement methods. Foot Ankle Int. 2013;34(10):1403–10.
32. Malhotra G, Cameron J, Toolan BC. Diagnosing chronic diastasis of the syndesmosis: a novel measurement using computed tomography. Foot Ankle Int. 2014;35(5):483–8.
33. Nault ML, Hebert-Davies J, Laflamme GY, Leduc S. CT scan assessment of the syndesmosis: a new reproducible method. J Orthop Trauma. 2013;27(11):638–41.
34. Miller AN, Carroll EA, Parker RJ, Boraiah S, Helfet DL, Lorich DG. Direct visualization for syndesmotic stabilization of ankle fractures. Foot Ankle Int. 2009;30(5):419–26.
35. Raasch WG, Larkin JJ, Draganich LF. Assessment of the posterior malleolus as a restraint to posterior subluxation of the ankle. J Bone Joint Surg Am. 1992;74(8):1201–6.
36. O'Connor TJ, Mueller B, Ly TV, Jacobson AR, Nelson ER, Cole PA. "A top" screw versus posterolateral plate for posterior malleolus fixation in trimalleolar ankle fractures. J Orthop Trauma. 2015;29(4):e151–6.
37. Geideman W, Early JS, Brodsky J. Clinical results of harvesting autogenous cancellous graft from the ipsilateral proximal tibia for use in foot and ankle surgery. Foot Ankle Int. 2004;25(7):451–5.
38. O'Keeffe Jr RM, Riemer BL, Butterfield SL. Harvesting of autogenous cancellous bone graft from the proximal tibial metaphysis. A review of 230 cases. J Orthop Trauma. 1991;5(4):469–74.
39. Raikin SM, Brislin K. Local bone graft harvested from the distal tibia or calcaneus for surgery of the foot and ankle. Foot Ankle Int. 2005;26(6):449–53.
40. Beals TC, Manoli II A. Late syndesmosis reconstruction: a case report. Foot Ankle Int. 1998;19(7):485–8.
41. Grass R, Rammelt S, Biewener A, Zwipp H. Peroneus longus ligamentoplasty for chronic instability of the distal tibiofibular syndesmosis. Foot Ankle Int. 2003;24(5):392–7.
42. Morris MW, Rice P, Schneider TE. Distal tibiofibular syndesmosis reconstruction using a free hamstring autograft. Foot Ankle Int. 2009;30(6):506–11.
43. Olson KM, Dairyko Jr GH, Toolan BC. Salvage of chronic instability of the syndesmosis with distal tibiofibular arthrodesis: functional and radiographic results. J Bone Joint Surg Am. 2011;93(1):66–72.

Ankle Arthrodesis

29

Jason A. Piraino and Chrisitne P. Miller

Introduction

Ankle arthrodesis has been a time-tested procedure for the treatment of a variety of ankle pathologies. It is still considered the gold standard for treatment of a painful ankle joint. While the procedure is not without its shortcomings, if performed successfully, the procedure can be rewarding for both patient and surgeon alike.

The history of ankle arthrodesis follows the scientific development of surgery through the centuries. Though there is evidence that some ancient cultures, namely, the Aztecs and Incas, utilized internal fixation devices, it is not until the nineteenth century where this surgical technique becomes more widely used [1].

In the United States, the Civil War drove the technical surgical advances of internal fixation consisting of metal wire and brass pins but with limited success largely due to the absence of infection control [2]. In 1877, Dr. Joseph Lister performed internal fixation of a patellar fracture with a wire while applying an antiseptic agent (carbolic acid) [3]. Austrian surgeon, Eduard Albert, first used the term "arthrodesis" in 1878, when he performed surgical fusions on both knees and ankles of a 14-year-old child with severe palsy [4]. Within the next decade, German surgeon, Carl Hansmann, performed the first internal plate fixation using a removable steel plate and nickel screws in 1886 [5].

By the twentieth century, the menace of postoperative infection was tamed with the discovery of penicillin in 1928 [6]. Throughout the rest of the century and still today, arthrodesis remains a reliable procedure to reduce joint pain and provide stability.

J.A. Piraino (✉) • C.P. Miller
Department of Orthopaedics-Division of Foot and Ankle, University of Florida College of Medicine-Jacksonville, 655 West 8th Street, Jacksonville, 32209 FL, USA
e-mail: Jason.piraino@jax.ufl.edu

While it may seem the incidence of ankle arthrodesis has decreased in recent years due to the advent of total ankle arthroplasty, some studies have shown little to no decrease in incidence. One recent study by Best, displayed a 58% increase in ankle arthrodesis from 1994 to 2006 [7]. Two trends in this particular study were apparent: the increased use of the arthroscopic-assisted ankle arthrodesis and a transition from inpatient to ambulatory procedures. Terrel reported an increased number of arthroplasties from 2004 to 2009, however no change in the percentage of arthrodesis procedures [8]. Arthroscopic ankle arthrodesis appears to be gaining popularity as the authors also found a significant increase in the arthroscopic technique over this time period. Anecdotally it appears within the last 5 years that total ankle arthroplasty has gained traction over ankle arthrodesis for the subset of patients with ankle osteoarthritis. This is likely to have a twofold effect on the arthrodesis procedure: (1) Complications of the arthroplasty procedure will require a much more technically demanding ankle arthrodesis, and (2) the more complicated patients that are not candidates for implant arthroplasty will require arthrodesis, which may contribute to making the procedure more challenging. These two factors have the potential to lead to increased complications, as increasing the complexity of any case often leads to increasing complication rates.

Successful osseous union relies on a variety of factors including high contact area, rigid immobilization, and increased compression at the site of arthrodesis [9].

Uncomplicated open ankle arthrodesis has been shown to be efficacious for the treatment of ankle arthritis with a reported complication rate as low as 9% [10]. Arthroscopic ankle arthrodesis has also been shown to be a safe an effective treatment option with nonunion rates reported in a systematic review by Roukis at 8.6% [11]. Overall the complication rate for any ankle arthrodesis has been reported between 15 and 20% [12]. While complications of ankle arthrodesis are uncommon, they can be equally devastating to both patient and surgeon alike. As surgeons, we must be ever more vigilant to identify and be prepared for any and all complications associated with the surgeries we perform.

M.S. Lee, J.P. Grossman (eds.), *Complications in Foot and Ankle Surgery*, DOI 10.1007/978-3-319-53686-6_29

Indications

Painful end-stage arthritis of the ankle joint is the leading indication for arthrodesis [13]. Arthritis, secondary to trauma, accounts for roughly 70% of patients undergoing ankle arthrodesis, while a smaller group (12%) had inflammatory arthritis [14]. It is important to distinguish between inflammatory and noninflammatory arthritis for proper pre-, peri-, and postoperative management [14]. Patients with rheumatoid arthritis (RA) require special consideration due to the progressive inflammatory nature of the disease which often leads to diminished bone stock and impaired ability to heal from the use of disease-modifying anti-rheumatic drugs (DMARDs) [15]. Neuropathic (Charcot) arthropathy in advanced cases causes aggressive joint destabilization where in an arthrodesis may be warranted.

The epidemic of obesity has been on the rise in this nation over the past 20 years with 54.4% of American adults exceeding the healthy weight standards [16]. The association between end-stage arthritis and elevated body mass index (BMI) is ever-relevant [16]. The use of ankle arthrodesis is a viable option to reduce pain and disability in this patient population [17]. Avascular necrosis of the talus (AVN) with associated degenerative arthritis can be challenging for surgical management due to impaired osseous healing potential and ankle deformity [18]. Selecting the best technique for ankle arthrodesis can be controversial depending on the condition of the talus, but arthrodesis remains a viable option to restore stability [19].

Other conditions that benefit from arthrodesis of the ankle include previous infection (septic joint), tumor resection, and salvage for failed total ankle arthroplasty (TAA) or open reduction internal fixation (ORIF) [20].

Contraindications

The list of contraindications for ankle arthrodesis is quite minimal. The presence of an active infection, lack of adequate blood supply, and insufficient bone stock to support fixation are the most common [20]. The severity of osteoporosis, a prominent feature in both the rheumatoid and alcoholic patient populations, is a major factor in surgical planning.

Pearls and Pitfalls

Dealing with a complication can often be a complex task. The greatest recommendation about the ankle arthrodesis procedure is a thorough patient assessment. It is most important to address why the complication occurred rather than shy away from it. Typically this author will perform a root cause analysis as to why the complication occurred. It is important to think through the complication critically, to identify who, what, when, where, and why the complication occurred. Inevitably it comes down to either patient-related issues, surgeon-related issues, or combination of both in most cases.

Patient Factors

While it may be easy to blame the patient for a complication, it is of the utmost importance to understand that the patient may not be fully at fault, or they may not have factors in their control.

Noncompliant Patient

The noncompliant patient is not uncommon to any surgeon. One of the most critically important aspects of a preoperative workup is a thorough history and physical examination including a socioeconomic understanding of the patient's home life. Ultimately it comes down to the patient's ability to be compliant with your postoperative regimen. Is the patient able to maintain a non-weight bearing status for your expected time frame if internal fixation is utilized? If external fixation is your fixation of choice, does the patient have the ability to maintain the appropriate pin care management? If you feel the patient is unable to achieve these postoperative goals, it is recommended that outside assistance be obtained. While there's been a shift to move ankle arthrodesis procedures into the outpatient setting, patients that you identify with these potential risks should be admitted to the hospital for evaluation with a case manager or social worker. While admission may not be popular, especially given the cost, if a patient is identified as being high risk for noncompliance, then the procedure should either not be performed or they should be given adequate access to ancillary services to help and protect them from themselves.

Diabetes

There has been a significant increase in patients with diabetes undergoing ankle arthrodesis in the past several years [21]. This is not surprising due to the increase in overall population with diabetes. That being said this author chooses not to perform any elective ankle arthrodesis on patients with a hemoglobin A-1 C of greater than 7. There is significant literature that supports this threshold for hemoglobin A-1 C [21]. That only with patients with controlled blood sugars biologically do better, it is also an indicator of compliance for the patient. Not only will patients with uncontrolled diabetes and elevated hemoglobin A-1 C levels be at risk for a nonunion but they will also be at risk for developing a Charcot event, which can inevitably lead to amputation. Even in patients with a controlled hemoglobin A1c, it is prudent to ensure tight blood sugar control during the preadmission-testing visit and immediately prior to surgery.

Obesity

Obesity in this country along with diabetes is an ever-evolving problem and the numbers continue to grow year by year. There is no end in sight to this trend as of now.

The morbidly obese patient is not only at a higher risk for complication but also has the potential to make the procedure more difficult for the surgeon. Patients with a BMI greater than 30 are five times more likely to suffer a major complication and six times more like to have a minor complication [22]. Aside from the increased complications, these patients often have difficulty maintaining non-weight bearing status, which can result in increased length of stay if admitted. Postoperative casting and/or splinting may be a challenge for the surgeon as well. When the patient is allowed to progress to weight bearing, there is significantly more force transmitted through the fused joint that may inevitably create a breakdown, especially if the fusion is not in the optimal position [23]. Many surgeons, including the author, implement a BMI limit of 30 on patients that are undergoing elective surgery especially fusions of the lower extremity and/or arthroplasties.

Smoking

Smoking in the United States, while it has diminished in certain areas of the country, is still quite popular, even with the advent of smoking cessation programs and a public media campaign highlighting the dangers of smoking that include death. The author advocates that current smokers not be operated on for elective surgery given the disparaging statistics especially with arthrodesis procedures. Specifically, patients that smoke compared to patients without any other risk factors are at 16 times the risk of nonunion [24]. Any patient that is a current smoker that has quit or a former smoker, it is the recommendation of this author to undergo nicotine level testing as well as cotinine testing. These labs as well as a thorough history and physical should be implemented in the preoperative planning portion of the procedure. In any patient that is a former smoker, care should be taken to carefully assess their vascular status as sequela of long-term smoking can often affect blood vessels especially in men. Long-term smokers will often undergo ankle-brachial index with pulse volume recordings and if needed angiography.

Insufficient Vascularity

Insufficient vascularity in patients is a relative contraindication to ankle arthrodesis procedure. As stated above patients that smoke and with diabetes should undergo ankle-brachial index with pulse volume recordings and again if needed angiography. Often patients with an insufficient vascularity to heal an incision will undergo either bypass surgery or stenting during angiography (Fig. 29.1). Once sufficent vascularity has returned to the patient's extremity, and a vascualr specialist has given clearance, surgical intervention is then warrented.

Soft Tissue Envelope

Almost equally important to the bone is the ability for patient to mend their soft tissue envelope. It is of the upmost importance that a thorough examination be performed to determine incision planning and tissue perfusion. Oftentimes, patients that are undergoing ankle arthrodesis procedures will have had one or multiple surgeries, or poor quality skin from previous high-energy trauma (Fig. 29.2). This edematous, non-pliable, fibrous skin may be at risk when performing incisional placement for the ankle fusion [25]. The author often utilizes fluorescence microangiography preoperatively to assess skin and tissue perfusion for incisional planning (Fig. 29.3). This has helped prevent skin and soft tissue closure complications including dehiscence and infection. An incisional wound vacuum-assisted closure device has also been useful in reducing pain, edema, and skin and soft tissue complications, especially when an angiosome may be at risk (Fig. 29.4).

Rheumatological Disease

The complex interaction between the skeletal system and immune system explains the joint destructive nature of rheumatoid arthritis [26]. It is estimated that 1.5 million adults in the United States have rheumatoid arthritis (RA) [27]. The effect of RA on bone mineral density (BMD) derives from the interference of the dynamic balance between osteoblastic and osteoclastic activity [28]. This imbalance leads to bone demineralization and is a serious concern in regard to using and maintaining proper fixation. If the patient's bone mineral density is adequate, ankle arthrodesis benefits overall stability. It has been demonstrated that when ankle arthrodesis is performed in the RA patient, it succeeds in decreasing pain and improves movement of the knee and hip joints as well [29].

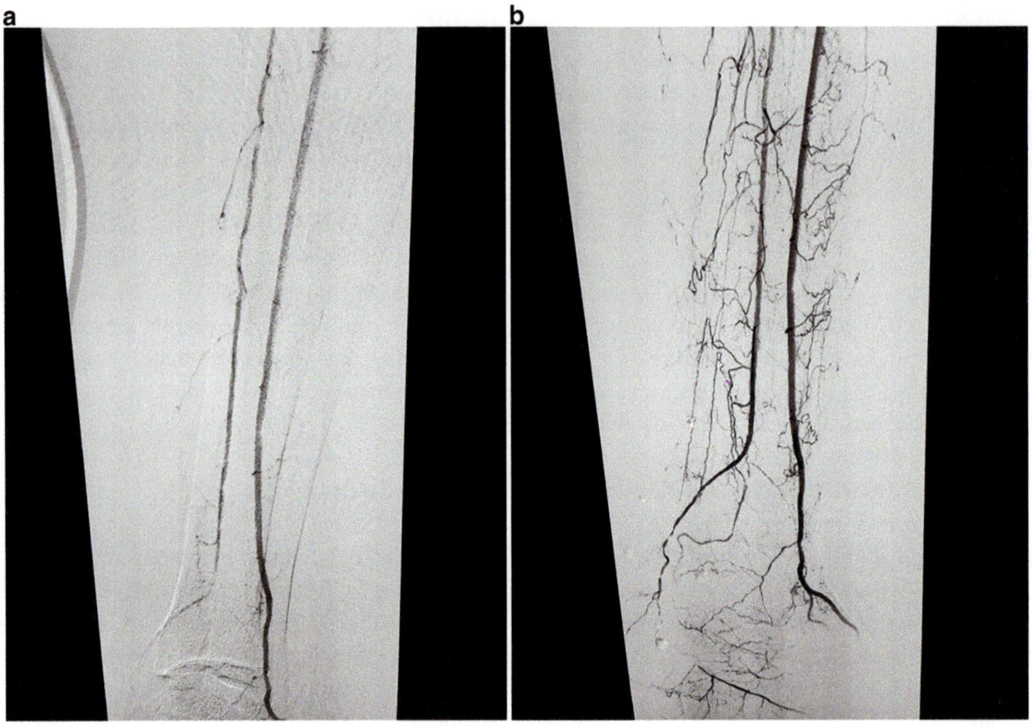

Fig. 29.1 (**a**) Preoperative TTC arthrodesis patient with diabetes sent for angiography. Confirmed occlusion of anterior tibialis artery. (**b**) Poststenting procedure showing significantly improved flow (Courtesy of Dr. Patrick Antoun)

Fig. 29.2 Patient with poor skin envelope. Multiple surgical interventions including skin grafting for open fracture following motor vehicle accident

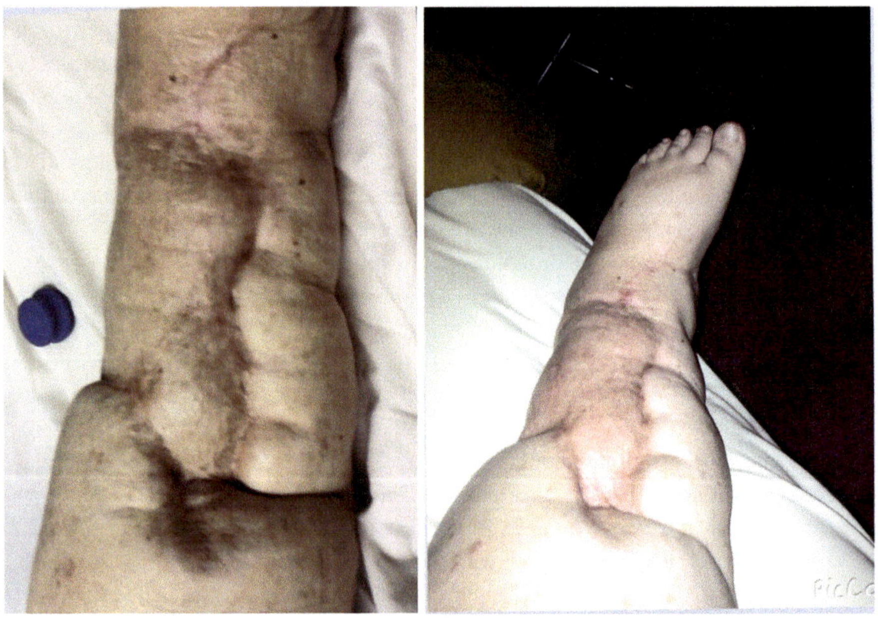

Alcohol Abuse

Alcohol abuse has also been reported to increase risk of nonunions in patients [30]. Excessive alcohol consumption can lead to an osteopenic state decreasing the ability to form bone across arthrodesis site. In an animal model, elevated levels of alcohol have been noted to decrease total bone mineral content with decreased bone formation at periosteal and cancellous sites [31].

Alcoholism and substance abuse in general have been linked to patient noncompliance as well. Thorough screening should be performed if alcoholism or drug dependency is

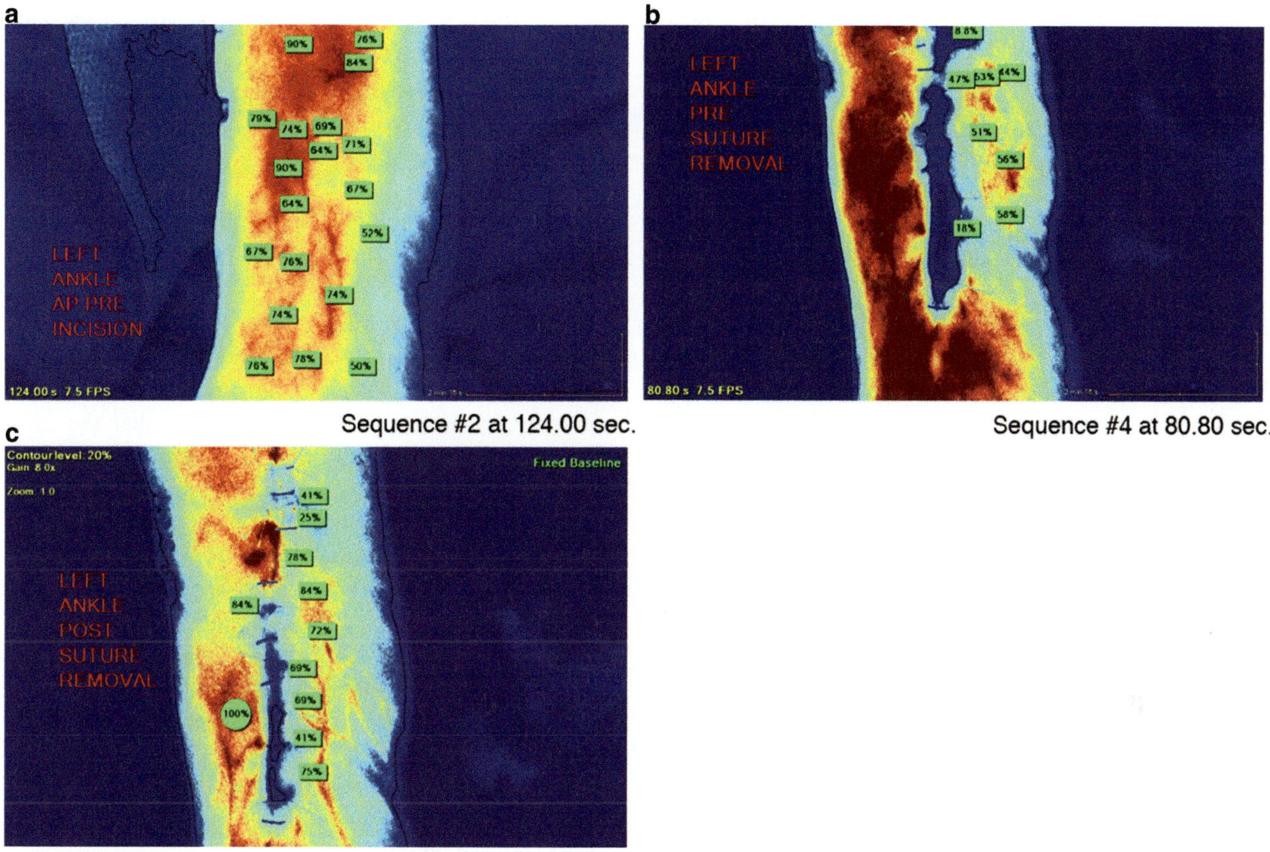

Fig. 29.3 (**a**) Fluorescence microangiography used preoperatively to assess skin perfusion and avoid areas of concern. (**b**) Postoperative microangiography displaying poor perfusion along the incision site; this indicates future tissue necrosis. (**c**) Removal of offending staples increasing perfusion to site

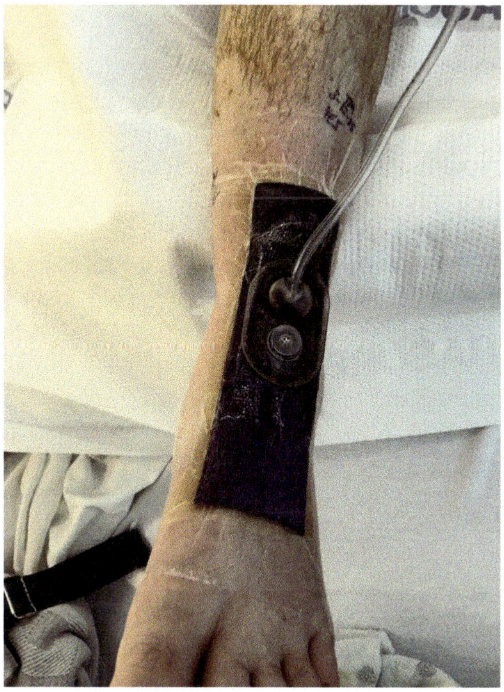

Fig. 29.4 Use of an incisional VAC to help prevent dehiscence

suspected. Although it is unclear at this time whether or not intervention can prevent noncompliance, it is beneficial for the overall health of the patient [32].

Surgeon Factors

As a surgeon it is sometimes difficult to own responsibility of a complication; however, during the process of the root cause analysis, it is essential to critically evaluate our own technique during the time of the surgery. The primary errors typically made by the surgeon include improper technique, in adequate fixation for the patient, and in proper patient selection.

Technique

Ankle arthrodesis is a technically demanding procedure and requires attention to detail. This begins with the dissection involved, which should be carefully carried out as to not create significant disruption of the neurovascular structures.

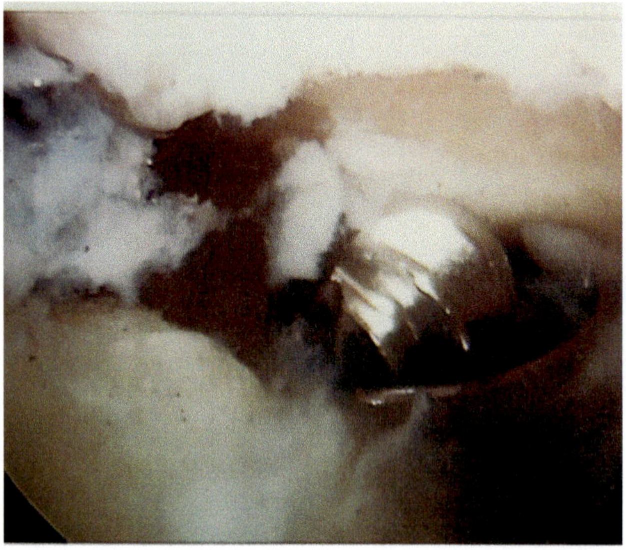

Fig. 29.5 Use of a rotary burr during arthroscopic ankle arthrodesis, joint preparation can be difficult to visualize utilizing the camera alone

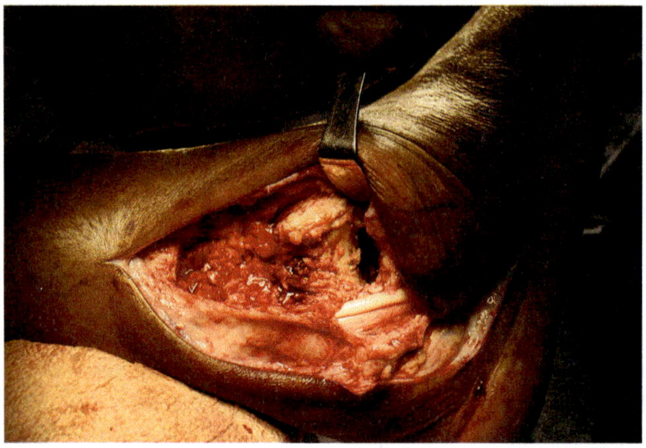

Fig. 29.6 Overaggressive retraction of soft tissue as well as stripping of vascular supply to the talus may lead to postoperative complications including dehiscence and avascular nonunions

Care must be taken around peritalar structures as not to disturb the vascularity of the talus as it is tenuous. Aggressive dissection has been known to lead to an avascular necrosis, or avascular nonunions (Fig. 29.5).

If the subchondral bone plate is not adequately removed or violated, no arthrodesis will ever be achieved. It is essential that the subchondral bone plate be removed during open and/or arthroscopic procedure (Fig. 29.6). Oftentimes it may be difficult to assess how much of the subchondral bone plate and/or surface of the tibiotalar joint has been resected during an arthroscopic procedure, especially for those new to this technique. Utilizing intraoperative arthroscopy and intraoperative fluoroscopy simultaneously can often be helpful to assess the area of resection. It has often been said that "position is everything" and "thou shall not varus," these tenants hold true especially in ankle arthrodesis where position can be considered one of the most vital aspects of the procedure, and one that is in complete control of the surgeon. Insuring a proper position of the tibiotalar arthrodesis will help prevent malunion and nonunion [33].

Fixation

Inadequate fixation can often lead to complications involving nonunion or malunion. Careful determination of the type fixation should be evaluated during preoperative evaluation. In a study by Hutchinson, he has shown that the ideal mechanical construct would be an anterior plate and with a lag screw (Fig. 29.7), which is similar to the biomechanical data for first MPJ arthrodesis [34]. It is important to note that lateral plate with compression screw was similar in stiffness. While this construct is sufficient for open procedures, it may not be relevant for arthroscopic procedures, which requires percutaneous fixation. It has been shown that when performing arthroscopic ankle arthrodesis in vivo, the fastest rate of union was achieved with three parallel screws placed medially from the distal tibia into the talus [35]. While this construct has shown to lead to a faster time to fusion, it has not been shown to be biomechanically more stable. In patients with a suspected infectious process, it may be advantageous to utilize external fixation, as internal fixation often will propagate the infectious process (Fig. 29.8).

Patient Selection

While the ankle arthrodesis is quite versatile with minimal contraindications, it is essential that as the surgeon, we critically analyze the patient to determine whether or not the procedure would be best for them. As stated above it is essential to perform not only a thorough history and physical but also a social and socioeconomic evaluation of the patient prior to surgery. Often complications can occur because we are focused more on the patient's radiographic findings and deformity rather than on the patient as a whole. It is the recommendation of this author that patients with multiple comorbidities be critically evaluated to determine whether or not they are candidates for elective ankle arthrodesis; it cannot be understated that a thorough history and physical examination should be performed prior to surgery. Laboratory testing to determine if an infection is present should be performed especially if the patient has sustained an open fracture or any type of trauma that is unknown, or history of surgery. All revision should be worked up for an infectious process. Circulatory, hematopoietic, metabolic, and nutritional profiles should be established and corrected to decrease healing deficits prior to any surgery.

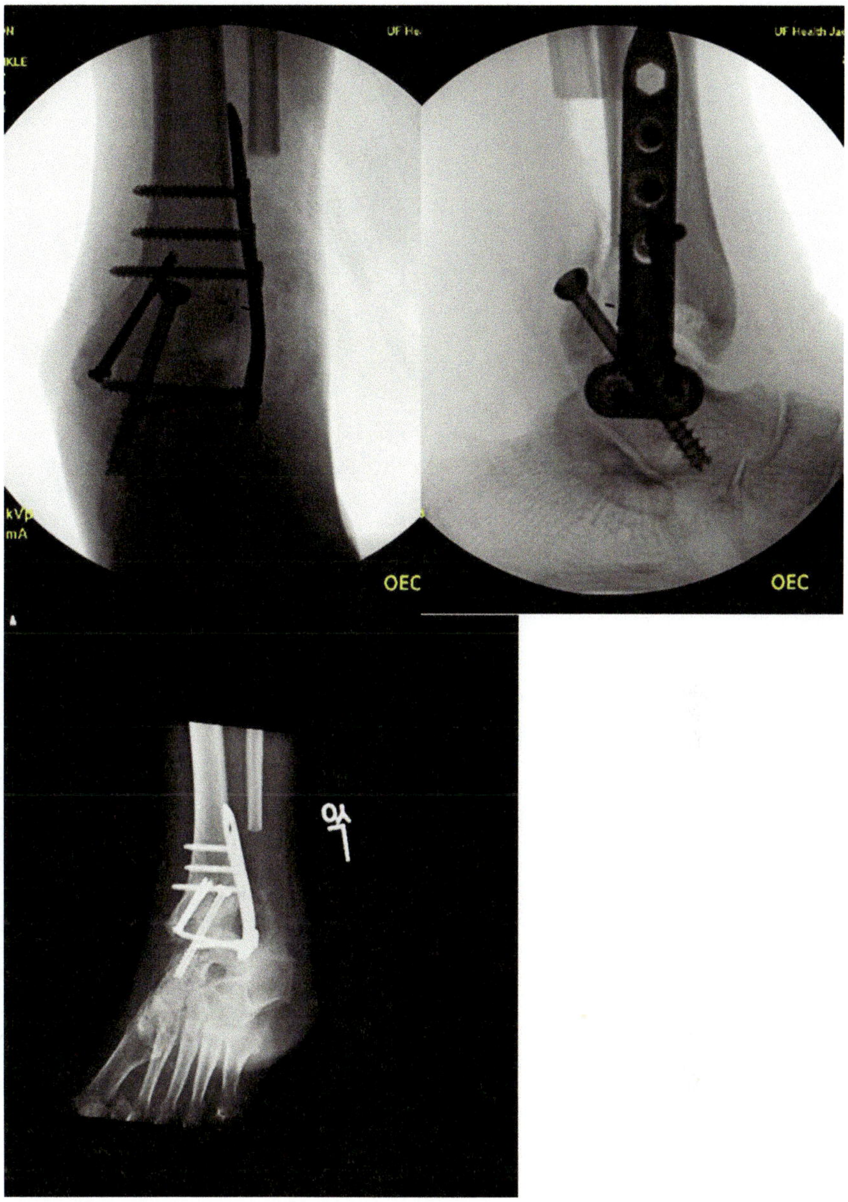

Fig. 29.7 Use of compression screw with locking plate leading to successful union

Nonunions

Nonunion is the most common complication of the ankle arthrodesis procedure (Fig. 29.9). It has been reported in the literature that the percentage of nonunions is anywhere between 10 and 30%. As discussed earlier, patient selection and comorbidities can play a significant role in the incidence of nonunion. Frey et al. found nonunion rates of 89% in patients with documented avascular necrosis of the talus, 83% in patients with open fractures, and 60% of patients with known infection. He also reported an 85% nonunion rate in patients with significant medical issues [36]. While nonunions are the most frequent complication of ankle arthrodesis, it has not been established which type of nonunion most commonly occurs with this procedure. Inevitably when revising nonunions, one should always suspect an infectious process. Appropriate blood work and even bone biopsy may be useful in determining if the process is infectious in nature. Not only infectious but also nutritional labs such as vitamin D levels should be checked with any nonunion diagnosis. Nonunions can often be subtle and sometimes difficult to assess radiographically due to hardware interference. Oftentimes a thorough physical examination will reveal pain and edema around the affected joint or surgical site, several months after the procedure. If a nonunion is inspected and not obviously detected on radiograph, it is imperative to order a CT scan to assess the fusion site.

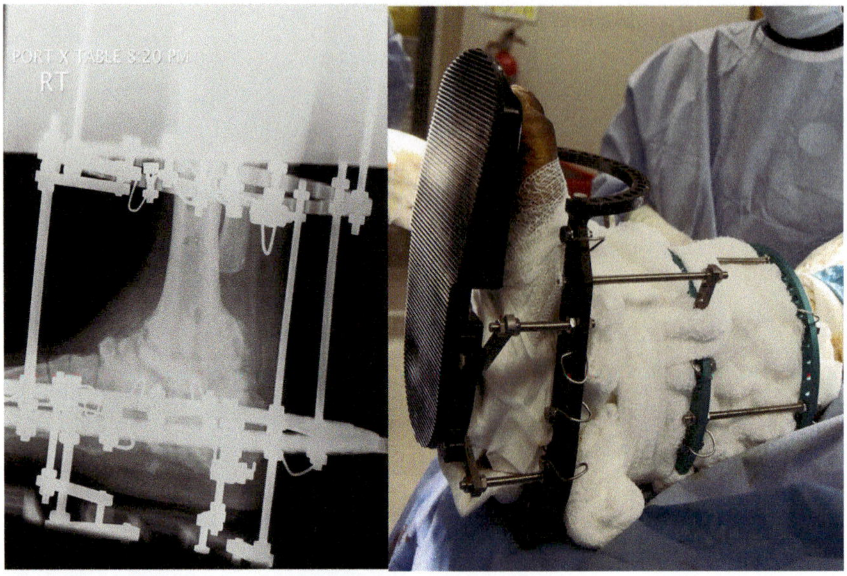

Fig. 29.8 Use of external fixation for septic nonunion

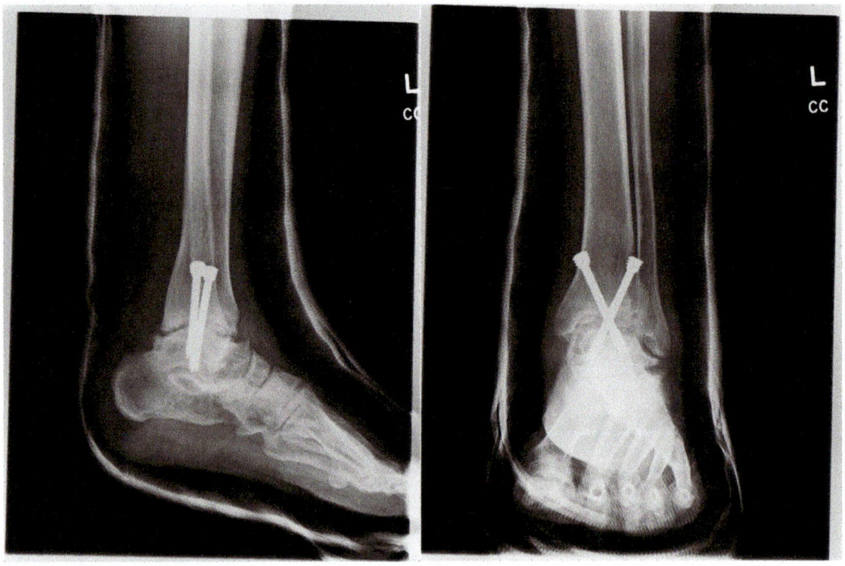

Fig. 29.9 Nonunion following arthroscopic ankle arthrodesis. The patient's failure to quit smoking and inadequate joint preparation likely combined to play a role in the failure

Surgical Treatment of Nonunions

Once the diagnosis of a nonunion has been made, it is vital to identify the cause. A root cause analysis may be performed to determine the etiology of the nonunion. Achieving this can prevent future surgical errors as well as prevent a reoccurrence nonunion. Identification of the type of nonunion is also helpful in creating a treatment plan. Treatment should also be based upon the patient's symptoms. Often a nonunion may not be painful; in this case, surgery is not indicated. In these cases the patient should be educated as to potential hardware failure, or other complications that may occur in the future. If the nonunion is asymptomatic and stable and the patient is neuropathic, a rigid brace should be prescribed to maintain correction [37].

The surgical plan should begin with the incisional approach. A thorough inspection of the soft tissue envelope should be performed as well as a review of vasculature in the potential surgical site. Often it is necessary to place the incision through the previous surgical site when percutaneous hardware removal cannot be achieved. If percutaneous hardware removal can be achieved, it may advantageous to plan an incision that will allow adequate access to the nonunion and through non-traumatized skin. Incision placement, when possible, should respect the angiosomes of the lower extremity. Anterior incision placement should be avoided if possible, as it may compromise this angiosome and is the reason for a 25% reported dehiscence rate in ankle arthroplasty [38].

Lateral or posterior incisional approaches tend to be safe and reliable. Hanson reported no complications in his series

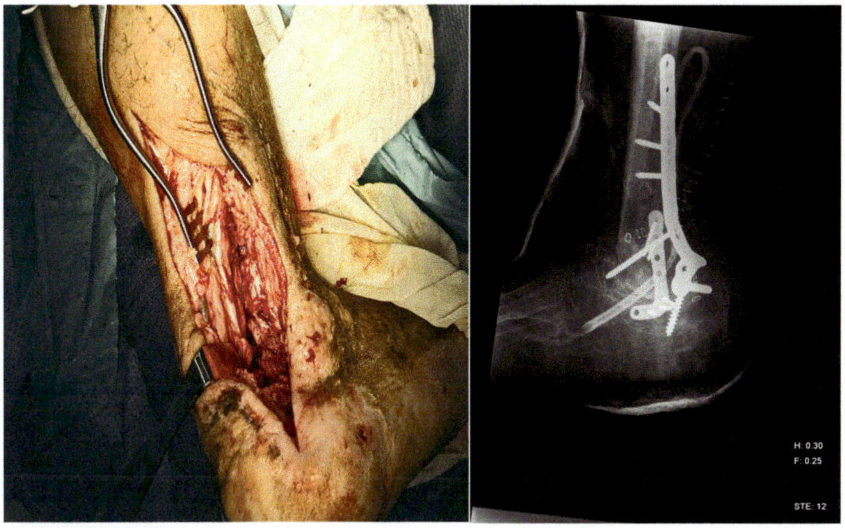

Fig. 29.10 Posterior approach to revision arthrodesis given multiple previous surgery performed through medial and lateral incisions

of ten patients undergoing pantalar arthrodesis through a posterior approach (Fig. 29.10).

Once the surgical approach has been determined, attention should be directed to the osseous component of the surgery. A plethora of fixation, biologic, and grafting options are available to the surgeon in preparation for surgery. There is no general consensus on which combination of options is most advantageous. The treatment plant should be patient specific and therefore may result in a variety of combinations of fixation, biologic, and nonbiologic augmentations as well as bone grafting. Typically if the nonunion is a simple hypertrophic type, without any other suspected pathology other than poor technique and/or fixation, the nonunion may be treated with takedown and aggressive resection followed by either bone grafting or biologic augmentation, with rigid internal fixation. If the patient has multiple comorbidities that may have contributed to the nonunion, it is recommended that the underlying malady be addressed. This might include tighter control of a patient's Hba1c, smoking cessation, weight loss, or discontinuation of DMARDS. Only once these issues are addressed, it is recommended to proceed with the surgical plan.

Fixation

There are over 40 documented fixation techniques described in the literature which fall into two major categories: internal fixation which is the most common and includes crossing screws, plate fixation, intramedullary nails, and combinations of these [39]. The other is external fixation, which is typically reserved for complex planar deformities, Charcot, and in patients who have suspected or known infection. When using screw fixation it has been advocated that a three-screw tripod technique be utilized. This technique is commonly employed for primary fusions; however, it is the opinion of the author that given the biomechanical data comparing screw with plate and screw fixation, the later technique be employed to ensure the most biomechanically stable construct. Patients who are identified with a nonunion may often have concomitant subtalar joint pain with degeneration of the joint. Use of intramedullary retrograde nail or precontoured anatomic tibiotalocalcaneal (TTC) locking plates should be considered in this patient population. A recent biomechanical evaluation of intramedullary nail versus locking TTC fusion plate with TTC augmentation screw in cadaveric models showed higher final rigidity in the locking plate group [40]. While plate fixation may be more biomechanically stable, it often requires a large exposure; therefore, it may not be optimal if there is concern for the soft tissue envelope. If possible a posterior approach with a posterior locking TTC plate would be an ideal approach if plate fixation is the choice of fixation. In cases where minimal exposure is desired, intramedullary nail fixation may be utilized successfully. In a retrospective review of ten cases of nonunion, a minimally invasive retrograde locking nail gave excellent results with a 90% union rate [41]. The use of a blade plate has also been advocated by many authors for complex ankle or TTC fusions with reported successful union rates as high as 90% [42]. Biomechanically this construct has been shown to be inferior to crossing screw constructs in a sawbone model [43] (Fig. 29.11).

External fixation can be a valuable tool for treatment of nonunions especially when infection is suspected. External fixation provides rigid immobilization with resistance to multiplane stresses especially torsional and axial load while allowing access to soft tissue defects and early weight bearing (Fig. 29.12). If there is significant bone loss after resec-

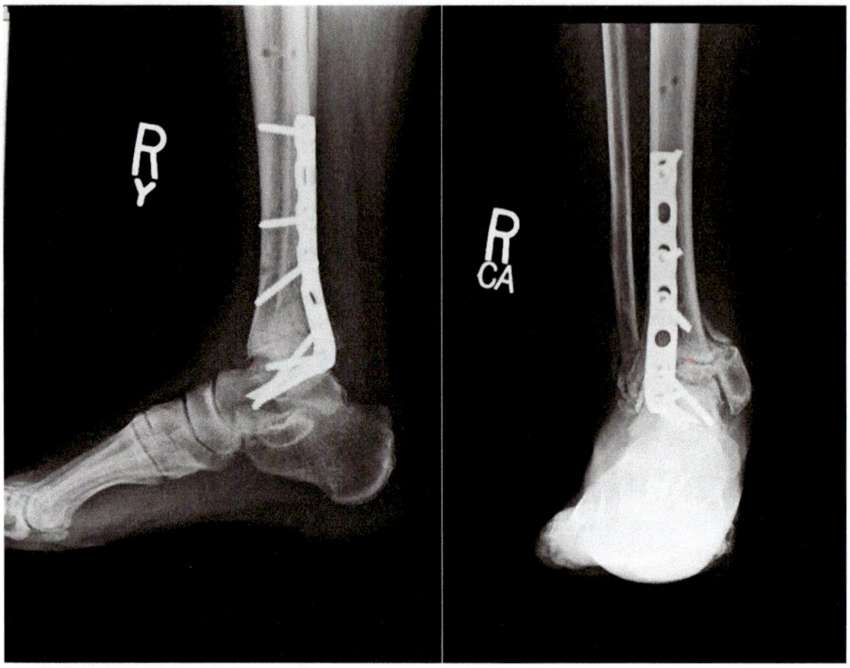

Fig. 29.11 Attempted ankle arthrodesis in an uncontrolled diabetic with a blade plate resulted in asymptomatic nonunion given the patients neuropathy. The patient was placed in a ridged brace to prevent breakdown

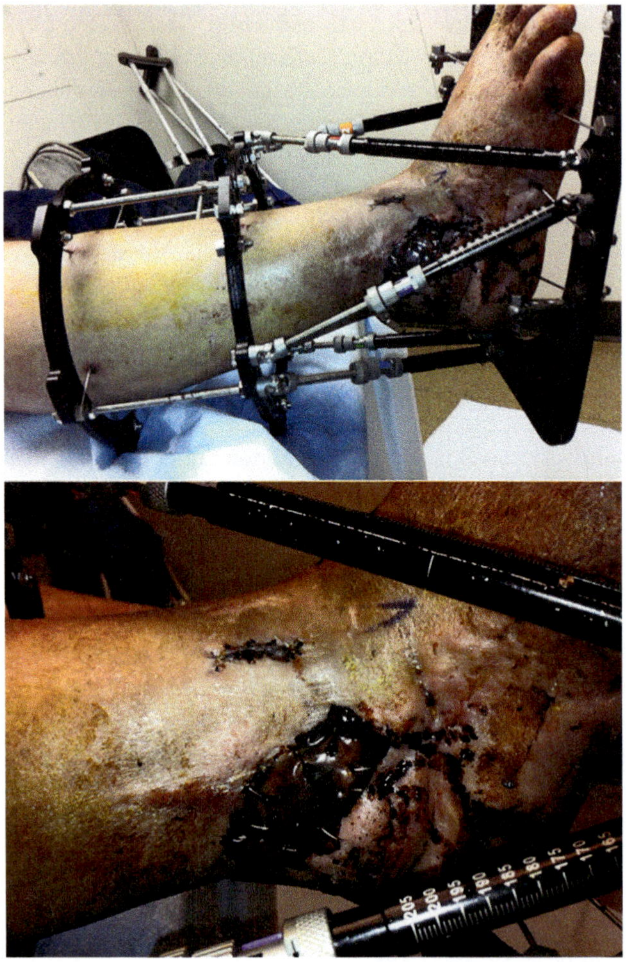

Fig. 29.12 Use of TSF for ankle malunion allowing access to the graft laterally

tion, external fixation may but utilize with proximal corticotomy and distraction osteogenesis to lengthen and then compression distally at the nonunion site. External fixation is the author's fixation of choice in treatment of septic nonunions. External fixation may be considered for aseptic nonunions as well; however, in a retrospective review of 26 nonunions treated with external fixation, Kitaoka reported a satisfactory result with only 77% of the nonunions going on to successful fusion and fair or poor results in nearly half the patients [44].

Biologics and Grafting

The past decade has seen significant advances in the field of orthobiologics. Bone biology may be manipulated to promote healing potential through osteoconductive or osteoinductive mediators. Osteoconductive products provide a scaffold for ingrowth of bone (Fig. 29.13). More recently research has been focused on osteoinductive products that stimulate osteoprogenitor stem cells to differentiate into osteoblasts. Bone morphogenetic protein (BMP) has been the most widely studied type of the osteoinductive cell mediators. Bibbo showed a 96% union rate in 108 high-risk fusion patients using recombinant human BMP-2 (rhBMP-2) [45]. Equally impressive, Fourman reported a 93% union rate in his rhBMP-2 group versus a 53% union rate in patients without the growth factor in complex ankle fusions [46]. Allogenic stem cells have also been reported in the literature as a safe and effective biologic augmentation, although it has not performed as well as autogenous grafting [47].

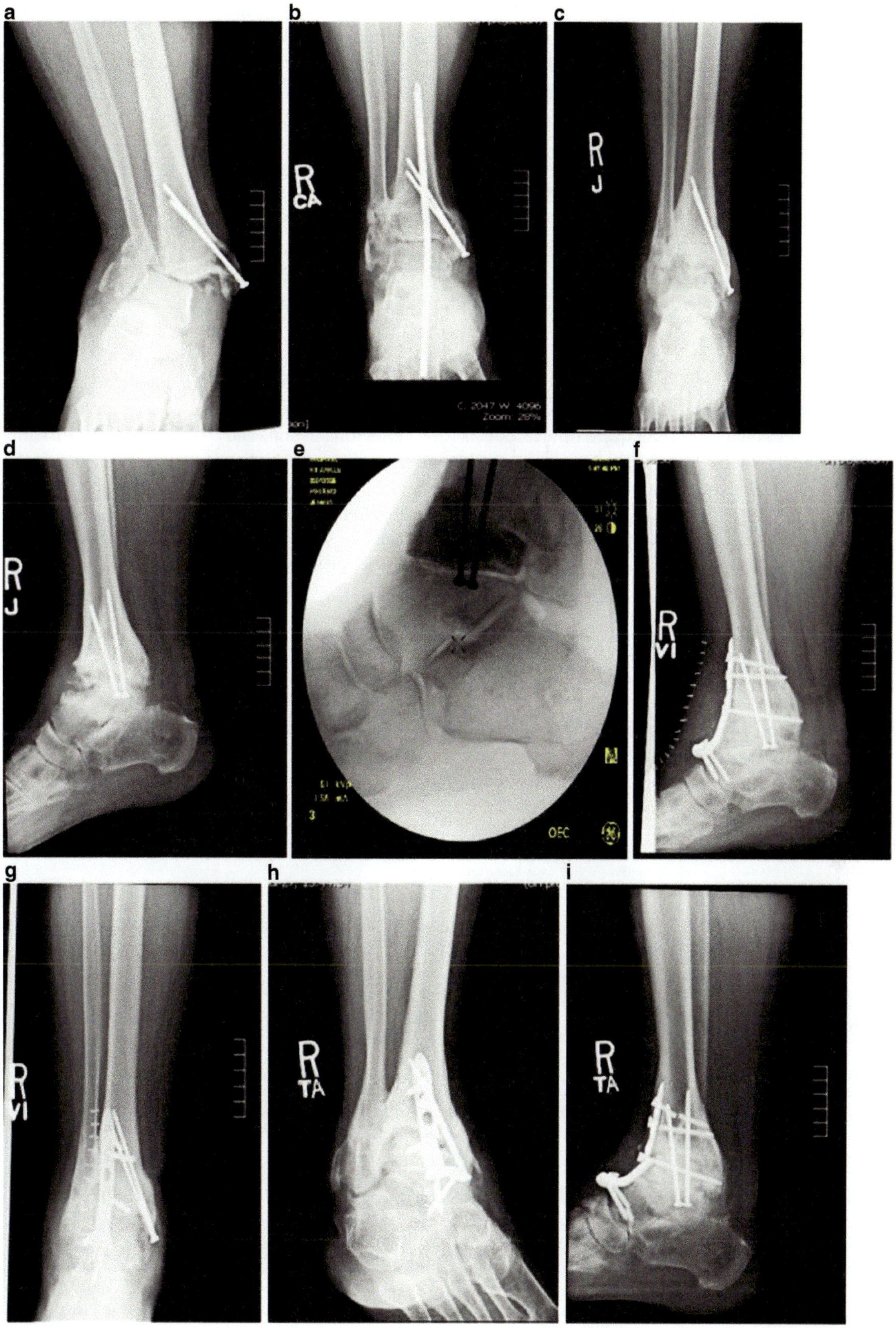

Fig. 29.13 Patient with open injury and subsequent fusion with osteoconductive bone grafting results in nonunion. (**a**) After ORIF patient reinjured site due to non-compliance resulting in an open injury. (**b**) Patient underwent pinning of ankle joint to prevent future dislocation. (**c, d**) Patient with resulting ankle deformity. (**e**) Patient underwent bone biopsy with antibiotic spacer placement. (**f, g**). After negative cultures patient underwent ankle arthrodesis with plate fixation and osteoconductive bone graft resulting in what appeared to be a successful union. (**h, i**) After being lost to follow-up after 1 year, patient returned to the office with subsequent nonunion and broken hardware

The gold standard for bone grafting is autograft. It possesses all properties needed to create bone: osteoconduction, osteoinduction, and osteoprogenitor stem cells. Bone graft has been harvested from a variety of sites including iliac crest, proximal tibia, distal tibia, and calcaneus. While harvesting graft can often be routine, it does expose the patient to an additional surgical site with associated potential complications. Most recently recombinant human platelet-derived growth factor-BB (rhPDGF-BB) has been shown to demonstrate comparable fusion rates with decreased pain and side effects when compared to autograft [48]. This would provide the surgeon with an alternative to bone graft harvest and the potential sequelae associated with the additional procedure. It has recently been approved for use specifically in rearfoot and ankle fusions.

Nonbiologic augmentation such as internal and external bone stimulation to aid with the failure of arthrodesis has also been shown to be beneficial. There are three modalities of bone stimulation available: internal direct current stimulation, pulsed electromagnetic, and low-intensity pulsed ultrasound. Of the three, only implantable direct current stimulators have sufficient evidence to suggest use as an adjunct to surgical correction of ankle nonunions [49].

While not acting directly at the site of the surgical nonunion, oral supplementation of medication may also play a role in reducing failure of a revision. As stated previously vitamin D levels preoperatively should be checked and if deficient supplementation may be useful in healing a secondary surgery. More interesting is the potential role of teriparatide in the use of nonunions. It has been shown in animal models and clinical trials to have an accelerated effect in fracture healing. There has been recent evidence to suggest the use in failed ankle arthrodesis in patients with Charcot [50].

Malunion

While malunion may not be the most common complication of ankle arthrodesis, it certainly can be one of the most complex to treat (Fig. 29.14). Position of the ankle arthrodesis is of upmost importance. A malunion has the potential to affect not only the ankle joint but also the corresponding proximal and distal joints significantly. Ideal position of the arthrodesis should be neutral position in the sagittal plane, slight valgus 0–5° in the frontal plane, midsagittal translation, slight posterior translation, and 5–10° of external rotation in the transverse plane [51]. Excessive plantarflexion in the sagittal plane has been shown to lead to clinically significant genu recurvatum of the knee [52]. Fusion of the ankle at neutral or slightly internally rotated leads to valgus stress of the knee resulting in ligamentous laxity of the medial collateral ligaments [52]. Casillas proposed a classification system for malunions of the ankle, which aids in facilitating surgical planning. They are broken down into angular, translation, rotation, or multiaxis deformities. They are further subclassified by the rigidity of the foot and the anticipated position of the foot after correction. Foot types include the following: type I, the supple foot; type II, the rigid foot with projected plantargrade position; and type III, the rigid foot with projected nonplantargrade position. Based on the classification

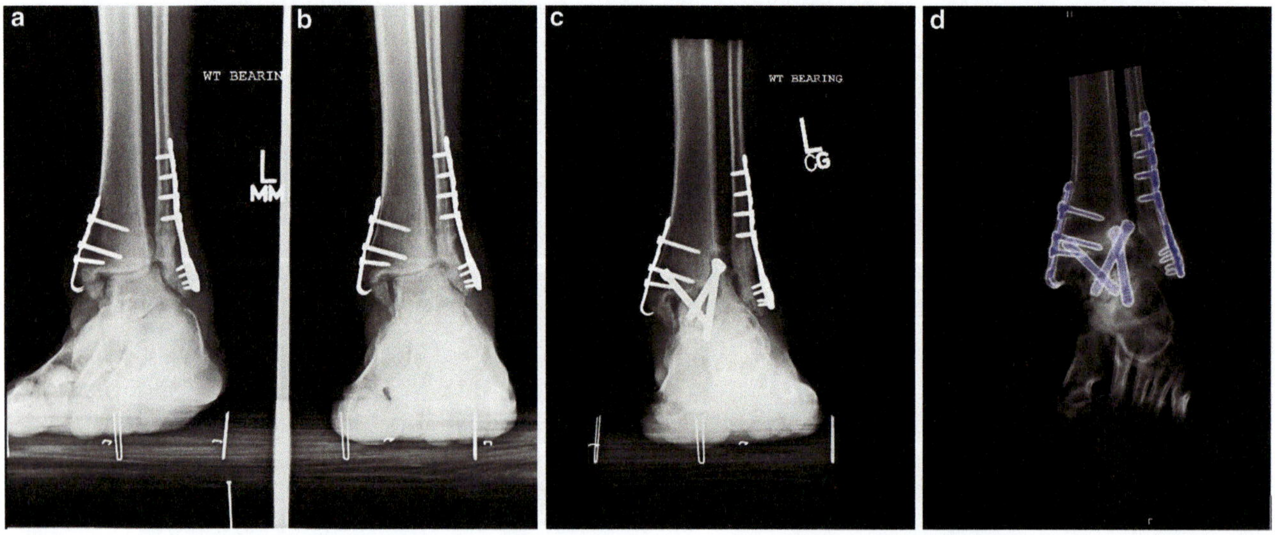

Fig. 29.14 (**a**, **b**) Diabetic patient with malunion ankle fracture. (**c**, **d**) Arthroscopic ankle arthrodesis was attempted and resulted in continued malunion. (**e**) CT scan with hardware addition demonstrating nonunion, subtraction may also be utilized

and subtype, the authors give recommendations for surgical treatments of the malunited ankle.

Treatments

Treatment should be based on the anatomical location and type of malunion. Using the Casillas and Allen classification, repair can be grouped into angular deformities, translational deformities, rotational deformities, and multiaxis deformities [53]. It is recommended that advanced imaging be obtained prior to surgical correction in order to facilitate an optimal surgical plan. Advanced CT scanners have the ability to subtract hardware and isolate areas of interest such as the deformity site. A careful preoperative plan including center of rotation and angulation (CORA) measurements should be obtained if warranted for correction. Care should be taken during these procedures as revision surgery can hold a higher risk of complication.

Angular deformities encompass varus, valgus, plantarflexion, or dorsiflexion of the arthrodesis site, while translational deformities include medial, lateral, anterior, posterior translation of the talus on the tibia and include shortening. Typically closing wedge osteotomies of the fusion site are utilized to correct the deformity with use of internal fixation. If there is a preexisting limb length discrepancy, opening wedge osteotomy may be more advantageous to correct the malalignment and prevent further length change (Fig. 29.15). Use of precut or custom titanium graft has been used in revision arthrodesis procedures with success [54]. Correction of translational deformities includes resection of the arthrodesis site and realignment in the corrected position. These are also performed with internal fixation of choice. If the subtalar joint is affected in patients with angular or translational deformity, the use of an intramedullary retrograde nail is recommended for fusion of both subtalar and ankle deformities.

Rotational deformities include internal and/or external rotation of the arthrodesis site. Correction of rotational deformity can be performed either at the original arthrodesis site or proximal through a supramalleolar osteotomy. If the original arthrodesis site is chosen and screw fixation was utilized, a percutaneous approach may be utilized. The screws may be backed out just past the level of the fusion site and either osteotomies or a Gigli saw may be carefully utilized to osteotomize the original fusion site. Once the correction is dialed in, a single screw may be used to hold the position and then the original screws may be reintroduced (Fig. 29.16). If a supramalleolar approach is chosen, a similar percutaneous approach may be utilized. If the subtalar joint is arthritic, the use of a retrograde intramedullary nail in either case would be recommended. Figure 29.10 shows a supramalleolar osteotomy performed with the previous hindfoot arthrodesis nail. The proximal screws from the nail were removed, the tibia was then osteotomized with a Gigli saw, the correction was achieved around the nail, and the position was locked in with the proximal screws being replaced in the new corrected position.

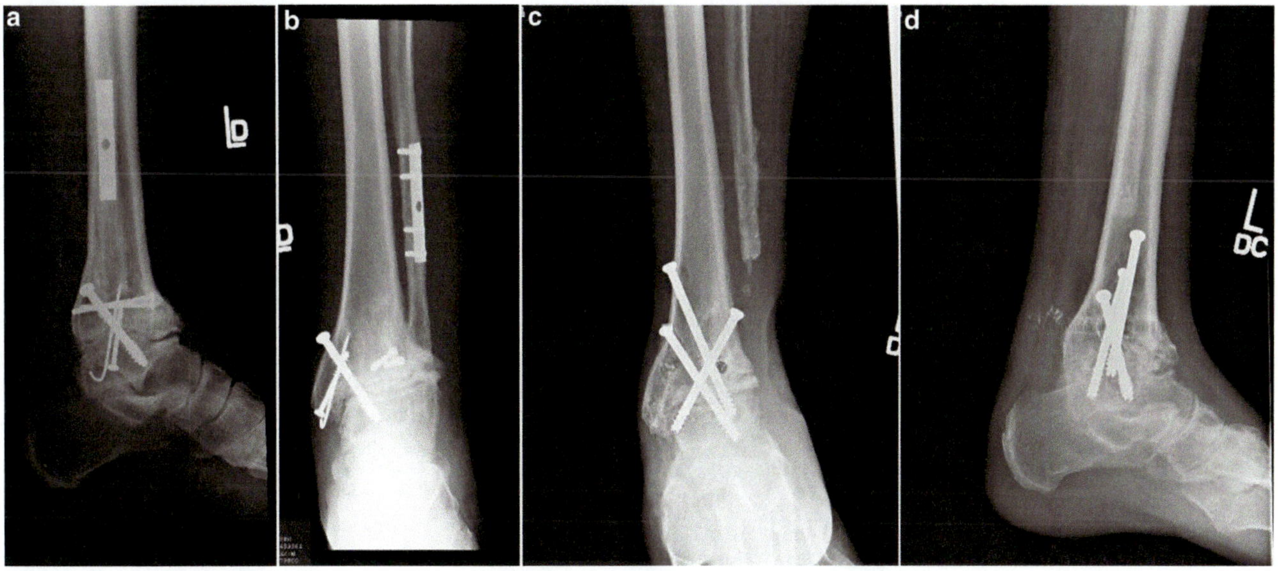

Fig. 29.15 (**a**, **b**). Patient underwent single screw attempted ankle arthrodesis resulting in a valgus malunion. (**c**, **d**) Revisional arthrodesis was performed using a portion of the fibula as a lateral opening wedge graft with crossing screws

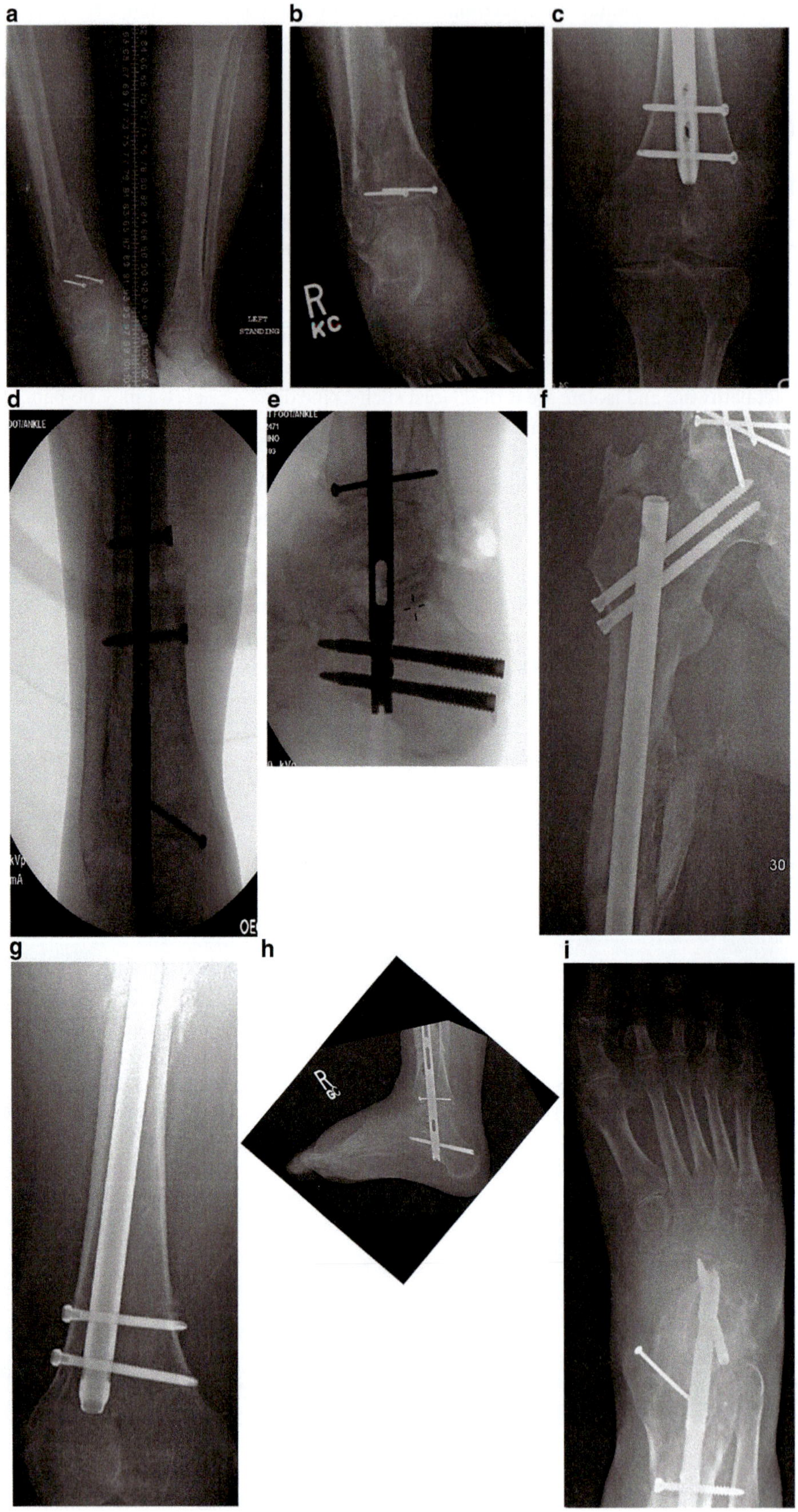

Fig. 29.16 (**a**) Patient sustained a polytrauma resulting in limb length discrepancy, arthritis, and drop foot. (**b**, **c**) Patient had fixed equinovarus with 20° of internal rotation. (**d**, **e**, **f**, **g**) Combination of Orthopedic trauma and Foot and Ankle Surgeons performed corrective surgery. (**d**, **e**) Ankle TTC fusion was performed and the ankle was externally rotated 20 degrees to zero and dorsiflexed to correct the deformity. (**f**, **g**) Unfortunately orthopedic surgery planned to internally rotate the femur 20 degrees with malunion correction resulting in a return to the original 20° of internal rotation. (**h**, **i**) Patient subsequently underwent correction of the rotational malunion with removal of proximal TTC screws, corticotomy with Gigli saw, external rotation to the corrected position, and reintroduction of the proximal screws to hold the position

According to Casillas, multiaxis deformity correction depends on soles on the foot type. Typically if the deformity requires a multiple plane deformity correction, the use of a Taylor spatial frame is warranted [55] (Fig. 29.12). If arthrodesis is not indicated in the foot, then wedge osteotomies may be used with the external fixator. If there is an indication for hindfoot arthrodesis, a combination of supramalleolar and/or wedge osteotomies may be used with external fixation or retrograde intramedullary nail fixation.

Skin and Soft Tissue Complications

Complications such as incisional dehiscence that lead to minor infectious processes are not uncommon with ankle arthrodesis especially in the open variety. Superficial infection and pin tract infections when external fixation is utilized have been reported in 40–50% of cases [56]. Care must be taken when handling soft tissues during the procedure, overaggressive retraction and strangulation of soft tissue can lead to wound dehiscence postoperatively (Fig. 29.6). Attention to angisomal circulation during incision planning is also vital. As stated previously the author utilizes fluorescence microangiography to assess skin perfusion preoperatively (Fig. 29.3). Postoperatively the use of an incisional vacuum-assisted closure (VAC) device is often used in at risk patients and incisions (Fig. 29.4). This device has been shown to reduce dehiscence and infection rates [57]. Most wound complications can be resolved with appropriate antibiotic therapy if superficial infection is present and wound care. If needed aggressive operating room debridement with grafting or wound VAC may be warranted if the wound persists.

Charcot

Charcot neuroarthropathy is one of the most difficult deformities the foot and ankle surgeon will face. When performing any operative procedure on a patient with diabetes, it is a potential complication most surgeons fear, especially in the rearfoot where it must be addressed. With most Charcot cases, if possible it is prudent to maintain a course of strict non-weight bearing until the patient has moved out of the active phase. This may be followed by total contact casting if ulcerations are present. In the event the deformity becomes unstable for the patient to ambulate, revisional surgery may be necessary. The use of intramedullary retrograde nail, external fixation, or a combination of both may be needed to revise the arthrodesis site. Prior to surgical correction, any infectious markers should be drawn, such as C-reactive protein, and sedimentation rate along with a white blood cell count assist with a potential diagnosis of infection.

Hardware-Related Complications

Typically hardware failures are related to nonunion. If motion is occurring across an arthrodesis site, it predisposes the hardware to failure (Fig. 29.13). Oftentimes this may complicate removal of the broken hardware for revision or in the case of infection. Although not as common, periprosthetic fracture may also become problematic, especially when using an intramedullary retrograde nail. The author advocates the use of a long IM nail when possible to extend proximal to the tibial isthmus, and this may aid in the prevention of tibial fracture from mechanical forces proximal to the nail (Fig. 29.17). Other less common occurrences may include stripped screws necessitating the need for trephine screw removal, or broken drill bits or k-wires that may difficult to retrieve (Fig. 29.18).

Infection

In the event of a suspected active infection at the fusion site, action should be taken immediately. It is recommended that the patient be admitted for intravenous antibiotics, and the patient be scheduled for hardware removal with bone biopsy and cultures along with aggressive debridement of suspected infections tissues. Recently we have had success with the use of ultrasonic debridement of bone and soft tissue in our infectious cases. The patient may be taken back for subsequent debridement as needed with use of antibiotic cement if applicable. In the event a retrograde nail was used in the arthrodesis site, the use of a cement retrograde nail may be employed (Fig. 29.19). Infectious disease consult is beneficial for duration and choice of antimicrobial therapy postinfection. The use of vancomycin powder has been advocated in patients with diabetes during closure and is common practice at our institution after any infectious case prior to closure [58].

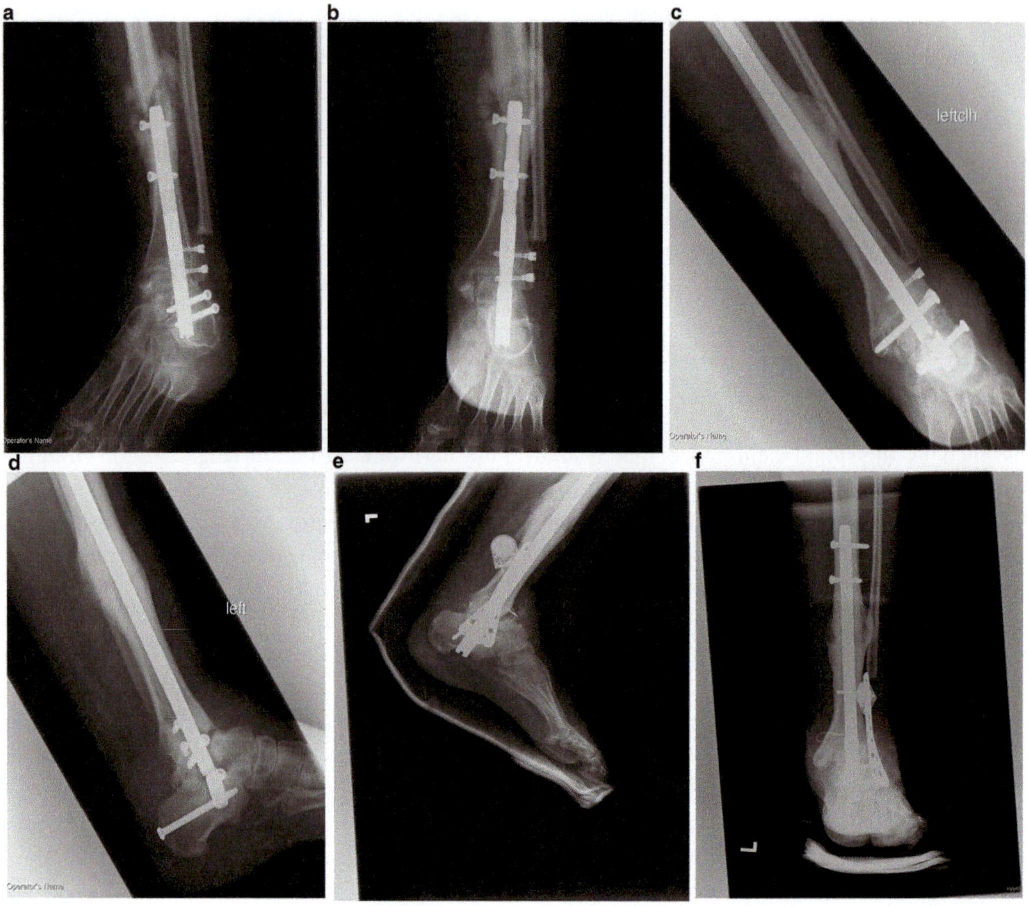

Fig. 29.17 (**a**, **b**) Patient underwent attempted TTC fusion with short intramedullary nail resulting in a midshaft tibial fracture after a fall. (**c**, **d**) Orthopedic trauma surgery was consulted who placed an anterograde nail across the nonunion which resulted in fracture of the IM nail at the nonunion site. (**e**, **f**) After subsequent removal of the nail, patient requested second opinion. A successful revision of the nonunion was performed with implantable bone stimulator, long TTC nail, and locking plate fixation

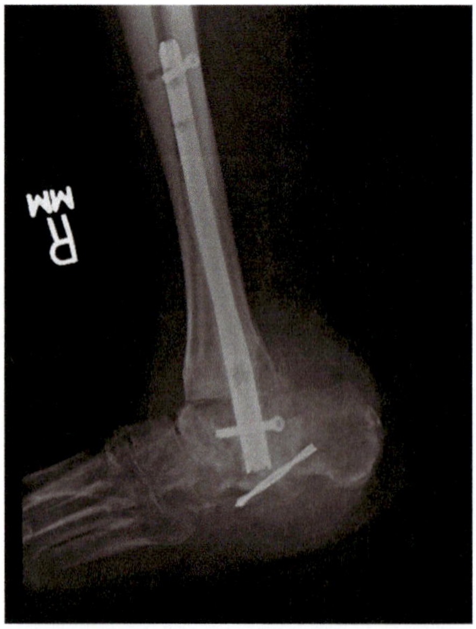

Fig. 29.18 Broken drill bit in patients calcaneus after TTC fusion

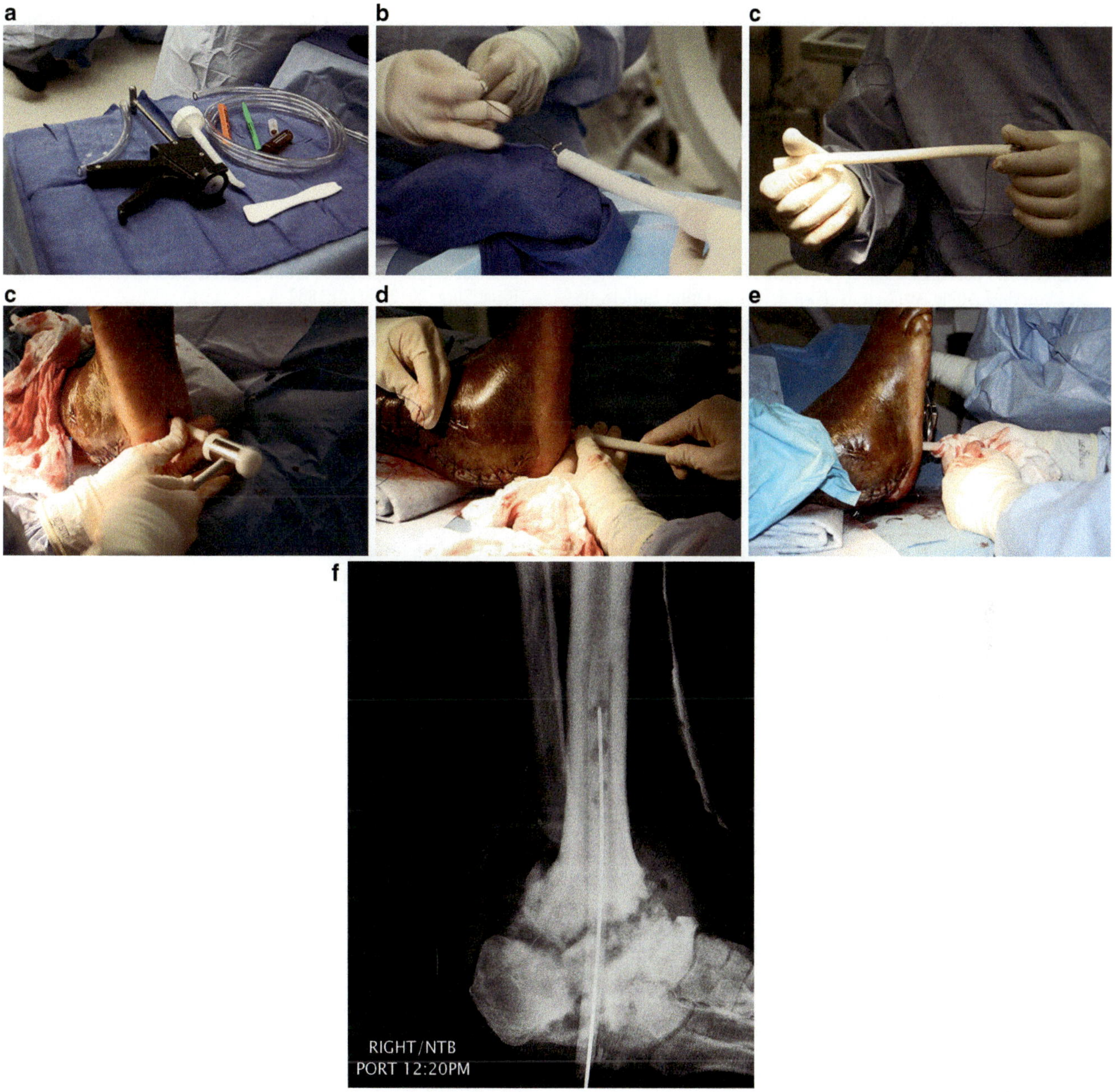

Fig. 29.19 (**a**) Antibiotic cement "gun" with chest tube to exchange infected intramedullary retrograde nail. (**b**, **c**) Use of suture and Steinmann pin centrally in the cement to assist with future removal. (**d**, **e**). Use antibiotic nail being introduced into the infected canal after ultrasonic debridement. (**f**) Antibiotic nail in place

References

1. Greenhagen RM, Johnson AR, Joseph A. Internal fixation: a historic review. Clin Podiatr Med Surg. 2011;28:607–18.
2. Miller C, Finn A, Delzell E. Battlefield injuries: saving lives & limbs throughout history. Lower Extremity Rev. 2013;5(10):16–23.
3. Greenhagen RM, et al. Internal fixation: a historic review. Clin Podiatr Med Surg. 2011;28(4):607–18.
4. Zwipp H, Rammelt S, Endres T, Heineck J. High union rates and function scores at midterm followup with ankle arthrodesis using a four screw technique. Clin Orthop Relat Res. 2009;468(4):958–68.
5. Roberts TT, Prummer CM, Papliodis DN, Uhl RL, Wagner TA. History of the orthopedic screw. Orthopedics. 2013;36(1):12–4.
6. Miller C, Finn A, Delzell E. Battlefield injuries: saving lives & limbs throughout history. Lower Extremity Rev. 2013;5(10):20.
7. Best MJ, Buller LT, Miranda A. National Trends in Foot and Ankle Arthrodesis: 17-year analysis of the National Survey of Ambulatory Surgery and National Hospital Discharge Survey. J Foot Ankle Surg. 2015;54(6):1037–41.
8. Terrell RD, Montgomery SR, Pannell WC, Sandlin MI, Inoue H, Wang JC, Soohoo NF. Comparison of practice patterns in total ankle replacement and ankle fusion in the United States. Foot Ankle Int. 2013;34(11):1486–92.

9. Kakarla G, Rajan DT. Comparative study of anthrodesis using crossing screws fixation versus anterior contoured plate plus cross screw fixation. Acta Orthop Belg. 2006;72:716–21.
10. Chalayon O, Wang B, Blankenhorn B, Jackson JB, Beals T, Nickisch F, Saltzman CL. Factors affecting the outcomes of uncomplicated primary open ankle arthrodesis. Foot Ankle Int. 2015;36(10):1170–9.
11. Abicht BP, Roukis TS. Incidence of nonunion after isolated arthroscopic ankle arthrodesis. Arthroscopy: J Arthroscopic Relat Surg. 2013;29(5):949–54.
12. Muir DC, Amendola A, Saltzman CL. Long-term outcome of ankle arthrodesis. Foot Ankle Clin. 2002;7(4):703–8.
13. Szatkowski J Ankle Arthrodesis. Foot & Ankle. Ortho Bullets, 05 Mar. 2016. Web. 09 Mar. 2016. <http://www.orthobullets.com/foot-and-ankle/7052/ankle-arthrodesis>.
14. Hayes BJ, Gonzalez T, Chioda CP, Bluman EM. Ankle arthritis: you can't always replace it. J Am Acad Orthop Surg. 2016;24(2):E29–39.
15. Rabinovich RV, Haleem AM, Robert Rozbruch S. Complex ankle arthrodesis: review of the literature. World J Orthop. 2015; 6(8):602–13.
16. Penner MJ, Pakzad H, Younger A, Wing KJ. Mean BMI of overweight and obese patients does not decrease after successful ankle reconstruction. J Bone Jt Surg Am. 2012;94(9):e57.
17. Penner MJ, Pakzad H, Younger A, Wing KJ. Mean BMI of overweight and obese patients does not decrease after successful ankle reconstruction. J Bone Jt Surg Am. 2012;94(9):e57.
18. Royer C, Brodsky JW. Arthrodesis techniques for avascular necrosis of the talus. Tech Foot Ankle Surg. 2002;1(1):50–9.
19. Royer C, Brodsky JW. Arthrodesis techniques for avascular necrosis of the talus. Tech Foot Ankle Surg. 2002;1(1):50–9.
20. Szatkowski J, Ankle arthrodesis, p. 1.
21. Shibuya N, Humphers JM, Fluhman BL, Jupiter DC. Factors associated with nonunion, delayed union, and malunion in foot and ankle surgery in diabetic patients. J Foot Ankle Surg. 2013;52(2):207–11.
22. Werner BC, Burrus MT, Looney AM, Park JS, Perumal V, Cooper MT. Obesity is associated with increased complications after operative management of end-stage ankle arthritis. Foot Ankle Int. 2015;36(8):863–70.
23. Thevendran G, Wang C, Pinney SJ, Penner MJ, Wing KJ, Younger ASE. Nonunion risk assessment in foot and ankle surgery: proposing a predictive risk assessment model. Foot Ankle Int. 2015;36(8):901–7.
24. Cobb TK, Gabrielsen TA, Campbell DC, Wallrichs SL, Ilstrup DM. Cigarette smoking and nonunion after ankle arthrodesis. Foot Ankle Int. 1994;15(2):64–8.
25. Pawar A, Dikmen G, Eragomen A, Rozbruch SR. Antibiotic-coated nail for fusion of infected chariot ankles. Foot Ankle Int. 2013;34:80–4.
26. Treadwell JR. Surgery on the rheumatoid ankle joint: efficacy versus effectiveness. Clin Podiatr Med Surg. 2010;27(2):275–93.
27. Barr, W.G., Scientific has arthritis on the run. In: Arthritis foundation-scientific strategy 2015–2020. Atlanta, GA: Arthritis Foundation; 2015. p. 7–57. <http://www.arthritis.org/Documents/arthritis-foundation-scientific-strategy.pdf>.
28. Treadwell JR. Surgery on the rheumatoid ankle joint: efficacy versus effectiveness. Clin Podiatr Med Surg. 2010;27(2):26.
29. Weiss RJ, Brostrom E, Stark A, Wick MC, Wretenberg P. Ankle/hindfoot arthrodesis in rheumatoid arthritis improves kinematics and kinetics of the knee and hip: a prospective gait analysis study. Rheumatology. 2007;46(6):1024–8.
30. Frey C, Halikus NM, Vu-Rose T, Ebramzadeh E. A review of ankle arthrodesis: predisposing factors to nonunion. Foot Ankle Int. 1994;15(11):581–4.
31. Berg KM, Kunins HV, Jackson JL, Nahvi S, Chaudhry A, Harris KA, Malik R, Arnsten JH. Association between alcohol consumption and both osteoporotic fracture and bone density. Am J Med. 2008;121(5):406–18.
32. Kleinsinger F. Working with the noncompliant patient. Perm J. 2010;14(1):54–60.
33. Casillas MM, Allen M. Repair of malunions after ankle arthrodesis. Clin Podiatr Med Surg. 2004;21(3):371–83.
34. Clifford C, Berg S, Mccann K, Hutchinson B. A biomechanical comparison of internal fixation techniques for ankle arthrodesis. J Foot Ankle Surg. 2015;54(2):188–91.
35. Yoshimura I, Kanazawa K, Takeyama A, Ida T, Hagio T, Angthong C, Naito M. The effect of screw position and number on the time to union of arthroscopic ankle arthrodesis. Arthroscopy: J Arthroscopic Relat Surg. 2012;28(12):1882–8.
36. Frey C, Halikus NM, Vu-Rose T, Ebramzadeh E. A review of ankle arthrodesis: predisposing factors to nonunion. Foot Ankle Int. 1994;15(11):582.
37. Pinzur MS. Current concepts review: charcot arthropathy of the foot and ankle. Foot Ankle Int. 2007;28(8):952–9.
38. Taylor GI, Corlett RJ, Dhar SC, Ashton MW. The anatomical (angiosome) and clinical territories of cutaneous perforating arteries: development of the concept and designing safe flaps. Plas Reconstr Surg. 2011;127(4):1447–59.
39. Rabinovich RV, Haleem AM, Robert Rozbruch S. Complex ankle arthrodesis: review of the literature. World J Orthop. 2015;6(8):605.
40. O'neill PJ, Logel KJ, Parks BG, Schon LC. Rigidity comparison of locking plate and intramedullary fixation for tibiotalocalcaneal arthrodesis. Foot Ankle Int. 2008;29(6):581–6.
41. Mader K, Verheyen CC, Gausepohl T, Pennig D. Minimally invasive ankle arthrodesis with a retrograde locking nail after failed fusion. Strategies Trauma Limb Reconstr. 2007;2(1):39–47.
42. Sowa DT, Krackow KA. Ankle fusion: a new technique of internal fixation using a compression blade plate. Foot Ankle Int. 1989;9(5):232–40.
43. Nasson S, Shuff C, Palmer D, Owen J, Wayne J, Carr J, Adelaar R, May D. Biomechanical comparison of ankle arthrodesis techniques: crossed vs. blade plate. Foot Ankle Int. 2001;22:575–80.
44. Kitaoka HB, Anderson PJ, Morrey BF. Revision of ankle arthrodesis with external fixation for non union. J Bone Joint Surg Am. 1992;74-A(8):1191–201.
45. Wang B, Saltzman CL, Chalayon O, Barg A. Does the subtalar joint compensate for ankle malalignment in end-stage ankle arthritis? Clin Orthop Relat Res. 2014;473(1):318–25.
46. Fourman MS, Borst EW, Bogner E, Robert Rozbruch S, Fragomen AT. Recombinant human BMP-2 increases the incidence and rate of healing in complex ankle arthrodesis. Clin Orthop Relat Res. 2013;472(2):732–9.
47. Anderson JJ, Boone JJ, Hansen M, Brady C, Gough A, Swayzee Z. Ankle arthrodesis fusion rates for mesenchymal stem cell bone allograft versus proximal tibia autograft. J Foot Ankle Surg. 2014;53(6):683–6.
48. Digiovanni CW. Recombinant human platelet-derived growth factor-BB and beta-tricalcium phosphate (rhPDGF-BB/β-TCP): an alternative to autogenous bone graft. J Bone Jt Surg Am. 2013;95(13):1184–92.
49. Midis N, Conti SF. Revision ankle arthrodesis. Foot Ankle Int. 2002;23:243–7.
50. Tamai K, Takamatsu K, Kazuki K. Successful treatment of nonunion with teriparatide after failed ankle arthrodesis for charcot arthropathy. Osteoporos Int. 2013;24(10):2729–32.
51. Mann RA, Van Manen JW, Wapner K, Martin J. Ankle fusion. Clin Orthop. 1991;268:49–55.
52. Buck P, Morrey BF, Chao EYS. The optimum position of arthrodesis of the ankle. J Bone Jt Surg Am. 1987;69-A(7):1052–63.
53. Casillas MM, Allen M. Repair of malunions after ankle arthrodesis. Clin Podiatr Med Surg. 2004;21(3):375.

54. Mulhern JL, Protzman NM, White AM, Brigido SA. Salvage of failed total ankle replacement using a custom titanium truss. J Foot Ankle Surg. 2016:1–6.
55. Casillas MM, Allen M. Repair of malunions after ankle arthrodesis. Clin Podiatr Med Surg. 2004;21(3):376.
56. Raikin SM, Rampuri V. An approach to the failed ankle arthrodesis. Foot Ankle Clin. 2008;13(3):401–16.
57. Ingargiola MJ, Daniali LN, Lee ES. Does the application of incisional negative pressure therapy to high-risk wounds prevent surgical site complications?: A systematic review. Eplasty. 2013;13:413–24.
58. Wukich DK, Dikis JW, Monaco SJ, Strannigan K, Suder NC, Rosario BL. Topically applied vancomycin powder reduces the rate of surgical site infection in diabetic patients undergoing foot and ankle surgery. Foot Ankle Int. 2015;36(9):1017–24.

Problems, Obstacles, and Complications of External Fixation in the Foot and Ankle

30

Bradley M. Lamm and Matthew J. Hentges

Introduction

External fixation has been used in the foot and ankle for acute trauma, reconstruction, lengthening, and limb salvage techniques. Traditionally, internal fixation constructs have been thought to provide more reliable fixation and fusion rates [1]. However, more recent biomechanical studies have shown that similar stability can be obtained using external fixation compared to internal fixation (compression screws, intramedullary nail, etc.) [2–4]. The general consensus is that the use of external fixation is complex; however, the use of external fixation has many advantages due to the modularity and adjustability of the components both intraoperatively and postoperatively. Most forms of external fixation allow for immediate weight bearing during the postoperative course. The dynamic nature of many external fixation constructs allows for adjustments to be made outside of the operative room, including correction of residual deformities and augmenting compressive forces through fusion sites. External fixation can also be used as an adjuvant to soft tissue reconstruction. The use of external fixation allows patients earlier mobilization and the ability to better perform their activities of daily living during the treatment phase [5].

The use of external fixation can be complex and has been thought of as high risk with the potential for complications. Many factors can influence these issues, including surgeon experience, patient compliance, patient comorbidities, type of external fixation utilized, and indication for the use of external fixation. Complications can arise intraoperatively, postoperatively, and after frame removal. Paley published a standardized classification of difficulties that can arise during distraction osteogenesis for limb lengthening [6]. Many of these adverse results that occur during the treatment phase are not true complications, as they do not affect the final outcome. Therefore, adverse results associated with external fixation can be classified as problems, obstacles, and complications [6, 7].

Problems are defined as adverse results that are anticipated but resolved by the end of treatment without surgical intervention. Obstacles are defined as adverse results that require surgical intervention but resolved by the end of treatment. Complications can be local or systemic adverse events, and the resultant sequelae remain unresolved at the end of treatment. Complications can be further divided into minor and major. Minor complications are considered to be of little significance and do not interfere with the end goals of treatment. Major complications interfere with the end goals of treatment and can cause increased morbidity [6, 7].

Adverse results and complications in the use of external fixation include pin site infections, length of time in the external fixator, neurologic and/or vascular injury, thermal necrosis of bone during wire/pin insertion, increased amount of follow-up care, and the increased burden on staff and family caring for patients with external fixators. These complications can be more or less common depending on the type of external fixator construct utilized. The two types that will be discussed in this chapter include circular external fixation and monolateral external fixation. Indications for the use of external fixation are discussed in Table 30.1. Guidelines on the prevention and management of complications will be discussed, as well as techniques for building a stable external fixation construct will also be presented.

Complications of External Fixation: Pin Site Infections

Pin site infections are the most common complication of circular external fixation. It is important to maintain a stable construct throughout the course of treatment because loosening of

B.M. Lamm (✉)
Foot and Ankle Deformity Center, Paley Orthopedic and Spine Institute, St. Mary's Medical Center & Palm Beach Children's Hospital, 901 45th Street, Kimmel Bldg, West Palm Beach, FL 33407, USA
e-mail: blamm@paleyinstitute.org

M.J. Hentges
The Foot and Ankle Institute of Western Pennsylvania, 4800 Friendship Avenue, Pittsburgh, PA 15224, USA
e-mail: matthew.j.hentges@gmail.com

M.S. Lee, J.P. Grossman (eds.), *Complications in Foot and Ankle Surgery*, DOI 10.1007/978-3-319-53686-6_30

Table 30.1 Indication for external fixation and conditions that external fixation can be of a distinct advantage in comparison to internal fixation

Indications for external fixation	Conditions treated with external fixation
• Nonunion/Malunion • Joint distraction • Callus distraction/ lengthening of bone • Off-loading of wound/flap • Osteotomy • Arthrodesis • Infection/Osteomyelitis • Soft tissue/skin contracture • Fracture	• Extensive scarring/contracture/burns • Previous infection • Osteopenia/osteoporosis • Charcot neuroarthropathy • Poor soft tissue quality • Large deformity • Open wounds • Patient unable to maintain non-weight bearing • Immune compromised host

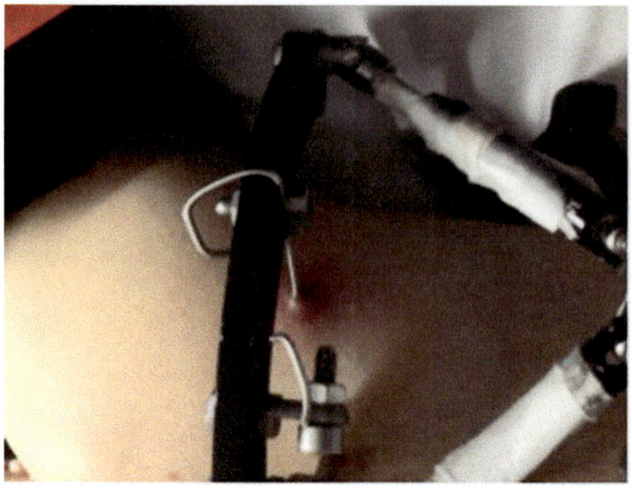

Fig. 30.1 Grade 1 pin site infection with soft tissue inflammation due to edema of the lower extremity. Treatment was successful with oral antibiotics and edema management (Reprinted with permission from the Rubin Institute for Advanced Orthopedics, Sinai Hospital of Baltimore)

the fixation can lead to inflammation of the surrounding soft tissue. An unstable external fixator can result in a higher likelihood of a pin site infection. Paley developed a simple grading system for pin site associated problems: Grade 1, soft tissue inflammation (Fig. 30.1); Grade 2, soft tissue infection (Fig. 30.2); Grade 3, bone infection (Fig. 30.3) [6]. As long as Grade 1 and 2 problems are addressed (usually with a 10-day course of orally administered antibiotics), progression of serious infection to Grade 3 usually does not occur. The recalcitrant infections that infect a joint or have prominent cellulitis might require pin removal in the office or in the operating room, with additional wire placement as needed to maintain stability. Pin site infections that fail to respond to oral antibiotics should be treated with intravenous antibiotics. Prompt action is required to prevent premature removal secondary to deep infection.

Patients and their families should be well educated before and after the application of the fixator that infection may occur more than once during treatment. It is important to clean the pins with saline daily and keep them dry. The authors allow non-neuropathic patients to shower daily as long as attention is made to dry the pin sites thoroughly. Neuropathic patients have a higher likelihood of pin tract infections, and therefore as long as the pin sites are stable, we do not recommend showering or daily care. However, if the pin sites become inflamed, infected and/or draining, we recommend daily saline cleansing of the pin sites with Q-tips and wrapping gauze on the affected sites to stabilize the soft tissue. Oral antibiotics are prescribed for pin site infections, along with advising the patient to limit weight-bearing activity until the infection resolves. Persistent pin site infections are treated with removal of the affected pin/wire. If proper care is initiated immediately upon the discovery of a pin site infection, the progression to osteomyelitis is rare.

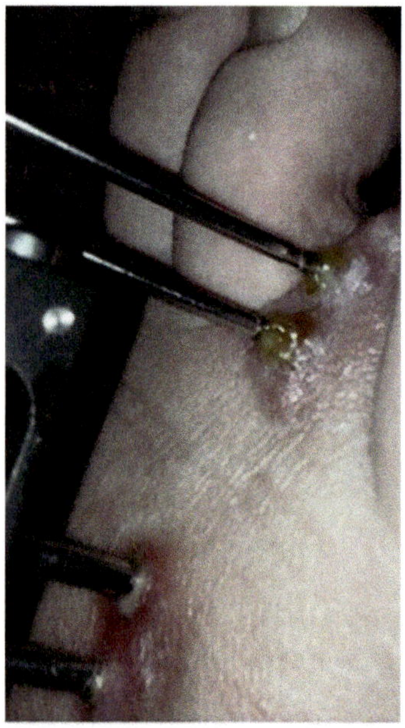

Fig. 30.2 Grade 2 pin site infection in a brachymetatarsia lengthening. Prompt pin care and oral antibiotics resolved this pin site infection (Reprinted with permission from the Rubin Institute for Advanced Orthopedics, Sinai Hospital of Baltimore)

Classification of Pin Site Infections

Problem—Pin site infection requiring removal of the half-pin or wire in the office and treatment with wound care and orally administered antibiotics.

Obstacle—Pin site infection requiring removal of the half-pin or wire and addition of a new half-pin performed in the operating room.

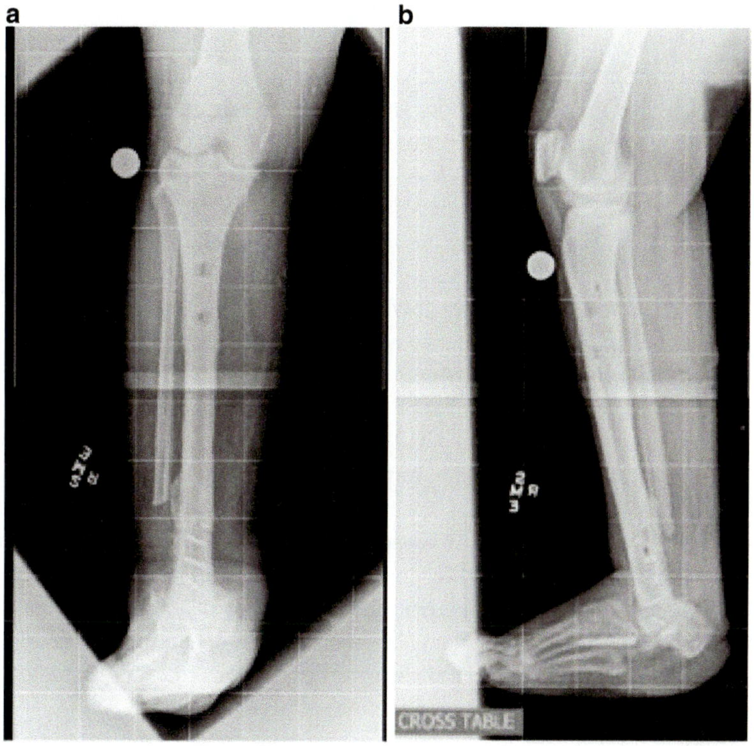

Fig. 30.3 Grade 3 pin site infection with radiographic evidence of proximal half-pin loosening and osteomyelitis formation in a neuropathic patient undergoing calcaneal-tibial arthrodesis for limb salvage (Reprinted with permission from the Rubin Institute for Advanced Orthopedics, Sinai Hospital of Baltimore)

Complication—Bone infection resulting from pin or wire site infection. Treatment of osteomyelitis consists of bone debridement and intravenously administered antibiotics.

Nerve and Vascular Injury

Injury to the major nerves and vessels of the lower extremity with the insertion of thin wire fixation and half-pin fixation is relatively rare. The surgeon must have intimate knowledge of the cross-sectional anatomy of the extremity and the safe zones for transosseous fixation. Nerve lesions manifest as pain in the anatomic distribution of the nerve. This is caused by nerve impingement from the percutaneous insertion of a wire or pin or during gradual deformity correction as a nerve becomes stretched or tethered. The best treatment is to remove the offending wire or pin and monitor the patient for improvement in symptoms. If symptoms do not improve, exploration of the nerve may be warranted.

Entrapment of the posterior tibial nerve can occur with external fixation during distal tibial/ankle deformity correction, especially when combined with lengthening. Prophylactic tarsal tunnel release should be considered for acute varus, equinus, or procurvatum ankle correction greater than 10° and gradual correction of deformity greater than 20° (Fig. 30.4) [8]. It is important to ensure complete decompression of the posterior tibial nerve, including the distal medial and lateral plantar nerve tunnels at the porta pedis. If tarsal tunnel decompression is not done prophylactically, it is important to monitor the patient closely for signs and symptoms of posterior tibial nerve entrapment postoperatively. Prompt intervention if symptoms arise will prevent irreversible nerve damage.

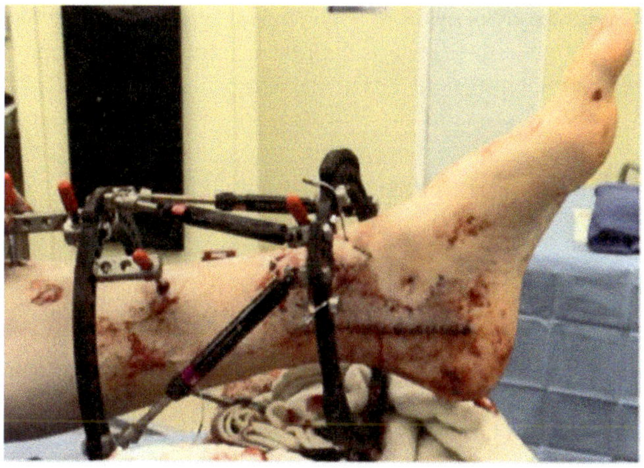

Fig. 30.4 Tarsal tunnel decompression performed prophylactically in a case of varus ankle deformity correction with ankle distraction. This was done prior to application of the multiplanar external fixator for correction of the deformity. Note the vertical nature of the incision so as not to disrupt healing during deformity correction (Reprinted with permission from the Rubin Institute for Advanced Orthopedics, Sinai Hospital of Baltimore)

Classification of Neurological Injury

Problem—Distraction and/or deformity correction results in numbness to the ankle/foot/toe. Decreasing the rate of correction allows the nerve compromise to resolve before the end of treatment.

Obstacle—Distraction results in numbness to the ankle/foot/toe; however, decreasing the rate of distraction does not resolve the numbness. Nerve decompression is then performed, and the nerve recovers before the end of treatment.

Complication—Intraoperative nerve injuries that result in slight numbness of the ankle/foot/toe but are not painful and do not affect the patient's function are minor complications. A major complication is a residual nerve insult that creates a neuropathic ankle/foot/toe that remains well after treatment and affects function.

Vascular injury is typically caused by a wire or pin introduced directly into a vessel. Bleeding will be noted with a vascular injury. The treatment is removal of the pin or wire and compression. Angiography may be necessary to determine what vessel has been injured and elucidate the sequelae. Edema throughout the treatment course is common as patients are often weight bearing as tolerated. To reduce edema, gauze is wrapped tightly around the pin sites between the skin and external fixator. Venous thromboembolism is uncommon in foot and ankle surgery; however, in patients with external fixation, proper prophylaxis should be considered based on the patient's risk factors.

Classification of Vascular Injury

Problem—Edema that is controlled with daily gauze wrapping. The daily gauze wrapping allows the edema to resolve before the end of treatment.

Obstacle—Vascular insult because of a misplaced pin/wire. The offending pin/wire should be removed and adjusted during a second surgery, which will allow the vascular insult to repair. This obstacle resolves before the end of treatment.

Complication—Non-repairable intraoperative vascular insult that affects vascularity to the foot is a minor complication. Intraoperative vascular insult, deep vein thrombosis, pulmonary embolism, and compartment syndrome are major complications.

Thermal Necrosis

Prevention of thermal necrosis is extremely important when placing wires and pins. Techniques used to reduce thermal necrosis include predrilling for half-pins and inserting by hand, use of sharp and non-cannulated drill bits, use of "on-off" drilling technique of pins and wires, tapping the wire through the soft tissues, deflation of the tourniquet to allow blood flow to cool the wires, and use of saline irrigation around the wires/pins during insertion. All cortical wires should be avoided due to rapid generation of heat during drilling. The prevention of thermal necrosis is vital because this can potentially lead to a stress riser and stress fracture in the bone or place the site at increased risk for developing later infection due to formation of a ring sequestrum.

Classification of Thermal Necrosis

Problem—Dense bone is noted during predrilling of half-pin. The drill bit is removed and flutes are cleaned. Drilling is continued with "on-off" technique to prevent further heat generation.

Obstacle—Pin/wire becomes loose postoperatively due to bone resorption from thermal necrosis. Pin/wire should be removed and replaced in a second surgery.

Complication—Thermal necrosis during pin insertion results in loosening of pin and forms a sequestrum leading to osteomyelitis. This is a minor complication if treatment leads to resolution prior to end of treatment. This is a major complication if it remains after treatment ends.

Stress Fractures/Fractures

Stress fractures and fractures can occur during treatment or following frame removal. The use of half-pins in neuropathic patients can increase the risk of this complication [9]. If this occurs during the treatment course, it is necessary to return to the operating room to extend the frame or increase the stability of the external fixation (Fig. 30.5). If this occurs following frame removal and the fracture is non-displaced, cast immobilization can be utilized. Most often, this does not affect the final result as long as the fracture heals. However,

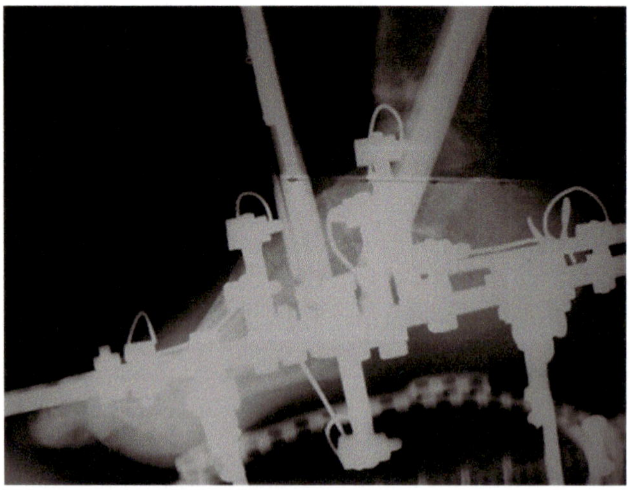

Fig. 30.5 Tibial diaphyseal fracture in a neuropathic patient (**a**), which required modification of external fixator for reduction and stabilization (**b**) (Reprinted with permission from the Rubin Institute for Advanced Orthopedics, Sinai Hospital of Baltimore)

it is important to adhere to proper principles of building a stable frame to reduce the stress placed on the lower extremity. The authors recommend the use of all wire fixation and avoiding fixation in the isthmus of the tibia in patients whenever possible. The tibial ring block fixation should be utilized to diminish the amount of stress placed on the fixation.

Classification of Stress Fracture/Fracture

Problem—Intraoperative stress fracture/fracture noted. Frame bridged across the fracture to stabilize.

Obstacle—Postoperative stress fracture/fracture necessitates return to surgery for modification of frame to bridge and stabilize fracture. Fracture healing does not prolong treatment course.

Complication—Stress fracture/fracture after removal of external fixator that necessitates return to surgery for fixation or further immobilization in cast. This is a minor complication if the fracture heals without residual functional loss. This is a major complication if results in residual deformity or loss of function.

Joint Subluxation

Subluxation or dislocation of the ankle joint or metatarsophalangeal (MTP) joint can be seen with gradual correction of ankle equinus (Fig. 30.6) and gradual lengthening of the metatarsals for brachymetatarsia, respectively. This adverse result is due to preexisting muscle imbalance, joint incongruity, or improper external fixation construct. In order to prevent joint subluxation/dislocation, it is important to plan for this preoperatively.

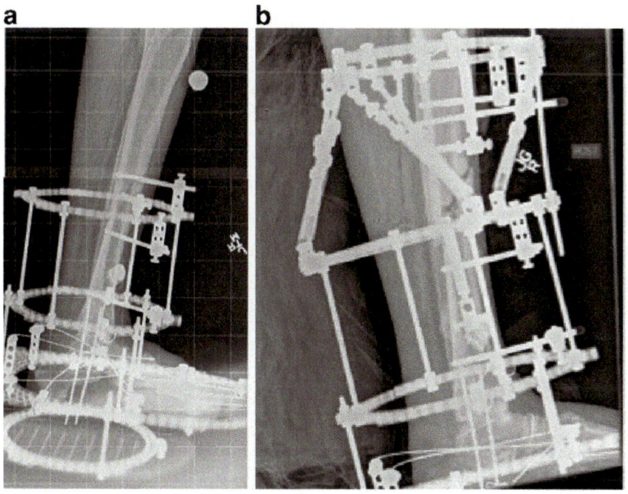

Fig. 30.6 Anterior ankle subluxation during gradual equinus correction requires modification of the axis of correction or insertion of additional talar fixation (Reprinted with permission from the Rubin Institute for Advanced Orthopedics, Sinai Hospital of Baltimore)

Correctly applying hinges at the axis of ankle joint motion and using two points of fixation in the talus will maintain ankle joint congruity while gradually correcting for equinus deformity. Relocation of the MTP joint and bridging of the external fixator across the MTP joint to the digit allows for maintenance of alignment during lengthening of the metatarsal. Pinning of the MTP joint with a Kirschner wire to maintain alignment has also been described, but in our experience, this causes a great amount of joint stiffness once the pin is removed. Treatment options for joint subluxation include physiotherapy, splinting, adjustment/modification of external fixation, revision surgery, decreasing the distraction rate, and isolated capsular release [7].

Classification of Joint Subluxation

Problem—Joint subluxation caused by rapid lengthening or correction of deformity. Decreasing the rate of distraction allows the tendon/capsule to elongate to resolve the joint subluxation.

Obstacle—Joint subluxation requiring modification or extension of the external fixation to relocate the subluxed joint and prevent recurrence. The subluxation resolves before the end of treatment.

Complication—Irreducible subluxation/dislocation of the joint after removal of the external fixator. This is a minor complication if the dislocation can be resolved with physical therapy. This is a major complication if residual subluxation creates pain and the foot/ankle loses function as compared with the preoperative function.

Length of Treatment

The length of time spent in the external fixator depends primarily on the indication for which it is used. In the case of acute trauma, the length of time can be a few weeks to a month if it is used as a temporary bridge to internal fixation. If circular or monolateral external fixation is used as the primary form of fixation, fracture healing, osteotomy, and soft tissue correction of any residual deformity determine the length of time in the fixator. Once there is evidence of healing of three cortices and the patient is clinically asymptomatic, the frame can be reduced in stiffness and subsequently removed. The principle of three cortices of healing works well in the long bones (i.e., tibia and femur); however, in the foot (i.e., metatarsals), this is more difficult to ascertain due to the superimposition of the metatarsals on a lateral radiograph.

Circular external fixation used for foot and/or ankle reconstruction or deformity correction has a much longer length of treatment. It is not uncommon for patients to have their fixator in place for up to three to six months or

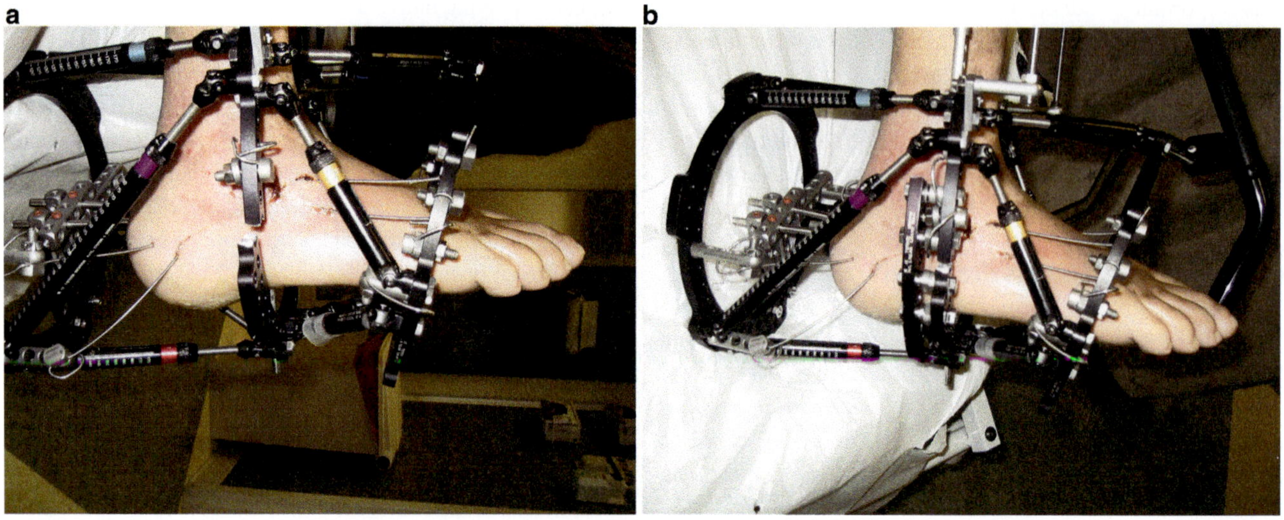

Fig. 30.7 Broken external fixation ring in a neuropathic patient (**a**) repaired by plating with additional ring (**b**) (Reprinted with permission from the Rubin Institute for Advanced Orthopedics, Sinai Hospital of Baltimore)

even greater than six months. Patients must be well educated prior to initiating treatment in regards to the possibility of returning to the operating room for fixator adjustments and modifications during the course of treatment (Fig. 30.7). The foot and ankle surgeon must ensure that the patient is psychologically able to tolerate the external fixator. The patient's home environment must also be conducive to treatment.

Patients who have external fixation of the foot and ankle are in need of increased amount of follow-up with their surgeon. These patients often have very complex pathology and close surveillance, weekly or biweekly, is important to prevent complications from occurring. If these adverse events do occur, it is vital to ensure that proper care and intervention is rendered. The surgeon must have a capable support staff to care for these patients and their needs. Dressing changes, frame checks, component changes, all can take a substantial amount of time. Having a well-educated staff is important for handling these difficult cases.

Patient and family education is of vital importance when embarking on treatment with external fixation. We regularly have training sessions with patients prior to their surgical reconstruction to familiarize them with the equipment and the aftercare necessary to have a successful outcome. We also supply the patient with a manual of external fixation, which provides them a variety of information. The ability of the patient to tolerate the length of treatment often needed to undergo such intervention is crucial. The ability of family members to be present at home with the patient for support and assistance is also important postoperatively. Setting realistic goals and expectations with patients and their families prior to intervention is essential. Having a nurse or assistant with experience in the use of external fixation acting as a "point person" can assist the surgeon in handling phone calls and messages regarding the status of patients after hospital discharge. Although it is difficult to answer many questions without seeing the patient, some care and reassurance can be offered.

Building a Stable Frame

Circular External Fixation

Creating a stable external fixation construct is important in reducing the amount of complications. It is vital to understand the biomechanics of external fixation, both monolateral and circular [10]. Circular fixators are made of ring blocks, which consist of two rings and at least four points of fixation to a bone segment. Rings are connected with at least three threaded connecting rods. The stability of the ring block will increase with increasing the number of rings, decreasing the distance between the rings, controlling the near and far segments of the bone segments, increasing the number of connections between each ring, and increasing the number of points of fixation to the bone segment. Smaller diameter rings are more stable than larger diameter rings when of the same thickness. The smallest ring that accommodates a patient's extremity should be utilized, allowing for approximately 2 cm of clearance between the skin and the inner surface of the ring. The distance between rings also influences frame stability. Increasing the distance between rings allows for motion between them. Utilizing a "dummy" ring (a ring with no osseous fixation) will shorten the length of the connecting rods and increase the stability. The use of thicker telescoping rods will also help impart stability as

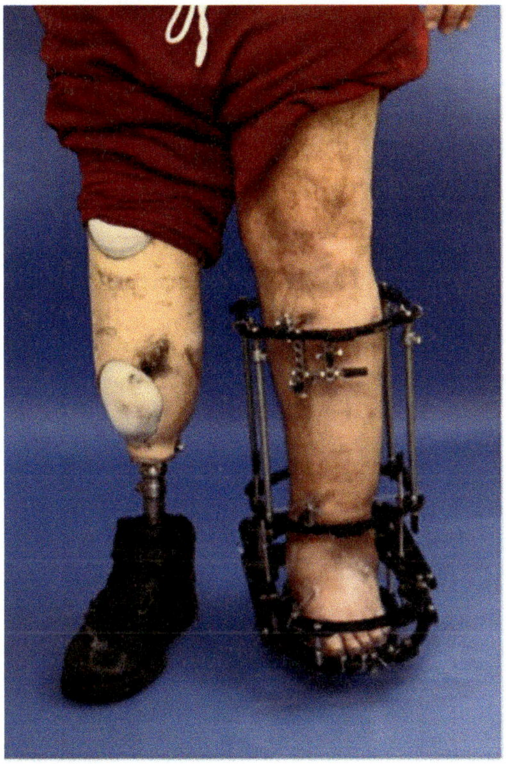

Fig. 30.8 Stable external fixation: a large tibial block allows for avoidance of placing fixation in the isthmus of the tibia, which is a high-risk zone for fracture. This strategy allows for increased stability of the tibia and disperses the stress of the fixation over a larger area. Note a foot ring block is used for increased stability (Reprinted with permission from the Rubin Institute for Advanced Orthopedics, Sinai Hospital of Baltimore)

they have superior bending strength when compared to threaded connecting rods (Fig. 30.8).

The type of fixation to the bone segment also affects frame stability. Each ring block should have a minimum of four points of fixation (each ring a minimum of two points). The use of thin wires versus half-pin fixation is per surgeon discretion, anatomic considerations, and biomechanical principles. Increasing the number of wires, placing wires above and below a ring, and inserting wires in difference planes (oblique wires) all enhance stability. Knowledge of anatomic safe zones is of vital importance when placing both half-pins and thin wires so as not to entrap neurovascular and musculotendinous structures. Proper tensioning of thin wires enhances stability. Wires in the distal tibia are tensioned to 130 kg, in the calcaneus 100 kg, and in the midfoot/forefoot region 90 kg. Careful attention should be paid to the ring during tensioning so as not to cause deflection (bending) of the ring. When utilizing a foot plate, make sure to close the foot plate before tensioning the foot wires so as not to distort the ring.

The use of half-pin fixation (4, 5, or 6 mm diameter) is common in limb lengthening and deformity correction. Their use in neuropathic patients should be done with caution as this may increase the risk for tibial stress fractures [9]. Increasing the diameter of the pins increases the rigidity of fixation. Half-pins should be predrilled with a sharp drill bit and inserted bicortical by hand. Unicortical half-pins increase the risk of fracture and should be avoided. We commonly use hydroxyapatite (HA)-coated half-pins, which increases the pull out strength of the fixation. The diameter of the half-pin should be no more than one-third the width of the bone diameter to minimize the risk of fracture. By increasing the half-pin diameter by 1 mm, the strength increases exponentially.

A stable circular external fixation construct will allow patients the ability to bear weight early. This will allow for axial loading of the fracture or osteotomy site and stimulate bone healing. It should be kept in mind that when weight bearing after midfoot/forefoot procedures, axial loading can cause cantilever loading. Patients with neuropathy should be educated on limiting their ambulation due to their diminished proprioception. Excessive weight bearing in neuropathic patients can lead to pin/wire loosening, pin tract infections, and broken fixation components.

Monolateral External Fixation

Constructing a stable monolateral (unilateral) external fixation device follow similar concepts to that of a circular external fixator. Monolataral devices can be divided into monobody designs and pin-to-bar fixators. The primary difference is the use of all half-pin fixation. These devices are commonly utilized for femoral, tibial, and metatarsal deformity correction. Stability of these devices increases by using larger diameter pins, decreasing the distance between the frame and the bone, controlling both the far and near ends of each bone segment, increasing the number of connecting rods, placing pins obliquely to one another, and adding an additional monolateral fixator for multiplanar stability. The primary downside to the use of monolateral external fixation is that the far cortex is more difficult to gain compression or distraction in comparison to the near cortex. Monolateral external fixators demonstrate cantilever bending when axial load is applied. Monolateral fixators are commonly used in our practice for gradual distraction of metatarsal deformities (i.e., brachymetatarsia). Protected weight bearing in a wooden bottom surgical shoe is important to prevent any acquired deformity of the regenerate bone.

Frame removal

Dynamization is an important concept to consider prior to frame removal. Dynamization allows for the stress of weight bearing to be gradually transferred from the external fixator to the bone. This is particularly important when regenerate bone is healing from procedures such as lengthening or gradual deformity correction. Dynamization has been shown to accelerate bone healing [11]. Once osteotomy or arthrodesis healing has been achieved, the frame is dynamized by reducing the stiffness through removal or detachment of fixation pins/wires from each ring. This allows the osteotomy or arthrodesis site to "mature" and accept full weight once the frame is entirely removed. During the dynamization process, the surgeon must be aware that delayed union, refracture, or development of secondary deformity may occur. Only weeks after dynamization does the bone completely heal.

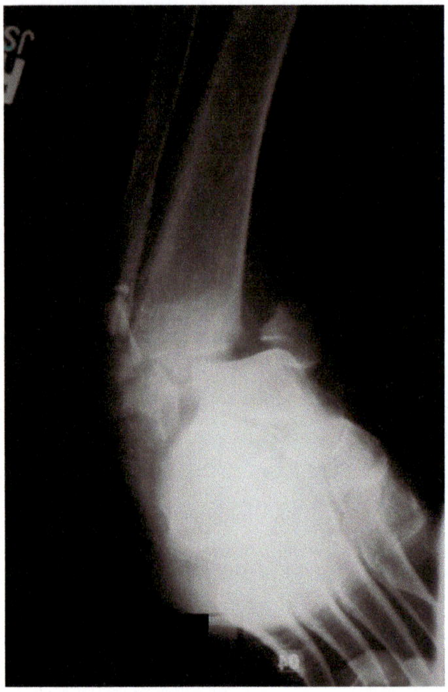

Fig. 30.9 Preoperative radiograph of trimalleolar ankle fracture dislocation (Reprinted with permission from the Rubin Institute for Advanced Orthopedics, Sinai Hospital of Baltimore)

Clinical Cases with Use of External Fixation

Case Example #1: Complex Ankle Arthrodesis

Sixty-two-year-old female referred after a failed ORIF of a right trimalleolar ankle fracture with subsequent ankle subluxation and development of ankle arthritis (Figs. 30.9 and 30.10). She had been diagnosed with idiopathic neuropathy. Circular external fixation was used because of concern for Charcot neuroathropathy of the ankle and severe osteopenia. She underwent successful fusion of the ankle joint with subtalar joint distraction (Figs. 30.11 and 30.12). A stable fusion was obtained with a plantigrade foot (Fig. 30.13). She was able to ambulate brace-free without an assistive device following the procedure.

Case Example #2: Equinus Deformity Correction

Forty-year-old male presented with severe fixed equinovarus deformity and post-polio syndrome without prior surgery (Figs. 30.14 and 30.15). Circular external fixation

a b c

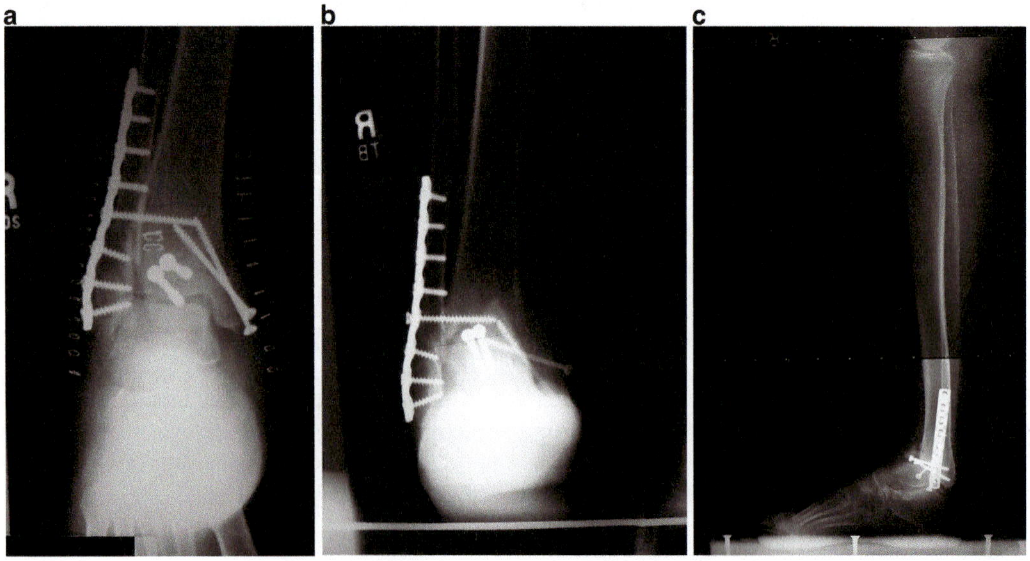

Fig. 30.10 Open reduction internal fixation of trimalleolar ankle fracture (**a**) and subsequent ankle degeneration and subluxation (**b**, **c**) (Reprinted with permission from the Rubin Institute for Advanced Orthopedics, Sinai Hospital of Baltimore)

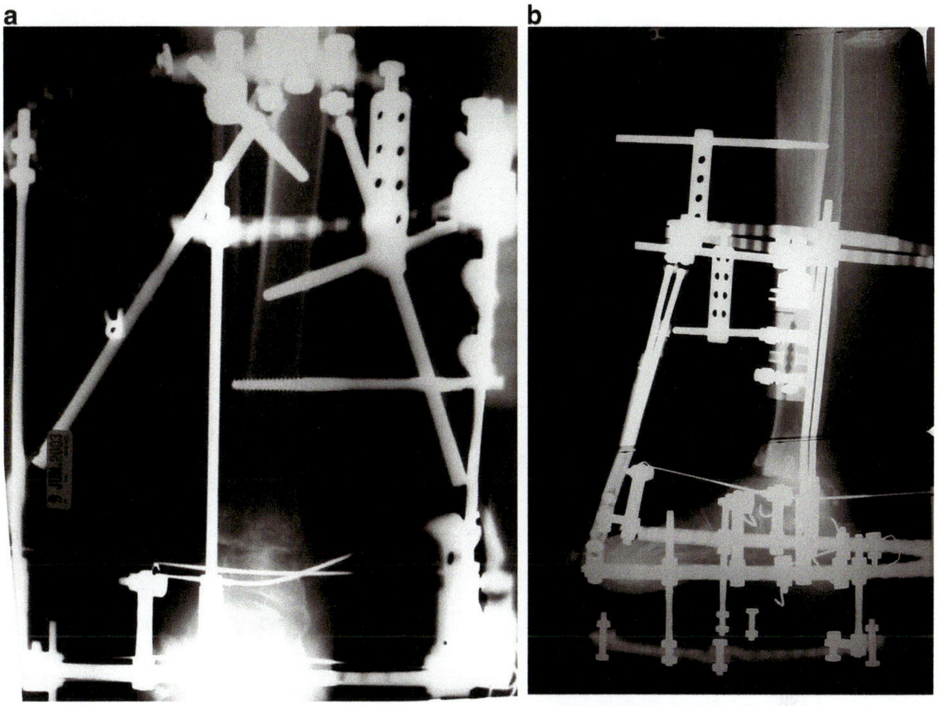

Fig. 30.11 Circular external fixation utilized for ankle arthrodesis and subtalar joint distraction (Reprinted with permission from the Rubin Institute for Advanced Orthopedics, Sinai Hospital of Baltimore)

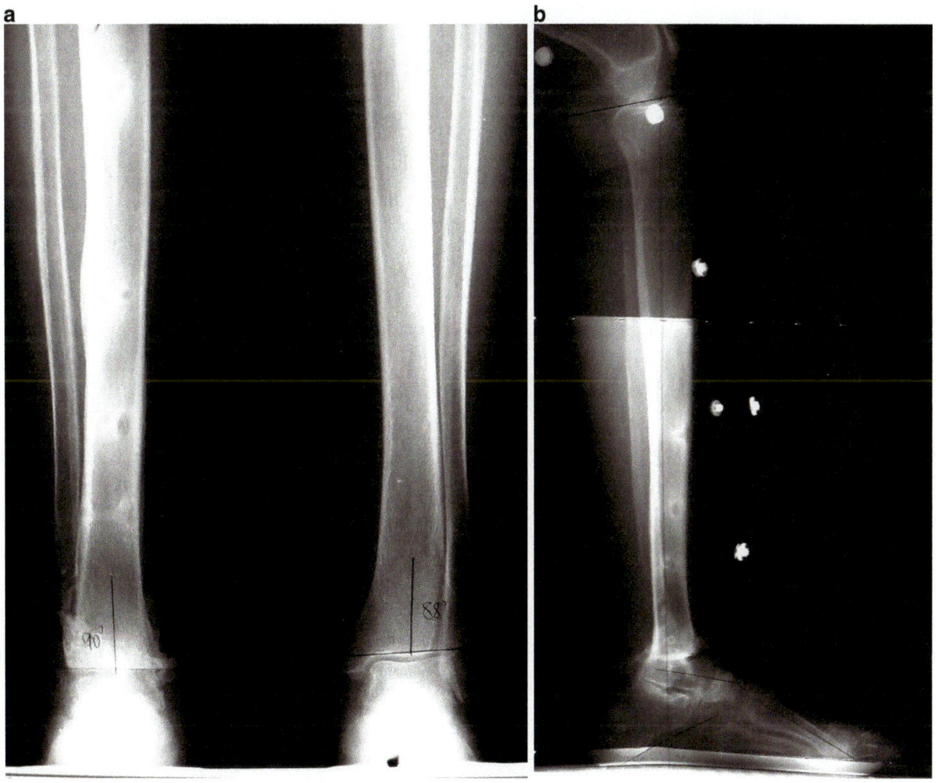

Fig. 30.12 Postoperative radiographic evaluation showing successful fusion of the subtalar joint and maintenance of the subtalar joint (Reprinted with permission from the Rubin Institute for Advanced Orthopedics, Sinai Hospital of Baltimore)

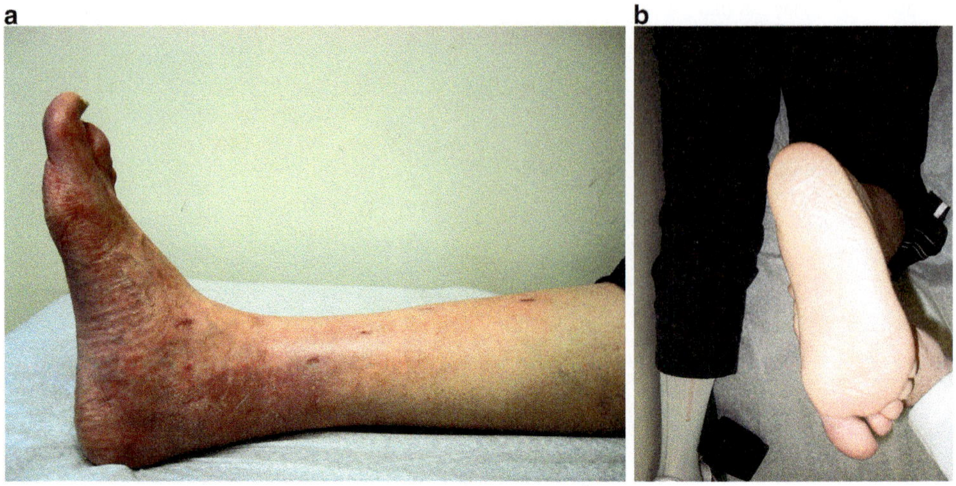

Fig. 30.13 Clinical photographs postoperatively showing a properly aligned ankle arthrodesis (Reprinted with permission from the Rubin Institute for Advanced Orthopedics, Sinai Hospital of Baltimore)

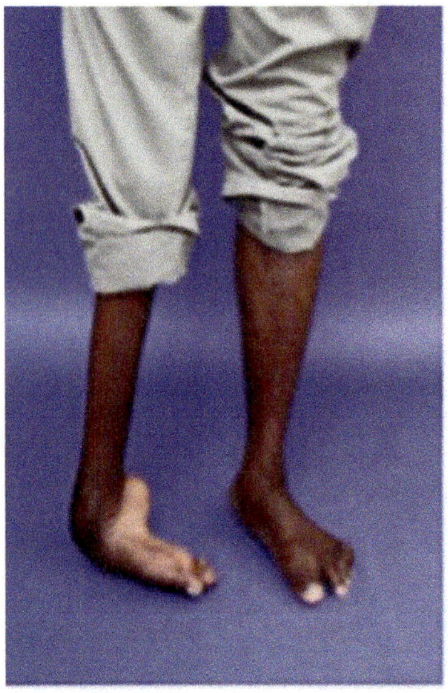

Fig. 30.14 Preoperative clinical presentation of severe equinovarus deformity (Reprinted with permission from the Rubin Institute for Advanced Orthopedics, Sinai Hospital of Baltimore)

was used for gradual soft tissue correction of the foot and ankle to a plantigrade position. The first stage included correction of the equinus contracture, followed by modification of the external fixator for the second stage correction of varus foot deformity (Figs. 30.16 and 30.17). The patient did also have a knee flexion contracture, which was treated with casting, bracing, and physical therapy. He has had no recurrence of the deformity and is walking with a plantigrade foot position 2 years following his surgery (Fig. 30.18).

Case Example #3: Charcot Midfoot Reconstruction

Forty-three-year-old male was referred with right midfoot Charcot deformity and chronic non-healing lateral column wound (Fig. 30.19). His condition was complicated by a history of kidney and pancreas transplant requiring immunosuppressant therapy. He had been treated with total contact cast immobilization without wound improvement. He underwent midfoot Gigli saw osteotomy (talar neck and calcaneal neck osteotomy) and gradual deformity correction with multiplanar external fixation (Fig. 30.20). The foot position was gradually corrected out of abduction and varus and then compressed for realignment arthrodesis of the midfoot osteotomy (Fig. 30.21). Due to the external fixation construct (butt frame) used to correct this patients deformity, he was unable to bear weight during his course of treatment. Only minimal incisions were made and the patient healed without any bone or soft tissue complications. He now walks with diabetic shoe gear and he is brace- and wound-free (Fig. 30.22).

Case Example #4: Gradual Distraction for Brachymetatarsia Correction

Thirty-two-year-old male presented with bilateral brachymetatarsia of the fourth metatarsal and hypoplastic fourth toe (Figs. 30.23 and 30.24). He underwent gradual distraction for correction of the bilateral brachymetatarsia. The external fixator construct included bridging to the fourth toe to reposition the fourth MTP joint and prevent joint subluxation/dislocation during the lengthening phase (Fig. 30.25). He underwent 33 days of lengthening to create a normal metatarsal parabola. Following consolidation of the regenerate bone, his bilateral fixators were removed in clinic approximately 4 months postoperatively (Fig. 30.26). Throughout his entire treatment, he was weight bearing as tolerated in wooden bottom surgical shoes.

Conclusion

External fixation is often utilized for high-risk, revisional, and complex cases because of its modularity, dynamic nature, and ability for patients to maintain weight bearing throughout the course of treatment. This inherently

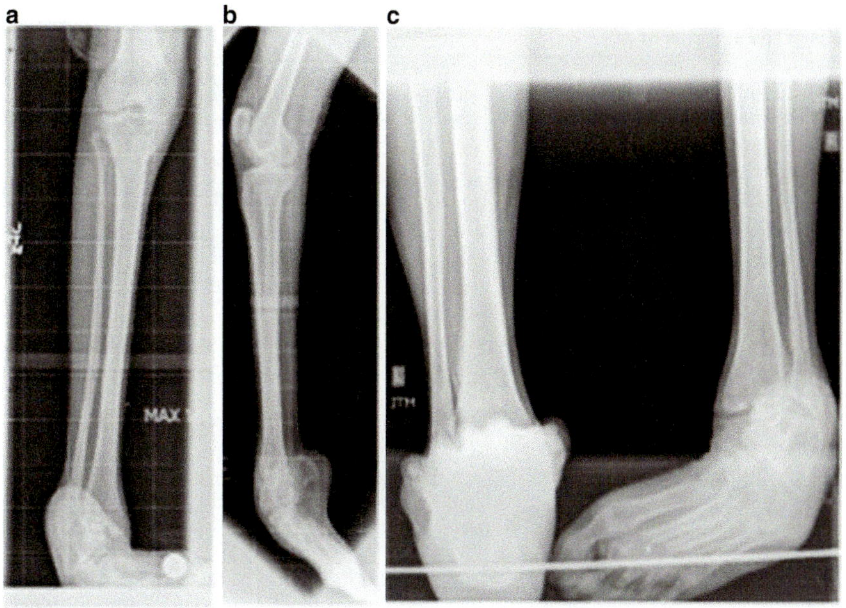

Fig. 30.15 Preoperative radiographic presentation of severe equinovarus deformity (Reprinted with permission from the Rubin Institute for Advanced Orthopedics, Sinai Hospital of Baltimore)

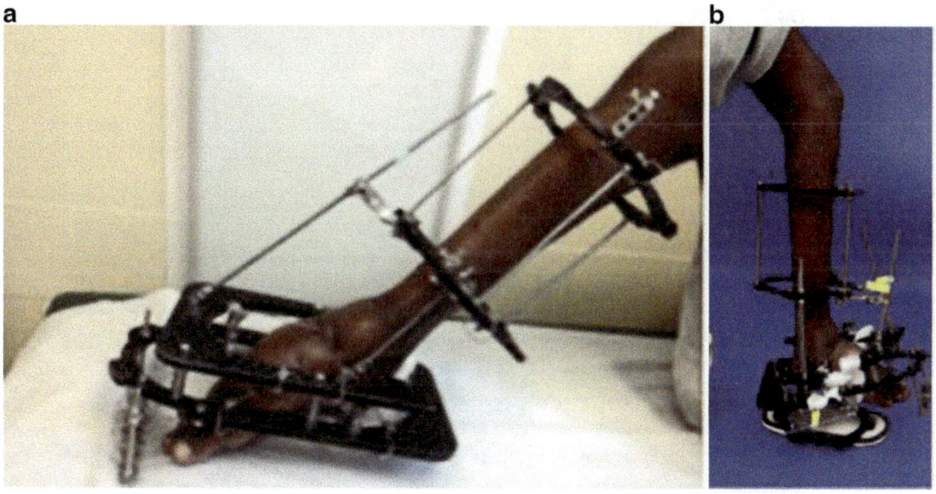

Fig. 30.16 Clinical pictures during treatment of severe equinovarus deformity with external fixation. Deformity correction was accomplished through gradual distraction with a semi-constrained construct. This two-stage approach included first correcting the equinus deformity of the ankle, followed by correction of the varus deformity of the foot (Reprinted with permission from the Rubin Institute for Advanced Orthopedics, Sinai Hospital of Baltimore)

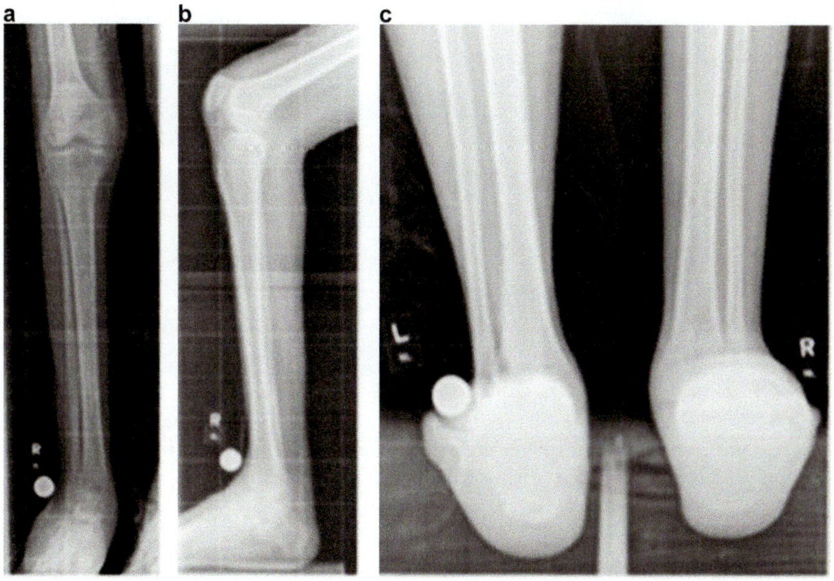

Fig. 30.17 Postoperative radiographic presentation of a plantigrade foot following gradual correction of severe equniovarus deformity (Reprinted with permission from the Rubin Institute for Advanced Orthopedics, Sinai Hospital of Baltimore)

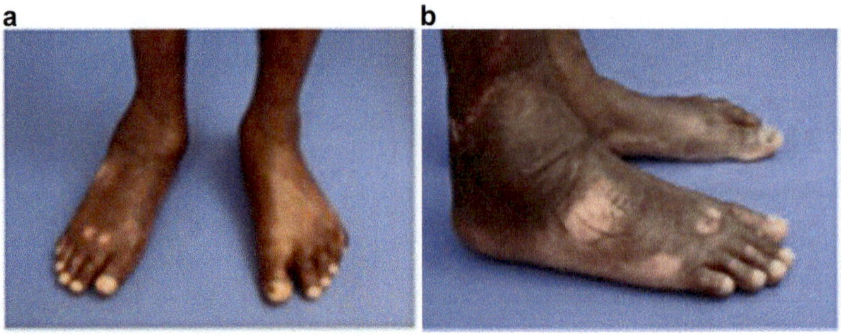

Fig. 30.18 Postoperative clinical presentation of a plantigrade foot following gradual correction of severe equniovarus deformity with circular external fixation (Reprinted with permission from the Rubin Institute for Advanced Orthopedics, Sinai Hospital of Baltimore)

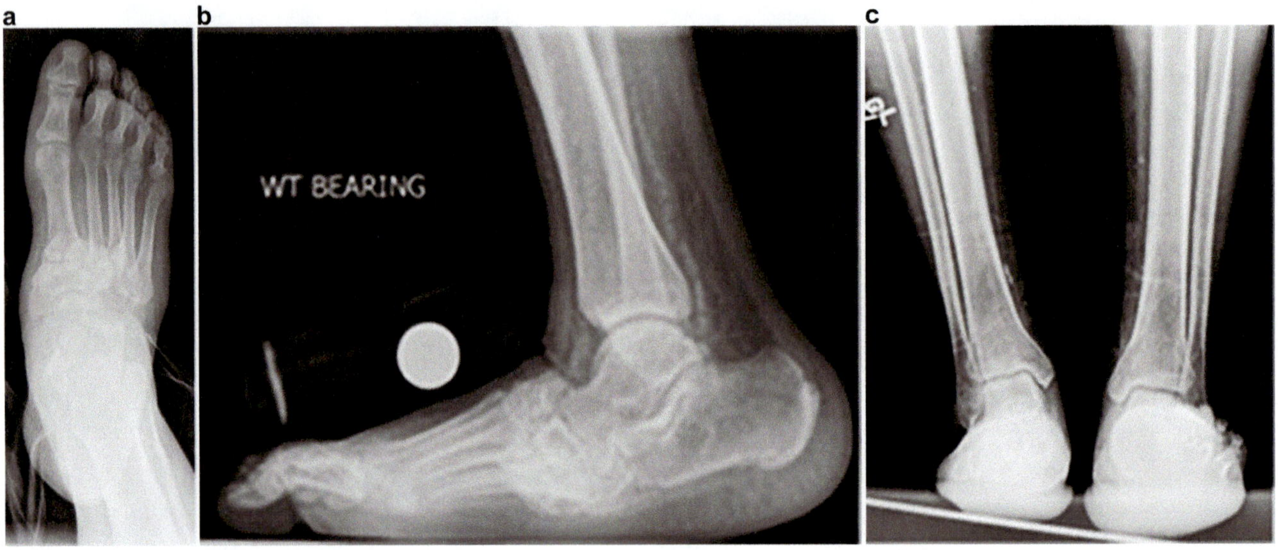

Fig. 30.19 Preoperative radiographic presentation of Charcot neuroarthropathy of the midfoot resulting in a rocker-bottom deformity and non-healing ulceration (Reprinted with permission from the Rubin Institute for Advanced Orthopedics, Sinai Hospital of Baltimore)

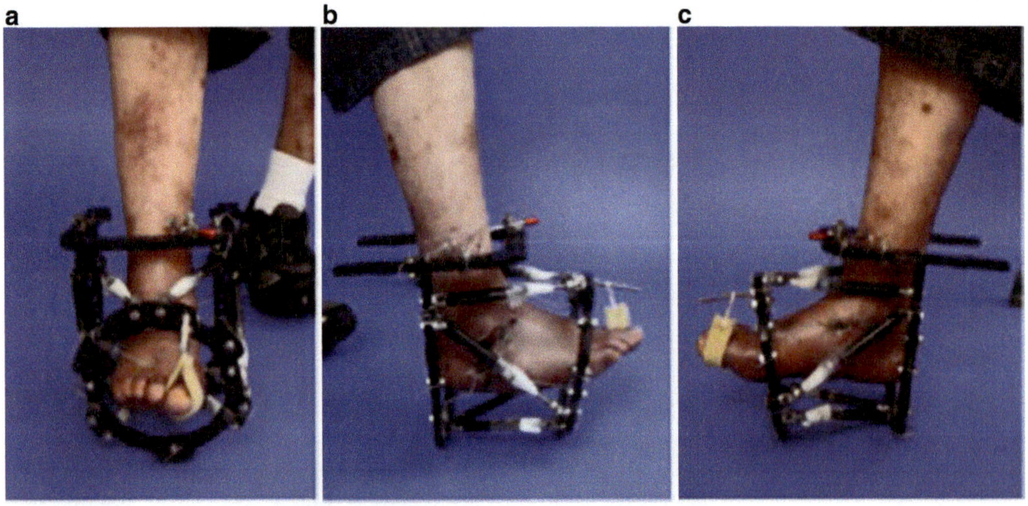

Fig. 30.20 Clinical presentation during treatment with six-axis correction construct used to obtain and maintain correction of the midfoot deformity following minimally invasive osteotomy (Reprinted with permission from the Rubin Institute for Advanced Orthopedics, Sinai Hospital of Baltimore)

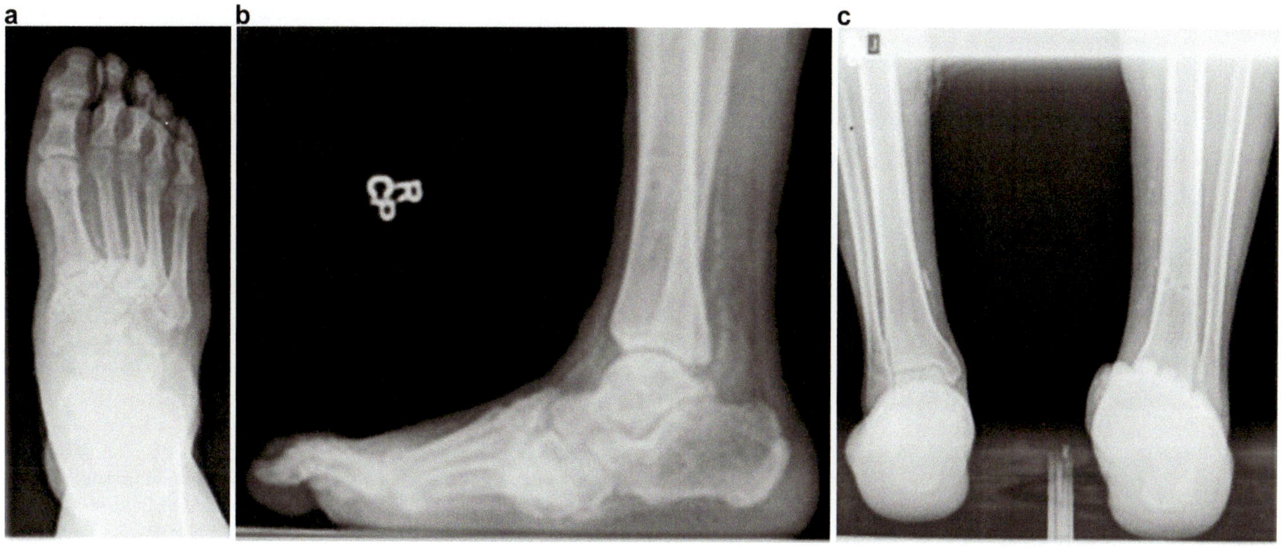

Fig. 30.21 Postoperative radiographic presentation following correction and stabilization of midfoot deformity (Reprinted with permission from the Rubin Institute for Advanced Orthopedics, Sinai Hospital of Baltimore)

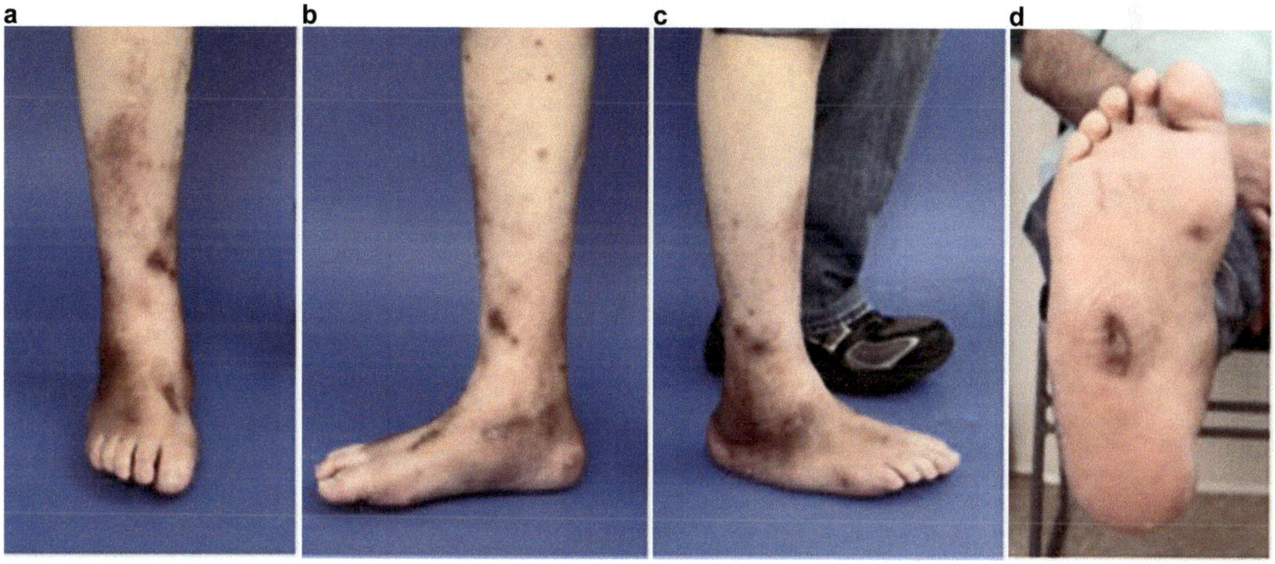

Fig. 30.22 Clinical presentation following correction of midfoot deformity shows a plantigrade foot and healed plantar ulceration (Reprinted with permission from the Rubin Institute for Advanced Orthopedics, Sinai Hospital of Baltimore)

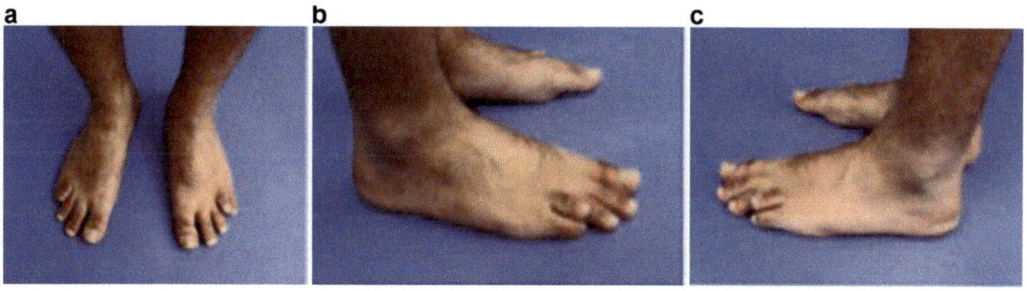

Fig. 30.23 Preoperative clinical presentation of bilateral fourth brachymetatarsia (Reprinted with permission from the Rubin Institute for Advanced Orthopedics, Sinai Hospital of Baltimore)

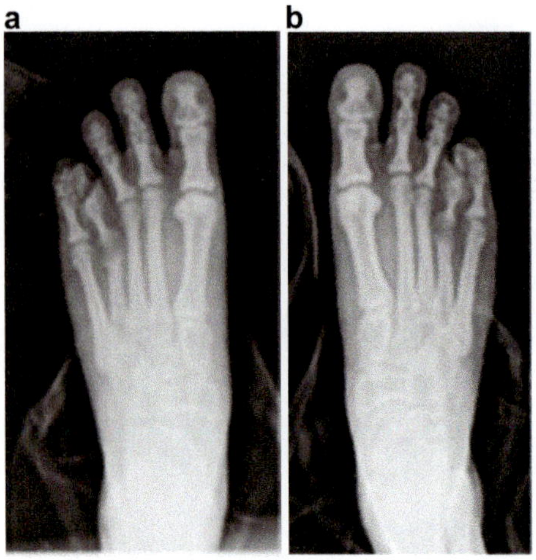

Fig. 30.24 Preoperative radiographic presentation of bilateral fourth brachymetatarsia and hypoplastic fourth digit. Note the subluxation of the fourth metatarsophalangeal joint (Reprinted with permission from the Rubin Institute for Advanced Orthopedics, Sinai Hospital of Baltimore)

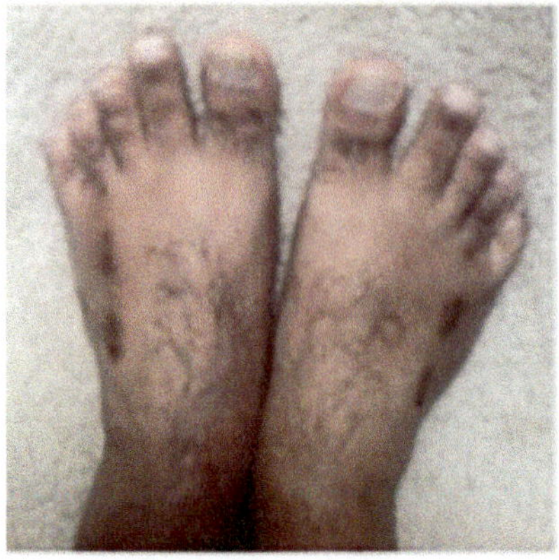

Fig. 30.26 Clinical presentation following gradual distraction for correction of brachymetatarsia (Reprinted with permission from the Rubin Institute for Advanced Orthopedics, Sinai Hospital of Baltimore)

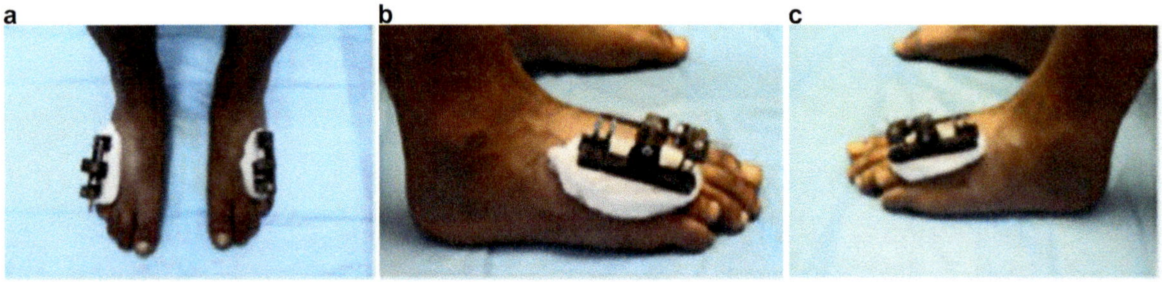

Fig. 30.25 Clinical presentation during gradual distraction for correction of fourth brachymetatarsia. Note the extension of the external fixator to the fourth digit to reduce and protect the metatarsophalangeal joint during the distraction process (Reprinted with permission from the Rubin Institute for Advanced Orthopedics, Sinai Hospital of Baltimore)

increases the likelihood of problems, obstacles, and complications. Not all adverse events are complications. Problems and obstacles are often encountered with external fixation without interfering with the goals of treatment. Patient education is of critical importance when preparing patients to undergo treatment with external fixation. Experience, training, and a thorough understanding of problems and obstacles complications decrease the risk of complications.

References

1. Thordarson DB, Markolf K, Cracchilo A. Biomechanical analysis of ankle arthrodesis comparing cancellous screws to an external fixator. J Bone Joint Surg Am. 1992;74:1050–5.
2. Santangelo JR, Glisson RR, Garras DN, Easley ME. Tibiotalocalcaneal arthrodesis: a biomechanical comparison of multiplanar external fixation with intramedullary fixation. Foot Ankle Int. 2008;29:936–41. doi:10.3113/FAI.2008.0936.
3. Ogut T, Glisson RR, Chuckpaiwong B, Le IL, Easley ME. External ring fixation versus screw fixation for ankle arthrodesis: a biomechanical comparison. Foot Ankle Int. 2009;30:353–60. doi:10.3113/FAI.2009.0353.
4. Fragomen AT, Meyers KN, Davis N, Shu H, Wright T, Rozbruch SR. A biomechanical comparison of micromotion after ankle fusion using 2 fixation techniques: intramedullary arthrodesis nail or Ilizarov external fixator. Foot Ankle Int. 2008;29:334–41. doi:10.3113/FAI.2008.0334.
5. McGarvey WC. The use of external fixation in arthrodesis and salvage of the foot and ankle. Foot Ankle Clin. 2002;7:147–73.
6. Paley D. Problems, obstacles, and complications of limb lengthening by the Ilizarov technique. Clin Orthop Relat Res. 1990;250:81–104.
7. Lamm BM, Gourdine-Shaw MC. Problems, obstacles, and complications of metatarsal lengthening for the treatment of brachymetatarsia. Clin Podiatr Med Surg. 2010;27:561–82. doi:10.1016/j.cpm.2010.06.006.
8. Lamm BM, Paley D, Testani M, Herzenberg JE. Tarsal tunnel decompression in leg lengthening and deformity correction of the foot and ankle. J Foot Ankle Surg. 2007;46:201–6.
9. Jones CP, Youngblood CS, Waldrop N, Davis WH, Pinzur MS. Tibial stress fracture secondary to half-pins in circular ring external fixation for charcot foot. Foot Ankle Int. 2014;35:572–7.
10. Fragomen AT, Rozbruch SR. The mechanics of external fixation. HSS J. 2007;3:13–29. doi:10.1007/s11420-006-9025-0.
11. Younger AS, Morrison J, MacKenzie WG. Biomechanics of external fixation and limb lengthening. Foot Ankle Clin. 2004;9:433–48.

Erratum to: Talar Fractures: The Injury, the Management, and the Aftermath

Justin J. Fleming, Kwasi Y. Kwaadu, and Michael W. Downey

Erratum to:
Chapter 18 in: M.S. Lee, J.P. Grossman (eds.), *Complications in Foot and Ankle Surgery*, DOI 10.1007/978-3-319-53686-6_18

The original version of this book was published without Michael W. Downey listed among the chapter authors in Chapter 18.

It has been corrected and updated as:

Justin J. Fleming, Kwasi Y. Kwaadu, and Michael W. Downey

The updated original online version for this chapter can be found at
https://doi.org/10.1007/978-3-319-53686-6_18

M.S. Lee, J.P. Grossman (eds.), *Complications in Foot and Ankle Surgery*, DOI 10.1007/978-3-319-53686-6_31

Index

M.S. Lee, J.P. Grossman (eds.), *Complications in Foot and Ankle Surgery*, DOI 10.1007/978-3-319-53686-6

D

O

P

R